SEVENTH EDITION

Articulation and Phonological Disorders
Speech Sound Disorders in Children

JOHN E. BERNTHAL
University of Nebraska–Lincoln

NICHOLAS W. BANKSON
James Madison University

PETER FLIPSEN JR.
Idaho State University, Meridian Health Sciences Center

PEARSON

Boston   Columbus   Indianapolis   New York   San Francisco   Upper Saddle River
Amsterdam   Cape Town   Dubai   London   Madrid   Milan   Munich   Paris   Montréal   Toronto
Delhi   Mexico City   São Paulo   Sydney   Hong Kong   Seoul   Singapore   Taipei   Tokyo

Executive Editor and Publisher: *Stephen D. Dragin*
Editorial Assistant: *Michelle Hochberg*
Marketing Manager: *Joanna Sabella*
Production Editor: *Mary Beth Finch*
Editorial Production Service: *Jouve North America*
Manufacturing Buyer: *Megan Cochran*
Electronic Composition: *Jouve India*
Interior Design: *Jouve North America/Jouve India*
Cover Designer: *Jennifer Hart*

Library of Congress Cataloging-in-Publication Data
Bernthal, John E.
   Articulation and phonological disorders : speech sound disorders in children / John E. Bernthal, Nicholas W. Bankson, Peter Flipsen Jr. — 7th ed.
      p. cm.
   Includes bibliographical references and index.
   ISBN-13: 978-0-13-261263-0
   ISBN-10: 0-13-261263-1
   1. Articulation disorders.   I. Bankson, Nicholas W.   II. Flipsen, Peter.   III. Title.
   RC424.7.B47 2013
   616.85'5—dc23

                                                                          2012020662

10 9 8 7 6 5 4 3 2 1

PEARSON

ISBN 13: 978-0-13-261263-0
ISBN 10:   0-13-261263-1

Contents

Preface   vii

1 Introduction to the Study of Speech Sound Disorders   1
by Nicholas W. Bankson, John E. Bernthal, and Peter Flipsen Jr.

2 Normal Aspects of Articulation   6
by Ray Kent

Structure of Language   7
Fundamentals of Articulatory Phonetics   11
Coarticulation: Interactions among Sounds in Context   42
Aerodynamic Considerations in Speech Production   47
Acoustic Considerations of Speech   50
Sensory Information in Speech Production   51
Summary of Levels of Organization of Speech   52
Concluding Note on Implications for Speech Acquisition   55
Questions for Chapter 2   57

3 Speech Sound Acquisition   58
by Sharynne McLeod

Relevance of Understanding Typical Speech Sound
Acquisition for SLPs   58
Models of Speech Acquisition   59
How Speech Acquisition Data Are Obtained   71
Overall Sequence of Speech Sound Acquisition   77
Phase 1: Laying the Foundations for Speech   77
Phase 2: Transitioning from Words to Speech   84
Phase 3: The Growth of the Inventory   87
Phase 4: Mastery of Speech and Literacy   106
Factors Influencing Typical Acquisition of Speech   107
Conclusion: Understanding and Applying Typical Speech Acquisition   112
Questions for Chapter 3   112

4 **Classification and Comorbidity in Speech Sound Disorders   114**
by Peter Flipsen Jr., John E. Bernthal, and Nicholas W. Bankson

Organically Based Speech Sound Disorders   115
Childhood Apraxia of Speech   125
Speech Sound Disorders of Unknown Origin   127
Summary of Classification   136
Comorbidity   136
Conclusion   142
Questions for Chapter 4   143

5 **Factors Related to Speech Sound Disorders   144**
by Peter Flipsen Jr., Nicholas W. Bankson, and John E. Bernthal

Structure and Function of the Speech and Hearing Mechanism   144
Motor Abilities   158
Cognitive-Linguistic Factors   164
Psychosocial Factors   172
Conclusion   179
Questions for Chapter 5   179

6 **Speech Sound Assessment Procedures   180**
by Nicholas W. Bankson, John E. Bernthal, and Peter Flipsen Jr.

Speech Sound Sampling   180
Screening for Speech Sound Disorders   181
Comprehensive Speech Sound Assessment: The Assessment Battery   184
Related Assessment Procedures   201
Conclusion   211
Questions for Chapter 6   211

7 **Determining the Need for Intervention and Target Selection   212**
by John E. Bernthal, Nicholas W. Bankson, and Peter Flipsen Jr.

Case Selection   212
Target Speech Sound Selection   228
Other Factors to Consider in Case Selection: Intervention Decisions   232
Computer-Assisted Phonological Analysis   234
Case Study   235
Conclusion   240
Questions for Chapter 7   241

8 Remediation Procedures 242
by Nicholas W. Bankson, John E. Bernthal, and Peter Flipsen Jr.

Basic Considerations 242
Making Progress in Therapy: Measuring Clinical Change 249
Facilitation of Generalization 254
Dismissal from Instruction 263
Questions for Chapter 8 266

9 Motor-Based Treatment Approaches 267
by Peter Flipsen Jr., John E. Bernthal, and Nicholas W. Bankson

Approaches to Intervention 267
The Published Evidence 268
Treatment Continuum 270
Motor Learning Principles 272
Teaching Sounds/Establishment 273
Beyond Individual Sounds 283
Remediation Guidelines for Motor Approaches 294
Core Vocabulary Approach 294
The Use of Nonspeech Oral-Motor Activities 296
Intervention for Childhood Apraxia of Speech 297
Case Study Revisited: Motor Perspective 303
Questions for Chapter 9 305

10 Linguistically Based Treatment Approaches 306
by Peter Flipsen Jr., Nicholas W. Bankson, and John E. Bernthal

Minimal Pair Contrast Therapy 307
Cycles Approach 314
Broader-Based Language Approaches 317
Remediation Guidelines for Linguistically Based Approaches 322
Case Study Revisited: Linguistic Perspective 323
Questions for Chapter 10 325

11 Language and Dialectal Variations 326
by Brian A. Goldstein and Aquiles Iglesias

Dialect 326
Characteristics of American English Dialects 328
Phonology in Speakers of Language Varieties Other than English 335
Phonological Development in Bilingual Children 343
Assessment Considerations for Children from Culturally and Linguistically Diverse Populations 345

Intervention for Speech Sound Disorders in Children from Culturally and Linguistically Diverse Populations 348
Summary 352
Questions for Chapter 11 353

12 Phonological Awareness: Description, Assessment, and Intervention 355
by Laura M. Justice, Gail T. Gillon, Brigid C. McNeill, and C. Melanie Schuele

What Is Phonological Awareness? 356
Phonological Awareness as Literacy Development 357
The Development of Phonological Awareness 358
Phonological Awareness Development and Reading 362
Phonological Awareness and Speech Sound Disorders 364
The Role of the Speech-Language Pathologist 367
Assessment 368
Intervention 372
Phonological Awareness Experiences for Preschool Children 376
Questions for Chapter 12 382

Appendix A 383

Appendix B 387

References 389

Index 433

Preface

We are pleased to share with you the seventh edition of our speech sound disorders text-book. We frequently hear the comment that this text is a "classic" in this area of speech-language pathology practice. Given that the first edition was published in 1981, this book has been utilized as a college text and "articulation" resource for more than 30 years. Our intention in each edition has been to provide the reader updated information while retaining a comprehensive summary of the literature in the area of speech sound disorders (articulation and phonology).

NEW TO THIS EDITION

In this seventh edition, we have retained the basic organization of information from the previous edition, but we have also:

1. Divided some chapters into shorter, more manageable units (for both students and instructors),
2. Added a separate chapter on the classification of speech sound disorders that also includes a substantial new section on comorbidity of speech sound disorders with several other disorders,
3. Included a revised focus on evidence-based practice with specific discussion of levels of evidence,
4. Identified and discussed the highest-level evidence available relative to the treatment approaches discussed in the new Chapters 9 and 10,
5. Expanded the discussion of childhood apraxia of speech, particularly relative to treatment, and
6. Added more on treatment application by discussing our case study (presented in Chapter 7) from both motor-based (Chapter 9) and linguistically based perspectives (Chapter 10).

As with previous editions, in all chapters we have attempted to synthesize the most up-to-date literature in the field while maintaining our "eclectic" perspective relative to the nature and treatment of articulation and phonological disorders. In the assessment and treatment chapters, you will continue to see some of our biases regarding clinical management. We continue, however, to defer to clinician judgment in deciding which assessment and treatment procedures are most useful to them and the clients they serve.

We are indebted to several professionals who have contributed their knowledge and expertise in specialized areas to this text. Ray Kent has once again authored the chapter on normal aspects of articulation. Sharynne McLeod has updated and modified her chapter on normal speech sound acquisition. Brian Goldstein and Aquiles Iglesias have revised their chapter on language and dialectal variations, and Laura Justice, Gail Gillon, and Melanie Schuele have added Brigid McNeill as an additional coauthor in their revision of the phonological awareness chapter. Each of these contributing authors is a recognized expert who is engaged in cutting-edge scholarship in the area about which they are writing, and we are fortunate to include their efforts in this text.

We'd like to thank the reviewers of this edition for their suggestions: HyeKyeung Seung, California State University, Fullerton; Jane Hilton, University of Virginia; Megan Overby, The College of Saint Rose; and Harriet B. Klein, New York University. We'd also like to thank reviewers of previous editions, including Brenda J. Beverly, University of South Alabama; Gina Keene, University of Mississippi; and Michael J. Moran, Auburn University.

As authors, we assume all responsibility for errors, oversights, and misconceptions that may appear in this book. Our hope is that this edition will provide you a comprehensive source of information on speech sound disorders and that it will be a valuable resource as you learn about and practice clinical phonology.

CHAPTER 1

Introduction to the Study of Speech Sound Disorders

NICHOLAS W. BANKSON
James Madison University

JOHN E. BERNTHAL
University of Nebraska–Lincoln

PETER FLIPSEN JR.
Idaho State University

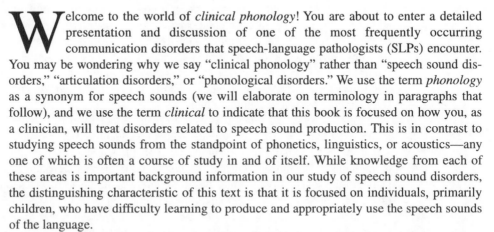

Welcome to the world of *clinical phonology*! You are about to enter a detailed presentation and discussion of one of the most frequently occurring communication disorders that speech-language pathologists (SLPs) encounter. You may be wondering why we say "clinical phonology" rather than "speech sound disorders," "articulation disorders," or "phonological disorders." We use the term *phonology* as a synonym for speech sounds (we will elaborate on terminology in paragraphs that follow), and we use the term *clinical* to indicate that this book is focused on how you, as a clinician, will treat disorders related to speech sound production. This is in contrast to studying speech sounds from the standpoint of phonetics, linguistics, or acoustics—any one of which is often a course of study in and of itself. While knowledge from each of these areas is important background information in our study of speech sound disorders, the distinguishing characteristic of this text is that it is focused on individuals, primarily children, who have difficulty learning to produce and appropriately use the speech sounds of the language.

The term presently accepted by the American Speech-Language-Hearing Association to identify those persons who have disorders related to saying the sounds of the language is *speech sound disorders*. Historically, these disorders were referred to as *articulation disorders*—a term still in widespread use. From the time the profession of speech-language pathology came into existence in the 1920s until the 1970s, the prevailing viewpoint related to speech sound disorders was that they reflected a client's inability to either auditorally perceive or discriminate a particular sound or sounds, and/or to motorically produce these sounds.

1

The role of the speech clinician was to teach a client to discriminate a sound auditorally, and then to say the sound followed by practicing the sound until the new motor behavior became habitual. When the first edition of this text was published in 1981, *Articulation Disorders* was used as the title of the book because that was still the prevailing term used to identify speech sound disorders. Beginning in the 1970s, as the first edition of this book was being written, the field of linguistics began to influence the perception of how our field viewed speech sound disorders. Linguists, who study how speech sounds are used in various languages, provided information that indicated that speech sound disorders should not be viewed only as motor production difficulties but also as a child's lack of knowledge regarding where to appropriately use sounds that he or she can produce. Said another way, the child might be having difficulty acquiring the phonological rules of the language. For example, a child may have difficulty in learning to use sounds contrastively (e.g., /s/ and /z/ are contrasted in *sue* versus *zoo*), or in learning that certain sounds need to be placed at the beginning or ends of words in order to communicate effectively (e.g., *at* versus *hat; go* versus *goat*). Disorders related to learning the phonological rules of the language were referred to as *phonological disorders*; thus, the term *phonology* was the second term (in addition to articulation) that moved into our vocabulary to identify speech sound disorders.

From the second edition of this book (1988) through the sixth edition (2009), the terms *articulation* and *phonological* were used in the title of the book (i.e., *Articulation and Phonological Disorders*). Some SLPs have differentiated these two terms for purposes of assessment and treatment of speech sound disorders. *Articulation* refers to production-based speech sound disorders, and *phonological* denotes speech sound errors that are rule based. However, in reality, it may be difficult to determine which of these concepts is most appropriate in describing a particular client's error productions. We must also recognize that there may be variables beyond motor production and rule acquisition that we need to attend to when we try to understand speech sound disorders. Presently, the term *speech sound disorder* is used as the umbrella term to refer to disorders that may be found in clients who have difficulty producing speech sounds. In this book we use the terms *articulation, phonology,* and *speech sound disorders* somewhat interchangeably, but will hold to the traditional differentiation we have referred to between *articulation* and *phonology* when we talk about assessment and treatment.

Speech sound disorders may be described as ranging from something as "mild" as a lisp (interdentalizing the /s̪/ sounds; sometimes identified as substituting a voiceless *th* sound for an /s/) to a disorder as significant as that found in an individual who is completely unintelligible. The terms *delay* and *deviant* are concepts that are often used to describe the nature of the sound errors produced by children. *Delay* refers to speech sound errors that are often noted as "normal" errors found in young children as they learn to properly use sounds (e.g., lisps, misarticulations of /r/ or the affricates). *Deviant* refers to errors not typically observed in young children's development (e.g., lateralization of sibilants, backing of alveolars, vowel errors). It should be noted that some scholars argue that the terms *delay* and *deviance* are not particularly useful because, in terms of overall language development (including speech sounds), delay often leads to deviance. This progression occurs because of the high degree of coordination involved in the development of all aspects of language (e.g., speech sounds, vocabulary, syntax). If one area is slow (i.e., delayed), it may lead to difficulties across several areas of development, which results in errors that we might then describe as "deviant."

Typically, speech sound disorders are found in children, and the pediatric population is the focus of this text. In 2003 Campbell and colleagues presented data suggesting that speech sound disorders occur in approximately 15.2% of 3-year-old children. Findings reported by Shriberg, Tomblin, and McSweeny (1999) suggest that by age 6 years, up to 3.8 percent of that group continues to have difficulty with speech sound production. The difference between these two percentages indicates that many of these problems are being resolved in the preschool period. Although a positive trend, it does not remove the need for continued services. This is seen most obviously in the report of Mullen and Schooling (2010), which indicated that up to 56 percent of the caseloads of school-based clinicians may involve work on speech sound production problems. Many of these disorders often co-exist with other aspects of communication (something we discuss in more detail near the end of Chapter 4). Most speech sound disorders occur in children under the age of 8 years, but speech sound production errors may persist past that point and occur in adults. Information contained in this book is relevant to the treatment of any client who faces difficulties producing speech sounds; however, adult speech sound disorders are often related to organic conditions, and thus you will need to review other materials in planning treatment for most adult clients.

As we begin our discussion of speech sound disorders, it is important to recognize that for most children, the cause of the disorder is unknown. Often it is assumed that many children do not say their sounds properly because of difficulty in language development that is reflected in learning speech sounds. In some instances the problem may be related to difficulty with other aspects of language (e.g., vocabulary, syntax). As will be discussed later, a number of variables have been studied as they relate to such learning problems (e.g., familial history, tongue thrust, speech sound discrimination). Research focused on giving us a better understanding of causality in speech sound disorders has been difficult to establish but is ongoing. Certainly, efforts to categorize or classify various types of speech sound disorders (e.g., speech delay related to otitis media with effusion, motor speech involvement, or genetic factors) is a step in the direction of helping us better understand those children with speech sound disorders of unknown origin. For some children, the cause of their disorder may be more obvious (e.g., hearing loss, cleft palate); however, even then the impact of an organic condition does not necessarily determine the type of speech sound disorder a client may have, nor how he or she will respond to treatment.

In order to better understand and appreciate the contents of this book, it is assumed that you, the student, will already have obtained skills related to phonetic transcription of the speech sounds of the language, knowledge related to the physiological production of various sounds, an introduction to the acoustical characteristics of speech sounds, and knowledge of speech sound development in children. Many of you will already have taken a separate course that covers each of these areas, or perhaps a course that covers two areas (e.g., physiology of sound productions and their transcription). If this is the case, the information we present in our introductory chapters may serve as a review for you. If you have not had courses in these areas, information included in the next two chapters of this text ("Normal Aspects of Articulation" and "Speech Sound Acquisition") will be especially helpful. These chapters will provide background information that you may wish to study further by consulting other texts and/or sources. For all students, the information will be something that you may want to refer to as you encounter some of the concepts included in these chapters as you delve into assessment and treatment of speech sound disorders.

In addition to the background information referred to in the last paragraph, it is important to recognize that speech sounds are a part of language. In this instance the sounds are identified as the phonology of the language. Other aspects of language include semantics (meaning attached to words, vocabulary); morphology (minimum meaningful units in the language), or the words and attachments to words such as plural markers (e.g., /s/ in *dogs*) and tense markers (e.g., *ed* in *walked*, indicating past tense), or parts of words (e.g., *doghouse* has two minimum meaningful units); syntax (grammatical rules for putting words together in phrases and sentences); pragmatics (using language appropriately in a social context); and discourse (ability to string sentences together in a meaningful manner while communicating with others). Each of these areas is acquired gradually and simultaneously by young children. Initially we are concerned that children learn to use meaningful utterances to express themselves, but soon thereafter we become concerned about how accurate sounds are because it is through accurate use of speech sounds that the child is understood by the listener, or, in other words, becomes intelligible. SLPs are initially concerned with a young child's acquisition of semantics and vocabulary, phonology, and grammatical rules (morphology and syntax). Concern over the other areas comes later because pragmatics and discourse are based on vocabulary and syntax. Thus, it is often older children for whom pragmatics and discourse may be targeted for instruction.

Increasingly it is being recognized that a normal sound system is important in learning to read and spell. A child's phonological awareness skills (or their ability to mentally manipulate the sounds and syllables in words) have been shown to impact literacy skills, and children with speech sound disorders are at risk for appropriate development of phonological awareness and later literacy. For this reason, clinicians have been drawn into using their knowledge of phonology as part of a child's literacy development. Chapter 12 will provide information related to the role of the clinician in terms of developing phonological awareness in children.

In our discussion of speech sound disorders, we need to recognize that some children use different speech sounds than those found in their environment because perhaps their first language is different from English, or maybe they are a part of a regional or cultural group that uses a less common dialect of English. Certainly, the increasing cultural diversity, the number of second language learners, and other languages spoken in the United States make us acutely aware of the fact that linguistic differences are a part of everyday communication. As speech-language pathologists, we are primarily focused on disorders that individuals may have in their speech sound productions. It is sometimes very challenging to determine what is a disorder and what is a difference when the clinician does not speak the language or dialect. Fortunately, there are some guidelines to help us, but the reality is that there is a need for clinicians who are bilingual and/or represent different language/dialect groups. All sound systems, whether they are part of a separate language or dialect, are legitimate and deserve acceptance. In some instances, the clinician may, however, help an individual learn the sound system of mainstream English when a client elects to do this, often for educational, business, or social reasons. Chapter 11 will present language variations often found in the United States and outline the role of speech-language pathologists as they assess and treat disorders, as well as provide instruction to those who wish to enhance their mainstream English speaking skills.

Often speech sound disorders is the first specific disorders course in a student's curriculum. Academicians have historically found that assessment and treatment of speech sound disorders is a good place to launch the development of clinical skills in beginning clinicians and thus, the frequent placement of this course early in a student's curriculum. The study of speech sound disorders lends itself to helping students come to recognize the processes involved in formulating assessment and treatment protocols. Thus, the knowledge and skills that you will acquire in the process of studying speech sound disorders can provide the basis for learning how to proceed with other types of communication disorders. Speech sound disorders and all the complexities they encompass are a challenging study but one that is critical to individuals who for one reason or another need assistance in learning the speech sounds of the language. For many children, learning to talk, including the learning of speech sounds, is difficult. For this reason, you need to be in a position to assist them so that communication is both effective and satisfying for them.

A final note in laying the groundwork for our study of speech sound disorders is to place it in its most current context. The dawn of the current millennium brought with it a new era of accountability. Those who pay for our services, whether they be taxpayers, school or hospital administrators, insurance executives, or our clients and their families, have begun to ask that we as a profession demonstrate that the services we provide are both effective (i.e., that they actually work) and efficient (i.e., that they do so in the most cost-effective way). No longer is it sufficient for us to simply say, "Trust us; we know what we're doing." We need to provide scientific evidence; put another way, we need to demonstrate that we are engaging in *evidence-based practice (EBP)*. This book is a step in that direction. In her 2007 book on EBP, Christine Dollaghan suggests that EBP requires

> the conscientious, explicit, and judicious integration of 1) best available *external* evidence from systematic research, 2) best available evidence *internal* to clinical practice, and 3) best available evidence concerning the preferences of a fully informed patient (p. 2, italics in original).

Relative to external evidence, this book has, since its first edition, been about presenting the best of the available scientific studies relating to working with children who have speech sound disorders. Relative to internal evidence, the section in Chapter 8, "Measuring Clinical Change," discusses how the conscientious clinician can and should generate his or her own evidence about whether what he or she is doing with each client is in fact resulting in meaningful change. Finally, relative to patient preferences, the last 20 years have yielded a long and varied menu of treatment approaches, many of which are highlighted in Chapters 9 and 10. It is no longer a matter of clinicians simply telling parents that we will "do artic therapy." Rather, parents of children with speech sound disorders need to be made aware of available treatment options, and EBP mandates that they be partners in determining which approach or instructional formats may be best prescribed for their child.

Each of the chapters in this text was developed with the thought of providing the student the latest information and research in clinical phonology. The breadth and depth of information presented is designed to provide a broad-based perspective of how the speech-language pathologist can go about helping children who face difficulties producing the sounds of the language.

CHAPTER 2

Normal Aspects of Articulation

RAY KENT

University of Wisconsin–Madison

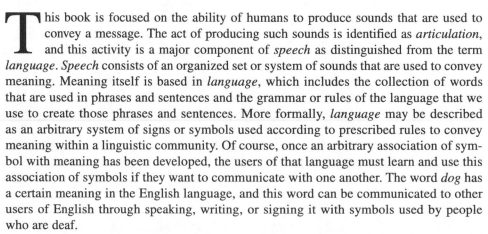

This book is focused on the ability of humans to produce sounds that are used to convey a message. The act of producing such sounds is identified as *articulation*, and this activity is a major component of *speech* as distinguished from the term *language*. *Speech* consists of an organized set or system of sounds that are used to convey meaning. Meaning itself is based in *language*, which includes the collection of words that are used in phrases and sentences and the grammar or rules of the language that we use to create those phrases and sentences. More formally, *language* may be described as an arbitrary system of signs or symbols used according to prescribed rules to convey meaning within a linguistic community. Of course, once an arbitrary association of symbol with meaning has been developed, the users of that language must learn and use this association of symbols if they want to communicate with one another. The word *dog* has a certain meaning in the English language, and this word can be communicated to other users of English through speaking, writing, or signing it with symbols used by people who are deaf.

Speech is but one modality for the expression of language; however, speech has special importance because it is the primary, first-learned modality for hearing language users. Speech is a system in the sense that it consistently and usefully relates the meanings of a language with the sounds by which the language is communicated.

Not all sound variations in speech are related to meaning. When a person suffers from a cold, he or she has a different way of talking, but so long as the cold is not so severe as to make speech unintelligible, the relation of sound to meaning is basically the same as when the person is healthy. The acoustic signal of speech—that is, the vibrations of air molecules in response to the energy source of human speech—carries more information than just the expression of meaning. As we listen to a speaker, we often make judgments not only about the intended meaning but also about the speaker's age and sex (if the speaker isn't visible), the speaker's mood, the speaker's state of health, and perhaps even the speaker's dialectal background. Thus, on hearing a simple question—"Could you tell me the time, please?"— we might deduce that the speaker is a young southern woman in a hurry, an elderly British gentleman in a cheerful mood, or a young boy quite out of breath.

STRUCTURE OF LANGUAGE

Speech sounds, then, may be viewed from two perspectives: (1) as motor production (speech) and (2) as units that facilitate the expression of meaning (language). When sounds are studied as part of the language system, they are called *phonemes*.

To derive a speaker's meaning, the listener is basically concerned with the phonemes in the speech message. From a linguistic perspective, phonemes are sound units related to decisions about meaning. In the list *cat hat mat bat sat fat that chat,* each word rhymes with every other word because all end with the same sounds (the vowel /æ/ and the consonant /t /). However, the words differ in their initial sounds, and these differences can change the meaning of the syllables. In fact, the linguist identifies the phonemes in a given language by assembling lists of words and then determining the sound differences that form units of meaning. The layperson usually thinks of words as the units of meaning, but the linguist recognizes a smaller form called the *morpheme*. For example, the linguist describes the words *walked* and *books* as having two morphemes: *walk + past tense* for *walked*, and *book + plural* for *books*. If two sounds can be interchanged without changing word meaning, or if they never occur in exactly the same combination with other sounds, then they are not different phonemes. Hence, phonemes are the minimal sound elements that represent and distinguish language units (words or morphemes).

A *phonemic transcription* (which is always enclosed in virgules / /) is less detailed than a *phonetic transcription* (which is enclosed in brackets [ ]). A phonetic transcription is sensitive to sound variations within a phoneme class. An individual variant of this kind is called an *allophone*. Thus, a phoneme is a family of allophones. Phonemes are the minimal set of sound classes needed to specify the meaningful units (words or morphemes) of the language. Allophones are a more numerous set of distinct sounds, some of which may belong to the same phoneme family. As a very simple example, the word *pop* begins and ends with the same phoneme but often begins and ends with a different allophone. If the final /p/ is produced by holding the lips together after they close, then this sound is the unreleased allophone of the /p/ phoneme. However, the initial /p/ must be released before the vowel is formed, so this sound is the released allophone of the /p/ phoneme. The /p/ phoneme also includes a number of other allophones, though perhaps not as obvious as these two.

To understand more clearly the difference between phonemes and allophones, say the following word-pairs to yourself as you try to detect a difference in the production of the italicized sounds.

*k*eep − *c*oop	(phoneme /k/)
m*a*n − b*a*t	(phoneme /æ/)
te*n* − te*n*th	(phoneme /n/)

In the first pair of words, the phoneme /k/ is articulated toward the front of the mouth in the first word and toward the back of the mouth in the second. Despite the differences in the place of tongue contact, the two sounds are heard by speakers of English to be the same phoneme. Speakers of other languages, such as Arabic, may hear the two sounds as different phonemes. The tongue-front and tongue-back versions are allophones of the /k/ phoneme in English.

In the next pair of words, *man* and *bat*, the pertinent difference might be more easily heard than felt through articulation. In the word *man*, the vowel is nasalized (produced with sound transmission through the nose) owing to the influence of the surrounding nasal consonants. But in the word *bat*, the vowel /æ/ is not normally nasalized. The phonetic environment of the vowel—that is, its surrounding sounds—determines whether the vowel is nasalized. The nasal and nonnasal versions of the vowel are allophones of the /æ/ phoneme.

Finally, in comparing /n/ in the words *ten* and *tenth*, you might notice that your tongue is more toward the front (just behind the upper front teeth) in the word *tenth*. The final *th* sound exerts an articulatory influence on the preceding /n/, causing it to be dentalized or produced at the teeth. Again, the two types of /n/ are simply allophones of the /n/ phoneme.

Allophonic variation is of two types: complementary distribution and free variation. In *complementary distribution*, two (or more) allophones never occur in exactly the same phonetic environment, so that the occurrence of one is complementary (nonoverlapping) to the occurrence of the other. For example, the front and back /k/ discussed above are in complementary distribution. The front /k/ occurs in the environment of vowels made in the front of the mouth, and the back /k/ occurs in the environment of vowels made in the back of the mouth. Similarly, the nasal and nonnasal allophones of /æ/ are in complementary distribution, determined by the presence or absence of nasals in the phonetic environment. The nasalized /æ/ occurs only when this vowel is preceded or followed by nasal sounds. Allophones are said to be in *free variation* when they can occur in the same phonetic context. For example, the released /p/ and the unreleased /p/ are in free variation in word-final position in words like *pop* or *map*. As previously indicated, the final /p/ can be released audibly with a small burst as the lips open. or it can be unreleased if the lip closure is maintained.

The discipline of linguistics is concerned primarily with the structure of language. The disciplines of psychology and speech-language pathology are concerned primarily with the processing of language—with its formulation and its reception. The linguistic study of language structure has influenced the study of language processing, and, to some degree, the reverse is true as well. Descriptions of language processing often use terms, such as *syntax, semantics, phonology*, and *phonetics*, that denote traditional areas of linguistic study. These terms have come to have a dual usage, one referring to structure and another to processing.

To briefly round out our discussion of the structure of language, we need to mention phonemes and morphemes. *Phonemes* are combined to produce meaningful units, called *morphemes*, which we usually identify as words. However, it should be recognized that a given word, such as *walked*, may actually be composed of two or more morphemes—in the case of *walked*, the morphemes are the verb *walk* and the past tense marker *ed*. *Morphemes* are combined into phrases and sentences according to the grammatical rules of the language, and these combinations are referred to as the *syntax* of the language. Thus, language includes a set of phonemes and morphemes that are combined according to certain rules to reflect the syntax of the language. Meaning that is ascribed to individual words is identified as the *semantics* of the language. In a sense, the components of language (phonology, morphology, syntax) are one side of the coin with semantics being the other side.

Figure 2.1 is a diagram of an information-processing model of verbal formulation and utterance production. The diagram attempts to show how different types of information

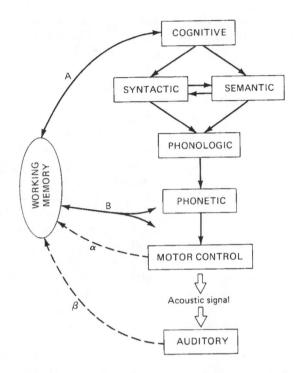

FIGURE 2.1 Information-processing model of verbal formulation production.

Source: Adapted from Bock (1982).

are processed in the act of speaking. The cognitive level is where a thought is initiated. This is a prelinguistic, propositional level that involves decisions such as the identification of participants and actions. For example, the cognitive processing that preceded formulation of the sentence, *The dog chased the cat*, involved the identification of a dog and a cat as participants and chasing or pursuit as an action. However, the specific words *dog*, *cat*, and *chased* were not actually selected. Rather, concepts that later lead to the identification of these words at the semantic level are established.

Information from the cognitive level is used to make decisions at the syntactic and semantic levels. Syntax involves the ordering of words in a sentence, and semantics involves the selection of words. Research on verbal formulation indicates that syntactic and semantic processing is interactive (hence, the arrows between them in the diagram). Deciding on a particular syntactic structure for a sentence can influence word selection, and selection of particular words can limit or direct syntactic decisions. The semantic level is sometimes called *lexicalization*, or the choice of lexical units. Lexicalization appears to be a two-stage process. The first stage is selection of a lexical concept, not a phonologically complete word. Phonologic specification—that is, specification of the word's sound pattern—is accomplished in the second stage of the process. The phonologic level in Figure 2.1 is the level at which the evolving sentence comes to have phonologic structure. Various decisions are made at this level to ensure that a sound pattern accurately represents the syntactic and semantic decisions made earlier. The phonologic information then directs decisions at the phonetic level, where the details of the sound pattern are worked out. We might think of the phonetic level as producing a detailed phonetic representation of the utterance.

The output of the phonetic level is sufficient to specify the phonetic goals to be satisfied in speech production. Actual motor instructions are determined by a motor control level. This level selects the muscles to be activated and controls the timing and strength of the muscle contractions. This is no small task. Speech requires rapid changes in the activation of about 100 muscles, which are controlled to meet exacting spatiotemporal goals. Once the muscles have done their work, the acoustic speech signal is produced. This signal is then processed by the speaker and the listener(s) as auditory information. For the speaker, the auditory processing completes a feedback loop.

One component that remains to be explained in Figure 2.1 is working memory and its connections to other parts of the diagram. Working memory is a speaker's operational memory, the memory that is used to keep track of the information involved in sentence production. But this memory is limited, so it is in the interest of efficient processing to minimize demands on it. Therefore, the theory goes, two kinds of processing are involved in utterance production. One is *controlled processing*; this kind makes demands on working memory. The other is *automatic processing*, which does not require allocation of working memory. Verbal formulation is performed with both controlled processing and automatic processing. Controlled processing can be identified in Figure 2.1 by the arrows labeled A and B. Note that syntactic, semantic, and phonologic processing are automatic; that is, the speaker does not have direct access to these operations. It is for this reason that slips of the tongue are not detected until they are actually spoken.

Feedback is provided by two channels, labeled α and β in Figure 2.1. Channel α represents information from touch and movement. Channel β represents auditory feedback.

Researchers have concluded that when a person ordinarily produces a sentence, he or she doesn't make all of the syntactic, semantic, and phonologic decisions before beginning to speak. Rather, it is likely that the individual will utter a few words and then formulate the remainder of the utterance.

According to this view of verbal formulation, producing a sentence involves highly interactive levels of processing and a complex time pattern for this processing. It would not be surprising, then, to discover that articulation is affected by syntactic, semantic, and phonologic variables.

The following discussion of articulatory phonetics presents basic information on speech sound production. For the student who has had a course in phonetics, this chapter will serve as a summary review. The student without such background should be able to acquire at least the basics of articulatory phonetics. The topics to be discussed are these:

The Speech Mechanism

Vowels
   Monophthongs (single vowels)
   Diphthongs

Consonants
   Stops
   Nasals

> Fricatives
> Affricates
> Liquids
> Glides

Suprasegmentals

Coarticulation

Aerodynamics

Acoustics

Sensory Information

Phonology

FUNDAMENTALS OF ARTICULATORY PHONETICS

The Speech Mechanism

The anatomy of the speech production system is not within the scope of this chapter, but some general anatomical descriptions are needed to discuss the fundamentals of articulatory phonetics. The basic aspects of speech production can be understood by an examination of six principal organs or subsystems, illustrated in Figure 2.2. The *respiratory system*,

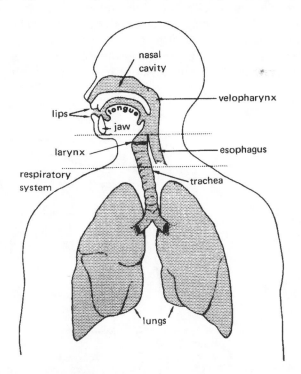

FIGURE 2.2 Organs of speech production.

consisting of the lungs, airway, rib cage, diaphragm, and associated structures, provides the basic air supply for generating sound. The *larynx,* composed of various cartilages and muscles, generates the voiced sounds of speech by vibration of the vocal folds, or it allows air to pass from lungs to the vocal tract (the oral and nasal cavities) for voiceless sounds. The *velopharynx*—the soft palate (or velum) and associated structures of the velopharyngeal port—joins or separates the oral and nasal cavities so that air passes through the oral cavity, the nasal cavity, or both. The *tongue*, primarily a complex of muscles, is the principal articulator of the oral cavity; it is capable of assuming a variety of shapes and positions in vowel and consonant articulation. For articulatory purposes, the tongue is divided into five major parts: the tip or apex, the blade, the back or dorsum, the root, and the body. These divisions are illustrated in Figure 2.3. The *lips*, along with the jaw, are the most visible of the articulators; they are involved in the production of vowels and consonants. The *jaw*, the massive bony structure and its associated muscles, supports the soft tissues of both tongue and lower lip. It participates in speech production by aiding tongue and lip movements and by providing skeletal support for these organs. Other anatomical features shown in Figure 2.2 provide general orientation or are relevant in a significant way to the processes of speech and hearing.

The respiratory system and larynx work together to provide the upper airway with two major types of air flow: a series of pulses of air created by the action of the vibrating vocal folds (for voiced sounds like the sounds in the word *buzz*) and a continuous flow of air that can be used to generate noise energy in the vocal tract (for voiceless sounds like the *s* in *see*). The basic function of the respiratory system in speech is to push air into the airway composed of the larynx and the oral and nasal cavities. The basic function of the larynx is to regulate the airflow from the lungs to create both voiced and voiceless segments. The upper airway, often called the *vocal tract*, runs from the larynx to the mouth or nose and is the site of what is commonly called *speech articulation.* For the most

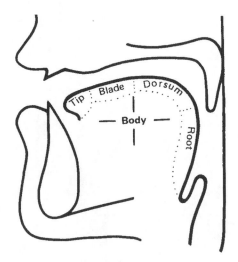

FIGURE 2.3 Divisions of tongue into five functional parts for speech articulation.

part, this process is accomplished by movements of the *articulators*: tongue, lips, jaw, and velopharynx. The vocal tract may be viewed as a flexible tube that can be lengthened or shortened (by moving the larynx up and down in the neck or by protruding and retracting the lips) and constricted at many points along its length by actions of tongue, velopharynx, and lips. Speech articulation is thus a matter of lengthening, shortening, and constricting the tube known as the *vocal tract.*

This entire process is controlled by the nervous system, which must translate the message to be communicated into a pattern of signals that run to the various muscles of the speech mechanism. As these muscles contract, a variety of things can happen: Air may be pushed out of the lungs, the vocal folds may start to vibrate, the velopharynx may close, the jaw may lower, or the lips may protrude. The brain has the task of coordinating all the different muscles so that they contract in the proper sequence to produce the required phonetic result. The margin for error is small; sometimes an error of just a few milliseconds in the timing of a muscle contraction can result in a misarticulation.

It is appealing to suppose that speech production is controlled at some relatively high level of the brain by discrete units, such as phonemes. However, a major problem in the description of speech articulation is to relate the discrete linguistic units that operate at a high level of the brain to the muscle contractions that result in articulatory movements. For example, to say the word *stop*, a speaker's brain must send nerve instructions, in the proper sequence, to the muscles of the respiratory system, larynx, tongue, lips, and velopharynx. The full understanding of speech production therefore involves a knowledge of *phonology* (the study of how sounds are put together to form words and other linguistic units), *articulatory phonetics* (the study of how the articulators make individual sounds), *acoustic phonetics* (the study of the relationship between articulation and the acoustic signal of speech), and *speech perception* (the study of how phonetic decisions are made from the acoustic signal).

Vowel Articulation: Traditional Phonetic Description

A vowel sound is usually formed as sound energy from the vibrating vocal folds escapes through a relatively open vocal tract of a particular shape. Because a syllable must contain a vowel or vowel-like sound, vowels sometimes are called *syllable nuclei.* Each vowel has a characteristic vocal tract shape that is determined by the position of the tongue, jaw, and lips. Although other parts of the vocal tract, like the velum, pharyngeal walls, and cheeks, may vary somewhat with different vowels, the positions of the tongue, jaw, and lips are of primary consequence. Therefore, individual vowels can be described by specifying the articulatory positions of tongue, jaw, and lips. Furthermore, because the jaw and tongue usually work together to increase or reduce the mouth opening (Figure 2.4), for general phonetic purposes, vowel production can be described by specifying the positions of just two articulators, tongue and lips. Usually the vocal folds vibrate to produce voicing for vowels, but exceptions, such as whispered speech, do occur.

The two basic lip articulations can be demonstrated with the vowels in the words *he* and *who*. Press your finger against your lips as you say first *he* and then *who*. You should feel the lips push against your finger as you say *who*. The vowel in this word is a rounded

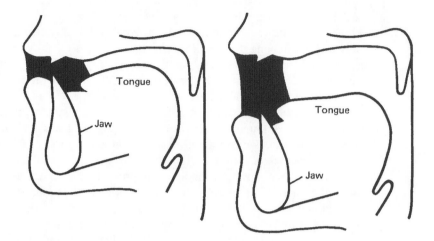

FIGURE 2.4 Variations in mouth opening (darkened area) related to lowering of jaw and tongue.

vowel, meaning that the lips assume a rounded, protruded posture. Vowels in English are described as being either rounded, like the vowel in *who*, or unrounded, like the vowel in *he*. Figure 2.5 illustrates the lip configuration for these two vowels.

The tongue moves in essentially two dimensions within the oral cavity, as shown in Figure 2.6. One dimension, front-back, is represented by the motion the tongue makes as you alternately say *he*, *who* or *map*, *mop*. The other dimension, high-low, is represented by

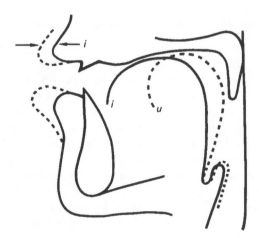

FIGURE 2.5   Vocal tract configurations for /i/ and /u/. Note lip rounding for /u/.

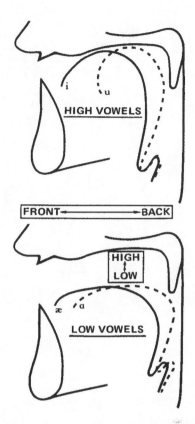

FIGURE 2.6 The two major dimensions of tongue position, front-back and high-low.

the motion the tongue makes as you say *heave-have* or *who-ha*. With these two dimensions of tongue movement, we can define four extreme positions of the tongue within the oral cavity, as shown in Figure 2.7. The phonetic symbols for these four vowels also are shown in the illustration. With the tongue high and forward in the mouth, the high-front vowel /i/ as in *he* is produced. When the tongue is low and forward in the mouth, the low-front vowel /æ/ as in *have* is produced. A tongue position that is high and back in the mouth yields the high-back vowel /u/. Finally, when the tongue is low and back in the mouth, the vowel is the low-back /ɑ/. The four vowels, /i/, /æ/, /u/, and /ɑ/, define four points that establish the *vowel quadrilateral*, a four-sided figure against which tongue position for vowels can be described. In Figure 2.8, the vowels of English have been plotted by phonetic symbol and key word within the quadrilateral. As an example, notice the vowel /ɪ/ as in *bit* has a tongue position that is forward in the mouth and not quite as high as that for /i/. The tongue position for any one vowel can be specified with terms such as low-high, front for /ɪ/ as in *bit*, low-mid, front for /ɛ/ as in *bet*, mid-central for /ɝ/ as in *Bert*, and low-mid, back for /ɔ/ as in *bought*.

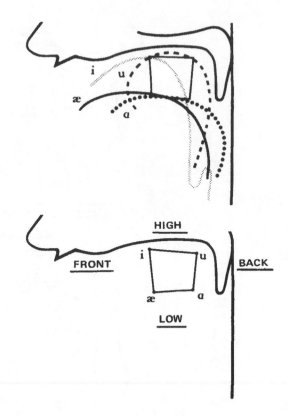

FIGURE 2.7 The four corner vowels /i/, /u/, /ɑ/, and /æ/ are shown at the top as tongue positions in the oral cavity and at the bottom as points of a quadrilateral.

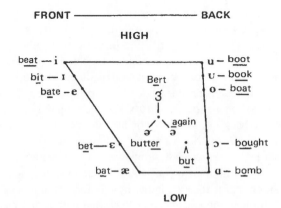

FIGURE 2.8 English vowels, identified by phonetic symbol and key word and plotted within vowel quadrilateral.

The vowels of English can be categorized as follows with respect to tongue position:

Front vowels:	/i/	/ɪ/	/e/	/ɛ/	/æ/			
Central vowels:	/ɝ/	/ʌ/	/ɚ/	/ə/				
Back vowels:	/u/	/ʊ/	/o/	/ɔ/	/ɑ/			
High vowels:	/i/	/ɪ/	/u/	/ʊ/				
Mid vowels:	/e/	/ɛ/	/ɝ/	/ʌ/	/ɚ/	/ə/	/o/	/ɔ/
Low vowels:	/æ/	/ɑ/						

The vowels can also be categorized with respect to lip rounding, with the following being rounded: /u/, /ʊ/, /o/, /ɔ/, and /ɝ/. All other vowels are unrounded. Notice that, in English, the rounded vowels are either back or central vowels; front rounded vowels do not occur.

Vowel production is also commonly described as *tense (long)* or *lax (short)*. Tense vowels are longer in duration and supposedly involve a greater degree of muscular tension. Lax vowels are relatively short and involve less muscular effort. One way of demonstrating the distinction between tense and lax is to feel the fleshy undersurface of your jaw as you say /i/ as in *he* and /ɪ/ as in *him*. Most people can feel a greater tension for /i/ (a tense vowel) than for /ɪ/ (a lax vowel). The tense vowels are /i/, /e/, /ɝ/, /u/, /o/, /ɔ/, and /ɑ/. The remaining vowels are considered lax, but opinion is divided for the vowel /æ/ as in *bat*.

In standard production, all English vowels are voiced (associated with vibrating vocal folds) and nonnasal (having no escape of sound energy through the nose). Therefore, the descriptors *voiced* and *nonnasal* usually are omitted. However, it should be remembered that vowels are sometimes devoiced, as in whispering, and nasalized, as when they precede or follow nasal consonants. For phonetic purposes it is usually sufficient to describe a vowel in terms of the three major characteristics of tenseness—laxness, lip configuration, and tongue position. Examples of vowel description are given as follows:

/i/	tense, unrounded, high-front
/o/	tense, rounded, high-mid, back
/ɝ/	tense, rounded, mid-central
/ʊ/	lax, rounded, low-high, back

Closely related to the vowels are the *diphthongs*, which, like vowels, are produced with an open vocal tract and serve as the nuclei for syllables. But unlike vowels, diphthongs are formed with an articulation that gradually changes during production of the sound. Diphthongs are dynamic sounds because they involve a progressive change in vocal tract shape. An example of the articulation of /aɪ/ is shown in Figure 2.9. Many phoneticians regard diphthongs as combinations of two vowels, one called the *onglide* portion and the other called the *offglide* portion. This vowel + vowel description underlies the phonetic

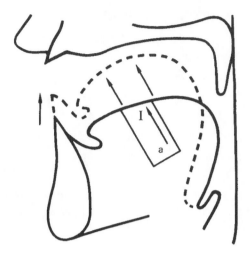

FIGURE 2.9   Articulation of diphthong /aɪ/ (as in eye), represented as onglide (/a/) and offglide (/ɪ/) configurations.

symbols for the diphthongs, which have the *digraph* (two-element) symbols /aɪ /, /aʊ/, /ɔɪ/, /eɪ/, and /oʊ/. Key words for these sounds are as follows:

/aɪ/   I, buy, why, ice, night

/aʊ/   ow, bough, trout, down, owl

/ɔɪ/   boy, oil, loin, hoist

/eɪ/   bay, daze, rain, stay

/oʊ/   bow, no, load, bone

Whereas the diphthongs /aɪ/, /aʊ/, and /ɔɪ/ are truly phonemic diphthongs, /eɪ/ and /oʊ/ are not; they are variants of the vowels /e/ and /o/, respectively. The diphthongal forms /eɪ/ and /oʊ/ occur in strongly stressed syllables, whereas the monophthongal (single-vowel) forms /e/ and /o/ tend to occur in weakly stressed syllables. For example, in the word *vacation*, the first syllable (weakly stressed) is produced with /e/ and the second syllable (strongly stressed) is produced with /eɪ/. Stressed syllables tend to be long in duration and therefore allow time for the articulatory movement of the diphthong. The diphthongs /aɪ/, /aʊ/, and /ɔɪ/ do not alternate with monophthongal forms. To produce a recognizable /aɪ/, /aʊ/, or /ɔɪ/, a speaker must use a diphthongal movement.

As shown in Figure 2.10, the onglide and offglide segments of the diphthongs are roughly located by the positions of the digraph symbols on the vowel quadrilateral. For example, in diphthong /aɪ/, the tongue moves from a low-back to nearly a high-front position. However, it should be noted that these onglide and offglide positions are only approximate and that substantial variation occurs across speakers and speaking conditions.

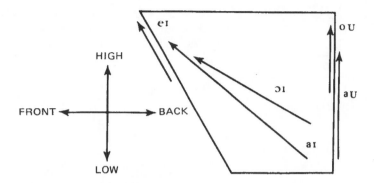

FIGURE 2.10 Diphthong articulation shown as onglide to offglide arrows in the vowel quadrilateral.

Vowel Articulation: Description by Distinctive Features

The phonetic descriptions considered to this point are one method of classifying vowel sounds. An alternative is a method relying on *distinctive features*, as defined by the linguists Noam Chomsky and Morris Hallé (1968). The distinctive features are a set of binary (two-valued) features designed to describe the phonemes in all languages of the world. A convenient example of a binary feature is nasality. In general terms, a given speech sound is either nasal or nonnasal, meaning that sound energy is transmitted through the nose (nasal) or is not (nonnasal). If nasality is described as a binary feature, then sounds can be classified as +nasal (indicating the nasal transmission of sound) or −nasal (indicating the absence of nasal transmission). Hence, a positive value (+nasal) means that the property is present or is relevant to description of the sound. In some ways, distinctive feature analysis is similar to the guessing game Twenty Questions in which the participants have to identify an object by asking questions that can be answered with only yes or no. Chomsky and Hallé proposed a set of 13 binary features, which, given the appropriate yes (+) or no (−) answers, can describe all phonemes used in the languages of the world.

In the Chomsky-Hallé system, the voiced vowels are specified primarily with the features shown in Table 2.1. First, notice the three major class features of *sonorant, vocalic,* and *consonantal.* A sonorant sound is produced with a vocal cavity configuration in which spontaneous voicing is possible. Essentially, the vocal tract above the larynx is sufficiently open so that no special laryngeal adjustments are needed to initiate voicing. For nonsonorants, or *obstruents,* the cavity configuration does not allow spontaneous voicing. Special mechanisms must be used to produce voicing during the nonsonorant sounds. Vocalic sounds are produced with an oral cavity shape in which the greatest constriction does not exceed that associated with the high vowels /i/ and /u/ and with vocal folds that are adjusted so as to allow spontaneous voicing. This feature, then, describes the degree of opening of the oral cavity together with the vocal fold adjustment. Finally, consonantal sounds have a definite constriction in the *midsagittal,* or midline, region of the vocal tract; nonconsonantal sounds do not. Vowels are described as +sonorant, +vocalic, and −consonantal. Taken together, these three features indicate that vowels are produced with a

TABLE 2.1 Distinctive Features for Selected Vowel Sounds (The Class Features Distinguish Vowels from Various Consonants; Therefore, All Vowels Have the Same Values for These Features)

Class Features	i	ɪ	ε	æ	ʌ	ɝ	u	ʊ	ɔ	ɑ
Sonorant	+	+	+	+	+	+	+	+	+	+
Vocalic	+	+	+	+	+	+	+	+	+	+
Consonantal	−	−	−	−	−	−	−	−	−	−
Cavity Features										
High	+	+	−	−	−	−	+	+	−	−
Low	−	−	−	+	−	−	−	−	+	+
Back	−	−	−	−	−	−	+	+	+	+
Rounded	−	−	−	−	−	+	+	+	+	−
Nasal	−	−	−	−	−	−	−	−	−	−
Manner of Articulation Feature										
Tense	+	−	−	+	−	+	+	−	+	+

relatively open oral cavity, with no severe constriction in the midsagittal plane, and with a vocal fold adjustment that allows for spontaneous vocal fold vibration.

Vowels are also described with respect to cavity features and manner of articulation features, some of which are shown in Table 2.1 (the others will be discussed with respect to consonants later in this chapter). The cavity features of primary concern in vowel description are:

> **Tongue Body Features: High-Nonhigh; Low-Nonlow; Back-Nonback (see Figure 2.11a, b, c)**
>
> High sounds are produced by raising the body of the tongue above the level that it occupies in the neutral (or resting) position, as shown in Figure 2.11a.
>
> Low sounds are produced by lowering the body of the tongue below the level that it occupies in the neutral position; see Figure 2.11b.
>
> Back sounds are produced by retracting the body of the tongue from the neutral position, as shown in Figure 2.11c.
>
> *Rounded–Nonrounded.* Rounded sounds have a narrowing or protrusion of the lips.
>
> *Nasal–Nonnasal.* Nasal sounds are produced with a lowered velum, so that sound energy escapes through the nose.

Table 2.1 shows that most vowels can be distinguished using the cavity features. For example, /i/ and /u/ differ in the back and rounded features, and /æ/ and /i/ differ in the high and low features. Most other distinctions can be made by referring to a manner of articulation called *tense–nontense*. Tense sounds are produced with a deliberate, accurate, maximally distinct gesture that involves considerable muscular effort. The

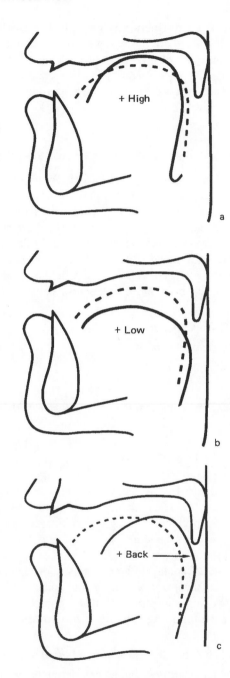

FIGURE 2.11 Vocal tract drawings illustrating the tongue body features (a) high, (b) low, and (c) back relative to the neutral tongue position (broken line).

tense–nontense distinction is best illustrated with the vowel pairs /i/–/ɪ/ and /u/–/ʊ/. Vowels /i/ and /u/ are tense vowels because they are lengthened and are produced with marked muscular effort. As mentioned earlier, the difference in muscular effort can be felt by placing your fingers in the fleshy area just under the chin, saying alternately /i/–/ɪ/. A greater tension occurs during production of the tense vowel /i/ than during the nontense vowel /ɪ/.

Consonant Articulation: Traditional Phonetic Description

The consonants generally differ from the vowels in terms of the relative openness of the vocal tract and the function they play within the syllable. Vowels are produced with an open vocal tract; most consonants are made with a complete or partially constricted vocal tract. Within a syllable, vowels serve as a nucleus, meaning that a syllable must contain one and only one vowel (the only exceptions to this rule are the diphthongs, which are like vowels plus vowel glides, and certain syllabic consonants to be discussed later). Consonants are added to the vowel nucleus to form different syllable shapes, such as the following, where V represents a vowel and C represents a consonant.

> VC shape: *on, add, in*
> CV shape: *do, be, too*
> CVC shape: *dog, cat, man*
> CCVC shape: *truck, skin, clap*
> CCCVCC shape: *screams, squint, scratched*

Consonants are described by degree or type of closure and by the location at which the complete or partial closure occurs. The *manner* of consonant articulation refers to the degree or type of closure, and the *place* of consonant articulation refers to the location of the constriction. In addition, consonants are described as *voiced* when the vocal folds are vibrating and *voiceless* when the vocal folds are not vibrating. Thus, an individual consonant can be specified by using three terms: one to describe *voicing*, one to describe *place*, and one to describe *manner*. Tables 2.2 and 2.3 show combinations of these terms used to specify the consonants of English.

Table 2.2 contains four columns, showing place of articulation, phonetic symbol and key word, manner of articulation, and voicing. The terms for place of articulation usually signify two opposing structures that accomplish a localized constriction of the vocal tract. Notice in the following definitions the two structures involved for the place terms.

> Bilabial: two lips (*bi* = *two* and *labia* = *lip*)
> Labial/velar: lips, and a constriction between the *dorsum* or back of the tongue and the velum
> Labiodental: lower lip and upper teeth
> Linguadental or interdental: tip of tongue and upper teeth (*lingua* = *tongue*)
> Lingua-alveolar: tip of tongue and the *alveolar ridge*

TABLE 2.2 Classification of Consonants by Manner and Voicing within Place

Place of Articulation	Phonetic Symbol and Key Word	Manner of Articulation	Voicing
Bilabial	/p/ (pay)	Stop	−
	/b/ (bay)	Stop	+
	/m/ (may)	Nasal	+
Labial/velar	/ʍ/ (which)	Glide (semivowel)	−
	/w/ (witch)	Glide (semivowel)	+
Labiodental	/f/ (fan)	Fricative	−
	/v/ (van)	Fricative	+
Linguadental	/θ/ (thin)	Fricative	−
(interdental)	/ð/ (this)	Fricative	+
Lingua-alveolar	/t/ (two)	Stop	−
	/ð/ (do)	Stop	+
	/s/ (sue)	Fricative	−
	/z/ (zoo)	Fricative	+
	/n/ (new)	Nasal	+
	/l/ (Lou)	Lateral	+
	/ɾ/ (butter)	Flap	+
Linguapalatal	/ʃ/ (shoe)	Fricative	−
	/ʒ/ (rouge)	Fricative	+
	/tʃ/ (chin)	Affricate	−
	/dʒ/ (gin)	Affricate	+
	/j/ (you)	Glide (semivowel)	+
	/r/ (rue)	Rhotic	+
Linguavelar	/k/ (back)	Stop	−
	/g/ (bag)	Stop	+
	/ŋ/ (bang)	Nasal	+
Glottal (laryngeal)	/h/ (who)	Fricative	−
	/ʔ/	Stop	+(−)

> Linguapalatal: blade of tongue and palatal area behind the alveolar ridge
>
> Linguavelar: dorsum or back of tongue and roof of mouth in the velar area
>
> Glottal: the two vocal folds

Each of these places of articulation is discussed more fully on the next several pages. To get a feeling for these different places of consonant articulation, concentrate on the first sounds in each word as you say the sequence: *pie, why, vie, thigh, tie, shy, guy, hi*. Notice

TABLE 2.3 Classification of Consonants by Place and Voicing within Manner

Manner	Place	Voiced	Voiceless
Stop	Bilabial	b	p
	Lingua-alveolar	d	t
	Linguavelar	g	k
	Glottal		
		-----------?-----------	
Fricative	Labiodental	v	f
	Linguadental	ð	θ
	Lingua-alveolar	z	s
	Linguapalatal	ʒ	ʃ
	Glottal		h
Affricative	Linguapalatal	dʒ	tʃ
Nasal	Bilabial	m	
	Lingua-alveolar	n	
	Linguavelar	ŋ	
Lateral	Lingua-alveolar	l	
Rhotic	Linguapalatal	r	
Glide	Linguapalatal	j	
	Labial/Velar	w	ʍ

from Figure 2.12 that the initial sounds constitute a progression from front to back in place of articulation.

Table 2.3 provides a breakdown of English consonants by place and voicing within manner classes. The manner of production associated with complete closure is the *stop*,

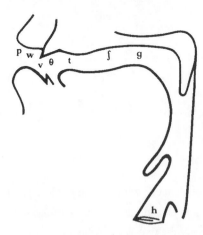

FIGURE 2.12 Places of articulation are marked by location of the phonetic symbols for the initial sounds in *pie, why, vie, thigh, tie, shy, guy, hi.*

which is formed when two structures completely block the passage of air from the vocal tract, building up air pressure behind the closure. Usually, when the closure is released, the air pressure built up behind the constriction causes a burst of escaping air. The burst is audible in words like *pie* and *two*.

Fricatives, like the initial sounds in *sue* and *zoo*, are made with a narrow constriction so that the air creates a noisy sound as it rushes through the narrowed passage.

Affricates, as in *church* and *judge*, are combinations of stop and fricative segments; that is, a period of complete closure is followed by a brief fricative segment. The stop + fricative nature of the affricates explain why these sounds are represented by the digraph symbols /tʃ/ and /dʒ/.

Nasals, as in the word *meaning* /minɪŋ/, are like stops in having a complete oral closure (bilabial, lingua-alveolar, or linguavelar) but are unlike stops in having an open velopharyngeal port so that sound energy passes through the nose rather than the mouth.

The *lateral* /l/ as in *lay* is formed by making a lingua-alveolar closure in the midline but with no closure at the sides of the tongue. Therefore, the sound energy from the vibrating folds escapes laterally, or through the sides of the mouth cavity.

The *rhotic* (or *rhotacized*) /r/ as in *ray* is a complex phoneme sometimes called *retroflex* in the phonetic literature. *Retroflex* literally means "turning" or "turned back" and refers to the appearance of the tongue tip, as viewed in X-ray films, for some /r/ productions. But in other productions of /r/, the tongue has a bunched appearance in the center or near the front of the mouth cavity. Because /r/ is produced in at least these two basic ways, the general term *rhotic* (Ladefoged, 1975) is preferable to the narrower term *retroflex*. This issue is discussed in more detail later in this chapter.

The /ʍ/, /w/, and /j/ sounds are said to have a *glide* (semivowel) manner of production. These sounds are characterized by a gliding, or gradually changing, articulatory shape. For example, in /ʍ/ and its voiced counterpart /w/, the lips gradually move from a rounded and narrowed configuration to the lip shape required by the following vowel simultaneously with a change in tongue position from high-back (like that for /u/) to the position for the following vowel. The glides always are followed by vowels.

In the following summary, manner of articulation is discussed for different places of articulation, proceeding from front to back.

Bilabial Sounds

In American English, the only consonant phonemes produced with a complete or partial closure (bilabial production) are the voiceless and voiced stops /p/ as in *pay* and /b/ as in *bay*, the nasal /m/ as in *may*, and the voiced and voiceless glides /w/ as in *witch* and /ʍ/ as in *which*. The vocal tract configurations for /p/, /b/, and /m/ are shown in Figure 2.13. These three sounds share a bilabial closure but differ in voicing and nasality. The stops /p/ and /b/ are called voiced and voiceless *cognates*, which means that they differ only in voicing. The production of these bilabial sounds is usually marked by a closed jaw position because the jaw closes somewhat to assist the constriction at the lips. The tongue is virtually unconstrained for /p/, /b/, and /m/, so that these bilabial sounds often are made simultaneously with the tongue position for preceding or following vowels. In other words, when we say words like *bee*, *pa*, and *moo*, the tongue

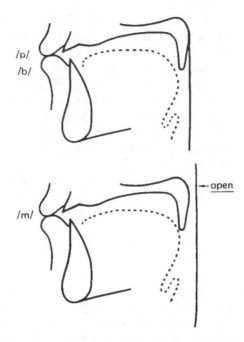

FIGURE 2.13 Vocal tract configurations for /p/, /b/, and /m/. Note labial closure for all three sounds and the open velopharynx for /m/.

is free to assume the required shape for the vowel during the closure for the bilabial, as illustrated in Figure 2.14.

The glides /w/ and /ʍ/ have a specified tongue position, roughly like that for the high-back vowel /u/, so these sounds cannot interact as freely with preceding or following sounds. Students (and even some practicing clinicians) sometimes fail to appreciate the importance of tongue articulation for /w/ and /ʍ/; for these sounds, both the tongue and lips execute gliding movements, as shown for the word *we* in Figure 2.15.

Labiodental Sounds

The voiceless and voiced *fricatives* /f/ as in *fan* and /v/ as in *van* are the only labiodental sounds in American English. The articulation is illustrated in Figure 2.16. Frication noise is generated by forcing air through the constriction formed by the lower lip and the upper teeth, principally the incisors. The noise is quite weak, very nearly the weakest of the fricatives. Like the labial sounds /p/, /b/, and /m/, the labiodentals allow the tongue to assume its position for preceding or following sounds. The jaw tends to close to aid the lower lip in its constricting gesture.

Interdental Sounds

There are only two interdentals, both fricatives: the voiceless /θ/ (e.g., *thaw*) and voiced /ð/ (e.g., *the*). They are illustrated in Figure 2.17. The frication noise is generated as air flows

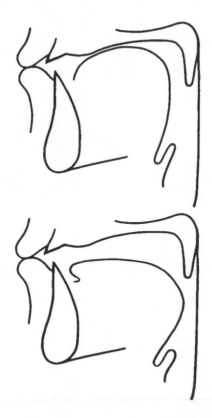

FIGURE 2.14 Variation in tongue position during a bilabial closure: (*top*) tongue position during *pea*; (*bottom*) tongue position for *pa*.

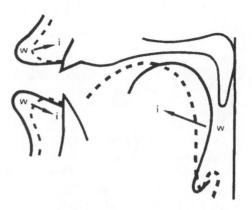

FIGURE 2.15 Illustration of gliding motion of tongue and lips for the word *we* (/wi/).

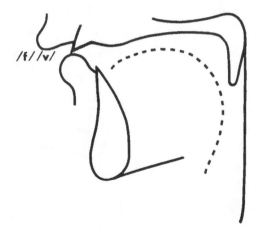

FIGURE 2.16 Vocal tract configuration for /f/ and /v/. Note labiodental constriction.

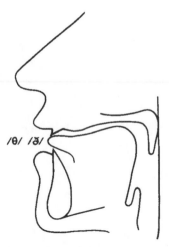

FIGURE 2.17 Vocal tract configuration for /θ/ and /ð/. Note linguadental (interdental) constriction.

through the narrow constriction created by the tongue tip and the edge of the incisors. The weak frication noise is not much different from that for /f/ or /v/. The weak intensity of these sounds should be remembered in articulation testing, and the clinician should include both visual and auditory information in evaluating this pair of sounds. Jaw position for /θ/ and /ð/ usually is closed to aid the tongue in making its constriction. These sounds may be produced with either an interdental projection of the tongue or tongue contact behind the teeth.

Alveolar Sounds

The alveolar place of production is used for two stops: the voiceless /t/ (e.g., *too*) and the voiced /d/ (e.g., *do*); a nasal: /n/ (e.g., *new*); a lateral: /l/ (e.g., *Lou*); and two fricatives: the voiceless /s/ (e.g., *sue*) and the voiced /z/ (e.g., *zoo*). Not surprisingly, given the frequent and diverse movements of the tongue tip in the alveolar region, motions of the tongue tip are among the fastest articulatory movements. For example, the major closing and release movement for the stops /t/ and /d/ is made within about 50 milliseconds, or a twentieth of a second. For /t/ and /d/, an airtight chamber is created as the tongue tip closes firmly against the alveolar ridge and the sides of the tongue seal against the lateral oral regions. The site of tongue tip closure actually varies to a limited degree with phonetic context. When /t/ or /d/ are produced before the dental fricatives /θ/ and /ð/, the stop closure is made in the dental region. This context-dependent modification of alveolar consonant production is termed *dentalization* and is illustrated for /t/ in Figure 2.18.

The nasal /n/ is similar in basic tongue shape and movement to the stops /t/ and /d/. But /n/ differs from both /t/ and /d/ in having an open velopharyngeal port, making /n/ nasalized. But /n/ further differs from /t/ in that /n/ is voiced; /t/ is not. Because /n/ and /d/ are very similar in lingual articulation and voicing, failure to close the velopharyngeal port for /d/, as might happen with some speech disorders, results in /n/. Like /t/ and /d/, /n/ is dentalized when produced in the same syllable and adjacent to a dental sound like /θ/; compare, for example, the /n/ in *nine* /naɪn/ with the /n/ in *ninth* /naɪnθ/.

The lateral /l/ is a *liquid* formed with midline closure and a lateral opening, usually at both sides of the mouth (see Figure 2.19). Because of the midline closure made by the tongue tip against the alveolar ridge, sound energy escapes through the sides of the oral cavity. Although /l/ is the only lateral sound in English, there are at least two major allophones. Historically, these allophones are termed *light* and *dark*, but phoneticians disagree as to exactly how these allophones are formed. Wise (1957a, 1957b) explained that the light /l/ is made with linguadental contact, whereas the dark /l/ is made with a lingua-alveolar

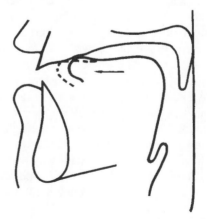

FIGURE 2.18 Dentalization of /t/. The normal alveolar closure is shown by the solid line, and the dental closure is shown by the broken line.

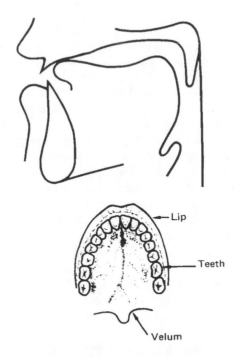

FIGURE 2.19   Articulation of /l/, shown in side view of a midline section (*top*) and as regions of tongue closure (*shaded areas*) against roof of mouth.

contact. However, Kantner and West (1960) contend that the light /l/ has a greater lip spread and a lower and flatter tongue position than the dark /l/. An important feature of /l/, presumably, is a raising of the tongue toward the velum or palate. Giles (1971) concluded from X-ray pictures of speech that for allophonic variations of /l/, the position of the tongue dorsum falls into three general groups regardless of phonetic context: prevocalic, postvocalic, and syllabic (with syllabic being similar to postvocalic /l/). The postvocalic allophones had a more posterior dorsal position than the prevocalic allophones. Tongue tip contact occasionally was not achieved for the postvocalic allophones in words like *Paul*. Otherwise, the only variation in tongue tip articulation was dentalization influenced by a following dental sound. Apparently, then, /l/ can be produced with either a relatively front (light /l/) or back (dark /l/) dorsal position, but the light and dark variants are perhaps just as well termed prevocalic and postvocalic. Lingua-alveolar contact is not essential at least for /l/ in postvocalic position, which explains why postvocalic /l/ in words like seal may sound like /o/ or /ʊ/. The fricatives /s/ and /z/ are made with a narrow constriction between the tongue tip and the alveolar ridge (see Figure 2.20).

Palatal Sounds

The palatal sounds include the voiceless and voiced fricatives /ʃ/ (e.g., *shoe*) and /ʒ/ (e.g., *rouge*), the voiceless and voiced affricates /tʃ/ (e.g., *chin*) and /dʒ/ (e.g., *gin*), the glide /j/

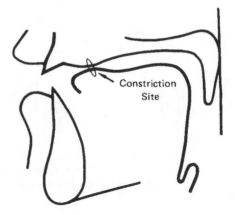

FIGURE 2.20 Vocal tract configuration or /s/ and /z/. Note lingua-alveolar constriction.

(e.g., *you*), and the rhotic or retroflex /r/ (e.g., *rue*). For these sounds, the blade or tip of the tongue makes a constriction in the palatal region, the area just behind the alveolar ridge (see Figure 2.21).

The fricatives /ʃ/ and /ʒ/, like /s/ and /z/, are sibilants associated with intense noisy energy. For /ʃ/ and /ʒ/, this noise is generated as air moves rapidly through a constriction formed between the blade of the tongue and the front palate. Similarly, the affricates /tʃ/ and /dʒ/ are made in the palatal area as stop + fricative combinations. The airstream is first

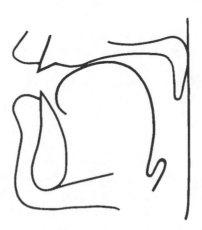

FIGURE 2.21 Vocal tract configuration for /ʃ/ and /ʒ/. Note linguapalatal constriction.

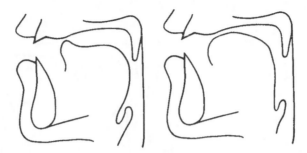

FIGURE 2.22   The two major articulations of /r/: (*left*) the retroflexed articulation; (*right*) the bunched articulation.

interrupted during the stop phase and then released during the fricative phase that immediately follows. In English, the only affricates are the palatal /tʃ/ and /dʒ/.

The glide /j/ is similar to the high-front vowel /i/ (as in *he*). The tongue is initially far forward and high in the mouth and subsequently moves toward the position for the following vowel. The similarity between /j/ and /i/ can be demonstrated by saying the biblical pronoun *ye* while noting the tongue position. Because the glide /j/ must be followed by a vowel, its articulation involves a gliding motion from the high-front position to some other vowel shape. The gliding motion can be felt during articulation of the words *you, yea, ya*.

As mentioned previously, the articulation of /r/ is highly variable. It sometimes is produced as a retroflexed consonant, in which case the tongue tip points upward and slightly backward in the oral cavity. But /r/ also can be produced with a bunching of the tongue, either in the middle of the mouth or near the front of the mouth. These basic articulations are illustrated in Figure 2.22. Some speakers also round their lips for /r/, and some constrict the lower pharynx by pulling the root of the tongue backward. Because /r/ is variably produced, it seems advisable to use *rhotic* or *rhotacized* (Ladefoged, 1975) rather than *retroflex* as a general articulatory descriptor. Given the complicated articulation of /r/, it is not surprising that it should present a major problem to children learning to talk. The variation in tongue shape and position also complicates a speech clinician's attempts to teach /r/ articulations to a child who misarticulates the sound.

Velar Sounds

A velar constriction, formed by elevation of the tongue dorsum toward the roof of the mouth, occurs for the voiceless and voiced stops /k/ and /g/ and for the nasal /ŋ/. This articulation is illustrated in Figure 2.23, which shows that the constriction can be made with the tongue relatively toward the front or relatively toward the back. The tongue placement is generally determined by the vowel context, with a front placement for velars adjacent to front vowels (e.g., /g/ in *geese*) and a back placement for velars adjacent to back vowels (e.g., /g/ in *goose*). The nasal /ŋ/ has a tongue constriction similar to that for /k/ and /g/ but has an open velopharyngeal port for nasalization. The velar and bilabial places of speech sound are similar in that both are used in English only for stops and nasals.

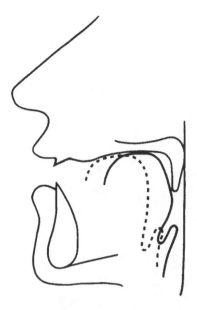

FIGURE 2.23 Vocal tract configurations for velar consonants. Note variation in site of closure.

Glottal Sounds

The glottis, or chink between the vocal folds, is primarily involved only with two sounds, the voiceless fricative /h/ and the stop /ʔ/ (a stoppage of air at the vocal folds). The fricative is produced with an opening of the vocal folds so that a fricative noise is generated as air moves at high speed through the glottis. A similar vocal fold adjustment is used in whisper.

It can be seen from Tables 2.2 and 2.3 that more types of sounds are made at some places of articulation than at others. Moreover, some sounds occur more frequently in the English language than others, contributing to a further imbalance in the use of places of articulation. Actual data on the frequency of occurrence of English consonants, grouped by place of articulation, are shown in Figure 2.24. In this circle graph, based on data from Dewey (1923), the relative frequencies of occurrence of different places of articulation are shown by the relative sizes of the pieces of the graph. Notice that alveolar sounds account for almost 50 percent of the sounds in English. The rank order of frequency of occurrence for place of articulation, from most to least frequent, is alveolar, palatal, bilabial, velar, labiodental, interdental, and glottal. Within each place-of-articulation segment in Figure 2.24, the individual consonants are listed in rank order of frequency of occurrence. For example, /n/ is the most frequently occurring alveolar consonant (in fact, it is the most frequently occurring of all consonants). Because of the differences in frequency of occurrence of consonants, a misarticulation affecting one place of articulation can be far more conspicuous than a misarticulation affecting another place. Therefore, statistical properties of the language are one consideration in the assessment and management of articulation disorders.

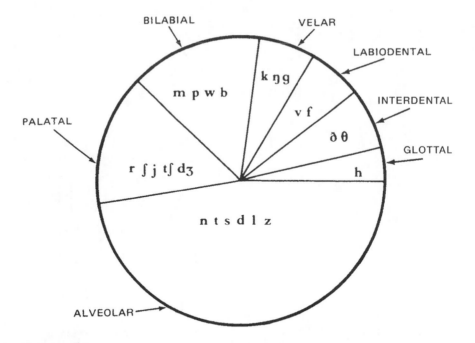

FIGURE 2.24 Circle graph showing relative frequency of occurrence of consonants made at different places of articulation.

Source: Based on data from Dewey (1923).

Consonant Articulation: Description by Distinctive Features

Distinctive features, discussed earlier with respect to vowels, can be used as an alternative to the place-manner chart to describe consonants. One simple example is the feature of voiced: All voiced consonants can be assigned the feature value of +voiced, and all voiceless consonants can be assigned the value of −voiced. Some important features for consonants are defined briefly below and are used for consonant classification in Table 2.4. These definitions are based on Chomsky and Hallé (1968).

Consonantal sounds have a radical or marked constriction in the midsagittal region of the vocal tract. This feature distinguishes the "true" consonants from vowels and glides.

Vocalic sounds do not have a radical or marked constriction of the vocal tract and are associated with spontaneous voicing. The voiced vowels and liquids are vocalic; the voiceless vowels and liquids, glides, nasal consonants, and obstruents (stops, fricatives, and affricates) are *nonvocalic* (that is, −vocalic).

Sonorant sounds have a vocal configuration that permits spontaneous voicing, which means that the airstream can pass virtually unimpeded through the oral or nasal cavity. This feature distinguishes the vowels, glides, nasal consonants, and

TABLE 2.4 Distinctive Feature Classifications for Selected Consonants

Feature	p	b	m	t	d	n	s	l	θ	k
Consonantal	+	+	+	+	+	+	+	+	+	+
Vocalic	−	−	−	−	−	−	−	−	−	−
Sonorant	−	−	+	−	−	+	−	+	−	−
Interrupted	+	+	−	+	+	−	−	−	−	+
Strident	−	−	−	−	−	−	+	−	−	−
High	(−)	(−)	(−)*	−	−	−	−	−	−	+
Low	(−)	(−)	(−)	−	−	−	−	−	−	−
Back	(−)	(−)	(−)	−	−	−	−	−	−	+
Anterior	+	+	+	+	+	+	+	+	+	−
Coronal	−	−	−	+	+	+	+	+	+	−
Rounded	−	−	−	−	−	−	−	−	−	−
Distributed	+	+	+	−	−	−	−	−	+	
Lateral	−	−	−	−	−	−	−	+	−	−
Nasal	−	−	+	−	−	+	−	−	−	−
Voiced	−	+	+	−	+	+	−	+	−	−

*Feature values enclosed in parentheses indicate that the feature in question may not be specified for this sound. For example, tongue position for /p/, /b/, and /m/ is not really specified because it is free to assume the position required for the following vowel.

lateral and rhotacized consonants from the stops, fricatives and affricates (the class of obstruents).

Interrupted sounds have a complete blockage of the airstream during a part of their articulation. Stops and affricates are +interrupted, which distinguishes them from fricatives, nasals, liquids, and glides. Sometimes the feature *continuant* is used rather than interrupted, with opposite values assigned, that is, +continuant sounds are − interrupted and vice versa.

Strident sounds are those fricatives and affricates produced with intense noise: /s/, /z/, /ʃ/, /ʒ/, /tʃ/, /dʒ/. The amount of noise produced depends on characteristics of the constriction, including roughness of the articulatory surface, rate of air flow over it, and angle of incidence between the articulatory surfaces.

High sounds are made with the tongue elevated above its neutral (resting) position (see Figure 2.11a).

Low sounds are made with the tongue lowered below its neutral position (see Figure 2.11b).

Back sounds are made with the tongue retracted from its neutral position (see Figure 2.11c).

Anterior sounds have an obstruction that is farther forward than that for the palatal /ʃ/. Anterior sounds include the bilabials, labiodentals, linguadentals, and lingua-alveolars.

Coronal sounds have a tongue blade position above the neutral state. In general, consonants made with an elevated tongue tip or blade are +coronal.

Rounded sounds have narrowed or protruded lip configuration.

Distributed sounds have a constriction extending over a relatively long portion of the vocal tract (from back to front). For English, this feature is particularly important to distinguish the dental fricatives /θ/ and /ð/ from the alveolars /s/ and /z/.

Lateral sounds are coronal consonants made with midline closure and lateral opening.

Nasal sounds have an open velopharynx allowing air to pass through the nose.

Voiced sounds are produced with vibrating vocal folds.

The feature assignments in Table 2.4 are for general illustration of the use of features. The features should be viewed with some skepticism because several different feature systems have been proposed, and any one system is subject to modification. It should be understood that distinctive features are one type of classification system. It should also be realized that distinctive features have an intended linguistic function that may not always be compatible with their application to the study of articulation disorders. The issue is beyond the scope of this chapter, but the interested reader is referred to Walsh (1974) and Parker (1976).

The relationship between the traditional place terms of phonetic description and the distinctive features is summarized here. For each traditional place term, the associated features are listed. As an example, a bilabial stop is +anterior, −coronal, and +distributed. (The placement of both features within brackets indicates that they are considered together in sound description.)

Bilabial
$$\begin{bmatrix} + \text{ anterior} \\ - \text{ coronal} \\ + \text{ distributed} \end{bmatrix}$$

Labiodental
$$\begin{bmatrix} + \text{ anterior} \\ - \text{ coronal} \\ - \text{ distributed} \end{bmatrix}$$

Interdental
$$\begin{bmatrix} + \text{ anterior} \\ + \text{ coronal} \\ + \alpha\text{distributed}^* \end{bmatrix}$$

Alveolar
$$\begin{bmatrix} + \text{ anterior} \\ + \text{ coronal} \\ - \alpha\text{distributed}^* \end{bmatrix}$$

Palatal
$$\begin{bmatrix} - \text{ anterior} \\ + \text{ high} \\ - \text{ back} \end{bmatrix}$$

Velar

$$\begin{bmatrix} -\text{coronal} \\ +\text{high} \\ +\text{back} \end{bmatrix}$$

---

*The symbol ɑ is a "dummy variable" and is used here to indicate that the Chomsky-Hallé features can distinguish the interdental and alveolar consonants only if they differ with respect to the feature *distributed*. Thus, if interdentals are regarded as −distributed, then alveolars must be +distributed. (See Ladefoged [1971] for development of this issue.)

Suprasegmentals

The phonetic characteristics discussed to this point are *segmental*, which means that the units involved in the description are the size of phonemes or phonetic segments. *Suprasegmentals* are characteristics of speech that involve larger units, such as syllables, words, phrases, or sentences. Among the suprasegmentals are stress, intonation, loudness, pitch level, juncture, and speaking rate. Briefly defined, the suprasegmentals, also called *prosodies*, or *prosodic features*, are properties of speech that have a domain larger than a single segment. This definition does not mean that a single segment cannot, at times, carry the bulk of information for a given suprasegmental; on occasion, a segment, like a vowel, can convey most of the relevant information. Most suprasegmental information in speech can be described by the basic physical quantities of amplitude (or intensity), duration, and fundamental frequency (f_0) of the voice. Stated briefly, *amplitude* refers to the perceptual attribute of loudness; *duration*, to the perceptual attribute of length; and *fundamental frequency*, to the perceptual attribute of vocal pitch.

Stress

Stress refers to the degree of effort, prominence, or importance given to some part of an utterance. For example, if a speaker wishes to emphasize that someone should take the *red* car (as opposed to a blue or green one), the speaker might say "Be sure to take the *red* car," stressing *red* to signify the emphasis. There are several varieties of stress, but all generally involve something akin to the graphic underline used to denote emphasis in writing. Although underlining is seldom used in writing, stress is almost continually used in speech. In fact, any utterance of two or more syllables may be described in terms of its stress pattern. Because it has influences that extend beyond the segment, stress usually is discussed with respect to syllables. The pronouncing guide of a dictionary places special marks after individual syllables to indicate stress. For example, the word *ionosphere* is rendered as (i-ɑn′ ə-sfer′), with the marks ′ and ′ signifying the primary and secondary stress for the syllables.

The International Phonetic Alphabet (IPA) uses a different stress notation from that commonly found in dictionaries. In IPA the stress mark precedes the syllable to which it refers, and the degree of stress is indicated by whether *any* stress mark is used and by the *location* of the stress mark in the *vertical* dimension. The strongest degree of stress is indicated by a mark above the symbol line: ′ɑn (rather like a superscript); the second degree of stress is indicated by a mark below the symbol line: 'aɪ (like a subscript); and the third degree of stress is simply unmarked: ə. The word *ionosphere* is rendered as /ˌaɪˈ ɑn ə ˌsfir/, with three degrees of stress marked.

Acoustically, stress is carried primarily by the vowel segment within a syllable. The acoustic correlates, roughly in order of importance, are fundamental frequency (especially with a rise in fundamental frequency on or near the stressed syllable), vowel duration (greater duration with increased stress), relative intensity (greater intensity with increased stress), sound quality (reduction of a vowel to a weaker, unstressed form, like /ɑ/ to /ə/, vowel substitution, and consonant changes), and disjuncture (pauses or intervals of silence) (Rabiner, Levitt, and Rosenberg, 1969).

Another form of unstressed (or weakly stressed) syllable is the syllabic consonant. This type of consonant, usually an /l/, /m/, or /n/ (but infrequently /r/), acts like a vowel in forming a syllable nucleus. Examples of syllabic consonants are the final sounds in the words *battle* /bætl̩/, *something* /sʌmʔm̩/, and *button* /bʌtn̩/. The syllabic function of a consonant is designated by a small vertical mark placed under the phonetic symbol. Syllabic consonants are most likely to occur when the consonant is *homorganic* (shares place of articulation) with a preceding consonant because it is economical or efficient simply to maintain the articulatory contact for both sounds. Additional information on stress will be provided following some basic definitions of related terms.

Intonation

Intonation is the vocal pitch contour of an utterance, that is, the way in which the fundamental frequency changes from syllable to syllable and even from segment to segment. Fundamental frequency can be affected by several factors, including the stress pattern of an utterance, tongue position of a vowel (high vowels have a higher f_0), and the speaker's emotional state.

Loudness

Loudness is related to sound intensity or to the amount of vocal effort that a speaker uses. Although loudness is ordinarily thought to be related to the amplitude or intensity of a sound, some evidence suggests that a listener's judgments of loudness of speech are related more directly to the perceived vocal effort, essentially the amount of work that a speaker does (Cavagna and Margaria, 1968). There is some evidence (Hixon, 1971; MacNeilage, 1972) that intensity variations in speech result mostly from respiratory activity, but variations of f_0 are easily accomplished at the level of the vocal folds.

Pitch Level

Pitch level is the average pitch of a speaker's voice and relates to the mean f_0 of an utterance. A speaker may be described as having a high, low, or medium pitch.

Juncture

Juncture, sometimes called *vocal punctuation,* is a combination of intonation, pausing, and other suprasegmentals to mark special distinctions in speech or to express certain grammatical divisions. For example, the written sentence "Let's eat, Grandma," has a much different meaning than the same sentence without the comma, "Let's eat Grandma!" A speaker can mark a comma vocally with a short pause and an adjustment in intonation. Juncture is also used to make distinctions between similar articulations, such as between the word *nitrate* and the phrase *night rate*. Intonation and pausing enable a speaker to indicate which alternative he or she wants to express.

Speaking Rate

The rate of speaking is usually measured in words per second, syllables per second, or phonemes per second. As speaking rate increases, segment durations generally become shorter, with some segments affected more than others. The segments most vulnerable to contraction as a speaker talks more rapidly are pauses, vowels, and consonant segments involving a sustained articulation (like fricatives). Apparently, most speakers do not really increase the rate of individual articulatory movement as they increase their rate of speaking. Rather, they reduce the duration of some segments and reduce the overall range of articulatory movement (Lindblom, 1963). As a result, the articulatory positions normally assumed during a slow rate of speaking may be missed at a faster rate. The "missing" of articulatory positions as speaking rate increases is called *undershoot*. This is why a speaker's words are apt to sound less distinct to you as the rate of speaking increases.

Vowel Reduction

Vowels are particularly susceptible to articulatory change as speaking rate is increased or stress is decreased. Such articulatory alterations are termed *reduction* and are schematized in Figure 2.25. The arrows between pairs of vowels show directions of reduction; for example, /i/ reduces first to /ɪ/ and then to /ə/, the ultimate reduced vowel. The scheme shows that, with reduction, all vowels tend toward /ə/ or /ʌ/.

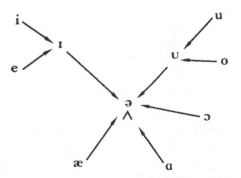

FIGURE 2.25 A scheme of vowel reduction. The arrows between vowel symbols show vowel changes resulting from reduction. For example, /i/ and /e/ reduce to /ɪ/, and /ɪ/ reduces to /ə/, which is the ultimate reduced vowel. Note that these changes occur within the quadrilateral defined by the corner vowels /i/, /æ/, /ɑ/, and /u/.

Clear versus Conversational Speech

There is considerable evidence to show that speakers alter their patterns of speech production depending on situation and listener. One variation is 'clear' versus 'conversational' speech. *Clear speech* is what speakers use when they are trying to be as intelligible as possible. Compared to more casual conversational speech, clear speech is (1) slower (with longer pauses between words and a lengthening of some speech sounds), (2) more likely to avoid modified or reduced forms of consonant and vowel segments (such as the vowel reduction described earlier), and (3) characterized by a greater intensity of obstruent sounds, particularly stop consonants (Picheny, Durlach, and Braida, 1986). When talkers want to be easily understood, they modify their speech to make it slower and more acoustically distinctive. Whereas vowels in conversational speech often are modified or reduced, therefore losing some of their acoustic distinctiveness, these sounds in clear speech are produced in distinctive forms. Similarly, word-final stops in conversational speech frequently are not released, so that the burst cue for their perception is eliminated. But in clear speech, stop consonants (and consonants in general) tend to be released, and this feature enhances their perception.

These differences are central to a hypothesis proposed by Lindblom (1990) that speakers vary their speech output along a continuum from *hypospeech* to *hyperspeech* (the H&H hypothesis). The basic idea is that speakers adapt to the various circumstances of communication to match their production patterns to communicative and situational factors. When a speaker believes that special care is required to be understood, he or she alters articulation accordingly. In Lindblom's view, clear speech (hyperspeech in his H&H hypothesis) is not simply loud speech but reflects an articulatory reorganization (Moon and Lindblom, 1989). Adams (1990), however, reported contrary evidence. He concluded from an X-ray microbeam study of speech movements that changes in speech clarity did not seem to reflect a reorganization of speech motor control. Adams observed that in clear speech, articulatory movements tended to be both larger and faster but there was no general indication that the speech patterns were organized differently than in conversational speech. The important point for clinical purposes is that speech articulation can be controlled by a speaker to enhance intelligibility when conditions warrant such deliberate effort. The primary articulatory change appears to be in the magnitude and speed of movement.

New versus Given Information

New information in a discourse is information that the listener would not be expected to know from the previous conversation or from the situation. Given information is predictable, either from the previous discourse or from the general situation. New information often is highlighted prosodically. For example, Behne (1989) studied prosody in a mini-discourse such as the following:

"Someone painted the fence."
"Who painted the fence?"
"Pete painted the fence."

In this exchange, the new information ("Pete") is lengthened and produced with a higher fundamental frequency. In effect, the speaker uses prosody to highlight the new information.

Contrastive Stress in Discourse

Another discourse-related prosodic effect is *contrastive stress*. Such stress can be given to almost any word, phrase, or clause that the speaker considers to contradict or contrast with one that was previously expressed or implied. For instance, a speaker who wants to emphasize that she took the red ball rather than the green or blue one, might say, "I took the *red* ball" (where the italicized word receives contrastive stress). Contrastive stress is sometimes used clinically to give prosodic variation to an utterance or to elicit a stressed form of a target element.

Phrase-Final Lengthening

At the syntactic level, juncture and pause phenomena are used to mark multiword units. For example, in English, *phrase-final lengthening* operates to lengthen the last stressable syllable in a major syntactic phrase or clause. For example, if we contrast the following two sentences:

1. Red, green, and blue are my favorite colors.
2. Green, blue, and red are my favorite colors.

the word *blue* will be longer in (1) than in (2) because in the former this word is at the end of the subject noun phrase and is therefore subject to phrase-final lengthening. This regularity can be exploited clinically to obtain durational adjustments for a target word. In addition, Read and Schreiber (1982) showed that phrase-final lengthening is helpful to listeners in parsing (that is, to recognize the structure of) spoken sentences. They also suggested that children rely more on this cue than adults do, and, moreover, that prosody assists the language-learner by providing structural guides to the complex syntactic structures of language.

Declination

Another effect at the syntactic level is *declination*, or the effect in which the vocal fundamental frequency contour typically declines across clauses or comparable units. Why this tilt in the overall fundamental frequency pattern occurs is a matter of debate (Cohen, Collier, and t'Hart, 1982), but it is a robust feature of prosody at the sentence or clause level. This pattern is helpful to listeners in recognizing the structure of discourse, such as in identifying sentence units.

Lexical Stress Effects

These effects operate at the level of the word. For example, English has many noun–verb pairs like *'import* versus *im'port*, or *'contrast* versus *con'trast*, in which the difference between the members of a pair is signaled primarily by stress pattern. Another common effect at the word level occurs with a distinction between compounds and phrases. For example, the compound noun *'blackbird* contrasts with the noun phrase *black 'bird* (a bird that is black).

Although the lay listener often thinks stress in English is just a matter of giving greater intensity to part of an utterance, laboratory studies have shown that stress is signaled by duration, intensity, fundamental frequency, and various phonetic effects (Fry, 1955). It is important to remember that stress affects segmental properties such as the articulation of vowels and consonants (de Jong, 1991; Kent and Netsell, 1972). Segments in stressed syllables tend to have larger and faster articulatory movements than similar segments in unstressed syllables. For this reason, stressed syllables often are favored in some phases of articulation therapy.

Because suprasegmentals like stress and speaking rate influence the nature of segmental articulation, some care should be taken to control suprasegmental variables in articulation tests and speech materials used in treatment. Vowels carry much of the suprasegmental information in speech, but stress, speaking rate, and other suprasegmentals can influence consonant articulation as well. The suprasegmental features of speech have been discussed by Crystal (1973), Lehiste (1970), and Lieberman (1967), and the reader is referred to these accounts for a more detailed consideration of this complex area.

COARTICULATION: INTERACTIONS AMONG SOUNDS IN CONTEXT

Convenient though it might be to consider phonemes as independent, invariant units that are simply linked together to produce speech, this simplistic approach does not really fit the facts. When sounds are put together to form syllables, words, phrases, and sentences, they interact in complex ways and sometimes appear to lose their separate identity. The influence that sounds exert on one another is called *coarticulation*, which means that the articulation of any one sound is influenced by a preceding or following sound. Coarticulation makes it impossible to divide the speech stream into neat segments that correspond to phonemes. Coarticulation implies nonsegmentation, or, at least, interaction of the presumed linguistic segments. Hockett (1955) provided a colorful illustration of the transformation from phoneme to articulation:

> Imagine a row of Easter eggs carried along a moving belt; the eggs are of various sizes, and variously colored, but not boiled. At a certain point, the belt carries the row of eggs between the two rollers of a wringer, which quite effectively smashes them and rubs them more or less into each other. The flow of eggs before the wringer represents the series of impulses from the phoneme source. The mess that emerges from the wringer represents the output of the speech transmitter. (p. 210)

Although this analogy makes the process of articulation sound completely disorganized, in fact the process must be quite well organized if it is to be used for communication. Phoneme-sized segments may not be carried intact into the various contractions of the speech muscles, but some highly systematic links between articulation and phonemes are maintained. Research on speech articulation has provided a clearer understanding of what the links are although the total process is far from being completely understood.

It often is possible to describe coarticulation in terms of articulatory characteristics that spread from one segment to another. Examine the following examples of coarticulation:

1a. He sneezed /h i s n i z d/ (unrounded /s/ and /s/)
1b. He snoozed /h i s n u z d/ (rounded /s/ and /n/)
2a. He asked /h i æ s k t/ (nonnasal /æ/)
2b. He answered /h i æ n s ɝ d/ (nasal /æ/)

The only phonemic difference between the first two items is the appearance of the unrounded vowel /i/ in 1a and the appearance of the rounded vowel /u/ in 1b. The lip rounding for /u/ in *He snoozed* usually begins to form during the articulation of the /s/. You might be able to feel this *anticipatory lip rounding* as you alternately say *sneeze* and *snooze* with your finger lightly touching your lips. In articulatory terms, the feature of lip rounding for the vowel is assumed during the /sn/ consonant cluster as the consequence of anticipating the rounding. The contrast between *sneeze* and *snooze* shows that the /sn/ cluster acquires lip rounding only if it is followed by a rounded vowel. This example of sound interaction is termed *anticipatory lip rounding* because the articulatory feature of rounding is evident before the rounded vowel /u/ is fully articulated as a segment.

Another form of anticipatory coarticulation occurs in 2b. Perhaps you can detect a difference in the quality of the /æ/ vowel in the phrases *He asked* and *He answered*. You should be able to detect a nasal quality in the latter because the vowel tends to assume the nasal resonance required for the following nasal consonant /n/. In this case, we can say that the articulatory feature of velopharyngeal opening (required for nasal resonance) is anticipated during the vowel /æ/. Normally, of course, this vowel is not nasalized. The contrasts between 1a and 1b and between 2a and 2b illustrate a type of coarticulation called *anticipatory*. Another type, *retentive*, applies to situations in which an articulatory feature is retained after its required appearance. For example, in the word *me,* the vowel /i/ tends to be nasalized because of a carryover velopharyngeal opening from the nasal consonant /m/. The essential lesson to be learned is that coarticulation occurs frequently in speech—so frequently, in fact, that the study of articulation is largely a study of coarticulation.

Phonetic context is highly important in understanding allophonic variation. For example, you should be able to detect a difference in the location of linguavelar closure for the /k/ sounds in the two columns of words below.

keen	*coon*
kin	*cone*
can	*con*

The point of closure tends to be more to the front of the oral cavity for the words in the first column than it is for the words in the second column. This variation occurs because, in English, the velar stops /k/ and /g/ do not have a narrowly defined place of articulation; all that is required is that the dorsum, or back, of the tongue touch the ceiling of the mouth. Therefore, the tongue is simply elevated at the position needed for the following vowel. When the tongue is in the front of the mouth (note that the vowels in the left column are front vowels), the dorsal closure is made in the front of the mouth, and when the tongue is in the back of the mouth (as it would be for the vowels in the right column), the point of closure is to the back of the velar surface.

Coarticulation arises for different reasons, some having to do with the phonology of a particular language, some with the basic mechanical or physiological constraints of the speech apparatus. Hence, some coarticulations are learned and others are the inevitable consequences of muscles, ligaments, and bones of the speech apparatus that are linked together and unable to move with infinite speed. Consider, for example, the closing and opening of the velopharyngeal port. This articulatory gesture is rather sluggish (compared to movements of the tongue tip), so it is not surprising that the velopharyngeal opening for a nasal consonant carries over to a following vowel, as in the word *no*. The extent of this carryover nasalization, however, varies with the phonologic characteristics of a particular language. In French, vowel nasalization is phonemic (that is, it can make a difference in meaning), but in English, vowel nasalization is only allophonic. Some aspects of coarticulation reflect universal properties of the human speech mechanism and hence affect all languages. Other coarticulations are governed by the phonemic structure of a particular language and are therefore learned with that language. Many coarticulatory effects are assimilatory in that a feature from one segment is adopted by an adjacent segment. For example, the nasalization of vowels by neighboring nasal consonants is nasal assimilation. Such effects may make speech production easier and faster because articulatory movements can be adapted to a particular phonetic and motor sequence. Assimilation is a general process in spoken language.

Another aspect of coarticulation is the overlapping of articulations for consonants in clusters. Quite often, the articulation for one consonant is made *before* the release of a preceding consonant in any two-consonant cluster. For example, in the word *spy* /spaɪ/, the bilabial closure for /p/ is accomplished shortly (about 10 to 20 msec) before the release of the constriction for /s/. This overlapping of consonant articulations makes the overall duration of the cluster shorter than the sum of the consonant durations as they occur singly; that is, the duration of /sp/ in *spy* is shorter than the sum of the durations of /s/ in *sigh* /s aɪ/ and /p/ in *pie* /p aɪ/. The overlapping of articulation contributes to the articulatory flow of speech by eliminating interruptions. The temporal structure of a /spr/ cluster, as in the word *spray*, is pictured schematically in Figure 2.26. Notice that the constrictions for /s/ and /p/ overlap by 10 to 20 msec and that the closure for /p/ overlaps with the tongue position for /r/ by a similar amount. Because consonants in clusters frequently present special difficulties to children (and adults) with articulation disorders, clinicians must know how such clusters are formed. Because clusters have overlapping articulations of the constituent consonants, in general, the cluster is a tightly organized sequence of articulatory gestures. The articulation of clusters is further complicated by allophonic variations, such as those listed in Table 2.5. In English, unaspirated released stops occur only when stops follow /s/, as in the words *spy*, *stay*, and *ski*. Otherwise, released stops are aspirated, meaning that the release is followed by a brief interval of glottal frication (an /h/-like noise). Similarly, the devoiced /l/ and /r/ normally occur only after voiceless consonants, as in the words *play* and *try*.

The examples of context-dependent articulatory modifications in Table 2.5 show the variety of influences that sounds exert on adjacent sounds. For a given sound, place of

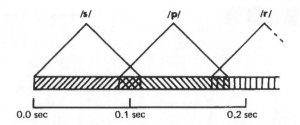

FIGURE 2.26 Schematic drawing of the articulatory organization of a /spr/ consonant cluster (as in the word *spray*), showing overlapping of consonantal articulations.

Source: Based on data from Kent and Moll (1975).

articulation, duration, voicing, nasalization, and rounding may vary with phonetic context, and these variations are noted with the special marks shown in Table 2.5.

Some aspects of coarticulation can be understood by knowing the extent to which individual sounds restrict the positions of the various articulators. Table 2.6 summarizes degrees of restriction on lips, jaw, and parts of the tongue for the different places of consonant articulation. A strong restriction is indicated by an X, a slight to moderate restriction by a –, and a minimal restriction by an O. Because this table shows which parts of the vocal tract are free to vary during articulation of a given consonant, it can be used to predict certain aspects of coarticulation. For example, because bilabial sounds do not restrict the tongue as long as it does not close off the tract, Os are indicated for all parts

TABLE 2.5 Examples of Context-Dependent Modifications of Phonetic Segments

Modification	Context Description
Nasalization of vowel	Vowel is preceded or followed by a nasal, e.g., [ɔ̃n]—*on* and [mæ̃n]—*man*
Rounding of consonant	Consonant precedes a rounded sound, e.g., [kʷwin]—*queen* and [tʷru]—*true*
Palatalization of consonant	Consonant precedes a palatal sound, e.g., [kiʂ ju]—*kiss you*
Devoicing of obstruent	Word-final position of voiced consonant, e.g., [dɔg̊]—*dog* and [liv̥]—*leave*
Devoicing of liquid	Liquid follows word-initial voiceless sound, e.g., [pl̥eɪ]—*play* and [tr̥i]—*tree*
Dentalization of coronal	Normally alveolar sound precedes a dental sound, e.g., [wɪd̪θ]—*width* and [naɪn̪θ]—*ninth*
Retroflexion of fricative	Fricative occurs in context of retroflex sounds, e.g., [haʂɚ]—*harsher* and [pɝʂɚ]—*purser*
Devoicing of sound	Consonant or vowel in voiceless context, e.g., [sɪ̥stɚ]—*sister*
Lengthening of vowel	Vowel preceding voiced sound, especially in stressed syllable, e.g., [ni : d]—*need*
Reduction of vowel	Vowel in unstressed (weak) syllable, e.g., [tæbjuleɪt] [tæbjəleɪt]—*tabulate*
Voicing of sound	Voiceless in voiced context, e.g., [æbs̬ɝd]—*absurd*
Deaspiration of stop	Stop follows /s/, e.g., [sp⁼aɪ]—*spy* vs. [pʰaɪ]—*pie*

TABLE 2.6 Coarticulation Matrix, Showing for Each Place of Consonant Articulation Those Articulators That Have Strong Restrictions on Position (Marked with X), Those That Have Some Restriction on Position (Marked with —), and Those That Are Minimally Restricted (Marked with O). For Example, the Bilabials /b/, /p/, and /m/ Strongly Restrict the Lips, Moderately Restrict the Jaw, and Leave the Tongue Essentially Free to Vary. The Glides /w/ and /ʍ/ Are Not Included Because They Involve Secondary Articulations. Lip Rounding, as Often Occurs for /r/, Has Been Neglected

Tongue Place	Lip	Jaw	Tip	Blade	Dorsum	Body
Bilabial /bpm/	X	—	O	O	O	O
Labiodental /vf/	X	—	O	O	O	O
Interdental /ðθ/	O	—	X	X	—	—
Alveolar /dtzsln/	O	—	X	X	—	—
Palatal /ʃ ʒ dʒ tʃ j r/	O	—	—	X	X	X
Velar /gkŋ/	O	O	O	—	X	X
Glottal /h/	O	O	O	O	O	O

of the tongue. Jaw position is shown as moderately restricted for most places of articulation because some degree of jaw closing usually aids consonant formation. The ability of jaw movement to aid tongue movement declines as place of articulation moves back in the mouth, so a velar consonant may not restrict jaw position as much as more frontal articulation (Kent and Moll, 1972). The only sound that allows essentially unrestricted coarticulation is the glottal /h/. Thus, /h/ usually is made with a vocal-tract configuration adjusted to an adjacent sound, such as the following vowel in the words *he* /hi/, *who* /hu/, *ham* /hæm/, and *hop* /hɑp/.

Investigators of speech articulation (Daniloff and Moll, 1968; Moll and Daniloff, 1971; Kent and Minifie, 1977) have shown extensive overlapping of articulatory gestures across phoneme-sized segments, causing debate about the size of unit that governs behavior. Some investigators propose that the decision unit is an allophone, others argue for the phoneme, and still others for the syllable. A popular syllable-unit hypothesis is one based on CV (consonant-vowel) syllables, with allowance for consonant clustering (CCV, CCCV, and so on). This hypothesis states that articulatory movements are organized in sequences of the form CV, CCV, CCCV, and the like, so that a word like *construct* would be organized as the articulatory syllables /kɑ/ + /nstrʌkt/. Notice the odd assembly of the second syllable. This issue is of more than academic importance. Discovery of the basic decision unit would have implications for speech remediation—for example, enabling a speech clinician to choose the most efficient training and practice items for correcting an error sound. In addition, syllabic structures may explain certain features of speech and language development as discussed by Branigan (1976).

Coarticulation also has clinical relevance, in that a sound might be more easily learned or more easily produced correctly in one context than in others. In other words, the phonetic context of a sound can facilitate or even interfere with correct production of the sound. The effect of phonetic context could explain why misarticulations are often incon-sistent, with correct production on certain occasions and incorrect productions on others. By judiciously selecting the phonetic context where an error sound is initially corrected, the clinician can sometimes enhance the efficiency of speech remediation. Such examples show why a thorough knowledge of articulatory phonetics is important to decisions in the management of articulation disorders.

AERODYNAMIC CONSIDERATIONS IN SPEECH PRODUCTION

Because the production of speech depends on the supply and valving of air, a knowledge of air pressure, flow, and volume is essential to an understanding of both normal and dis-ordered speech. Many abnormalities of speech production are caused by irregularities or deficiencies in the supply and valving of air, and a number of clinical assessment tech-niques rely on measures of air pressure, flow, or volume. To understand the regulation of air pressures and flows in speech, it is important to recognize that (1) air flows only in one direction—from a region of greater pressure to one of lesser pressure—and (2) whenever the vocal tract is closed at some point, the potential exists for the buildup of air pressure behind the closure.

English speech sounds are normally *egressive*, meaning that, in sound production, air flows from the inside (usually the lungs) to the outside (the air around us). The basic energy needed to produce sound is developed in the lungs. After air is inspired by enlargement of the lung cavity, the muscle activation changes so that the lung cavity returns to a smaller size. If the airway above is closed, the same volume of air is enclosed in a smaller space. Because the same amount of air is contained in a smaller cavity, the air pressure within the lungs increases. This overpressure (relative to atmosphere) in the lungs is the source of the regressive air flow for all speech sounds. It is a fact of clinical importance that the air flow requirements for speech are not much greater than the requirements for ordinary breathing; that is, the volume of air inspired and expired in speaking is not much different from that in quiet respiration.

The regulation of air pressure and flow for speech is diagrammed in Figure 2.27, a simple model of the vocal tract. This model, in the form of the letter F, shows the three general areas where constriction (narrowing or closure) can occur: the laryngeal, oral, and nasal sections. The first site of constriction for egressive air is in the larynx. If the vocal folds close tightly, no air can escape from the lungs. If the folds are maximally open, then air passes through the larynx readily. If the folds are closed with a moderate tension, then the buildup of air pressure beneath them eventually blows them apart, releasing a pulse of air. After the folds are blown apart, they quickly come together again through the action of various physical restoring forces. This alternation of closed and open states, occurring many times per second, is called *voicing*. Successive pulses of air from the vocal folds are a source of acoustic energy for all voiced sounds, such as vowels.

The F-shaped vocal tract model shown in Figure 2.27a illustrates the air flow for vowel sounds. The vocal folds are shown as being partly closed to represent the vibratory pattern of opening and closing. The nasal tube is tightly closed because vowels in English are nonnasal unless they precede or follow nasal consonants. The oral tube is widely open

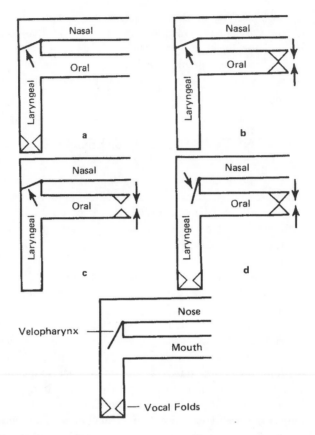

FIGURE 2.27 Simple models of vocal tract for major sound classes: (*a*) vowels, liquids, and glides; (*b*) voiceless stops; (*c*) voiceless fricatives; (*d*) nasals. The major parts of the model are shown at the bottom of the figure.

to represent the open oral cavity in vowel articulation. Because the nasal tube is closed, the acoustic energy from the vibrating vocal folds passes through the oral tube.

The configuration of the vocal tract for a voiceless stop like /p/, /t/, or /k/ is diagrammed in Figure 2.27b. The constriction at the larynx is shown as completely open because air from the lungs passes readily through the larynx and into the oral cavity. The constriction at the velopharynx is shown as closed to indicate that no air flows through the nasal tube. The oral constriction is closed to represent the period of stop closure. After this period, the oral constriction opens rapidly to allow a burst of air to escape from the oral pressure chamber. Assuming a stop closure of suitable duration, the air pressure developed within the oral cavity can be nearly equal to that in the lungs because the open vocal folds permit an equalization of air pressure in the airway reaching from the lungs up to the oral cavity. Therefore, voiceless stops have high intraoral air pressures. Also, it should be noted that children may use *greater* intraoral air pressures than adults (Subtelny, Worth, and Sakuda, 1966; Bernthal and Beukelman, 1978; Netsell, Lotz, Peters, and Schulte, 1994).

The model for voiceless fricatives in Figure 2.27c is like that for voiceless stops, but instead of a complete oral constriction, the model has a very narrow constriction, required for fricative noise. Because the velopharyngeal constriction is tightly closed and the laryngeal constriction is open, voiceless fricatives like /s/ and /ʃ/ have high intraoral air pressures. The voiceless stops and fricatives are sometimes called *pressure consonants*.

Voiced stops and fricatives differ from voiceless stops and fricatives in having vibrating vocal folds. Therefore, the models in Figures 2.27b and Figure 2.27c would have a partial laryngeal constriction to represent voicing of these sounds. Because a certain amount of air pressure is lost in keeping the vocal folds vibrating (that is, pressure across the glottis drops), the voiced stops and fricatives have smaller intraoral air pressures than their voiceless cognates.

Finally, the model for nasal consonants is depicted in Figure 2.27d. A partial constriction at the larynx represents the vibrating vocal folds, and a complete oral constriction represents the stoplike closure in the oral section of the vocal tract. For nasal consonants, the acoustic energy of voicing is directed through the nasal cavity. Very little air pressure builds up within the oral chamber.

Liquids and glides can be modeled in essentially the same way as vowels (Figure 2.27a). Because the oral constriction for these sounds is only slightly greater than that for vowels, there is very little intraoral air pressure buildup.

Pressures and flows can be used to describe the function of many parts of the speech system. For example, a normal efficient operation of the larynx can often be distinguished from inefficient pathological states by the excessive air flow in the latter conditions. This excessive flow, or air wastage, may be heard as breathiness or hoarseness. Velopharyngeal incompetence can be identified by recording air flow from the nose during normally nonnasal segments. Frequently, velopharyngeal incompetence is signaled both by inappropriate nasal air flow (for example, air flow during stops or fricatives) and by reduced levels of intraoral air pressure. Sometimes more than one pressure or flow must be recorded to identify the problem. For example, reduced levels of intraoral air pressure for consonants can be related to at least three factors: (1) respiratory weakness, resulting in insufficient air pressure; (2) velopharyngeal dysfunction, resulting in a loss of air through the nose; or (3) an inadequacy of the oral constriction, allowing excessive air to escape.

Clinically, aerodynamic assessment is especially important when dealing with a structural defect (such as cleft palate) or a physically based control problem (as in cerebral palsy, vocal fold paralysis, and other neurologic disorders). Young children may use greater intraoral air pressure than adults for consonant production, so normative pressure data obtained from adults should be used with caution in clinical evaluation of children. Moreover, the higher pressures in children's speech mean that children must close the velopharyngeal port even more tightly than adults to prevent nasal loss of air during stop or fricative consonants. Speech and language clinicians who do not possess equipment for aerodynamic recordings of speech should nonetheless be aware of the pressure and flow requirements in speech production. These requirements have important implications for the diagnosis and evaluation of communicative problems and for the design of remediation programs.

ACOUSTIC CONSIDERATIONS OF SPEECH

It is far beyond the scope of this chapter to consider in any detail the acoustic structure of speech sounds, but it is possible to draw here a few major conclusions about the acoustic signal of speech. Acoustic signals can be described in terms of three fundamental physical variables: frequency, amplitude, and duration. *Frequency* refers to the rate of vibration of a sound. Generally, the faster the rate of vibration, the higher the pitch heard. In other words, frequency is the most direct physical correlate of pitch. *Amplitude* refers to the strength or magnitude of vibration of a sound. The higher the magnitude of vibration, the louder the sound heard. Amplitude is the most direct physical correlate of loudness. Because the actual amplitude of vibration is minute and, therefore, difficult to measure, sound intensity or sound pressure level is used instead when making actual speech measurements. *Duration* refers to the total time over which a vibration continues. Duration is the most direct physical correlate of perceived length.

Virtually all naturally occurring sounds, speech included, have energy at more than a single frequency. A tuning fork is designed to vibrate at a single frequency and is one of the very few sound sources with this property. The human voice, musical instruments, and animal sounds all have energy at several frequencies. The particular pattern of energy over a frequency range is the *spectrum* of a sound. Speech sounds differ in their *spectra*, and these differences allow us to distinguish sounds perceptually.

Table 2.7 is a summary of the major acoustic properties of several phonetic classes. The table shows the relative sound intensity, the dominant energy region in the spectrum, and the relative sound duration for each class. Vowels are the most intense speech sounds, have most of their energy in the low to mid frequencies, and are longer in duration than other sounds (although the actual duration of vowel sounds may range from about 50 msec to half a second). Because vowels are the most intense sounds, they typically determine the overall loudness of speech. The most intense vowels are the low vowels and the least intense, the high vowels.

The glides and liquids are somewhat less intense than the vowels and have most of their energy in the low to mid frequencies. The duration of the glides /w/ and /j/ tends to be longer than that of the liquids /l/ and /r/.

The strident fricatives and affricates (/s, z, ʃ, ʒ, tʃ, dʒ/) are more intense than other consonants but considerably weaker than vowels. The stridents have energy primarily at the

---

TABLE 2.7   Summary of Acoustic Features for Six Phonetic Classes

Sound Class	Intensity	Spectrum	Duration
Vowels	Very strong	Low-frequency dominance	Moderate to long
Glides and liquids	Strong	Low-frequency dominance	Short to moderate
Strident fricatives and affricates	Moderate	High-frequency dominance	Moderate
Nasals	Moderate	Very low frequency dominance	Short to moderate
Stops	Weak	Varies with place of articulation	Short
Nonstrident fricatives	Weak	Flat	Short to moderate

high frequencies and, therefore, are vulnerable to high-frequency hearing loss. A good tape recording of the stridents requires a recorder with a wide-frequency response. Stridents tend to be relatively long in duration, especially compared to other consonants, and fricatives typically are longer than affricates.

The nasals are sounds of moderate intensity, low-frequency energy, and brief to moderate duration. The nasals have more energy at very low frequencies than do other sounds.

The stops are relatively weak sounds of brief duration. The burst that results from release of a stop closure can be as short as 10 msec The primary energy for stops varies over a wide range of frequencies—from low to high; bilabials have relatively low-frequency energy whereas velars and alveolars have most of their energy in, respectively, the mid and mid-to-high frequencies.

The nonsibilant fricatives /f, v, θ, ð/ are weak sounds of typically moderate duration. They tend to have a flat spectrum, meaning that the noise energy is distributed fairly uniformly over the frequency range. Of all sounds, /θ/ usually is the weakest—so weak that it can barely be heard when produced in isolation at any distance from a listener.

Finally, two points should be made concerning acoustic implications for clinical assessment and management. First, the absolute frequency location of energy for speech sounds varies with speaker age and sex. Men have the lowest overall frequencies of sound energy, women somewhat higher frequencies, and young children the highest frequencies. This relationship follows from the acoustic principle that an object's resonance frequency is inversely related to its length. The longest pipe in a pipe organ has a low frequency (or low pitch) and the shortest pipe a high frequency (high pitch); similarly, the adult male vocal tract is longer than a woman's or a child's and therefore has resonances of lower frequency. This difference has practical implications. Historically, most acoustic data were reported for men's speech, but more recent studies have provided substantial datasets for women's and children's speech, so that acoustic data are now available for speakers of both sexes and of many different ages, including infants. Modern methods of acoustic analysis make it easier to adjust measurement parameters to make them optimal for different speakers. For example, because the speech of women and children has a wider range of frequencies than men's speech, it is usually advisable to extend the range of frequencies when analyzing speech patterns for women and children, especially for fricatives and affricates.

Second, because speech sounds vary widely in intensity, dominant energy region, and duration, they are not equally discriminable under different listening situations. The acoustic differences summarized in Table 2.7 should be kept in mind when testing articulation or auditory discrimination.

SENSORY INFORMATION IN SPEECH PRODUCTION

As speech is produced, a number of different kinds of sensory information is generated. The types of information include tactile (touch and pressure), proprioceptive (position sense), kinesthetic (movement sense), and auditory. The total sensory information is genuinely plurimodal—that is, available in several modalities. Most authorities agree that the rich sensory information associated with speech production is particularly important in speech development and in the management of some speech disorders as when a child must learn a new articulatory pattern. A clinician therefore should be knowledgeable about the kinds and characteristics of sensory, or afferent, information.

The major characteristics of the sensory systems in speech were reviewed by Hardcastle (1976) and later by Kent, Martin, and Sufit (1990). Tactile receptors, which consist of free nerve endings and complex endings (for example, Krause end-bulbs and Meissner corpuscles), supply information to the central nervous system on the nature of contact (including localization, pressure, and onset time) and direction of movement. Remarkably, the oral structures are among the most sensitive regions of the body. The tongue tip is particularly sensitive and can therefore supply detailed sensory information. Tactile receptors belong to a more general class of receptors called *mechanoreceptors* (which respond to mechanical stimulation). These receptors respond not only to physical contacts of articulatory structures but also to air pressures generated during speech.

The proprioceptive and kinesthetic receptors include the muscle spindles, Golgi tendon organs, and joint receptors. Muscle spindles provide rich information on the length of muscle fibers, degree and velocity of stretch, and the direction of movement of a muscle. Golgi receptors relay information on the change of stretch on a tendon caused by muscular contraction or by other influences, including passive movement. Joint receptors, located in the capsules of joints, inform the central nervous system on the rate, direction, and extent of joint movement. Even a relatively simple movement, such as closing the jaw and raising the tongue, supplies a variety of afference to the central nervous system.

The auditory system supplies information on the acoustic consequences of articulation. Because the purpose of speech is to produce an intelligible acoustic signal, auditory feedback is of particular importance in regulating the processes of articulation. Interestingly, when an adult suffers a sudden and severe loss of hearing, speech articulation usually does not deteriorate immediately, but only gradually. The other types of sensory information are probably sufficient to maintain the accuracy of articulation for some time.

Many tactile receptors are comparatively slow acting because the neural signals travel along relatively small fibers in a multisynaptic pathway (a pathway composed of several neurons). Much of the tactile information is available to the central nervous system after the event to which it pertains. This information is particularly important to articulations that involve contact between articulatory surfaces, such as stops and fricatives. Obviously, prolonging an articulation helps to reinforce its sensory accompaniment. When the mucosal surfaces of the articulators are anesthetized, one of the most disturbed class of sounds is the fricatives.

SUMMARY OF LEVELS OF ORGANIZATION OF SPEECH

Various levels of organization of speech are shown in Table 2.8, beginning with the syllable and working down to the acoustic sequence that might be seen on a spectrogram or visual representation of sounds. Although *syllable integrity* is the highest level shown, the table could have begun with an even higher level, such as a phrase or a sentence. However, for our purposes here, it is sufficient to consider only the levels presented in the table. The syllable is an organizational unit that consists of one or more phonemes; in this case, the syllable /pa/ includes the phonemes /p/ and /a/. Because phonemes are abstract, a

TABLE 2.8	Levels of Organization of Speech
Syllabic integrity	/p a/
	SYL
Phonemic composition	/p/ + /a/
Phonetic properties	[pʰa:]
Note: stop /p/ is aspirated and vowel /a/ is length ended	
Segmental features	[p] — +Stop
	+Labial
	+Consonantal
	−Nasal
	−Voice
	[a] — +Syllabic
	−Consonantal
	−Front
	+Low
	−Round
	−Nasal
	+Voice
Articulatory sequence	Closure of velopharynx
	Abduction of vocal folds
	Adjustment of tongue for /a/
	Closure of lips
	Opening of lips and jaw
	Adduction of vocal folds
	Final abduction of vocal folds
Acoustic sequence	Silent period during /p/ closure
	Noise burst for /p/ release
	Aspiration period as folds close
	Voiced period after folds close, with distinct resonant shaping

phonemic description does not touch on a number of details of phonetic organization and speech behavior. Some of these details are shown in the level of *phonetic properties*. The phoneme /p/ has as its phonetic representation the aspirated [pʰ], and the phoneme /a/ has as its phonetic representation the lengthened [a:]. These phonetic representations are, of course, allophones of the /p/ and /a/ phonemes. The English phoneme /p/ is always aspirated in syllable-initial position, and the phoneme /a/ frequently is lengthened when uttered in an open monosyllable (that is, a CV syllable).

Segmental features comprise the next level of the table. These features are phonetic dimensions or attributes by which sounds may be described. For example, the consonant

[p] is defined by its inclusion in the classes of *stops, labials*, and *consonantals* and by its exclusion from the classes of *nasals* and *voiced sounds*. These features are similar to the distinctive features discussed earlier in this chapter, but they are intended to be more phonetic in character. Even without rigorous definitions of the features suggested, it should be clear that each feature defines an articulatory property of the sound in question; for example, vowel [a] is a syllable nucleus, is not a consonant, is low back and unrounded, and is a voiced nonnasal sound.

The features are less abstract than phonemes but still must be interpreted by the motor control system of the brain to provide proper neural instructions to the speech muscles; that is, the features listed for [p] and [a] must be translated into a pattern of muscle contractions that yields the articulatory sequence shown in the next to last level of the table. The –*nasal* feature of [p] requires that the velopharynx be closed, and the –*voice* feature of the same segment requires that the vocal folds be abducted (open). In this way, each feature requirement is given an articulatory interpretation, accomplished by the contraction of muscles.

Finally, as the consequence of muscle contractions, a series of speech sounds is uttered. In this *acoustic sequence*, the last level of the table, one can see acoustic segments of the kind visible on a spectrogram. Notice that one acoustic segment does not necessarily correspond to a single phoneme. The phoneme /p/ is associated with at least three acoustic segments: a silent period corresponding to the bilabial closure, a noise burst produced as the lips are rapidly opened, and an aspiration interval related to a gradual closure of the vocal folds in preparation for voicing the following vowel.

Although Table 2.8 is fairly detailed, it represents only part of the complexity of speech. In the linguistic-phonetic organization of speech behavior, we need to consider three major components: the *segmental* (or *phonetic*) component, the *suprasegmental* (*prosodic*) component, and the *paralinguistic* component. The first two already have been discussed in this chapter. The paralinguistic component is similar to the prosodic component in that it might be called nonsegmental. This component includes those aspects of speech represented by terms such as *emotion* and *attitude*. A speaker who plans an utterance must decide not only about phonetic sequencing but also about prosodic structure and emotional and attitudinal content (that is, the "tone of voice"). The segmental component includes words, syllables, phonemes, and features. The suprasegmental or prosodic component includes stress, intonation, juncture, rate, loudness, and pitch level. The paralinguistic component is made up of tension, voice quality, and voice qualifications (Crystal, 1969).

The complexity of speech behavior can be illustrated by listing the various types of information represented in the speech signal. A *partial* listing (mostly from Branigan, 1979) is

1. A set of articulatory targets or goals corresponding to the intended phonetic sequence
2. Assignment of stress to the syllables that make up the sequence
3. Adjustments of syllable duration to stress, phonetic composition, and position of the syllable in the utterance
4. Specification of junctural features, including transitions between elements and terminal juncture at the end of the utterance
5. Internal ordering of words reflecting syntactic form to convey semantic intentions (meaning)

6. Determination of other prosodic features such as speaking rate, pitch, level, and loudness
7. Use of paralinguistic features to convey emotion or attitude

It is important to remember that even an apparently simple aspect of speech behavior can be influenced by a host of variables. For example, the duration of a vowel is determined by tongue height, tenseness or laxness, consonant context, stress pattern, frequency of occurrence of the word in which the vowel occurs, syntactic ordering of the word in which the vowel appears, and rate of speaking (Klatt, 1976).

CONCLUDING NOTE ON IMPLICATIONS FOR SPEECH ACQUISITION

Speech articulation has its early roots in the vocalizations of infants. Just how the coos and babbles of the first year of life relate to the development of speech is not well understood, but there is growing evidence that early vocalizations prepare the child for acquisition of a phonetic system. The syllable appears to be an important unit in early sound patterns, and the development of syllabic organization of sounds may be a major framework of speech development. If so, it is of interest to chart the way in which syllabic structures develop during the first year of life. The following account is based on several chapters in *Precursors of Early Speech Development*, edited by Bjorn Lindblom and Rolf Zetterström (1986) and *The Emergence of the Speech Capacity* by Oller (2000).

The major phases in syllable development are as follows: (1) Continuous phonation in a respiratory cycle provides the basic phonatory pattern from which refinements in articulation can develop; (2) intermittent phonation within a respiratory cycle breaks the basic pattern of continuous phonation and, thus, is a precursor of syllable units; (3) articulatory (supraglottal) movements interrupting or combined with phonation provide early experience in the control of co-occurring phonation and articulation; (4) marginal syllables (in isolation or in sequence) are early syllabic forms that, although lacking the detailed structure of adult syllables, prefigure the basic syllable shape; (5) canonical syllables (in isolation or in sequence) anticipate important structural properties of adult speech and may be particularly important in relating an infant's perceptions of adult speech with his or her own productive patterns; and (6) reduplicated babble (repeated syllable patterns) gives the infant experience with both prosody (especially rhythm) and sequences of articulations. It is on this vocal bedrock that speech develops. For a time, babbling and early words co-exist, sharing some phonetic properties but, perhaps, differing in others.

The CV syllable, occurring in virtually all of the world's languages, has long been recognized as a preferred basic unit of speech articulation. It appears to be an optimal unit for learning perceptual discriminations in infancy. Infants younger than 4 months old can discriminate segments contained in sequences of the form CV, CVC, VCV, and CVCV (Bertoncini and Mehler, 1981; Jusczyk and Thompson, 1978; Trehub, 1973); and an alternating CV pattern seems to enhance the infant's ability to discriminate variations in place, manner, and voicing. Because redundant syllable strings, such as [ba ba ba ba] (Goodsitt, Morse, and Ver Hoeve, 1984), further enhance this performance, we can conclude that the

CV syllable train characterizing reduplicated babble is an excellent perceptual training ground for the infant.

The advantage of the CV syllable applies to production as well. This syllable form is one of the earliest to be identified in infant vocalizations; the vocalizations of 1-year-olds are, predominantly, simple V or CV syllables and their elaborations, for example, VCV or CVCV (Kent and Bauer, 1985). Branigan (1976) regarded the CV syllable as a training ground for consonant formation. Most consonants are produced first in the initial position of CV syllables and then, later, in postvocalic (e.g., VC) position.

The importance of the canonical CV syllable as a unit for perceptuomotor integration is indicated by its long-delayed appearance in the vocal development of infants with hearing impairments (Kent, Osberger, Netsell, and Hustedde, 1987; Oller, 1986). There is also evidence that early CV syllable production is correlated, in a developmental chain, to the early word production and to the development and use of word-final consonants (Menyuk, Liebergott, and Schultz, 1986).

Speech acquisition is a complex process, one that involves learning a language (its syntax, semantics, and phonology)—a speech code that relates meaning to sound, and a motor skill by which the speech organs are controlled to produce rapid and overlapping movements. The layperson often characterizes developing speech in the child by reference to frequently occurring substitutions (as when the child says *wabbit* for *rabbit* or *thee* for *see*) or other common misarticulations. But developing speech differs from adult speech in other ways.

First, children's speech generally is slower than adult speech. For example, McNeill (1974) reported speaking rates of slightly over 3 words per second for adults, about 2.5 words per second for 4- to 5-year-olds, and 1.6 words per second for children of about age 2. Not surprisingly, then, the durations of individual segments are longer in children's speech (Naeser, 1970; Smith, 1978; Kent and Forner, 1980). Smith reported that the durations of nonsense utterances were 15 percent longer for 4-year-olds than for adults and 31 percent longer for 2-year-olds than for adults. Similarly, when Kent and Forner measured durations of phrases and short sentences, they found them to be 8 percent longer for 12-year-olds than for adults, 16 percent longer for 6-year-olds than for adults, and 33 percent longer for 4-year-olds than for adults. Some individual segments, such as the duration of stop closure, were observed by Kent and Forner to be twice as long in children's speech as in adult speech. The speaking rates of children have implications for both the production and perception of speech. It has been shown that children more successfully imitate sentences spoken at a rate nearer their own than at slower or faster rates (Bonvillian, Raeburn, and Horan, 1979).

Second, children's speech differs from adult speech in its variability. When children make the same utterance several times, the duration of individual segments varies more than for adults (Eguchi and Hirsh, 1969; Tingley and Allen, 1975; Kent and Forner, 1980). This difference in reliability of production may be an index of the child's linguistic and neuromotor immaturity. In general, a young child's speech patterns are less well controlled than an adult's, and there is growing evidence that the control continues to improve until adolescence (Kent, 1976; Walsh and Smith, 2002). It can be concluded that motor control for speech has a protracted period of refinement, well beyond the ages at which phonemic mastery is demonstrated. Similar protracted development is observed for the maturation of neural pathways (Paus et al., 1999) and the anatomic development of the structures of the vocal tract (Vorperian et al., 2009). A third difference between the speech of children and adults is in patterns of coarticulation. Data on this difference are not abundant, but Thompson and Hixon (1979) reported that with increasing age, a higher proportion of their subjects showed nasal air flow beginning at the midpoint of the first vowel in /ini/. They interpreted this to mean that anticipatory coarticulation occurred earlier for progressively older subjects. In other words, more mature speakers show increased anticipation in producing a phonetic sequence.

In summary, young children differ from adults not only in their obvious misarticulations but also in their slower speaking rates, greater variability (error) in production, and reduced anticipation in articulatory sequencing.

QUESTIONS FOR CHAPTER 2

1. Discuss the relationship among the following concepts: *morpheme, phoneme,* and *allophone*. For example, explain why a morpheme is relevant to identifying phonemes and why phonemes are relevant to identifying allophones.

2. This chapter summarized two ways of describing vowel articulation: traditional phonetic description and distinctive features. Discuss the similarities and differences between these two approaches.

3. Using Table 2.2 as a guide, classify all of the consonants in the phrase *Good morning, take a ticket, and get in line* according to place of articulation, manner of articulation, and voicing. Note that in all of the words containing two or more consonants, the consonants share a phonetic feature. What is this feature for each word?

4. What is coarticulation and why does it occur?

CHAPTER 3

Speech Sound Acquisition

SHARYNNE McLEOD
Charles Sturt University, Australia

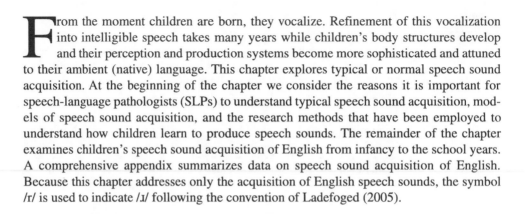

From the moment children are born, they vocalize. Refinement of this vocalization into intelligible speech takes many years while children's body structures develop and their perception and production systems become more sophisticated and attuned to their ambient (native) language. This chapter explores typical or normal speech sound acquisition. At the beginning of the chapter we consider the reasons it is important for speech-language pathologists (SLPs) to understand typical speech sound acquisition, models of speech sound acquisition, and the research methods that have been employed to understand how children learn to produce speech sounds. The remainder of the chapter examines children's speech sound acquisition of English from infancy to the school years. A comprehensive appendix summarizes data on speech sound acquisition of English. Because this chapter addresses only the acquisition of English speech sounds, the symbol /r/ is used to indicate /ɹ/ following the convention of Ladefoged (2005).

RELEVANCE OF UNDERSTANDING TYPICAL SPEECH SOUND ACQUISITION FOR SLPS

An understanding of typical speech sound acquisition is akin to having solid foundations under a house. In pediatric SLP practice, decisions whether a child's speech is typical or not occurs daily. This decision making is guided by knowledge of research data as well as clinicians' experience. Studies of children's typical speech sound acquisition are the primary research data used by SLPs to make these decisions.

Seven main areas of SLP practice are informed by a comprehensive understanding of speech sound acquisition:

1. *Referral.* Providing advice to parents, educators, and health professionals regarding whether a child should be referred for a speech assessment.
2. *Assessment.* Deciding which assessment tools are appropriate to examine speech behaviors that are relevant for the age of the child. For example, if the child is 1;6, an inventory of consonants, vowels, and syllable shapes should be determined. If the child is 7;0, polysyllabic words and phonological awareness skills also should be assessed.

3. *Analysis.* Analyzing the speech sample in order to decide whether the child's speech is age-appropriate on a range of measures.
4. *Diagnosis.* Determining whether a child has a delay or disorder and whether his or her areas of difficulty warrant speech sound intervention.
5. *Selecting intervention targets.* There are two major schools of thought regarding how to use knowledge of typical speech sound acquisition to select intervention targets. Proponents of the *traditional developmental approach* suggest intervention targets should focus on errors on the production of early developing sounds (cf. Davis, 2005; Shriberg and Kwiatkowski, 1982b). Proponents of the *complexity approach* (also called *nontraditional approach* and *least knowledge approach*) select later-developing sounds; the aim of such an approach is to produce a systemwide change (cf. Gierut, Morrisette, Hughes, and Rowland, 1996).
6. *Intervention.* Adapting teaching and feedback to an age-appropriate level, and determining that a child has achieved his or her goals to the expected level.
7. *Dismissal/discharge.* Deciding whether a child's speech is within normal limits for his or her age (Tyler, 2005) and whether his or her speech sound intervention should be concluded for other reasons e.g. the child has progressed as far as he/she is going to and no longer is making progress or child lacks motivation for continued therapy.

The goal of this chapter is to assist SLPs in all these areas by providing basic or foundational knowledge for working with children with speech sound disorders.

MODELS OF SPEECH ACQUISITION

The acquisition of speech and language is a complex process whose precise nature is not known. Many models of acquisition have been proposed. Each model provides a different insight into how the process might work. Thus, it is useful for SLPs working with children to have knowledge of a range of models. Barlow and Gierut (1999, p. 1482) recommend that when considering models of speech acquisition, an adequate model must account for "(a) the actual facts of children's productions and the mismatches between a child's output and the adult input forms; (b) the generalities that span children's sound systems, as well as associated variability within and across developing systems; and (c) the changes that occur in children's grammars over time." They also indicated that an adequate model must be "testable and falsifiable." With these premises in mind, a range of models of speech acquisition will be presented. For a comprehensive account, see Ball and Kent (1997).

Traditionally, SLPs used a behaviorist model to explain how children learn the sounds of the language. More recently, linguistic-based models have evolved based on theories of generative phonology, natural phonology, nonlinear theory, optimality theory, and sonority. Such approaches not only provided SLPs with insight into children's developing speech systems but also extended and enhanced guidelines for assessment, analysis, and intervention. Most linguistic theories maintain that innate or natural mechanisms govern a child's phonological system. These are expressed as *distinctive features* in generative phonology, *phonological processes* (or *patterns*) in natural phonology, *multitiered* representations in nonlinear phonology, and *constraints* in optimality theory. However, although linguistic-based models provided descriptions of children's phonology, they failed to provide explanations of the underlying cognitive mechanisms involved in the perception and production of speech. Consequently, the most recent explanations are psycholinguistic models of speech development.

Traditional Models of Speech Acquisition

Behaviorist Models

Behaviorism focused on describing overt and observable behaviors. Behaviorism was proposed by Watson (1913/1994, p. 248) in his article "Psychology as a Behaviorist Views It" and was described as an "objective experimental branch of natural science that can be studied without references to consciousness." The most influential proponent of behaviorism was B. F. Skinner. Skinner's operant conditioning can be traced back to the stimulus-response psychology of the Russian physiologist Pavlov, who trained a dog to respond by salivating when hearing the stimulus of a bell ringing. Skinner created the concept of operant or instrumental conditioning to focus on controlling acts by changing the consequences that occur immediately following the act (Skinner, 1972; Thomas, 2000). In a behaviorist approach, consequences can be described either as positive or negative, reinforcement or punishment. Skinner's behaviorism has been applied to a wide range of ages, cultures, and behaviors (including physical, social, and emotional). Behaviorist principles have been applied throughout SLP practice, particularly from the 1950s to the 1970s.

Application to Typically Developing Children. When behaviorist models have been applied to speech acquisition, the focus has been on observing environmental conditions (stimuli) that co-occur and predict overt verbal behaviors (responses). For example, Olmsted (1971) suggested that sounds that were easy to discriminate would be learned first; however, his order of discrimination has not been supported by subsequent research. Behaviorist researchers documented normative behaviors of large groups of children during the speech acquisition period. Speech-language pathologists described speech development as correct pronunciation of speech sounds. Age-of-acquisition data were collected to provide descriptive normative information (e.g., Templin, 1957).

A major criticism of the application of behaviorism to children's speech acquisition is that children master speech and language acquisition more quickly than they could if they had to depend on stimulus-response mechanisms to learn each element. That is, there is no capacity for parental/environmental reinforcement of all speech behaviors, leading to mastery of such a complex skill as speech and language. Another criticism is that acquisition of speech and language is too complex to be explained solely by reinforcement.

Application to Speech-Language Pathology Practice. Although behaviorism as an explanation for sound acquisition has not been supported, behavioral principles have had a significant impact on SLP practice for children with speech sound disorders. Speech production for many years was considered a motor activity, and analysis of speech was conducted using segmental error analysis. Speech was analyzed as a series of sounds, and the function of sound differences to signal meaning differences was not taken into consideration (e.g., Van Riper and Irwin, 1958). The stimulus-response paradigm was the basis of traditional articulation intervention. Using this behavioral approach, a child was presented with a sound or word that he or she was required to say and then received positive reinforcement in the form of praise, a sticker, or a token on a set schedule (cf. Winitz, 1969).

Linguistic Models of Speech Acquisition

In the traditional models of speech acquisition, there was limited consideration of the patterns, structures, and contexts of misarticulations (with exceptions such as McDonald, 1964b) or of the cognitive dimension of linguistic knowledge. This gave rise to the linguistic models of speech acquisition.

Generative Phonology

Generative phonology is a theory of the sound structure of human languages and was developed by Noam Chomsky. The key principles of generative phonology were illustrated in the landmark study of English phonology presented in Chomsky and Hallé's (1968) book, *The Sound Pattern of English*. Generative phonology moved away from the traditional phonemic analysis and introduced two major concepts:

1. Phonological rules map underlying representations onto surface pronunciations.
2. Phonological descriptions depend on information from other linguistic levels.

Although generative phonology incorporates consideration of semantic and syntactical aspects of language (concept 2), most phonology texts focus on concept 1. The area of generative phonology that has received the most attention is the description of phonological relationships that are expressed by proposing an abstract underlying representation and a set of phonological rules. To provide an example, generative phonology can be used to explain the way that English-speaking adults nasalize vowels before nasal consonants. In generative phonology, this concept is written as the following rule:

$$\begin{bmatrix} +\text{Vowel} \\ -\text{Consonant} \end{bmatrix} \rightarrow [\text{Nasal}]/ - \begin{bmatrix} +\text{Consonant} \\ +\text{Nasal} \end{bmatrix}$$

The information to the left of the arrow indicates the segments that conform to the rule. The arrow means "is realized as." Only the relevant rules are included to the right of the arrow. Other features are assumed to remain as they were. The diagonal slash means "in the context of." The dash and information that follow provide the context of the segment described by the rule. Thus, this generative phonology rule reads: Vowels are realized as nasal in the context of (in this case, specifically just before) nasal consonants.

Application to Typically Developing Children.   Generative phonology has been applied to the understanding of children's speech acquisition (cf. Grunwell, 1987) as it enabled description of the relationship of children's productions to adult pronunciation in terms of phonological rules. Grunwell indicated that generative phonology has been readily applied to children's speech because generative phonological rules can explain substitutions, distortions, omissions, additions, metathesis, and coalescence (for examples, see Grunwell, pp. 176–197).

Some of the premises of generative phonology have received criticism in subsequent research. For example, there has been criticism of the premise that the child's underlying representation of the sound is adultlike (this viewpoint will be discussed later when we consider psycholinguistic theories). Additionally, there has been criticism of the premise that the rules that were applied had a corresponding reality to the processing and production systems of the child (i.e., it is not clear that we actually apply such rules in our heads when we comprehend and produce speech).

Application to Speech-Language Pathology Practice.   As a theory, generative phonology has not seen broad application in the field of speech-language pathology. Hodson (2007b) describes generative phonology as the "first steps into phonologically based clinical analysis" (p. 55); however, additional knowledge gained from the theory of natural phonology (below) leads to the identification of patterns in phonological analysis procedures.

Natural Phonology

The theory of natural phonology (Stampe, 1969, 1979) formed the basis of the phonological process approach to assessment and treatment of speech sound disorders and is regarded as the phonological model that has had the greatest impact on the field of SLP (Edwards, 2007). *Natural processes* (or *patterns*) are those that are preferred or frequently used in phonological systems and are identified in two ways: those that are universal across languages and those that are frequently used by young children. According to Stampe, a phonological process is a "mental operation that applies in speech to substitute for a class of sounds or sound sequences presenting a common difficulty to the speech capacity of the individual, an alternative class identical but lacking the difficult property" (1979, p. 1), and phonological processes merge "a potential opposition into that member of the opposition which least tries the restrictions of the human speech capacity" (1969, p. 443).

In Stampe's view, the child's underlying representations are akin to adult forms. Natural (or innate) phonological processes apply to these underlying representations resulting in the child's productions (or surface forms). For example, it is assumed that children have the adult form of a word, such as *tree* /tri/, in their underlying representation. However, natural processes such as cluster reduction are applied because the child (at least temporarily) has some limitation to produce a particular sound or group of sounds. In this case, the surface form (child's production) would most likely be [ti]. Later, in the discussion of psycholinguistic models, we will critique the notion that children's underlying representations are akin to the adult form.

Application to Typically Developing Children.   Natural phonology has provided insight to the understanding of typical speech acquisition. Natural processes are described as innate rules that are systematically applied to speech production until children learn to suppress them. Because these rules are universal, they are meant to apply to all children speaking all languages. Thus, speech acquisition is a progression from these innate speech patterns to the pronunciation system of the language(s) learned by the child. By applying natural phonology to English speech acquisition, Grunwell (1987) presented a table of the ages of suppression of phonological processes by typically developing children, such as cluster reduction, fronting, and stopping. Other researchers have also provided lists of natural phonological processes (e.g., Ingram, 1976; Shriberg and Kwiatkowski, 1980). Shriberg and Kwiatkowski advocated the clinical use of eight "natural processes": (a) final consonant deletion, (b) velar fronting, (c) stopping, (d) palatal fronting, (e) liquid simplification, (f) cluster reduction, (g) assimilation, and (h) unstressed-syllable deletion.

Application to Speech-Language Pathology Practice. The phonological pattern/process approach to assessment and intervention based on natural phonology transformed the way that SLPs viewed children's speech sound errors. Since Ingram's (1976, 1989a) seminal work on phonological impairments in children, SLPs increasingly have applied descriptive linguistic-based models to their clinical activities. Ingram's application of natural phonology was widely accepted by SLPs in the 1970s and 1980s and remains popular for directing the assessment, analysis, and intervention of children with speech sound disorders (Bankson and Bernthal, 1990a; Khan, 1982; Shriberg and Kwiatkowski, 1980; Weiner, 1979). Assessment approaches were developed to specifically assess subgroups of sounds within a given phonological pattern (e.g., *Bankson-Bernthal Test of Phonology* [*BBTOP*], Bankson and Bernthal, 1990a). Phonological processes were also described as part of a broader analysis procedure for several speech-sampling tools (e.g., *Phonological Assessment of Child Speech* [*PACS*], Grunwell, 1985) and as stand-alone analyses to be applied to conversational speech (e.g., *Natural Process Analysis*, Shriberg and Kwiatkowski, 1980). One of the goals of intervention based on natural phonology is "to teach children to suppress innate simplification processes" (Hodson, 2007b, p. 55).

Limitations of the application of natural phonology to SLP practice have been identified. First, although most SLPs can readily describe children's nonadult productions using phonological process terms such as *cluster reduction* and *fronting*, SLPs' use of phonological processes are descriptive rather than an application of the theoretical tenets of natural phonology. Shriberg (1991, p. 270) described this as an "atheoretical use of process terminology." Second, natural phonology does not account for "nonnatural" simplifications in children's speech (Hodson, 2007a). Many children with highly unintelligible speech produce speech sounds in a way that cannot be classified using natural phonology. Terms such as *backing* and *initial consonant deletion* are in the literature to describe phonological processes that are not seen in children with typical speech acquisition (Dodd, 1995b).

One question that remains unresolved with natural phonology is whether the process labels being applied actually represent mental operations going on inside the head of the child. However because such labels do capture "patterns" of errors being observed, the term *phonological patterns* is frequently used in place of *phonological processes*. For example, the title of the most recent version of a popular assessment tool in this area is now the *Hodson Assessment of Phonological Patterns* (Hodson, 2004).

Nonlinear Phonology

Nonlinear phonology refers to a collection of theories that focus on the hierarchical nature of the relationships between phonological units. Goldsmith introduced nonlinear phonology in his doctoral dissertation (1979) and later expanded upon it (Goldsmith, 1990). These theories include autosegmental theory, metrical theory, moraic theory, feature geometry theory, and underspecification theory. Nonlinear phonology attempts to account for the idea that production of speech involves more than just production of a line of phonemes; it takes into account many elements (features, segments, syllables, feet, words, and phrases) both independently and in relation to one another, hence, the term *non*linear. There are two main tiers in nonlinear phonology:

1. The *prosodic tier* focuses on words and the structure of words and includes a number of levels: word tier, foot tier, syllable tier, onset-rime tier, skeletal tier, and segmental tier (see Figure 3.1).
2. The *segmental tier* focuses on the segments or speech sounds and the features that make up those sounds (see Figure 3.2).

In the prosodic tier, the *word tier* simply denotes words. Immediately below the word *tier* is the *foot tier*, which refers to grouping of syllables, and syllables may be either strong (S) or weak (w). A foot can contain only one strong syllable (but can also contain other weak syllables). A foot that includes a weak syllable can be either Sw (left prominent, or trochaic), or wS (right prominent, or iambic). Below the foot is the *syllable tier*. A syllable consists of

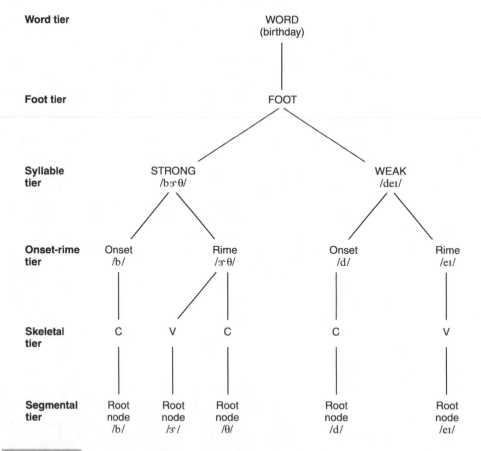

FIGURE 3.1 An example of the prosodic tier representation for the word *birthday*.

one prominent phoneme (the peak), which is usually a vowel and less prominent phonemes (generally consonants) that can appear before or after the peak. Consonants that appear before the vowel are known as *onsets,* and consonants that appear after the vowel are *codas.* The peak and the coda together make up the *rime.* All languages allow syllables without a coda (e.g., CV), but some do not allow a syllable to have a coda (e.g., CVC). A syllable with a coda is called a *closed syllable.* Across the world's languages, open syllables occur more often than closed. Below the syllable tier is the *skeletal tier,* which includes slots for the individual speech sounds.

In the *segmental tier,* features are described according to three nodes: the root node, the laryngeal node, and the place node (see Figure 3.2). The root node [sonorant] and [consonantal] defines the segment as a vowel/glide or a consonant. The features [continuant] and [nasal] define the classes of stops, fricatives, and nasals. The laryngeal node includes the features of [voice] and [spread glottis] and differentiate vowels as well as voiced from voiceless consonants. The place node designates the oral cavity characteristics of the segment and includes labial [round], coronal [anterior], [distributed], dorsal [high], [low], and [back]. Default nodes are generally the most frequent features (unmarked) and the easiest features for a child to use. In English, the default consonant is /t/ because it is coronal but not continuant, not lateral, not nasal, and not voiced.

Application to Typically Developing Children. Two of the major benefits of nonlinear phonology to the understanding of typical phonological development are (1) the concept of links between the segmental and suprasegmental tiers and prosodic variables that highlight the interaction between speech sounds and other speech-language domains and (2) the view that development is progressive or additive, which is in contrast to the negative progression

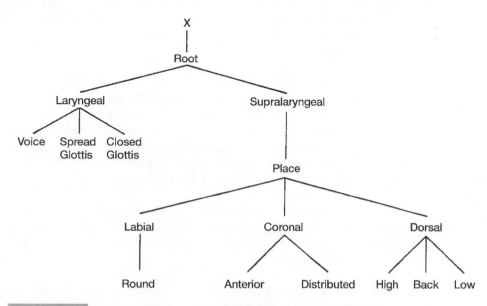

FIGURE 3.2 Hierarchical tree structure (segmental tier).

suggested by a phonological process approach whereby children learn to "undelete" deleted final consonants (Bernhardt and Stoel-Gammon, 1994). Bernhardt (1992a) discussed these developmental implications of nonlinear phonology and highlighted the importance of considering children's representations instead of the negative progression of rules of generative grammar. Bernhardt suggested that children's representations (or simple syllable templates such as CV units and stop consonants) account for a large proportion of young children's speech production and that children add to these representations as they mature. Nonlinear phonology also enables consideration beyond the acquisition of consonants, as it also addresses vowels, syllable shapes, words, and stress.

Application to Speech-Language Pathology Practice.   Bernhardt, Stemberger, and their colleagues have been major proponents of the use of nonlinear phonology in SLP practice. Bernhardt and Stoel-Gammon (1994) presented an excellent overview of the benefits of nonlinear phonology to SLPs. Bernhardt and Stemberger developed a theoretical text (1998), a workbook for clinicians (2000), and a computerized assessment and analysis (*CAPES: Computerized Articulation and Phonology Evaluation System*) (Masterson and Bernhardt, 2001). Additionally, Bernhardt and Stemberger have applied principles of nonlinear phonology to goal setting and intervention for children with speech sound disorders (Bernhardt, 1992b; Bernhardt et al., 2010). In the assessment of children's speech using nonlinear phonology, not only is attention paid to production of consonants but vowels, syllables, word shapes, and stress patterns are also important. Nonlinear intervention goals focus on utilizing established sounds in new syllable shapes and new sounds in established syllable shapes.

Optimality Theory

Optimality theory was first described by Prince and Smolensky (1993) in their report *Optimality Theory: Constraint Interaction in Generative Grammar*. Optimality theory originally was developed to describe adult languages. Its basic units are constraints, which are of two major types:

1. *Markedness constraints* (also called *output constraints*) capture limitations on what can be produced (or the output). Output is simplified by markedness constraints that are motivated by the frequency and distribution of sounds in the ambient language as well as perceptual and articulatory characteristics of the sounds. Sounds that are difficult to pronounce or perceive are marked.
2. *Faithfulness constraints* capture the features to be "preserved," prohibiting addition and deletion that violates the ambient language.

Constraints are assumed to be universal to all languages (Barlow and Gierut, 1999). There is a reciprocal relationship between faithfulness and markedness constraints (Kager, 1999). Faithfulness can result in the inclusion of phonological features whereas markedness can result in their exclusion.

Application to Typically Developing Children and Speech-Language Pathology Practice. Optimality theory has been applied to the understanding of the typical development of children's speech (see Barlow and Gierut [1999] for an overview). The aim during development is for the output to match the adult target, which is achieved by promoting faithfulness constraints and demoting markedness constraints. One example of the application of optimality theory has been to develop a model of children's acquisition of polysyllabic words (James, van Doorn, and McLeod, 2008). The model proposes five stages, each of which elucidates relevant faithfulness constraints. In stage 1 (ages 1;0 to 2;3), children are faithful to the stressed syllable and the duration of the whole word. Stage 2 (ages 2;4 to 3;11) focuses on faithfulness to the number of syllables in a word. That is, during this stage, children reduce the occurrence of weak syllable deletion, cluster reduction, and final consonant deletion. Stage 3 (ages 4;0 to 6;11) highlights faithfulness to all the phonemes in the words and can co-occur with a period of dysprosody (e.g., word rhythm is disrupted). Stage 4 (ages 7;0 to 10;11) emphasizes faithfulness to word rhythm with accurate delineation between stressed and unstressed syllables. The final stage (age 11;0 and older) represents adultlike production of polysyllabic words.

Optimality theory also has been applied to SLP practice with children with speech sound disorders (Barlow and Gierut, 1999). Children's possible productions of words are placed into a constraint table and violations of constraints are identified. Fatal violations (involving a highly ranked constraint) are also identified. The optimal constraint (the form most likely to be produced by the child) is the one that violates the least number of constraints, or the lowest-ranking constraints. As children's speech systems mature, they re-rank constraints until eventually their productions match the adult form (Edwards, 2007).

Sonority Hypothesis

Sonority, first described in 1865 (see Clements, 1990), refers to the relative loudness of a sound relative to other sounds with the same pitch, stress, and length (Ladefoged, 1993). The sonority of a sound depends on the degree of voicing and the amount of opening (stricture) involved in producing the sound. Voiced sounds are more sonorous than voiceless sounds. Sounds with open articulation (e.g., vowels and liquids) are highly sonorous whereas sounds with closed articulation (e.g., stops and fricatives) are less sonorous. Phonemes are allocated a numerical value to represent their degree of sonority. A number of different value hierarchies have been proposed with the one by Steriade (1990) being the one most commonly used within SLP (e.g., Gierut, 1999; Ohala, 1999). Steriade proposes that voiceless stops (value of 7) are the least sonorous phonemes and vowels (value of 0) are the most sonorous sounds.

The Sonority Sequencing Principle (SSP) is a "presumed universal which governs the permissible sequence of consonants within syllables" (Gierut, 1999, p. 708). Thus, phonemes with low sonority values are found at the syllable margins, and sounds with high sonority values are located toward the center of the syllable (Clements, 1990; Roca and Johnson, 1999). In the word *drink*, for example, the vowel /I/ has high sonority; therefore, it is found in the middle of the syllable. The next most sonorous sounds are liquids (such as /r/) and nasals (such as /n/); hence, they are found on either side of the vowel. The least sonorous sounds are stops (such as /d/ and /k/). These are found at the syllable margins.

Application to Typically Developing Children. In accordance with the SSP, it has been proposed that children reduce word-initial consonant clusters in a manner that produces a maximal rise in sonority and that word-final consonant clusters are reduced to produce a minimal fall in sonority. This pattern of reduction is termed the *sonority hypothesis*. Ohala (1999) considered the application of the sonority hypothesis when he described the productions of consonant clusters in nonsense words produced by 16 typically developing children ages 1;9 to 3;2. When the children reduced word-initial fricative + stop clusters (e.g., /sp/) and word-initial fricative + nasal clusters (e.g., /sn/), the remaining consonant was consistently the least sonorous element. Additionally, when the children reduced word-final fricative + stop consonant clusters (e.g., /-st/), the remaining consonant was consistently the most sonorous element. Wyllie-Smith, McLeod, and Ball (2006) analyzed the production of word-initial consonant clusters of 16 typically developing 2-year-old children over two occasions for each child. Overall, the sonority hypothesis was adhered to when the children reduced a consonant cluster by producing one of the target elements; however, reductions to nontarget consonants were inconsistent (some adhered to and some violated the sonority hypothesis). Yavaş (2006) led an international study to examine children's use of the sonority hypothesis. The hypothesis was upheld across children with typical speech acquisition who spoke languages as diverse as Turkish, Norwegian, and Israeli Hebrew.

Application to Speech-Language Pathology Practice.   Sonority has been used as a theoretical basis for making clinical decisions regarding target selection with children who have a speech sound disorder (Anderson, 2000; Baker, 2000; Ball and Müller, 2002; Gierut, 1998, 1999; Gierut and Champion, 2001). It has been used to analyze children's phonemic awareness skills (Yavaş, 2000; Yavaş and Core, 2001; Yavaş and Gogate, 1999) and productions of consonant clusters of children with speech sound disorders (Anderson, 2000; Baker, 2000; Chin, 1996; Gierut, 1998, 1999; Gierut and Champion, 2001; Wyllie-Smith et al., 2006; Yavaş and McLeod, 2010).

Psycholinguistic Models

Although linguistic applications are useful for the *description* of children's phonological systems, psycholinguistic applications provide the potential for the *explanation* of children's phonology. A psycholinguistic model draws on the fields of psychology and linguistics and attempts to account for psychological processes or mental mechanisms involved in the "perception, storage, planning and production of speech as it is produced in real time in real utterances" (McCormack, 1997, p. 4). At the simplest level, a psycholinguistic model describes the distinction between underlying representations of words and their production (Fee, 1995). It is used to map interactions between auditory input, underlying cognitive-linguistic processes, and speech production output (Dodd, 1995a). In doing so, psycholinguistic models attempt to provide explanations for the descriptive or symptomatic information derived from linguistic-based assessments (Stackhouse and Wells, 1993). An example of such a model is presented in Chapter 4 (Figure 4.1).

Application to Typically Developing Children.   Numerous authors have been involved in the construction of psycholinguistic models of speech development. These include Smith (1973, 1978); Menn and colleagues (Kiparsky and Menn, 1977; Menn, 1971, 1978; Menn and Matthei, 1992; Menn, Markey, Mozer, and Lewis, 1993); Macken (1980a, 1980b); Spencer (1986, 1988); Hewlett and colleagues (Hewlett, 1990; Hewlett, Gibbon, and

Cohen-McKenzie, 1998); and Stackhouse and colleagues (Pascoe, Wells, and Stackhouse, 2006; Stackhouse and Wells, 1993, 1997). A number of useful historical accounts and critiques of psycholinguistic models exist (e.g., Bernhardt and Stemberger, 1998; Maxwell, 1984; Menn and Matthei, 1992; Vihman, 1996).

In a psycholinguistic model, the first point of the speech process is the *input,* which is the speech signal the child hears. The final point of the speech process is the *output,* which is the speech signal (usually words) actually produced/spoken by the child. The possible events that occur between input and output are the focus of psycholinguistic models. Menn (1994) describes psycholinguistic modeling as a "black box approach" whereby input and output are examined to construct a mechanism, which can explain the effects seen.

input → black box → output

Within the "black box" different levels of representation of knowledge are hypothesized. *Underlying representation* refers to "the basic unaltered pronunciation before any processes have had a chance to operate" (Spencer, 1996, p. 50). Thus, the underlying representation is the phonological information that is stored in the speaker's mind about the words known and used.

input → underlying representation → output

The child's underlying representation is stored in the *lexicon* or "mental dictionary" (Maxwell, 1984, p. 18). Depending on the theoretical model being considered, the lexicon may contain semantic or meaning-based information (Bernhardt and Stemberger, 1998) and/or phonological information (e.g., Menn, 1978; Smith, 1973). Stackhouse and Wells (1997) suggest the lexicon contains phonological, semantic, grammatical, orthographic, and motor programming information. Definitions of the storage, nature, and number of underlying representations differ among researchers.

Initially, *single-lexicon models* of the speech process were posited, whereby children were considered to have an adultlike underlying representation of speech (e.g., Smith, 1973). The lexicon was synonymous with the underlying representation and contained information about the adult pronunciation of words. Development of single-lexicon models continued through the 1970s (Braine, 1979; Macken, 1980a; Smith, 1978). However, this was subsequently revised because evidence did not support Smith's (1973) original assumption that the child's perception was always adultlike. Consequently, Smith (1978) revised his model by adding a perceptual filter to account for the possibility that the child may have inaccurate perception.

Early single-lexicon models could not account for variable pronunciations, in particular, for instances when different tokens of a word could be pronounced in different ways, and when one phoneme could be pronounced differently in different words (Bernhardt and Stemberger, 1998). Consequently, *two-lexicon models* in which two levels of underlying representation exist—the input and output lexicons— were proposed. The *input lexicon* refers to the perceptually based phonological representations that enable the child to perceive speech, or "all the child's knowledge that permits him or her to recognize a word" (Menn and Matthei, 1992, p. 214). The *output lexicon* refers to the articulatorily based phonological representations that enable the child to produce speech. Menn (1983) described the output lexicon as "ways-to-say-words." If it exists independently, the input lexicon is almost certain to be richer in contrasts than the output lexicon (Hewlett, 1990), and some suggest that the input lexicon contains the same information as the adult surface representations (Spencer, 1988).

$$\text{input} \rightarrow \text{input lexicon} \rightarrow \text{outputlexicon} \rightarrow \text{output}$$

Two-lexicon models allowed for the notion that young children may have underlying representations that are unique to their own system. That is, the output (production) lexicon was able to hold underlying representations that were not adultlike (for a complete discussion, see Maxwell, 1984).

In a two-lexicon account, the child stores underlying adultlike perceptual representations in the input lexicon. These perceptual representations are then modified off-line through the application of rules or processes to create underlying production representations in the output lexicon. Once a child has stored a word in the output lexicon, subsequent productions are accessed from the output lexicon rather than from the input lexicon and modified on-line.

Although two-lexicon models provided a way of accounting for the variability in children's speech, there are three primary criticisms of the two-lexicon accounts (Bernhardt and Stemberger, 1998; Chiat, 1994; Menn and Matthei, 1992; Vihman, 1996). First, with the potential for duplication of lexical items, particularly in the output lexicon, the models fail to explain how children select one representation over another or how representations change to being more adultlike. That is, the models do not explain when and how old forms are deleted (Bernhardt and Stemberger; Dinnsen, Barlow, and Morrisette, 1997; Vihman). A second criticism concerns the "continuity hypothesis" (Bernhardt and Stemberger; Menn, 1994). Developmentalists argue that there should not be one model that applies to children and another for adults because accounting for the shift between the two models is difficult. It has been suggested that a child's output lexicon will eventually match his or her input lexicon because the forms within the output lexicon will become adultlike; thus, adults may have only a single lexicon. The third major criticism is that both single- and two-lexicon models were designed to describe single-word production and do not take into account constraints that occur between words in connected speech (Hewlett, 1990; Vihman, 1996).

Hence, two-lexicon accounts thus have a number of limitations. Consequently, single-lexicon theories are currently being postulated with the notion that input and output forms are represented in some way (e.g., Hewlett et al., 1998). Furthermore, the hard-walled "boxes" of the two-lexicon accounts are now being represented by connectionist models (Bernhardt and Stemberger, 1998; Menn and Matthei, 1992; see Baker, Croot, McLeod, and Paul [2001] for a description). Connectionist models use computer modeling to test a cognitive task, such as speech production. Networks of nodes connect the input and output, and during computer simulations, the probability of the activation of each node is tested. Connectionist models can be run many times to provide the probability of a specific output occurring, thus enabling testing of hypotheses of speech and language acquisition.

Application to SLP Practice.   The earliest authors in the field of speech-language pathology to suggest consideration of children's underlying representation were Shriberg and Kwiatkowski (1980) and Edwards (1983). Since then, consideration of underlying representation has been presented in speech-language pathology intervention case studies (e.g., Bryan and Howard, 1992; McGregor and Schwartz, 1992; Stackhouse, Pascoe, and

Gardner, 2006). Baker, Croot, McLeod, and Paul (2001) provide a tutorial of the application of psycholinguistic models to SLP practice, and an important series of books has been written for speech-language pathologists on assessment and intervention for speech and literacy within a psycholinguistic framework (Stackhouse and Wells, 1997, 2001; Pascoe, Wells, and Stackhouse, 2006; Stackhouse, Vance, Pascoe, and Wells, 2007).

The first part of this chapter included several models of speech sound acquisition that we related to clinical practice. As stated earlier, each has its strengths with some perhaps being more helpful than others to one's understanding of how sounds are acquired. In the section that follows, we shift our attention from theories to how to gather data to inform us about how speech sound acquisition has been observed, recorded, and analyzed.

HOW SPEECH ACQUISITION DATA ARE OBTAINED

It is important for SLPs to be well acquainted with typical speech sound development. Later in this chapter, a wide range of speech acquisition data, important to clinical practice is presented. Before getting to the actual developmental data, it is beneficial to understand how these speech acquisition data were obtained because some are based on small samples of children taken over a long period of time whereas other data are based on large groups of children seen during a relatively short period of time. Three major techniques have been used for collecting speech acquisition data: diary studies, large cross-sectional group studies, and longitudinal studies.

Historically, research into typical speech sound acquisition was conducted using *diary studies*. Famous historical diary studies include descriptions of the speech of children such as Amahl (Smith, 1973), Hildegarde (Leopold, 1947), and Joan (Velten, 1943). With the influence of behaviorism, *large cross-sectional group studies* became prevalent. Wellman, Case, Mengurt, and Bradbury (1931), Poole (1934), and Templin (1957) conducted the earliest cross-sectional group studies relating to English-speaking children's speech sound acquisition. More recently, *longitudinal studies* comprising a smaller group of participants have complemented the large-scale cross-sectional studies to enhance the understanding of speech acquisition (e.g., Carroll, Snowling, Hulme, and Stevenson, 2003; Dodd, 1995a; McLeod, van Doorn, and Reed, 2001b; Walker and Archibald, 2006; Watson and Scukanec, 1997a, 1997b). Each of these methodologies has strengths and weaknesses. A primary difference is in the trade-off between the extent of data analyzed and reported versus the number of participants.

To summarize our discussion of research methods of typical English speech sound acquisition, an overview of key studies is presented later in this chapter. You are encouraged to access the original sources in order to utilize the full range of information offered by these researchers. For a wide-ranging overview of speech acquisition in a range of English dialects and languages other than English, see *The International Guide to Speech Acquisition* (McLeod, 2007a) and a summary in McLeod (2010). Note that most speech acquisition studies have used either cross-sectional or longitudinal data collection methods. Those that used a cross-sectional design typically used single-word sampling. Those that used a longitudinal design typically used connected speech sampling. Each of these research techniques is described in detail next.

Diary Studies of Typical Speech Sound Acquisition

Diary studies were the initial major source of data about children's speech and language development. Typically, a parent who was a linguist or psychologist kept a comprehensive diary of his or her child's speech and/or language development over a period of time. An early diary study of a child's language development was that of Humphreys (1880). Famous diary studies which have focused on speech development include Leopold's (1939–1949) four-volume account of his daughter Hildegarde, Velten's (1943) study of his daughter Joan, and Smith's (1973) extensive analysis of his son Amahl's speech.

The parental diary study has continued to be used as a method for data collection but more specifically to collect data on a specific issue rather than general speech and language development. For example, Berg (1995) collected data from his German-speaking daughter on a daily basis from the age of 3;4 to 4;3. He presented data on interword variation in the development of velars. Other examples of diary studies of typical phonological development include Menn's (1971) report on her son's early constraints on sound sequences, the account by Elbers and Ton (1985) of Elbers's son's words and babbling within the first-word period, Stemberger's (1988) account of his eldest daughter's between-word processes and his (1989) account of both daughters' nonsystemic errors within and across phrases, French's (1989) account of her son's acquisition of word forms in the first 50-word stage, and Lleo's (1990) report of her daughter's use of reduplication and homonymy as phonological strategies.

The diary study methodology also has been used to study typical speech acquisition of children where the researchers are not the parents (e.g., Bernstein-Ratner, 1993; Fey and Gandour, 1982). An extension of diary studies is the single case study methodology that has been particularly beneficial for the documentation of intervention effects on children with speech sound disorder (e.g., Camarata, 1989; Camarata and Gandour, 1985; Crosbie, Pine, Holm, and Dodd, 2006; Crystal, 1987; Grunwell and Yavaş, 1988; Leonard and Leonard, 1985; McGregor and Schwartz, 1992; Pascoe, Stackhouse, and Wells, 2005).

Advantages and Disadvantages of Diary Studies

The primary advantage of diary studies is that they contain some of the most detailed accounts of speech acquisition. The depth and breadth of detail enables examination of descriptive, exploratory, and explanatory intent. The detail places change into context because diary studies allow for the retention of the holistic and meaningful characteristics of the child's real-life events (Yin, 1989).

Although general trends about speech acquisition cannot be derived from diary study data, the rich source of data (often contained in appendices) has been used to test and retest statements and hypotheses long after the original reason for collecting the data has been superseded. For example, the extensive data Smith (1973) provided in his appendices have been reexamined by Braine (1979) and Macken (1980a) to find evidence against Smith's earlier conclusion that the child's underlying representations must be adultlike. Similarly, Greenlee (1974) reexamined data from a number of cross-linguistic diary studies to describe a sequence of development for consonant clusters.

Using diary studies as the only means to understand children's speech acquisition has a number of disadvantages. First, it is easy to assume that the single child under study is typical unless reference is made to other normative studies. An example can be seen with Leopold's daughter Hildegarde, who replaced word-initial /f/ with a [w] or [v] (Leopold, 1947). These substitutions are atypical according to Ingram, Christensen, Veach, and Webster (1980), who did not find a single such instance in their study of the typical acquisition of fricatives in 73 children. Second, the fact that the children studied are primarily those of linguists suggests that these children may be precocious or at least different in their acquisition from the general population, whether as a result of genetic endowment or environment. Other disadvantages of using diary studies include potential randomness and lack of structure in data collection and potential observer bias because the parent is often the researcher (Ingram, 1989b). Until recently, many diary studies relied on on-line transcription, making it impossible to determine transcription reliability. Some of these problems were overcome with the introduction of the large-group cross-sectional study and the longitudinal study.

Large-Group Cross-Sectional Studies of Typical Speech Sound Acquisition

From the 1950s to 1970s, behaviorism was a major theoretical paradigm for considering speech sound acquisition, and the emphasis in data collection in the fields of psychology, linguistics, and speech-language pathology moved from diary studies to cross-sectional methodology. Using this methodology, researchers attempted to describe typical behavior by establishing developmental norms through the observation of large numbers of children. Commonly, children were placed into selected age groupings, and each child underwent the same testing procedure. Possible confounding influences such as gender, socioeconomic status, language background, and intelligence were controlled. The results of these experiments were presented as proportions and percentages, often in large tables indicating the age of acquisition of phonemes or the age of decline of certain phonological processes or patterns.

The majority of research describing the typical acquisition of English speech sounds uses large-group cross-sectional methodology (Anthony, Bogle, Ingram, and McIsaac, 1971; Arlt and Goodban, 1976; Bankson and Bernthal, 1990b; Chirlian and Sharpley, 1982; Dodd et al., 2002; Flipsen, 2006a; Haelsig and Madison, 1986; Ingram, Pittman, and Newman, 1985; Irwin and Wong, 1983; James, 2001; Kilminster and Laird, 1978; Lowe, Knutson, and Monson, 1985; McLeod and Ariuli, 2009; Olmsted, 1971; Paynter and Petty, 1974; Poole, 1934; Prather, Hedrick, and Kern, 1975; Preisser, Hodson, and Paden, 1988; Smit, 1993a, 1993b; Smit et al., 1990; Templin, 1957; Wellman et al., 1931).

Wellman and colleagues (1931) and Poole (1934) conducted the pioneering large-group studies of typical speech acquisition. However, the most famous study was conducted in 1957 when Templin undertook a comprehensive study of the speech development of 480 children aged 3;0 to 8;0. She provided comprehensive text, 71 tables, and 9 figures to explain children's acquisition of articulation, discrimination, sentence development, and vocabulary as well as academic performance. Templin presented the age of acquisition at which 75 percent of children could produce each speech sound in initial-, medial-, and final-word positions. Templin's classic study has been quoted as an authoritative source on speech development by researchers (e.g., Powell and Elbert, 1984; Smit, 1986; Stockman and Stephenson, 1981;

Young, 1987) and speech-language pathologists (e.g., Stewart and Weybright, 1980) for many years. Templin's study was considered to need updating in 1976 by Arlt and Goodban, who noted "expanding effects of television, earlier schooling . . . the accelerating effects of developments in education" and suggested that "for purposes of revalidation it seems appropriate to update or examine such norms at 10-year intervals" (Arlt and Goodban, 1976, p. 173). Their suspicions possibly were confirmed when they found that "33% of the sounds tested in this investigation were produced correctly by 75% of the children at least 1 year earlier than would be expected from previously established norms" (p. 176).

The largest and most currently cited cross-sectional study of American English was undertaken by Smit and colleagues (1990), who studied 997 children's productions of consonants and consonant clusters. They not only reported age of acquisition of phonemes but they also presented graphical data (cf. Sander, 1972) that indicated the progression of development from age 3;0 to 9;0. These graphs described the trajectory for boys' and girls' speech acquisition. As shown in Table 3.3, the data collected by Smit and associates either mirror Arlt and Goodban's data or fall between their data and those of Templin, possibly indicating the relevance of data collection methods and context. Other large cross-sectional studies of speech acquisition include those by Kilminster and Laird (1978), who studied the speech acquisition of 1,756 Australian English-speaking children; Nagy (1980), who studied the speech acquisition of 7,602 Hungarian children; and Nakanishi, Owada, and Fujita (1972), who studied the speech acquisition of 1,689 Japanese children. The largest studies of Spanish-speaking children were conducted by Acevedo (1993) and Jimenez (1987), who each studied 120 Mexican children.

Advantages and Disadvantages of Large-Group Cross-Sectional Studies

The primary advantage of large-group cross-sectional studies is that they provide normative information by which to compare children. Such norms are beneficial to SLPs in the identification of impairment. It is assumed that if enough participants are selected for each age group, then typical behavior is observed. Consequently, general trends are ascertained from summary tables provided by such studies. Another advantage of large-group cross-sectional studies is that the emphasis on methodology encourages systematic observation of behavior (Ingram, 1989b). All participants are studied for the same amount of time for the same behaviors. The third advantage of large-group cross-sectional studies is that there is an emphasis on standardized measurement tools so that studies can be replicated.

Disadvantages of such studies include the facts that (1) they typically are collected using single-word, not connected, speech samples; (2) they often used imitated (rather than spontaneous) productions; (3) they collect data in specific geographical regions that may have dialectical variants; and (4) the experience and reliability of examiners is not always reported (Smit, 1986). Additionally, Peña, Spaulding, and Plante (2006) recently questioned the assumptions behind the selection of children for participation in large-group cross-sectional studies. They argued that, traditionally, children were excluded from cross-sectional studies if they were not experiencing typical development. However, Peña and colleagues indicated that this strategy was akin to "shooting ourselves in the foot." They concluded that if the purpose of a normative study is to identify children who are not developing typically, then the normative sample should include children who are not developing typically. Although their study addressed the area of children's language, their claims are likely to also be true for children's speech.

To conclude, the major strengths of the large-group cross-sectional studies are also a weakness. The grouping of data for statistical analyses means that the data collected for individual children are not reported. The only glimpse of individual variation can be found in the standard deviations from the mean. Longitudinal studies, a third approach, can elucidate individual variability and provide additional insights into children's speech acquisition.

Longitudinal Studies of Typical Speech Sound Acquisition

The possibility that children follow different paths and strategies in typical speech and language acquisition prompted a shift in focus from the large-group studies to longitudinal studies of smaller groups of children. Ingram (1989b) expressed the concern that many of the diary and large-group studies considered only superficial issues, such as the timing of the occurrence of particular features in children's speech. Quotes such as this from Khan (1982, p. 78) occur commonly within the literature from the mid-1970s, expressing the need for "controlled, longitudinal examination of large numbers of children."

Longitudinal studies of speech sound acquisition are characterized by the study of groups of children at repeated intervals. These studies are usually conducted for specific purposes that are beyond describing the age of acquisition of phonemes, such as writing rules and explaining the acquisition process. Longitudinal studies share a number of characteristics with diary case studies, in that they study the same children over time. However, there have three primary differences. First, the researcher is independent (recall that diary studies often were conducted by the parent of the child). Second, instead of only one or two children, a small group typically is studied. Third, children in longitudinal studies usually are studied for a set period of time each week or month instead of daily or at random intervals. Thus, longitudinal studies have the potential to capitalize on the strengths of both diary and large-group studies.

Ferguson and Farwell (1975) conducted one of the earliest and most influential longitudinal studies of speech development. They studied the emergence of words and sounds in early language development, plotting the progress of three young children and the point of 50 words in the children's vocabularies. The data for one of the children were extracted from the diary of Leopold's (1947) Hildegarde; Ferguson and Farwell personally studied the other two children and presented phone trees of data to demonstrate individual learning strategies undertaken by these children.

Since Ferguson and Farwell's original work, a number of longitudinal studies considering different aspects of the development of young children's phonology have been conducted (e.g., Anderson, 2004; Dodd, 1995b; Dyson, 1986, 1988; Dyson and Paden, 1983; Fee and Ingram, 1982; McLeod et al., 2001b; Otomo and Stoel-Gammon, 1992; Robb and Bleile, 1994; Schwartz, Leonard, Wilcox, and Folger, 1980; Stoel-Gammon, 1985; Vihman and Greenlee, 1987; Walker and Archibald, 2006; Watson and Scukanec, 1997a, 1997b). For example, Robb and Bleile conducted a comprehensive longitudinal study of the consonant inventories of seven children aged 8 to 25 months and were able to present valuable individualized data on the sequence of development over time. Similarly, Selby, Robb, and Gilbert (2000) studied the development of vowels in five children aged 15, 18, 21, 24, and 36 months of age.

Advantages and Disadvantages of Longitudinal Studies

There are two major advantages of conducting longitudinal studies of a select group of children. First, studying a small group of children allows researchers to capture individual variations in approaches to learning that may be masked by a large-group study. Knowing about these individual differences increases the likelihood of creating successful individualized teaching and learning experiences for SLP clients. Second, longitudinal studies allow for the reporting of developmental trends (Macken, 1995). For example, Lleo and Prinz (1996) reported that German- and Spanish-speaking children produced word shapes in the following developmental sequence: CV → CVC → CVCC → CCVCC. Knowing about typical developmental sequences enhances the ability of SLPs to assess whether their clients are delayed or disordered and may yield a more accurate understanding of the learning process, which could be replicated in intervention strategies.

Interestingly, despite the unique data that result from longitudinal studies, not all such studies report individual developmental information. For example, Dyson and Paden (1983) conducted a longitudinal study of 40 children and reported grouped findings from the first and eighth observations; however, they did use their data to propose sequences of development.

Longitudinal studies have three major disadvantages. First, longitudinal studies frequently use small numbers of children. As a result, the findings may not be representative of the general population. Second, longitudinal studies generally have regularly scheduled intervals of weeks or months between visits. Such scheduling may allow the child to show considerable change between observations. On the other hand, possible crucial periods of change may occur over a day or two, and a flexible schedule may be more appropriate to allow "emergency visits" when alerted by parental reports of change (Ingram, 1989b). Finally, researchers using longitudinal methodology often prepare stimulus materials for elicitation; thus, a picture of the child's natural speech may not be obtained (French, 1989).

Combined Data-Collection Procedures

To obtain the advantages of both cross-sectional and longitudinal methodologies, a number of researchers have developed combined methodologies. Some fundamentally cross-sectional studies have assessed children more than once, thus gaining some longitudinal continuity in their data. For example, Roberts, Burchinal, and Footo (1990) utilized a combination of cross-sectional and longitudinal methodology in their examination of 145 children between the ages of 2;6 and 8;0. Over the six-year period, 13 of these children were examined six times, 24 were tested five times, and so on with 32 being tested only once. Similarly, Stoel-Gammon (1985) studied 33 children's development of phonetic inventories; 7 children were studied at age 15 months, 19 children at age 18 months, 32 children at age 21 months, and 33 children at age 24 months. Neither of these studies presented individualized longitudinal results.

Another approach is to undertake a longitudinal study in which children are studied over time, but different cohorts of children are studied at different ages (e.g., Chervela, 1981; Dyson, 1988). For example, Chervela conducted a "longitudinal and cross-sectional study" (p. 63) of the development of medial consonant clusters in four children ages 1;6 to 3;0. He selected one child at each of the ages of 1;6, 2;0, 2;6, and 3;0. The data were collected for each child once a month for six months. A combination of data-collection methodologies enables researchers to manipulate the advantages and disadvantages of each methodology to provide more comprehensive findings about the typical developmental sequence. As Stokes, Klee, Carson, and Carson (2005, p. 828) recommend: "Large-scale longitudinal studies, combined with statistical analyses, would provide the best possible view of the nature of phonemic development." With this understanding of data-collection procedures, we next explore data that have been collected on children's speech acquisition.

OVERALL SEQUENCE OF SPEECH SOUND ACQUISITION

It takes a child many years to progress from the first cries at birth to intelligible speech incorporating adultlike production of vowels, consonants, syllable structures, and prosody (including tones, if applicable). The four phases of speech acquisition (adapted from Bleile, 2004) are:

> *Phase 1.* Laying the foundations for speech (birth to 1 year)
>
> *Phase 2.* Transitioning from words to speech (1 to 2 years)
>
> *Phase 3.* The growth of the inventory (2 to 5 years)
>
> *Phase 4.* Mastery of speech and literacy (5+ years)

During the first year, the child produces sounds, first reflexively and then more purposefully. Children cry, coo, and babble during their first year, and toward the end of this time, they produce their first words. Within phase 2, children's communicative focus is on transitioning from words to speech. During their second year, they can produce a small vocabulary with a simplified phonological structure. During phase 3, from 2 to 5 years of age, children learn to produce the majority of speech sounds and syllable structures as well as grammatical and syntactical structures. Finally, phase 4 is a period of mastery that includes the sophistication of timing, prosody, and accurate production of polysyllabic words and consonant clusters. Additionally, sounds are conveyed through writing (reading and spelling) and are no longer only in the spoken domain.

PHASE 1: LAYING THE FOUNDATIONS FOR SPEECH

Development of the Structure and Function of the Oral Mechanism

An interrelationship exists between the ability to produce intelligible speech and the development of a child's oromotor, neurological, respiratory, and laryngeal systems (Kent, 1976). The development of oral structure and function begins in the fetus, starts to approximate the adult configuration at age 6 years, and is finished at approximately 18 years of age (Kent and Tilkens, 2007). The development of the anatomical structures and functions that support speech acquisition are described next.

Anatomical Structures Supporting Speech Acquisition

The vocal tract of the newborn differs both in size and shape from that of an adult. The vocal tract of the newborn is three times smaller than that of the adult and is considered to be similar to a single tube to facilitate coordination between breathing, sucking, and swallowing (Kent and Tilkens, 2007; Vorperian, Kent, Gentry, and Yandell, 1999). The adult vocal tract is considered to be akin to two tubes with the oral tube enabling a wide variety of articulations and the laryngeal tube facilitating coordination between breathing and swallowing. The newborn's larynx is located between the first and fourth cervical vertebrae; however, by 6 years of age, it has descended to the adultlike position between the fourth and seventh vertebrae (Kent and Tilkens). From puberty onward, there is a significant sex difference in the overall vocal tract length and the proportions of the pharyngeal and oral cavities (Fitch and Giedd, 1999).

In infancy, the respiratory system consists of a "bellows-like displacement of the diaphragm" (Kent and Tilkens, 2007, p. 9), and infants' breathing rate at rest is between 30 to 80 breaths per minute. By age 6 months, the infant's rib cage is horizontal and by 1 year of age, respiration for speech and breathing is differentiated. Respiration matures at approximately 7 years of age when the lung architecture is similar to that of an adult (Kent and Tilkens). However, during speaking tasks, children still have greater subglottal air pressure than adults. Low birth weight is a major factor in poor adult respiratory function as identified in a large prospective longitudinal birth cohort study conducted by Canoy and associates (2007).

Neurological development is also important for speech acquisition, and significant neurological development occurs over the life span (Sowell, Thompson, and Toga, 2004). Ruben (1997) described flexibility of the central auditory nervous system, stating, "The critical/sensitive period of phonology is from the 6th month of fetal life through the 12th month of infancy" (p. 202). Between infancy and adolescence, brain weight and intracranial space grows by approximately 25 percent and then declines in late adulthood to brain volumes similar to those of young children (Courchesne et al., 2000). In a longitudinal study, Sowell, Thompson, Leonard, et al. (2004) studied children between the ages of 5 and 11 years and found that brain growth progressed at a rate of between 0.4 to 1.5 mm per year. They also found that significant thickening was restricted to left Broca's and Wernicke's areas; gray matter thickness was correlated with changing cognitive abilities. Additionally, rapid myelination occurs during the first year of life (Barkovich, Kjos, Jackson, and Norman, 1988) and is important for gross- and fine-motor movements, including speech (Bleile, 2007).

Anatomical Functions Supporting Speech Acquisition

Precision of articulatory movements of the lip, jaw, and tongue commence in infancy and continue to develop well into adolescence (Walsh and Smith, 2002). Green, Moore, and Reilly (2002) examined vertical movements of the upper lip, lower lip, and jaw during speech for children and adults. They found that jaw movements matured before lip movements with 1- and 2-year-old children's jaw movements being similar to adults' jaw movements. However, the upper and lower lip movements were more variable and became more adultlike with maturation. Steeve et al. (2008) found that different mandibular control for sucking, chewing, and babble matured as children progressed from 9 months to 12 months to 15 months of age. Cheng and colleagues have conducted a number of studies of the maturation of tongue control for speech in children, adolescents, and adults using electropalatography (EPG) and electromagnetic articulography (EMA) (Cheng, Murdoch, and Goozee, 2007; Cheng, Murdoch, Goozee, and Scott, 2007a, 2007b). Using EPG, Cheng and colleagues (2007a) found that children's tongue/palate contact for the sounds /t/, /l/, /s/, and /k/ largely resembled those of adults; however, the children ages 6 to 11 years displayed increased palatal contact and an excessively posterior tongue placement compared with adults. The researchers also indicated that the maturation of the speech motor system was nonuniform and that significant changes in the maturation of tongue control occurred until 11 years of age. During adolescence, tongue control was continually refined. Cheng and associates (2007b) used EMA to consider the coordination of tongue and jaw. They found that maturation continued until 8 to 11 years of age with continual refinement into adolescence. The relationship between the tongue-tip and tongue-body movement with the jaw differed. The tongue-tip became increasingly synchronized with jaw movement, but the tongue-body retained movement independence with the jaw.

Speech and articulation rates also have been studied in children (Flipsen, 2002a; Ozanne, 1992; Robb, Gilbert, Reed, and Bisson, 2003; Robb and Gillon, 2007; Robbins and Klee, 1987; Williams and Stackhouse, 1998, 2000) and are relevant to our consideration of the maturation of oral functioning. Increasing rate may serve as an indicator of improving control over the articulators. Williams and Stackhouse (1998) suggested that typically developing children ages 3 to 5 years increased their accuracy and consistency but not rate of production during diadochokinetic (DDK) tasks. Williams and Stackhouse (2000) suggested that rate was not as useful a predictor as accuracy and consistency of response. Similarly, Walker and Archibald (2006) conducted a longitudinal study of articulation rates in children 4, 5, and 6 years old. They found that articulation rate did not increase significantly with age. However, Flipsen (2002a) reviewed a series of studies of articulation rate and concluded that rate does increase across the developmental period.

Infant Perception

Another important foundation of speech acquisition is infant perception.

Infant Auditory Perception

Humans are able to perceive sound well before birth (Lasky and Williams, 2005). For example, in a study of 400 fetuses at 16 weeks gestation, it was found that they were able to respond to pure tone auditory stimuli at 500Hz (Shahidullah and Hepper, 1992). In a follow-up study, Hepper and Shahidullah (1994) described the progression of the fetuses' responses to different sound frequencies:

- *19 weeks gestation.* Fetuses responded to 500Hz.
- *27 weeks gestation.* Fetuses responded to 250 and 500Hz (but not 1,000 and 3,000Hz).
- *33 to 35 weeks gestation.* Fetuses responded to 250, 500, 1,000, and 3,000Hz.

As the fetuses matured, they required a lower intensity of sound (20 to 30 dB) in order to respond. Hepper and Shahidullah (1994, p. F81) concluded that "the sensitivity of the fetus to sounds in the low frequency range may promote language acquisition." Another study demonstrated that fetuses demonstrate the ability not only to hear but also to perceive differences in sounds. DeCasper et al. (1994) asked mothers to recite a nursery rhyme to their fetus three times a day for 4 weeks between 33 and 37 weeks gestation. They found that the fetuses responded with a change in heart rate when presented with a recorded version of the nursery rhyme but not when presented with an alternative rhyme. They concluded that by the third trimester, "fetuses become familiar with recurrent, maternal speech sounds" (DeCasper et al., 1994, p. 159).

After birth, infants demonstrate sophisticated perceptual skills. Traditionally, the main experimental technique that was used to ascertain infants' ability to discriminate sounds is called the *high amplitude sucking technique* developed by Siqueland and Delucia (1969). Using this technique, infants sucked on a nonnutritive nipple that was equipped to detect changes in pressure. Experimenters found that infants sucked vigorously when a new sound was played, but as they became familiar with it, their sucking decreased in frequency and intensity. When a new sound was played, their sucking again became vigorous and then diminished with familiarity with the signal. More recently, *event-related potentials (ERPs)* have been used to determine infants' ability to discriminate aspects of communication (e.g., Shafer, Shucard, Shucard, and Gerken, 1998). Event-related potentials are low-amplitude neurophysiological responses that follow presentation of a stimulus and are typically recorded via electrophysiological instrumentation such as electroencephalograms (EEG) or electromyograms (EMG). ERPs are suitable for studying infants' perceptions because they are noninvasive and require no overt response. Using both of these techniques (high amplitude sucking, ERPs), researchers have discovered that infants prefer voices and have the ability to discriminate speech sounds.

The fact that infants demonstrate a preference for voices, particularly their mothers' voices has been shown by a number of researchers (Augustyn and Zuckerman, 2007). For example, DeCasper and Fifer (1980) demonstrated that by 3 days of age, children can distinguish their mothers' voices from a stranger's voice and show a preference for their mothers' voices. Infants appear to prefer child-directed speech (also called *motherese*) to adult-directed speech. Cooper and Aslin (1990) found that this held true for children as young as 2 days old and was still apparent in children who were 1 month old.

Infants also have been shown to be able to discriminate both place and voicing features of consonants. For example, Eimas (1974) showed that children who were 2 months old could discriminate between the place contrast of /d/ and /g/. Similarly, Aslin and colleagues (1983) showed that children could discriminate between /f/ and voiceless *th* phonemes that also differ by place. A number of authors have demonstrated that infants can discriminate between voiced and voiceless consonants. Eimas, Siqueland, Jusczyk, and Vigorito (1971) showed that infants who were 1 and 4 months old could discriminate between synthesized voiced and voiceless contrasts such as in the stimuli /pa/ and /ba/. Similarly, Eilers, Wilson, and Moore (1977) demonstrated that 6-month-old infants could discriminate /sa/ and /za/.

As children are exposed to their native language and reach the end of their first year, some authors suggest that their ability to discriminate nonnative sounds diminishes. For example, Ruben (1997, p. 203) describes this juxtaposition: "By at least 2 days of age, the neonate has an ability to discriminate language specific acoustic distinctions. . . . The

12 month old human has developed the capacity to categorize only those phonemes which are in its native language." However, more research is needed prior to confirming this view (Rvachew, 2007a) because we do not know whether all infants can discriminate all phonetic inputs, nor do we know that all infants lose the ability to discriminate language-specific inputs. Recent research indicates that infants may retain the ability to discriminate vowels without supporting input (Polka and Bohn, 2003), whereas other children may lose the ability to perceive contrasts despite receiving supporting input (Nittrouer, 2001). A significant relationship exists between infants' speech perception and subsequent language skills at 2 to 3 years (Tsao, Liu, and Kuhl, 2004) and vocabulary and receptive language skills in older children (Edwards, Fox, and Rogers, 2002; Vance, Rosen, and Coleman, 2009).

Infants' Visual Perception

In addition to auditory perception, visual speech perception plays a critical role in infants' learning of language. It has long been known that infants prefer looking at faces compared with objects and are even able to discriminate and imitate facial expressions (Field, Woodson, Greenberg, and Cohen, 1982). Recently, it has been discovered that infants are able to distinguish between familiar and unfamiliar languages using only visual cues (Weikum et al., 2007). Weikum and colleagues found that infants of 4 and 6 months of age were able to distinguish between English (familiar) and French (unfamiliar) using a video (without auditory input) of an adult; however, by 8 months of age, this ability had been lost.

Infant Production

Developmental Summaries of Early Speech Production

Infants enter the world being able to vocalize through crying. Throughout their first months, the repertoire of sounds and prosodic features increases. Two developmental summaries of early speech production will be presented, one based on the work by Stark and colleagues and the other based on the work by Oller and colleagues.

Stark's Typology of Infant Phonations. The *Stark Assessment of Early Vocal Development–Revised* is based on work by Stark and colleagues (Nathani, Ertmer, and Stark, 2006; Stark, Bernstein, and Demorest, 1983). This typology includes five levels of development of infant vocalizations (see Box 3.1). The first level comprises *reflexive* sounds, including *quasi-resonant nuclei (Q)*, defined as "faint low-pitched grunt-like sounds with muffled resonance" (Nathani et al., 2006, p. 367). Reflexive vocalizations are common between 0 and 6 weeks of age (Stark, Bernstein, and Demorest, 1983) and include fussing and crying. McGlaughlin and Grayson (2003) indicated that the mean amount of crying within a 24-hour period fell from 90 minutes when children were 1 to 3 months of age to 60 to 65 minutes from 4 to 9 months of age and then went back to 86 minutes from 10 to 12 months of age. However, McGlaughlin and Grayson reported that other studies show a decrease in crying after 10 months of age.

The second level of the *Stark Assessment of Early Vocal Development–Revised* is called *control of phonation*. During this level, *fully resonant nuclei (F)* occur and are

BOX 3.1 Two typologies of infants' vocalizations

Typology 1: _Stark Assessment of Early Vocal Development–Revised_ (Nathani, Ertmer, and Stark, 2006)

1. _Reflexive (0 to 2 months):_ Vegetative sounds, sustained crying/fussing, quasi-resonant nuclei (Q) ("faint low-pitched grunt-like sounds with muffled resonance"(p. 367))
2. _Control of phonation (1 to 4 months):_ Fully resonant nuclei (F), two or more Fs, closants (consonantlike segments: raspberry, click, isolated consonant), vocants (vowel-like segments), closant-vocant combinations, chuckles, or sustained laughter
3. _Expansion (3 to 8 months):_ Isolated vowels, two or more vowels in a row, vowel glide, ingressive sounds, squeals, marginal babbling
4. _Basic canonical syllables (5 to 10 months):_ Single consonant-vowel syllable, canonical babbling, whispered productions, consonant-vowel combination followed by a consonant (CV-C), disyllables (CVCV)
5. _Advanced forms (9 to 18 months):_ Complex syllables (e.g., VC, CCV, CCVC), jargon, diphthongs

Typology 2: Oller's typology of infant phonations (Oller, 2000; Oller, Oller, and Badon, 2006)

1. Non-speechlike vocalizations
   a. _Vegetative sounds:_ Burps, hiccups
   b. _Fixed vocal signal:_ Crying, laughing, groaning
2. Speechlike vocalizations (protophones)
   a. _Quasi-vowels (0 to 2 months):_ Vowel-like productions without shaping of the articulators
   b. _Primitive articulation stage (2 to 3 months):_ Vowel-like productions produced by shaping the articulators
   c. _Expansion stage (3 to 6 months):_ Marginal babbling comprising a consonantlike and a vowel-like sound
   d. _Canonical babbling (6+ months):_ Well-formed syllables such as [baba]

defined as "vowel-like sounds . . . that have energy across a wide range of frequencies (not restricted to low frequencies like Q)" (_Q_ refers to the quasi-resonant nuclei as defined above) (Nathani et al., 2006, p. 367). Additionally, _closants_ (consonantlike segments such as a raspberry, click, or isolated consonant) and _vocants_ (vowel-like segments) are produced during the second level. During the third level, _expansion,_ infants produce isolated vowels, two or more vowels in a row, vowel glide combinations, ingressive sounds, squeals, and marginal babbling. Marginal babbling comprises a series of closant and vocant segments. Additionally, Gratier and Devouche (2011) showed that 3-month-old infants and their mothers selectively imitated a variety of prosodic contours during vocalization. The fourth level, _basic canonical syllables_, occurs between 5 and 10 months of age. Infants during this level produce canonical babbling, single consonant-vowel syllables, whispered productions, disyllables (CVCV), and a consonant-vowel combination followed by a consonant (CV-C). *Canonical babbling* is seen as an important stage in the transition from babbling to speech. Nathani and associates (2006) define canonical babbling as including both reduplicated babbling (e.g., [baba]) and nonreduplicated babbling (e.g., [badu]). It is important for SLPs to pay attention to infants' babbling because late onset of canonical babbling may be a predictor of later speech sound disorders. For example, Oller, Eilers, Neal, and Schwartz (1999) found children who had late onset of canonical babbling had smaller production vocabularies at 1;6, 2;0, and 3;0 years of age.

The fifth and final levels of the *Stark Assessment of Early Vocal Development–Revised* are titled *advanced forms*. This level typically occurs between 9 and 18 months of age. During this time, children produce complex syllables (e.g., VC, CCV, CCVC), jargon, and diphthongs. Nathani and colleagues (2006) applied the *Stark Assessment of Early Vocal Development–Revised* to 30 infants in a mixed cross-sectional and longitudinal design spanning five age ranges from 0 to 20 months of age. They found that as the children increased in age, speechlike utterances increased in frequency while non-speechlike utterances decreased in frequency. Productions typically associated with levels 1 and 2 decreased with age whereas productions associated with level 4 were rarely produced before 9 months of age. Level 5 vocalizations occurred only 10 percent from 0 to 15 months, but jumped to 20 percent by 16 to 20 months of age.

Oller's Typology of Infant Phonations.   Oller and colleagues (Oller, 2000; Oller, Oller, and Badon, 2006) indicated that infants' vocalizations can be classified into being non-speechlike and speechlike (see Box 3.1). Non-speechlike vocalizations include *vegetative sounds*, such as burps and hiccups, and *fixed vocal signals*, such as crying, laughing, and groaning. Speechlike vocalizations are then classified into four phases of development: quasi-vowels, primitive articulation stage, expansion stage, and canonical babbling. From 0 to 2 months of age, children phonate and produce quasi-vowels (vowel-like productions) and glottals (Oller, Eilers, Neal, and Schwartz, 1999). The phase between 2 and 3 months of age (the primitive articulation stage) (Oller et al.) is where children begin to produce vowel-like sounds that are sometimes called *gooing* (Oller et al.), or cooing (Stark et al., 1983). From 3 to 6 months of age (the expansion stage), children expand their repertoires, producing full vowels and raspberries (Oller et al.). They also begin to produce syllablelike vocalizations (Stark et al.) or marginal babbling (Oller et al.). From 6 months of age onward, infants produce canonical babbling—that is, well-formed canonical syllables (e.g., [babababa]) (Oller et al.).

Babbling and Speech

The developmental typologies mentioned earlier indicate that children's babble consists of a series of consonants and vowels. However, over the years there have been differing views on the importance of babbling to children's speech acquisition. Some time ago, Jakobson (1968, p. 24) described babbling as "purposeless egocentric soliloquy" and "biologically orientated 'tongue delirium'" and contrasted babbling with the production of words in the following way: "In place of the phonetic abundance of babbling, the phonemic poverty of the first linguistic stages appear, a kind of deflation which transforms the so-called 'wild sounds' of the babbling period into entities of linguistic value" (p. 25). More recent researchers have opposed Jakobson's extreme views that babbling and speech are discontinuous. Indeed, most researchers now believe that there is continuity between babbling and early speech (Davis and MacNeilage, 1995; Storkel and Morrisette, 2002) and suggest that babbling and early words share consonants (such as /m, n, p, b, t, d/) and vowels.

There are differences between the babbling of children who are typically developing and those who have additional learning needs. For example, researchers compared the babbling of children with hearing loss to children who were typically developing (Oller and Eilers, 1988; Stoel-Gammon and Otomo, 1986). They found that babies with hearing loss babbled later, babbled less frequently, used fewer syllables, were more likely to use single syllables than repeated syllable combinations, and used a disproportionate number of glides and glottal sequences. Morris (2010) reviewed studies of the babbling of 207 infants and found that late talking (defined as talking that begins at 24 months) could be predicted by a lower-than-expected mean babbling level. The babbling of late talkers has also been found to be different from typically developing children. Stoel-Gammon (1989) indicated that less canonical babbling was produced by late talkers from 9 to 21 months than for typically developing children.

As children near their first birthdays, they utter their first words. These words are to be distinguished from babbling and from phonetically consistent forms (PCF). Owens (1994) suggested two indicators that designate production of true words:

1. The child's utterance must have a phonetic relationship to an adult word (i.e., it sounds somewhat similar).
2. The child must use the word consistently in the presence of a particular situation or object.

Therefore, if a child babbled "mama" but his or her mother was not present, this would not qualify as a word because there was no referent. Similarly, phonetically consistent forms that children regularly produce that do not have a relationship to an adult word (e.g., "taka" for *dog*) are not true words because they do not meet the first indicator.

PHASE 2: TRANSITIONING FROM WORDS TO SPEECH

Children's First Fifty Words

Children's pronunciation in the first 50-word stage appears to be constrained by their physiology, ambient language, and child-specific factors (Vihman, 1992). There is much individual and phonetic variability during this stage (Grunwell, 1982). First words typically consist of one or sometimes two syllables and are of the following shapes: CV, VC, CVCV. Consonants produced at the front of the mouth predominate (e.g., /p, b, d, t, m, n/) (Robb and Bleile, 1994). Final consonants are typically omitted or followed by a vowel (e.g., *dog* may be produced as "do" or "doggy"). Young children also produce a limited repertoire of vowels. According to Donegan (2002), children favor low, nonrounded vowels during their first year and produce height differences in vowels before they produced front-back differences. Common phonological processes (or patterns) produced by young children include reduplication, final consonant deletion, and cluster reduction.

It has been suggested that young children use selection (preferences) and avoidance strategies in the words they produce. Possible selection patterns are the size and complexity of syllables and the sound types included (Ferguson, 1978). Early words are thought to be learned as "whole word patterns." Homonyms are common in children's early words (e.g., "tap" for *tap*, *cap*, *clap*; "no" for *no*, *snow*, *nose*). Researchers suggest that children can approach homonyms in two ways: Sometimes they use them to increase their lexicon, and at other times they appear to limit the number of homonyms to be intelligible. As children mature, the number of homonyms decreases (McLeod, van Doorn, and Reed, 1998, 2001a).

Two different learning styles have been suggested for children learning to speak. Vihman and Greenlee (1987) conducted a comprehensive longitudinal study comparing the speech development of 10 typically developing children between 9 and 17 months and then examined them again at age 3. They reported wide individual variation, particularly for specific segment substitutions and cluster reductions. They described two differing learning styles that were evident in their children at 1 year and remained at 3 years of age. They proposed a continuum of "tolerance for variability" on which they could place their children as being either "systematic (and stable)" or "exploratory (and variable)" (Vihman and Greenlee, 1987, p. 519). These two learning styles are reminiscent of the research into the learning styles used by young children in language acquisition (Bates, Dale, and Thal, 1995). Bates and associates described children with learning style 1 as being word oriented and having high intelligibility, a segmental emphasis, and consistent pronunciation across word tokens. In contrast, children with learning style 2 were described as intonation oriented, having low intelligibility, a suprasegmental emphasis, with variable pronunciation across word tokens.

Young Children's Consonant Inventories

Children's early consonant inventories have nasal, plosive, fricative, approximant, labial, and lingual phonemes (Grunwell, 1981). As children grow older, the number of consonants in their inventories increases. In a large study of more than 1,700 children, Ttofari-Eecen, Reilly, and Eadie (2007) reported that by age 1;0, children had an average of 4.4 consonants in their inventories (median = 4; range = 0–16), and typically these were /m, d, b, n/. Robb and Bleile (1994) conducted a longitudinal study of seven children, examining phonetic inventories from ages 0;8 to 2;1. The most frequent manner of articulation was stops, and the most frequent places of articulation were toward the front of the mouth: labials and alveolars. Their findings, summarized in Table 3.1, demonstrate the broader range of consonants produced in syllable-initial compared with syllable-final position. For example, at 8 months of age, the children produced 5 syllable-initial consonants (typically /d, t, k, m, h/) and 3 syllable-final consonants (typically /t, m, h/). By age 2;1, children produced 15 syllable-initial consonants and 11 syllable-final consonants.

Phonological Knowledge and Vocabulary Acquisition

A close relationship appears to exist between young children's phonological knowledge and their acquisition of vocabulary (Storkel, 2006; Stoel-Gammon, 2011). According to Storkel, phonological knowledge can be defined in terms of three phonotactic constraints:

1. *Inventory constraints.* Inventory of sounds that are produced by the child
2. *Positional constraints.* Sounds that are produced in different syllable positions
3. *Sequence constraints.* Restrictions on the co-occurrence of sounds

TABLE 3.1   Summary of Studies of English-Speaking Children's Consonant Inventories

Age	Number of Syllable-Initial Consonants	Number of Syllable-Final Consonants
0;8	5	3
0;9	5	2
0;10	6	4
0;11	4	2
1;0	5	2
1;1	6	2
1;2	10	2
1;3	6	2
1;4	6	2
1;5	9	3
1;6	6	3
1;7	11	6
1;8	10	5
1;9	9	4
1;10	11	3
1;11	12	5
2;0	10	4
2;1	15	11

During the first year of life, children learn words that are consistent with phonotactic constraints within their babbling. According to Locke (2002, p. 249), "The sounds babbled most frequently are produced more accurately by English-learning 2-year-olds, and appear more often in the languages of the world, than other sounds."

Sounds within a child's inventory are sometimes described as IN sounds, and those not used within their inventories are described as OUT sounds. Much research has been conducted on the perception and production of IN and OUT sounds for infants who have learned fewer than 50 words. These young children appear to have opposite preferences for perception and production. Infants tend to listen to OUT sounds longer than to IN sounds (Vihman and Nakai, 2003, cited in Storkel, 2006). However, when infants are taught to produce new words, they tend to learn words containing IN sounds more quickly than OUT sounds (Schwartz and Leonard, 1982). Storkel (2005, 2006) extended this work by considering the role of IN and OUT sounds in word learning for preschool children beyond the 50-word stage. She found that these older children were more accurate in learning words containing OUT sounds than they were in learning words containing IN sounds. This finding held for both typically developing children and children with speech impairment and was counter to the finding for the younger children in the first 50-word stage.

PHASE 3: THE GROWTH OF THE INVENTORY

This section discusses the third phase of speech acquisition and focuses on typical acquisition of aspects of speech sound production beyond approximately 2 to 5 years of age. Traditionally, many speech-language pathologists' understanding of typical speech sound acquisition has been informed by normative data on the age of acquisition of phonemes (e.g., Smit et al., 1990) and the age at which phonological processes disappear (e.g., Grunwell, 1981). These measures typically address the final product—that is, the age of mastery of certain phonemes and phonological processes. In addition to such data, however, many other data on typical speech sound acquisition are available and should be used in clinical decision making. For example, data on the route of development include typical range of "errors" of phonemic, phonetic, and syllable inventories. This shift in emphasis to include both the endpoint and the route of development equips SLPs with information to identify children with impaired speech at a younger age than we have historically been able to.

A comprehensive overview of typical speech sound acquisition includes many facets (see Box 3.2). Each of these areas is described and speech sound acquisition data are summarized according to children's ages. Additionally, under each heading in the next section, a table highlights the findings from the available research studies. Data from a range of studies are presented in the columns to enable comparison of findings and encourage consideration of diversity and individuality across studies and children. However, rates of development vary among typically developing children. When possible, data from more than one study are presented for each category at each age to allow for comparison and to encourage consideration of diversity and individuality.

Intelligibility

Intelligibility has been described as "the single most practical measurement of oral communication competence" (Metz et al., 1985). A speaker's intelligibility can be affected by articulatory, phonological, suprasegmental, and other linguistic features. For example,

---

BOX 3.2 Components of a comprehensive overview of typical English speech acquisition

---

1. Intelligibility
2. Comparison of the child's speech sounds with the adult target
   a. *Acquired sounds.* Consonants, consonant clusters, vowels
   b. *Percent correct (percent error).* Consonants, consonant clusters, vowels
   c. *Common mismatches.* Consonants, consonant clusters, vowels
   d. Phonological patterns/processes
3. Abilities of the child (without comparison to the adult target)
   a. *Phonetic inventory.* Consonants, consonant clusters, vowels
   b. *Syllable structure*
4. Prosody
5. Metalinguistic/phonological awareness skills

Vihman (1988) indicated that at 3 years of age, children who used more complex sentences were more difficult to understand. Additionally, intelligibility is affected by the speaker's relationship with the listener; for example, differences occur according to whether the listener is the child's parent, a stranger, or a person trained in phonetic transcription (e.g., see Flipsen, 1995; McLeod, Harrison, and McCormack, 2012.

Kent, Miolo, and Bloedel (1994) provide a comprehensive review of procedures for the evaluation of intelligibility, including a range of commercially available instruments. Recently, Flipsen (2006b) discussed several variations of the Intelligibility Index (II) (Shriberg et al., 1997a). The Intelligibility Index is "the percentage of words in the entire sample that the transcriber could reliably understand" (Flipsen, 2006b, p. 306). Flipsen reported data from 320 children ages 3;1 to 8;0 and found gradual increases across this age range (see Table 3.2).

TABLE 3.2   Summary of Studies of English-Speaking Children's Intelligibility

Age	Roulstone et al. (2002)	Weiss (1982)	Coplan & Gleason (1988)	Vihman (1988)	Gordon-Brannan (1993, cited in Gordon-Brannan, 1994)	Flipsen (2006b)
	Intelligibility to the Children's Parents	Intelligibility	Parental estimates of Intelligibility to Strangers	Intelligibility Judged by Three Unfamiliar Listeners	Intelligibility in Conversational Speech with Unfamiliar Listeners	Percent of Words That Could Be Reliably Understood by the Transcriber*
2;0	87.3%	26–50%	50% (22 months)			
2;6		51–70%				
3;0		71–80%	75% (37 months)	73% (50–80%)		95.68% (88.89–100.00)
4;0			100% (48 months)		93% (73–100%)	96.82% (88.42–100.00)
5;0					Intelligible	98.05% (89.84–100.00)
6;0						98.43% (91.67–100.00)
7;0						99.51% (97.36–100.00)
8;0						99.01% (97.07–100.00

* = Intelligibility index – original (for more details, see Flipsen, 2006b).

The results reported several studies of children's intelligibility, summarized in Table 3.2, demonstrate that as children grow older, the percentage of intelligible words increases. The extent of intelligibility is also influenced by the children's relationship with the person to whom they are speaking. Roulstone et al. (2002) conducted the largest study of 2-year-olds' intelligibility. As a result of their study of 1,127 children who were 25 months of age, the researchers reported that "children were mostly intelligible to their *parents* with 12.7% parents finding their child difficult to understand and only 2.1% of parents reporting that they could rarely understand their child" (p. 264). In contrast, studies that considered children's intelligibility to *strangers* demonstrated that 2-year-old children's speech was 50 percent intelligible to strangers (Coplan and Gleason, 1988; Vihman, 1988), and by 3 years of age, children's speech was around 75 percent intelligible to strangers (Coplan and Gleason; Vihman). Whereas at 3 years of age 95 percent of words could be reliably understood by a *transcriber* (Flipsen, 2006b), Bernthal and Bankson (1998, p. 272) concluded that "a client 3 years of age or older who is unintelligible is a candidate for treatment and intelligibility expectations increase with age." Between 4 and 5 years of age, children's speech is considered to be intelligible.

Age of Acquisition of Speech Sounds

One of the major techniques for considering speech sound acquisition has been to compare children's development with the adult target. *Age of acquisition* refers to the age at which a certain percentage of children have acquired a speech sound. Large-group cross-sectional studies have predominantly been used for this purpose. Consonants have been the primary focus of these studies; however, some studies have examined consonant clusters and vowels. Age-of-acquisition data have had a long history of credence within the SLP profession. Well-known U.S. studies include those by Templin (1957) and, more recently, Smit et al. (1990). However, studies examining age of acquisition of speech sounds have been published for English dialects beyond American English and many languages around the world, including Arabic, Cantonese, Dutch, Finnish, German, Greek, Hungarian, Hebrew, Japanese, Korean, Maltese, Norwegian, Portuguese, Putonghua, Spanish, Thai, Turkish, and Welsh (see McLeod, 2007a).

When considering the age-of-acquisition findings for consonants, consonant clusters, and vowels, it is important to remember the methodological constraints of these data. The samples in these studies have been elicited from single words (not conversation) and often only one word has been elicited for each speech sound in each word position. Thus, the samples may not be fully representative of typical speaking situations, and variability in production has not been considered. Some studies have scored productions as either correct or incorrect and have not considered phonological development (hence, readers also need to consider additional data such as phonological processes, mismatches, etc.).

Another issue with these studies is that they vary in terms of the criterion for determining age of acquisition. For example, Templin (1957) indicated that a sound had to be acquired in the initial-, medial-, and final-word positions, whereas others have used only initial- and final-word positions (e.g., Prather et al., 1975; Smit et al., 1990). In addition, a range of standards (e.g., 50 percent, 75 percent, 90 percent, and 100 percent) have been used as criteria for age of acquisition. Tables 3.3 to 3.5 provide the criterion adopted by each researcher. In 1972, Sander emphasized the importance of presenting age-of-acqui-sition data using a continuum rather than a definite age at which phonemes are acquired. Consequently, a number of more recent authors (e.g., Smit et al., 1990) have adopted this approach and have presented graphical displays of acquisition for each speech sound over the different ages.

Consonants

Table 3.3 provides a summary of studies of English-speaking children's age of acquisi-tion of consonants. It includes studies of English dialects as spoken in the United States, England, Scotland, and Australia. As the table indicates, the majority of English consonants are acquired by the age of 3 to 4 years. As Porter and Hodson (2001, p. 165) indicated, "3-year-olds had acquired all major phoneme classes, except liquids . . . sibilant lisps were still common until the age of 7 years." However, the findings in Table 3.3 suggest that acquisition of all singleton consonants in English does not conclude until 8 or 9 years of age. It should be noted as well that in each study, the youngest and oldest ages of acquisi-tion are affected by the age range that has been studied. For example, only three studies included in Table 3.3 assessed the speech of children who were 2 years old (Chirlian and Sharpley, 1982; Prather et al., 1975; Paynter and Petty, 1974; thus, it could be that children acquire some sounds even earlier, as evidenced by studies of languages other than English (e.g., Cantonese) (So and Dodd, 1995).

While considering Table 3.3, notice the differences in the age of acquisition of con-sonants provided from these studies. Dodd, Holm, Hua, and Crosbie (2003), for example, reported a higher number of consonants acquired by age 3;0 than most of the other studies. This finding was probably influenced by their inclusion of children's spontaneous *and imitated* productions of speech sounds in defining age-appropriate production whereas many other studies have been based on only spontaneous productions. The age of acquisi-tion for the fricatives /s/ and /z/ appears to vary more than any other speech sounds. For example, some authors suggest that /z/ is acquired at age 3 years (Dodd, Holm, Hua, and Crosbie, 2003), others at 4 years (Arlt and Goodban, 1976), others at 5 years (Kilminster and Laird, 1978; Anthony et al., 1971; Smit et al., 1990 [females]), others at 6 years (Smit et al., 1990 [males]), others at 7 years (Templin, 1957), and others after 9 years (Chirlian and Sharpley, 1982). Similarly, the age range for the acquisition of /s/ extends from age 3 (Dodd, Holm, Hua, and Crosbie, 2003; Prather, Hedrick, and Kern, 1975) to age 7 (Poole, 1934). There are at least three possible reasons for the variability in the age of acquisition of /s/ and /z/. The first concerns whether children who had lost their central incisor teeth but had not yet acquired their adult dentition were included. Such an absence might well affect their ability to produce a fully correct /s/. The second possibility concerns differ-ences in the definition of an adultlike /s/, particularly whether dentalized /s/ sounds are considered to be correct (Smit et al., 1990). The final possibility relates to the methodol-ogy employed within the studies, including the complexity of the words elicited and the criterion for acquisition associated with such data.

Another approach to the consideration of the age of acquisition is that taken by Shriberg (1993), who created a "profile of consonant mastery" based on the average per-cent correct in continuous conversational speech. Using data from 64 children, ages 3 to

TABLE 3.3 Summary of Studies of English-Speaking Children's Age of Acquisition of Consonants

	Dodd, Holm, et al. (2003)	Smit et al. (1990) (females)	Smit et al. (1990) (males)	Chirlian & Sharpley (1982)	Kilminster & Laird (1978)	Arlt & Goodban (1976)	Prather et al. (1975)	Paynter and Petty (1974)	Anthony et al. (1971)	Templin (1957)
Age range tested	3;0–6;11	3;0–9;0	3;0–9;0	2;0–9;0	3;0–9;0	3;0–6;0	2;0–4;0	2;0–2;6	3;0–6;0	3;0–8;0
Criterion	90%	75%	75%	75%	75%	75%	75%	90%	90%	75%
Country	England & Australia	USA	USA	Australia	Australia	USA	USA	USA	Scotland	USA
2;0				m, n, h			m, n, ŋ, h, p	h, w		
2;4							j, d, k, f			
2;6				p, ŋ, w, d, g				p, b, t, m		
2;8							w, b, t			
3;0	p, b, t, d, k, g, m, n, ŋ, f, s, z, h, w, l, j	m, n, h, w, p, b, t, d, k, ŋ, f, s*	m, n, h, w, p, b, t, d, k, g	j, k, f, ʃ,	p, b, m, n, ŋ, h, w, j, t, d, k, g, ʒ*	p, b, t, d, k, g, m, n, ŋ, h, f, w	g, s		p, b, m, t, d, n, w, j	m, n, ŋ, p, f, h, w
3;4							l, r			
3;6	tʃ	j	f, j	b, t, tʃ, dʒ	f	v			k, g, ŋ, f, v, h	j
3;8				ʃ, tʃ						
4;0	ʒ, dʒ	v, ð, ʃ, tʃ	dʒ	l, ʒ, s	l, ʃ, tʃ,	s, z, ʒ, tʃ, dʒ, l	ð, ʒ		k, b, d, g, r	

(continued)

92

TABLE 3.3 (Continued)

	Dodd, Holm, et al. (2003)	Smit et al. (1990) (females)	Smit et al. (1990) (males)	Chirlian & Sharpley (1982)	Kilminster & Laird (1978)	Arlt & Goodban (1976)	Prather et al. (1975)	Paynter and Petty (1974)	Anthony et al. (1971)	Templin (1957)
Age range tested	3;0–6;11	3;0–9;0	3;0–9;0	2;0–9;0	3;0–9;0	3;0–6;0	2;0–4;0	2;0–2;6	3;0–6;0	3;0–8;0
Criterion	90%	75%	75%	75%	75%	75%	75%	90%	90%	75%
Country	England & Australia	USA	USA	Australia	Australia	USA	USA	USA	Scotland	USA
4;6	dʒ, l*	v			dʒ, s*, z*	ʃ	v, θ, z		l	s, ʃ, tʃ
5;0	ʃ	z*	s*, ʃ, tʃ	r,	r	θ, ð, r	dʒ			
5;6		ŋ, θ,	ð, r						s, z, ʃ, ʒ	t, θ, v, l
6;0	r	r	ŋ, θ, z, l	v						
6;6									θ, ð, tʃ	
7;0	θ, ð								dʒ, r	ð, z, ʒ, dʒ
7;6				ð, θ						
8;0					ð					
8;6				v	θ					
9;0										
9; 0+				z						
Not tested					j					

* = Reversal occurs at a later age group.

6 years with speech delays, Shriberg suggested that there were three stages of phoneme acquisition:

1. Early 8 [m, b, j, n, w, d, p, h]
2. Middle 8 [t, ŋ, k, g, f, v, tʃ, dʒ]
3. Late 8 [ʃ, θ, s, z, ð, l, r, ʒ]

Shriberg (1993) tested the validity of these three stages against four studies of speech sound acquisition (see Shriberg, Table 8): Sander (1972), Prather and colleagues (1975), Hoffmann (1982) (articulation and connected speech samples), and Smit and colleagues (1990). Shriberg reported that there were a number of differences between studies of typical development and his speech-delay data. For example, in the comparison with the Sander (1972) report, 15 of the 24 consonant ranks fell within their assumed groups on the consonant mastery profile. However, overall Shriberg (p. 122) concluded, "Thus, as a cross-sectional estimate of the rank-order of consonant mastery in speech-delayed children, the reference consonant mastery profile agrees quite well with estimates of the developmental order of consonant acquisition." Shriberg's profile of consonant mastery has received a large amount of attention within the SLP profession (e.g., Bleile, 2006), but it should be remembered that its basis is the mastery of phonemes by children with speech delays.

Consonant Clusters

The age of acquisition of consonant clusters for English-speaking children is summarized in Table 3.4, which includes three comprehensive studies (Anthony et al., 1971; McLeod and Arciuli, 2009; Smit et al., 1990; Templin, 1957) and one more narrowly focused study that considered the acquisition of three /s/ clusters (Higgs, 1968). Olmsted (1971) also has data on the acquisition of consonant clusters; however, his data were not included as the definition of initial and final positions related to the sentence rather than a word. McLeod, van Doorn, and Reed (2001a) presented an extensive literature review of the acquisition of consonant clusters. They indicated that 2-year-olds are able to produce at least some consonant clusters correctly; however, complete mastery may take until 9 years of age. Typically, two-element consonant clusters (e.g., /sp, st, sk/) are mastered before three-element consonant clusters (e.g., /spr, str, skr/). Clusters containing fricatives (e.g., /fl/) usually are more difficult than clusters containing stops (e.g., /kl/). To date, Templin (1957) and Anthony and associates are the only researchers to study the acquisition of word-final consonant clusters in English (see Table 3.4). It is important to consider the influence of morphological structures on the acquisition of word-final consonant clusters. For example, Templin reported that /kt/ was acquired at 8 years of age; however, this consonant cluster occurs both in monomorphemic contexts such as *act* and morphophonemic contexts such as *lacked* created by the past tense morpheme. It is possible that morphophonemic clusters may be acquired later due to their complexity.

Vowels

The description of the age of acquisition of vowels has received much less attention than that for consonants. One reason for this is that vowels are influenced by the accent or dialect spoken by the child. For example, General American English has either 18 or 19 vowels

TABLE 3.4 Summary of Studies of English-Speaking Children's Age of Acquisition of Consonant Clusters

Word Position	Smit et al. (1990) 3;0–9;0 (females) 90% Word Initial	Smit et al. (1990) 3;0–9;0 (males) 90% Word Initial	McLeod & Arciuli (2009) 5;0–12;11 90% Word Initial	Templin (1957) 3;0–8;0 75% Word Initial	Higgs (1968) 2;6–5;6 75% Word Initial	Anthony et al. (1971) 3;0–5; 75% Word Initial	Templin (1957) 3;0–8;0 75% Word Final	Anthony et al. (1971) 3;0–5;6 75% Word Final
3;0							ŋk	nt
3;6	tw, kw	tw, kw					rk, ks, mp, pt, rm, mr, nr, pr, kr, br, dr, gr, sm	
4;0	pl, bl, kl			pl, pr, tr, tw, kl, kr, kw, bl, br, dr, gl, sk, sm, sn, sp, st		kw	lp, rt, ft, lt, fr	
4;6	sp, st, sk, sw*, gl, fl, kr*, skw*	gl		gr, fr	sp, st, sk	kr, fl	lf	
5;0		sp, st, sn*, bl, dr*	br, tr, dr, kr, gr, fr, sp, st, sk, sm, sn, sl, sw, skw, skr, str	fl, str		gl*, tr, kl, br	rp, lb, rd, rf, rn, ʃr, mbr	
5;6	sm, sn	pl, kl, fl, pr, tr, kr, gr, fr				sl		dz, mps, ŋgz
6;0	sl, pr, br, tr, dr, gr, fr, spl	sk, sw, br		skw		θr, sm, st, str, sp	lk, rb, rg, rθ, nt, nd, ðr, pl, kl, bl, gl, fl, sl, str, rst, ŋkl, ŋgl, rdʒ, ntθ, rtʃ	sk
7;0	θr	sm, sl, θr, skw, spl,	spl	θr, ʃr, sl, sw, skr, spl, spr			lz, zm, tθ, sk, st, skr, kst, dʒd	

TABLE 3.4	(Continued)							
	Smit et al. (1990)	**Smit et al. (1990)**	**McLeod & Arciuli (2009)**	**Templin (1957)**	**Higgs (1968)**	**Anthony et al. (1971)**	**Templin (1957)**	**Anthony et al. (1971)**
Age Range Tested; Criterion: Word Position	**3;0–9;0 (females) 90% Word Initial**	**3;0–9;0 (males) 90% Word Initial**	**5;0–12;11 90% Word Initial**	**3;0–8;0 75% Word Initial**	**2;6–5;6 75% Word Initial**	**3;0–5; 75% Word Initial**	**3;0–8;0 75% Word Final**	**3;0–5;6 75% Word Final**
8;0	spr, str, skr	spr, str, skr					kt, tr, sp	
>8;0			pr, θr, spr, skr				lfθ tl	

* A reversal occurs in older age groups.

(depending on whether /ɔ/ is included) and 3 or 4 diphthongs (depending on whether /ju/ is included) (Smit, 2007). In contrast, there are 12 vowels and 8 diphthongs in English spoken in England (Howard, 2007), Australia (McLeod, 2007b), and New Zealand (Maclagan and Gillon, 2007), although there are differences between the exact vowels produced in each dialect. Scottish English has only 10 vowels and 3 diphthongs (Scobbie, Gordeeva, and Matthews, 2007). Howard and Heselwood (2002) provide a discussion of the sociophonetic variation between vowel productions for speakers of different dialects.

There are two aspects of acquisition of vowels: paradigmatic and syntagmatic acquisition (James, van Doorn, and McLeod, 2001). The *paradigmatic* aspect to mastering vowel production refers to learning to produce vowels in isolation or in simple monosyllabic words. Children attempt the paradigmatic aspects of vowel production at a very young age. In the first year, low, nonrounded vowels are favored, and height differences appear before front-back vowel differences (Donegan, 2002). Otomo and Stoel-Gammon (1992) conducted a longitudinal study of six children's acquisition of the unrounded vowels between 22 and 30 months of age and found that /ɪ/ and /ɛ/ were mastered early, then /e/ and /æ/ whereas /ɪ/ and /ɛ/ were least accurate. Children master the paradigmatic aspects of vowels by the age of 3 (Donegan; Selby, Robb, and Gilbert, 2000; Vihman, 1992) or 4 years (Dodd, Holm, et al., 2003). Statements such as the following are plentiful throughout the literature on typical speech acquisition:

- "By the age of 3 years, all normal children have evolved a stabilized vowel system" (Anthony et al., 1971, p. 12).
- "The literature on vowel development suggests that vowels are acquired early, both in production and perception. There is considerable variability in their production, but most studies suggest that vowel production is reasonably accurate by age 3, although some studies call this into question" (Donegan, p. 12).

However, these comments refer to the mastery of vowels in a paradigmatic context.

The second aspect of acquisition of vowels is called the *syntagmatic* acquisition (James et al., 2001). It refers to the ability to produce sequences of vowels within syllables and words in conjunction with other phonological variables such as stress. Knowledge of the syntagmatic aspect of vowel production is particularly apparent in the ability to produce schwa correctly in polysyllabic words. According to James and colleagues, children acquire at least some of the syntagmatic aspects of vowels between 3 to 5 years of age; however, mastery of vowels in polysyllabic words and stressed syllables extends beyond 3 years of age (Allen and Hawkins, 1980; James et al.; Selby, Robb, and Gilbert, 2000; Stoel-Gammon and Herrington, 1990). For example, Allen and Hawkins found that children mastered vowels in stressed syllables by 3 years of age but did not master vowels in unstressed syllables until they were 4 to 5 years old.

Percentage Sounds Correct/Percentage Sounds in Error

Consonants

Another index of speech sound acquisition is percentage of consonants correct (PCC), which considers the number of consonants produced correctly divided by the total number of consonants. Table 3.5 summarizes data from a range of studies detailing PCC at different

TABLE 3.5 Summary of Studies of English-Speaking Children's Percent of Consonants Correct (PCC)

	Pollock (2002)	Stoel-Gammon (1987)	Watson & Scukanec (1997b)	Dodd, Holm, et al. (2003)	James, van Doorn, and McLeod (2002)	Waring, Fisher, & Atkin (2001)
1;6	53%					
2;0	70%	70%	69.2% (53–91)			
2;3			69.9% (51–91)			
2;6	81%		75.1% (61–94)			
2;9	92%		82.1% (63–96)			
3;0			86.2% (73–99)	82.11%	76.77% (MSW)	
3;6	93%				76.41% (PSW)	85.2%
4;0	93%			90.37%	83.97% (MSW)	88.5%
4;6	94%				82.45% (PSW)	
5;0	93%				89.54%(MSW)	93.4%
5;6	96%			95.86%	88.36% (PSW)	
6;0	97%				93.74% (MSW)	95.1%
6;6	93%				90.76% (PSW)	
7;0					93.93% (MSW)	98.4%
7;6					90.99% (PSW)	

MSW = monosyllabic words; PSW = polysyllabic words.

ages. As can be seen, when children reach 2 years of age, it is typical for around 70 percent of their consonants to be produced correctly. For example, Watson and Scukanec (1997b) described longitudinal PCC data for 12 U.S. children. The mean PCC for the children at age 2;0 was 69.2 percent, and by age 3;0 it had climbed to 86.2 percent. As children age, their PCC increases. For example, Dodd, Holm, and associates (2003) found that children ages 5;6 to 6;6 produced 95.9 percent of consonants correctly.

Although Shriberg and Kwiatkowski's (1982a) original recommendations for computing PCC refers to connected speech samples, different sampling techniques have been applied to this metric. James, van Doorn, and McLeod (2002) demonstrated that there are significant differences between PCC scores depending on the speech-sampling task. Significantly higher PCCs were found for children's productions of monosyllabic versus polysyllabic words (see Table 3.5). The PCC will be discussed in Chapter 7 as a data analysis procedure employed in speech sound assessment.

Consonant Clusters

A few researchers have described children's percentage of consonant clusters correct at different ages (see Table 3.6). Roulstone and colleagues (2002) indicated that 1,127 children who were 25 months of age had an error rate of 78 percent (22 percent correct) for production of consonant clusters. In a longitudinal study of Australian 2-year-olds, McLeod, van Doorn, and Reed (2002) reported that overall 31.5 percent of consonant clusters were produced correctly in connected speech. Word-final consonant clusters (e.g., /nd/ in *hand*) were more likely to be correct (48.9 percent of the time), followed by word-initial

TABLE 3.6 Summary of Studies of English-Speaking Children's Percent of Consonant Clusters Correct (PCCC)

	Roulstone et al. (2002)	McLeod, van Doorn, & Reed (2002)	Waring, Fisher, & Atkin (2001)
2;0	22%*		
2;6		31.5%	
3;0			86.4%
3;6			
4;0			88.4%
4;6			
5;0			94.9%
5;6			
6;0			96.6%
6;6			
7;0			98.3%
7;6			

* Conversion from mean error rate of 78%.

fricative clusters (e.g., /sn/ in *snail*) (38.5 percent) and word-initial stop clusters (e.g., /bl/ in *blue*) (24.3 percent). Waring, Fisher, and Atkin (2001) presented cross-sectional data on Australian children's productions of consonant clusters in single words. They found that children ages 3;5 to 3;11 were able to produce 51 of a total of 59 (86 percent) consonant clusters correctly. By ages 7;0 to 7;11, most consonant clusters were produced correctly (58/59 to 98 percent). McLeod and Arciuli (2009) studied consonant cluster production by 74 children between the ages of 5 and 12 years. They found that 2-element /s/ clusters were produced correctly 96.8% of the time followed by 2-element /r/ clusters at 94.0% and 3-element /s/ clusters 92.0% of the time. The children's ability to produce consonant clusters changed from 92.4% at 5–6 years to 98.8% at 11–12 years.

Vowels

A summary of studies of the percentage of vowels produced correctly by children at different ages is provided in Table 3.7. Pollock and colleagues (Pollock and Berni, 2003; Pollock, 2002) have conducted the most extensive study of U.S. children's acquisition of rhotic (vowels with r-coloring such as ɝ) and nonrhotic vowels. They demonstrated that the nonrhotic vowels are more likely to be correct than rhotic vowels for a child of the same age. The studies by Dodd, Holm, et al. (2003) and James and associates (2001) were

TABLE 3.7 Summary of Studies of English-Speaking Children's Percent of Vowels Correct (PVC)

	Pollock (2002)	Pollock and Berni (2003)	Dodd, Holm, et al. (2003)	James, van Doorn, & McLeod (2001)
	Rhotic	Nonrhotic	Nonrhotic	Nonrhotic
1;6	23.52%	82.19%		
2;0	37.54%	92.39%		
2;6	62.52%	93.90%		
3;0	79.24%	97.29%	97.39%	94.90% (MSW)
3;6	76.50%	97.19%		88.28% (PSW)
4;0	90.11%	98.06%	98.93%	95.20% (MSW)
4;6	86.80%	98.20%		92.08% (PSW)
5;0	88.21%	99.21%		94.80% (MSW)
5;6	80.31%	99.38%	99.19%	94.30% (PSW)
6;0	77.20%	98.5%		95.39% (MSW)
6;6		99.19%		94.86% (PSW)
7;0				95.10% (MSW)
7;6				95.44% (PSW)

MSW = monosyllabic words; PSW = polysyllabic words.

conducted on nonrhotic vowels because rhotic vowels are not present in English produced in England and Australia. The data from Australian and English children are similar to those from Pollock and Berni regarding nonrhotic vowels. James and associates (2001) indicated that the accuracy of vowel production decreased with an increase in the number of syllables in the word: There was higher accuracy for vowels in monosyllabic words compared with polysyllabic words.

Phonological Patterns/Processes

Bankson and Bernthal (1990b, p. 16) defined p*honological processes* as "simplification of a sound class in which target sounds are systematically deleted and/or substituted." As mentioned in the section on natural phonology, the notion of systematicity was introduced to the field of linguistics by Stampe (1969) and then adapted and called *phonological processes* by authors such as Ingram (1976). Since that time, many authors have provided differing lists of phonological processes. Table 3.8 provides a summary of definitions and

TABLE 3.8 Definitions and Examples of Commonly Occurring Phonological Processes/Patterns

Overarching Description	Phonological Process	Definition	Example
Assimilation processes: When one sound in the word becomes similar to another sound in the word	Assimilation (consonant harmony)	One sound is replaced by another that is the same or similar to another sound within the word	*dod* instead of *dog*
Substitution processes: When one sound is substituted by another sound in a systematic fashion	Fronting	Velars are realized as sounds produced further forward in the oral cavity (typically alveolars)	*tar* instead of *car*
	Gliding	Liquids /l, r/ are replaced by a glide /w, j/ or another liquid	*wabbit* instead of *rabbit*
	Stopping	Fricatives and/or affricates are realized as stops	*tun* instead of *sun*
	Depalatization	Palatal sounds are realized as sounds produced further forward in the oral cavity (typically alveolars)	*fis* instead of *fish*

(continued)

TABLE 3.8	(Continued)

Overarching Description	Phonological Process	Definition	Example
	Deaffrication	Affricates are realized as fricatives	*shursh* instead of *church*
Syllable structure processes: Phonological processes that affect the syllable structure	Final consonant deletion	Deletion of the final consonant in the word	*do* instead of *dog*
	Cluster simplification/ reduction	Deletion of one element of the cluster	*pane* instead of *plane*
	Weak syllable deletion	Deletion of the unstressed syllable	*nana* instead of *banana*

Source: Adapted from Bankson and Bernthal (1990b), pp. 16–19.

examples of commonly occurring phonological processes. Recall, as mentioned earlier, that the term *pattern* is now more typically used than the term *process*.

In 1981, Grunwell presented a graphical display of the chronology of phonological processes that has been used widely as a means for identifying the age at which phonological processes are typically suppressed. Since that time, a number of other researchers have presented the age of suppression of phonological processes (e.g., Bankson and Bernthal, 1990b; Dodd, 1995a; Haelsig and Madison, 1986; James, 2001; Roberts, Burchinal, and Footo, 1990; Pressier, Hodson, and Paden, 1988). A summary of these studies is presented in Table 3.9. Some of the findings from these studies indicate that the most prevalent processes for young children (18 to 29 months) were cluster reduction (e.g., *spoon* – [pun]) and liquid deviation (e.g., *leaf* – [wif]) (Pressier et al.). According to Roberts and colleagues, there was a marked decline in the usage of phonological processes between 2;6 and 4;0 years with the most prevalent processes during these years being final consonant deletion, cluster reduction, fronting, stopping, and liquid gliding.

In 1999, James, McCormack, and Butcher presented data on 240 children's (ages 5;0 to 7;11) use of phonological processes. Among other findings, they reported four clusters of phonological process use from those that were rarely present (cluster 1) to those that were present in a majority of possible occurrences (cluster 4):

Cluster 1. Context sensitive voicing, early stopping, final consonant deletion, nasal assimilation

Cluster 2. Later stopping, velar assimilation, velar fronting

Cluster 3. Deaffrication and palatal fronting

Cluster 4. Cluster reduction, cluster simplification, fricative simplification, liquid simplification, and liquid deletion

James (2001) presented further data on the use of phonological processes by 365 children ages 2;0 to 7;11 years. She found that the major decline in the use of phonological

TABLE 3.9 A Summary of Studies of Children's Use of Phonological Processes/Patterns

Age	Dodd, Holm, et al. (2003)	Grunwell (1981, 1987)	Preisser et al. (1988)	Watson & Scukanec (1997b)	Lowe, Knutson, & Monson (1985)	James (2001)	Haelsig & Madison (1986)
2;0		**Present:** Weak syllable deletion; final consonant deletion, cluster reduction, fronting of velars, stopping, gliding, context-sensitive voicing **Declining:** Reduplication, consonant harmony	**Most prevalent:** Cluster reduction, liquid deviations (gliding)	**Present:** Final consonant deletion, liquid simplification, later stopping, cluster reduction, vowelization			
2;6		**Present:** Weak syllable deletion; cluster reduction, fronting of velars, fronting /ʃ/, stopping /v, θ, ð, tʃ, d, ʒ/, gliding, context-sensitive voicing **Declining:** Final consonant deletion			23% fronting	**Declining:** Affrication, depalatalization, gliding, meathesis, prevocalic voicing, vowel changes	
3;0	**Present:** Gliding, deaffrication, cluster reduction, fronting,* weak syllable deletion, stopping	**Present:** Weak syllable deletion; stopping /v, θ, ð/, fronting /ʃ, tʃ, dʒ/, gliding **Declining:** Cluster reduction		Later stopping, cluster simplification		**Declining:** Backing, cluster reduction, deaffrication, final consonant deletion, final devoicing, initial consonant deletion, labial assimilation, palatalization, stopping, unstressed syllable deletion, fricative simplification	Gliding of liquids, weak syllable deletion, glottal replacement, alveolar & labial assimilation, cluster reduction, stopping, vocalization, final consonant deletion

(continued)

TABLE 3.9 *(Continued)*

Age	Dodd, Holm, et al. (2003)	Grunwell (1981, 1987)	Preisser et al. (1988)	Watson & Scukanec (1997b)	Lowe, Knutson, & Monson (1985)	James (2001)	Haelsig & Madison (1986)
3;6	**Present:** Gliding, deaffrication, cluster reduction, fronting,[†] weak syllable deletion	**Present:** Stopping /θ, ð/ **Declining:** Weak syllable deletion, cluster reduction, gliding					
4;0	**Present:** Gliding, deaffrication, cluster reduction (3-element clusters)	**Present:** /θ/ → [ð], /ð/ → [d, v], depalatization of /ʃ, tʃ, dʒ/, gliding **Declining:** Cluster reduction				**Declining:** Depalatalization, gliding, glottal replacement	Weak syllable deletion, vocalization, gliding of liquids (20% criterion)
4;6	**Present:** Gliding, deaffrication	**Declining:** Stopping /θ, ð/, gliding /r/					
5;0	**Present:** Gliding	**Declining:** Stopping /θ, ð/, gliding /r/				**Declining:** Deaffrication, epenthesis, metathesis, fricative simplification (v/ð)	
5;6	**Present:** Gliding						

* Voicing pattern not present at any age.

† Fronting of /k, g/ ended at age 3;11 whereas fronting of /ŋ/ continued until 5;0 in the word *fishing*.

processes was between the ages of 3 to 4 years. However, some processes had fluctuating distributions. For example, gliding declined by 50 percent or more between 2 and 3 years and then again between 4 and 5 years.

Common Mismatches

As well as the identification of the age at which children generally learn to produce sounds, it is useful to have data to describe the typical "errors," or mismatches, children make in their attempts to produce the adult form of sounds. Phonological processes provide typical patterns of errors, but Smit (1993a, 1993b) has taken this further by presenting errors children make when attempting individual speech sounds. Smit reanalyzed the data from Smit and associates (1990) and provided tables of data containing frequent to rare errors children make in their attempts to produce consonants (Smit, 1993a) and consonant clusters (Smit, 1993b) (for a summary, see Table 3.10). Readers are encouraged to consult Smit (1993a, 1993b) to use the exhaustive information provided therein.

In Smit's analysis, two sounds warranted extra attention: /s/ and /r/. Smit (1993a) indicated that when children were ages 2;0 and 2;6, they were more likely to produce word initial /s/ as [t] or [d]; however, for children from 3;0 to 9;0 years the most common error in the word-final context was dentalization. Lateralized [ʂ] productions were rare, which could be interpreted that SLPs should consider that lateral production of /s/ warrants intervention regardless of the child's age. Smit (1993a) also indicated that the most common

TABLE 3.10 Children's Common Errors in Producing Consonants and Consonant Clusters (Errors Occurred > 15%)

Age	Smit (1993a) Consonants	Smit (1993b) Two-Element Consonant Clusters	Smit (1993b) Three-Element Consonant Clusters
2;0	ŋ → n	pr → p, pw	skw → k, t, kw, gw
	j → θ	br → b, bw	spl → p, b, pl, pw
	l → w	tr → t, tw	spr → p, pw, pr, sp
	r → w	dr → d, dw	str → t, d, st, tw, sw
	v → b	kr → k, kw	skr → k, w, kw, gw, fw
	θ → f	gr → g, gw	
	ð → d	fr → f, fw	
	s → dentalized*	θr→f, θ w	
	z → d	sw → w	
	ʃ → s	sm → m	
	tʃ → t/d	sn → n	
	ʒ → d	sp → p, b	

(continued)

TABLE 3.10 (*Continued*)

Age	Smit (1993a) Consonants	Smit (1993b) Two-Element Consonant Clusters	Smit (1993b) Three-Element Consonant Clusters
		st → t, d	
		sk → k	
3;0	ŋ → n	pr → pw	skw → θ kw
	r → w	br → bw	spl → θpl, spw
	v → b	tr → tw	spr → θpr, spw
	θ → f	dr → dw	str → θtr, stw
	ð → d	kr → kw	skr → θkr, skw
	s → dentalized	gr → gw	
		fr → fw	
		θr → fr	
		st → θt	
4;0	θ → f	pr → pw	skw → θkw
	s → dentalized	br → bw	spl → θpl, spw
		tr → tw	spr → θpr, spw
		dr → dw	str → θtr, stw
		kr → kw	skr → θkr, skw
		gr → gw	
		fr → fw	
		θr → fr	
		st → θt	
5;0	Nil	pr → pw	
5;6	Nil	br → bw	skw → θkw
		tr → tw	spl → θpl, spw
		dr → dw	spr → θpr, spw
		kr → kw	str → θtr, stw
		gr → gw	skr → θkr, skw
6;0	Nil	tr → tw	skw → θkw
			spl → θpl
			spr → θpr, spw
			str → θtr, stw
			skr → θkr, skw

* Smit (1993b) used dentalized (dnt); whereas /θ/ was used in the present table.

error production for word-initial /r/ was [w]. Less commonly, children used derhotacized and labialized productions.

Perception

Earlier in this chapter, we considered infants' perceptual capabilities. As children's speech develops, so does the link between their production and perceptual capabilities. This link was described in our consideration of the psycholinguistic models of speech acquisition. Although some authors believe that perception for speech is achieved in infancy, Rvachew (2007a, p. 28) suggests that there are three stages of development of "adult-like acoustic, phonological and articulatory representations" and that these stages are clinically relevant:

1. The child is unaware of the phonological contrast and can produce realizations that are acoustically and perceptually similar.
2. The child is aware of the phonological contrast and may produce acoustically different realizations that are not perceptible to adult listeners.
3. The child is aware of the phonological contrast and can produce different realizations that are acoustically and perceptually accurate.

Rvachew suggests that children's perceptual capabilities continue to develop into late childhood. For example, Hazan and Barrett (2000) found that children from 6 to 12 years of age showed increasing mastery in the ability to discriminate synthesized differences in place, manner, and voicing but had not yet achieved adultlike accuracy.

Suprasegmentals/Prosody

Prosody refers to the suprasegmental aspects of speech production, including stress, intonation, and rhythm. Gerken and McGregor (1998) present a helpful overview of prosody and its development in children, and Wells and Peppé (2003) provide a helpful overview of prosody in children with speech and language impairment. There appears to be a close interaction between suprasegmentals, "motherese," and early language development.

Intonation develops before stress. For example, Snow (1994) found that young children acquire skills that control intonation earlier than final-syllable timing skills. At 6 months of age, children use intonation, rhythm, and pausing in their speech (Crystal, 1986). By 1 to 2 years of age, children use intonation and stress to reduce homonyms and to differentiate between commands, requests, and calling (Dore, 1975).

Kehoe (1997) studied the ability of 18 children, ages 22, 28, and 34 months, to produce three- and four-syllable words. She found that there was a significantly higher number of stress errors in SwS words (S = strong, w = weak), and a tendency for a higher number of stress errors in SwSw words. Stress errors were more frequent in imitated than spontaneous productions. She suggested that stress errors may be associated with articulatory and phonetic-control factors. Omission of unstressed and nonfinal syllables is common in young children whereas stressed and final syllables are usually preserved (Kehoe, 2001;

James, 2007). Gerken and McGregor (1998) suggest that children leave an "acoustic trace" of the omitted syllable; that is, although changes cannot be detected by the human ear, spectrographic analysis can reveal changes in factors such as voice onset time and vowel length.

PHASE 4: MASTERY OF SPEECH AND LITERACY

When children attend school, refinement of their speech production and perception skills continues until eventually they reach adultlike mastery. This refinement occurs in a number of domains, including prosody, phonotactics, and their production of speech segments. As illustrated in the tables of speech acquisition previously presented in this chapter, studies show continued growth in skill until 8 to 9 years of age. A major area of attention during the school years is the development of literacy—specifically, reading and spelling. In the psycholinguistic model discussed earlier in this chapter authors such as Stackhouse and Wells (1993) closely link speech and literacy in input–storage–output pathways. Phonological awareness is a skill that is closely associated with speech and literacy and will be discussed in detail in Chapter 12.

Phonological Awareness

Phonological awareness is "the ability to reflect on and manipulate the structure of an utterance as distinct from its meaning" (Stackhouse and Wells, 1997, p. 53) and is essential for the development of reading and spelling (Gillon, 2004). Children's phonological awareness skills also affect their perception of salient auditory cues (Mayo, Scobbie, Hewlett, and Waters, 2003). Children with speech difficulties typically find phonological awareness tasks difficult. Severity and type of speech impairment have been suggested as a significant predictor of performance of phonological awareness tasks (Holm, Farrier, and Dodd, 2007; Leitão and Fletcher, 2004; Rvachew, 2007b; Stackhouse and Wells, 1997; Sutherland and Gillon, 2007). Phonological awareness skills (particularly phoneme isolation) were improved during a randomized controlled trial for children with speech impairment (Hesketh, Dima, and Nelson, 2007).

Phonological awareness includes rhyme knowledge, blending and segmentation, and manipulation of syllables, clusters, and phonemes. Although syllable segmentation and knowledge of nursery rhymes has been found to be a good predictor of literacy outcome, the best predictors are suggested to be phoneme segmentation and phoneme manipulation.

Rhyme Knowledge

Rhyme knowledge reflects an understanding of the constituents of a syllable; that is, a syllable is created with an onset + rime (see earlier discussion of nonlinear phonology). Words that rhyme differ in their onsets (e.g., *cat, mat, brat, splat*). There are three main rhyme knowledge tasks: rhyme judgment (*fan-van; fan-fin*), rhyme detection (*fan-van-pin*), and rhyme production (words that rhyme with *fan*).

Blending and Segmentation

During blending tasks, children are presented with elements of a word and are asked to put them together to produce a word. Thus, an example of syllable blending is *com-put-er* = *computer* and an example of phoneme blending is *f-i-sh* = *fish*. Segmentation tasks are the reverse; a child is asked to segment a word into either syllables or phonemes.

Manipulation

Manipulation of syllables, clusters, and phonemes requires children to respond to tasks such as the following: "Say *clap*, now say it again without the 'l'" = *cap*. The ability to manipulate syllables, clusters, and phonemes requires sophisticated understanding of onsets, rimes, and codas.

Acquisition of Phonological Awareness

Children's acquisition of phonological awareness is said to consist of three stages. Goswami and Bryant (1990) proposed that the three stages are (1) awareness of syllables and words, (2) awareness of onsets and rimes, and (3) awareness of phonemes. Carroll and associates (2003) conducted a longitudinal study of 67 preschool-age children and assessed them at the following average ages: 3;10, 4;2, and 4;9 years. They recommended a revised series of stages: (1) early implicit large-segment sensitivity (associated with vocabulary knowledge), (2) sound similarity, and (3) explicit awareness of phonemes.

A number of researchers have considered English-speaking children's acquisition of phonological awareness skills, and their results are summarized in Table 3.11. The results listed in this table demonstrate that children have emerging skills from 3 to 4 years of age. As Dodd and Gillon (2001, p. 142) reported, "The majority of 4-year-old children . . . will not exhibit phonological awareness other than syllable segmentation and the emergence of rhyme awareness." By 5 years of age, the following skills are established: syllable segmentation, rhyme awareness, alliteration awareness, phoneme isolation, and letter knowledge. Phoneme segmentation is one of the latest skills to be established when children are 6 to 7 years old.

FACTORS INFLUENCING TYPICAL ACQUISITION OF SPEECH

Many factors influence typical acquisition of speech. The tables in this chapter clearly indicate that one of the major influences is the age of the child. As children mature, so does their accuracy of all aspects of speech production. However, within the literature, there is discussion of other aspects that may influence speech acquisition. These include gender, socioeconomic status, and concomitant language development.

TABLE 3.11   Summary of Studies of English-Speaking Children's Acquisition of Phonological Awareness

	Lonigan, Burgess, Anthony, & Barker (1998)	Burt, Holm, & Dodd (1999)	Dodd & Gillon (2001)	Gillon & Schwarz (2001)	Carroll, Snowling, Hulme, & Stevenson (2003)
	USA	UK	UK & Australia	New Zealand	UK
2;0	Wide variability; some children could perform above the level of chance on rhyme oddity detection, alliteration oddity detection, blending, and elision				
3;0			Emerging skills		Easiest to most difficult: 1. Rime matching 2. Syllable matching 3. Initial phoneme matching
4;0		Awareness of the concepts of syllable, onset, and rime, but not awareness of individual phonemes	Awareness of syllable segmentation and rhyme awareness	Easiest to most difficult: 1. Generation of rhyming words 2. Phoneme blending 3. Phoneme segmentation	Easiest to most difficult: 1. Rime matching 2. Syllable matching 3. Initial phoneme matching
4;6					Easiest to most difficult: 1. Rime matching 2. Initial phoneme matching 3. Phoneme completion 4. Phoneme deletion
5;0	Syllable blending established for middle-income but not lower-income children		Established skills: Syllable segmentation, rhyme awareness, phoneme isolation, letter knowledge		

TABLE 3.11	(Continued)				
	Lonigan, Burgess, Anthony, & Barker (1998)	Burt, Holm, & Dodd (1999)	Dodd & Gillon (2001)	Gillon & Schwarz (2001)	Carroll, Snowling, Hulme, & Stevenson (2003)
	USA	UK	UK & Australia	New Zealand	UK
5;6			Established skills: Phoneme segmentation		
6;0			**Australia 6;0–6;5** Established skills: Syllable segmentation, rhyme awareness, alliteration awareness, phoneme isolation **Australia 6;6–6;11** Established skills: Phoneme segmentation Established skills: Syllable segmentation, rhyme awareness, alliteration awareness, phoneme isolation, letter knowledge, phoneme segmentation		

Gender

There is a range of differing evidence regarding the effect of gender on the age of acquisition of speech sounds. However, one generalization can be made: If a gender difference is reported, girls are found to acquire speech more quickly than boys. Kenney and Prather (1986) found that boys made significantly more speech sound errors than girls at ages 3;0, 3;6, 4;0, 4;6, and 5;0, but not at 2;6. Smit and colleagues (1990) reported that boys and girls had different ages of acquisition for 11 sounds with significant differences between genders at ages 4;0, 4;6, and 6;0. All consonants except for /dʒ/ were acquired earlier by the girls. Dodd, Holm, et al. (2003) found no gender differences in speech acquisition for children ages 3;0 to 5;5; however, girls outperformed the boys at ages 5;6 to 6;11 in areas such as production of interdental fricatives and consonant clusters. Similarly, Poole (1934) indicated that girls acquired sounds earlier than boys after 5;6 years, whereas their development was similar at younger ages. In a study of the occurrence of phonological processes,

McCormack and Knighton (1996) reported that boys age 2;6 had more final consonant deletion, weak syllable deletion, and cluster reduction than girls. In a study of phonological awareness, Gillon and Schwarz (2001) found that 6-year-old girls performed significantly better than boys. The suggestion that boys differ from girls in speech acquisition is consistent with the reports of more boys than girls being identified as having a speech sound disorder (Campbell et al., 2003; Law et al., 1998; McKinnon, McLeod, and Reilly, 2007)

Socioeconomic Status

The effect of socioeconomic status (SES) on speech sound acquisition is not straightforward because of the range of different ways that SES can be measured (income, education, occupation, urban/suburban/rural, etc.) and the level of inference that is made about factors such as home language environment (Dodd, Holm, et al., 2003). In some large-scale studies, SES has not been found to affect age of acquisition of speech (Dodd, Holm, et al.; Smit et al., 1990); however, in others, children from a high SES background performed better than those from a low one (Templin, 1957). Socioeconomic status background has been found to have a significant effect on the acquisition of phonological awareness skills with children from mid to high SES backgrounds outperforming children from low SES backgrounds (Burt, Holm, and Dodd, 1999; Gillon and Schwarz, 2001; Lonigan et al., 1998). For example, Lonigan and associates found that at 5 years of age, 89 percent of children from a middle-income background performed above chance on syllable blending tasks whereas only 27 percent of children from a lower-income background performed above chance on the same task.

Language Development

Speech and language acquisition are intimately connected during the early stages of language acquisition (Paul and Jennings, 1992; Roulstone et al., 2002; Stoel-Gammon, 1991). For example, Roulstone and colleagues reported an interrelationship between speech and language for 1,127 children age 25 months. Although these children were of the same age, they had differing levels of expressive language. The number of phonological errors decreased as the level of language increased. For instance, for the production of velar consonants, children at the single-word stage had 57 percent errors, children at the two-word utterance stage had 37 percent errors, and children at the three- to four-word utterance stage only had 24 percent errors. This pattern was repeated for fricatives (single-word, 61 percent; two-word, 48 percent; three- to four-word, 30 percent); liquids (75 percent, 66 percent, 51 percent, respectively); postvocalic consonants (48 percent, 33 percent, 15 percent, respectively); and consonant clusters (88 percent, 80 percent, 66 percent, respectively).

Smith, McGregor, and Demille (2006) also studied the interaction between language and speech for 2-year-old children. Their study compared the phonological development in lexically precocious (advanced vocabulary) 2-year-olds with age-matched and language-matched (2 1/2-year-old) peers. They found that the phonological skills of the lexically precocious 2-year-olds were similar to the language-matched peers and superior to the age-matched peers, again supporting the correlation between speech and language learning in the early years.

Individual Variability

Within the literature, variability is generally used in two ways: between individuals and within individuals. First, we examine *variability between individuals*—that is, variability in individuals' rates and/or sequences of development. Variability between individuals is also referred to as "individual differences" (e.g., Bleile, 1991; Ferguson and Farwell, 1975) and occurs when different children of the same age or stage of development have different realizations for speech sounds for the same words. Variability between individuals also describes different rates of development, different patterns of consistency in repetitions of words, and different styles of learning. Most researchers agree that no two children follow identical paths to development. Progress beyond the first 50 words has been understood as a period of significant transition for children developing language. For example, Vihman and Greenlee (1987) studied 10 typically developing children at 1 and 3 years of age. Significant differences were reported between the children's rate of vocabulary acquisition, phonological maturity, and general approach to learning.

Alternatively, variability is sometimes used to describe differences *within individuals* (e.g., Barlow, 1996; Berg, 1995; Bernhardt and Stemberger, 1998; French, 1989; Leonard, Rowan, Morris, and Fey, 1982) and occurs in two different forms. First, variability occurs when a child has different realizations of a particular speech sound for different lexical items. For example, /s/ may be realized as [s] in *sea*, but [t] in *seat*. Second, variability occurs when a child has different realizations for multiple productions of the same lexical item. For example, a child with variable repeated productions of *sleep* may realize /sl/ as [sl] in [sli:], simplify /sl/ by substituting [sw] in [swip], reduce /sl/ to [s] in [sip], and omit /sl/ entirely in [ip]. Leonard and colleagues described some of the reasons for variable productions of words: "Variable words are most often those which have more advanced canonical forms or sounds" and "Word shape as well as consonant composition may play a role in intra-word variability" (p. 56).

There are numerous examples of variability within the production of speech sounds by typically developing children. Ferguson and Farwell (1975) described a child age 1;3 who produced the word *pen* in 10 different ways. Vogel Sosa and Stoel-Gammon (2006) conducted a longitudinal study of four typically developing children between 1 and 2 years of age. They found high overall variability as well as a peak in variability that corresponded to the onset of combinatorial speech. Stoel-Gammon (2004) conducted a longitudinal study examining the speech of five children ages 21 to 33 months and found high rates of variability, even in CVC words. Dyson and Paden (1983) conducted a longitudinal study over a 7-month period to consider phonological acquisition strategies used by 2-year-olds. Comparisons of each child's productions of target words across time led them to comment, "This period of roughly two to three-and-one-half years of age seems to be one of extreme variability with subjects 'trying out' a variety of strategies to approximate the adult model" (Dyson and Paden, p. 16). Menn and Stoel-Gammon (1995, pp. 340–341) indicated that early words are "extremely variable in pronunciation." Similarly, in a longitudinal study of typically developing 2- to 3-year old children, McLeod and Hewett (2008) examined variability in the production of words containing consonant clusters produced in spontaneous speech. Half (53.7 percent, range = 42.4 to 77.6 percent) of all repeated words were produced variably. As the children reached age 3, they increased the accuracy and decreased the variability of their productions; however, variability between and within individuals continued to occur. Holm, Crosbie, and Dodd (2007) considered the variability of the speech of 405 typically developing children ages 3;0 and 6;11 on a single-word task that contained many polysyllabic words. The younger children demonstrated the highest levels of variability (13 percent) and their variable productions predominantly reflected maturational influences.

As will be noted in later chapters, variability has been considered a diagnostic marker of speech sound disorder (see, for example, the discussion in Chapter 4 on "Childhood Apraxia of Speech"; also see Holm et al., 2007). However, the presence of high degrees of variability in typically developing children's speech should be taken into account (Stoel-Gammon, 2007). If the speech of typically developing children is highly variable, then the extent and nature of variability must be defined when it is used as a diagnostic marker of speech impairment (McLeod and Hewett, 2008). From the studies examined here, there is much variability between children in the acquisition of speech. Additionally, there is variability within the speech of individuals. Variability within individuals is more likely to occur with younger children and in spontaneous speech contexts.

CONCLUSION: UNDERSTANDING AND APPLYING TYPICAL SPEECH ACQUISITION

As speech-language pathologists, we use information on typical speech acquisition as the foundation of our clinical decision making. Thomas (2000) suggests that there are two ways of understanding normal speech acquisition: (1) knowledge of statistical similarity (typical acquisition) and (2) understanding of attitudes and desirability within the child's speech and language culture (acceptable acquisition). The majority of this chapter has examined the literature on typical speech acquisition and has described ages of attainment of a wide range of measures. The tables presented will be useful as a resource in your SLP practice. However, you are also encouraged to think as an anthropologist in terms of the communities and clients with whom you are working. Such understanding underlies notions of "correctness" and "acceptability" appropriate to a given child's speech and language behaviors. Chapter 11 discusses these understandings in more detail.

QUESTIONS FOR CHAPTER 3

1. Describe how the following models of speech acquisition add to our overall picture of how children acquire speech: behaviorism, generative phonology, natural phonology, nonlinear phonology, sonority, optimality theory, and psycholinguistic theory.

2. Describe the advantages and disadvantages of the three major research methods employed to examine speech acquisition.

3. Delineate the stages of infant vocal production from birth to age 1.

4. How do perception and production interact in infants?

5. Describe the characteristics and accomplishments of the transition stage of speech acquisition.

6. Review the large-scale normative data for English and identify early, mid, and late developing sounds.

7. What are phonological patterns/processes? Describe young children's use of phonological patterns.

8. How would a child at age 2 years and 5 years with typical speech say *cheese, hat, spoon, caterpillar, running,* and *three*? To answer this question consider:

   a. What phonemes are in the words? When are they normally mastered?

   b. Which word position are they in?

   c. What syllable shapes are represented? Would a child of this age typically produce these syllable shapes?

   d. What phonological patterns normally operate at this age?

   e. What are normal mismatches for a child of this age?

9. What is the importance of the acquisition of phonological awareness in school-age children?

10. How are children similar and different in speech acquisition?

CHAPTER 4

Classification and Comorbidity in Speech Sound Disorders

PETER FLIPSEN JR.
Idaho State University

JOHN E. BERNTHAL
University of Nebraska–Lincoln

NICHOLAS W. BANKSON
James Madison University

In Chapter 1, we defined in a broad sense what we mean by speech sound disorders. In recognition of the many variations of these problems that are seen in children, speech-language pathologists have often sought to classify or group various types of disorders. Although our knowledge in this area remains limited, progress has been made on this issue, and in this chapter, we attempt to outline the ongoing research in this area. Following that, we also explore the question of comorbidity, or co-existing, disorders.

Relative to classification, for many years speech-language pathologists have divided the population of children with speech sound disorders into two relatively large groups. The first, often referred to as the *organically based disorders,* includes those children whose difficulty with speech sounds can be readily linked to an obvious etiology or cause. This group includes subgroups based on specific causes. The second large group is those for whom *there is no obvious cause.* This latter group has been much more elusive and more difficult to identify and classify. These speech sound disorders (SSDs) have been called many things over the years, including *functional articulation disorders, developmental phonological disorders, idiopathic speech sound disorders,* and *speech delay of unknown origin.*

ORGANICALLY BASED SPEECH SOUND DISORDERS

The following discussion is not meant to be all-inclusive. This discussion is meant only to be a representative sample of organically based speech sound disorders. The information is also not intended as an exhaustive coverage of any of the particular groups that are identified. Entire textbooks have been devoted to discussions of the assessment and treatment of the speech sound problems experienced by some of these populations (e.g., Bzoch, 2004).

Major Structural Variations of the Speech Mechanism

Speech-language pathologists should recognize that significant anomalies of the oral structures are frequently associated with specific speech problems. Oral structural anomalies may be congenital (present from birth) or acquired. Cleft lip and/or palate is perhaps the most common congenital anomaly of the orofacial complex. Acquired structural deficits may result from trauma to the orofacial complex or surgical removal of oral structures secondary to oral cancers. For individuals with orofacial anomalies, the course of habilitation or rehabilitation often includes surgical and/or prosthetic management, and therefore the speech clinician must work closely with various medical and dental specialists.

Lips

Surgical repair of clefts of the lip can result in a relatively short and/or immobile upper lip. Although this might be expected to adversely affect articulation skills, this is not generally the case. A retrospective study by Vallino, Zuker, and Napoli (2008) reported that only 12/90 (13 percent) of children with an isolated cleft lip would qualify as having a speech sound disorder. Note the similarity of that percentage with the 15 percent of preschool children overall who have speech sound disorders that we highlighted in Chapter 1. The fact that the numbers are so similar suggests that having an isolated cleft lip does not increase the chances of having a speech sound disorder. Earlier studies (e.g., Laitinen et al., 1998; Riski and DeLong, 1984) have reported similar percentages and thus support this conclusion.

Tongue

The tongue is a muscular structure capable of considerable changes in length and width. Because the tongue is such an adaptable organ, speakers are frequently able to compensate for extensive amounts of the tongue missing and still maintain intelligible speech. A glossectomy is a surgical procedure involving removal of some or all of the tongue. Clinical investigators have repeatedly reported intelligible speech production following partial glossectomies (see Leonard, 1994). One early case study (Backus, 1940) recorded the speech pattern of a 10-year-old boy with an undersized tongue after excision of the tongue tip and the left half of the tongue. Initially, the child's speech sound skills were characterized by numerous consonant substitutions, but after a period of treatment, he was able to produce all consonants with little identifiable deviation.

For many patients, however, speech production is affected to varying degrees when all or part of the tongue is excised. Furia et al. (2001) reported pretreatment and post-treatment intelligibility scores for 27 glossectomy (6 total, 9 subtotal, 12 partial) patients. Those in the partial group demonstrated the best speech intelligibility after surgery. A study by Skelly et al. (1971) noted a similar outcome pattern. The Furia et al. study also included 3–6 months of therapy following surgery, but only the total and subtotal groups made significant intelligibility improvements. In their study, Skelly et al. noted that the compensatory articulatory patterns differed depending on the extent of the surgery. Partial glossectomy patients utilized the residual tongue stump to modify articulation; total glossectomy patients made mandibular, labial, buccal, and palatal adjustments during speech production. Skelly et al. also noted that unilateral tongue excision required fewer speech adaptations than tongue tip excisions.

Leonard (1994) reported a study in which listeners were asked to evaluate consonants produced by 50 speakers with various types of glossectomy. She indicated that fricatives and plosives were most frequently judged to be inaccurate, whereas nasals and semivowels appeared more resistant to perceptual disruption.

For partial glossectomy patients, the specific surgical procedure used and/or the particular muscles removed may impact speech outcomes (Bressmann, Sader, Whitehill, and Samman, 2004; Sun et al., 2007). After surgery, improvements in speech production skill have been reported for some interventions. These include the use of a *palatal augmentation prosthesis (PAP)* in which "the palatal vault is re-established at a lower level than normal, requiring less bulk and mobility of the tongue for appropriate palatolingual contacts during speech" (Marunick and Tselios, 2004, p. 67) and the addition of artificial grafts (Terai and Shimahara, 2004).

The result of a glossectomy is having less than a complete tongue. At the opposite extreme is the individual with macroglossia, or a tongue that is too large. A distinction must be made here between *true macroglossia,* in which the tongue is larger than expected and *relative macroglossia,* in which a normal size tongue occurs with an oral cavity that is too small (Vogel, Mulliken, and Kaban, 1986). True macroglossia is thought to reflect either an active growth process such as a tumor or a vascular malformation, or it may reflect certain genetic conditions such as *Beckwith-Wiedemann syndrome (BWS)* (Van Lierde, Mortier, Huysman, and Vermeersch, 2010). A well-known example of relative macroglossia is seen in individuals with Down syndrome (DS). In either type of macroglossia, speech may be affected because the tongue essentially has less room within which to move. A survey by Van Borsel, Van Snick, and Leroy (1999), for example, indicated articulation difficulties in 29/40 (73 percent) individuals with macroglossia associated with BWS. Reduced intelligibility is a common issue in individuals with DS (Kumin, 1994), and their relative macroglossia is assumed to be a major factor.

In cases of true macroglossia a glossectomy procedure may be performed and can lead to improved speech skills (Van Lierde, Mortier, Huysman, and Vermeersch, 2010); each case must be considered individually. Glossectomy is not usually indicated in cases of relative macroglossia, in part because studies of glossectomy outcomes in individuals with Down syndrome have generally revealed poor outcomes (Klaiman, Witzel, Margar-Bacal, and Munro, 1988; Margar-Bacal, Witzel, and Munro, 1988; Parsons, Iacono, and Rozner, 1987). If the surgery is not performed, individuals with macroglossia must learn to compensate (Stephens, 2011; Van Borsel, Morlion, Van Snick, and Leroy, 2000).

Hard Palate

The removal of any part of the maxilla, which includes the hard palate (e.g., necessitated by oral cancer), if not restored surgically or prosthetically, creates a serious problem for the speaker. Most patients receive palatal closure through a prosthetic (dental) appliance sometimes called an *obturator*. Sullivan and colleagues (2002) reported results from 32 cancer patients who had palatal defects because of surgical removal of a portion of the palate as a result of cancer of the maxillar sinus and alveolar ridge. The maxillectomy patients had their defects obturated with a dental appliance. Testing was conducted one month after obturation on measures of speech intelligibility, speaking rate, nasality, and communication effectiveness. With the obturator removed, mean speech intelligibility was 61 percent, speaking rate was 138 words per minutes, and nasality was 5.8 on a 0–7 point scale where 7 is hypernasal and 0 is hyponasal. With the obturator inserted, mean speech intelligibility was 94 percent, speaking rate was 164 words per minute, and nasality was rated 1.6. The mean self-perception of communication effectiveness by patients was 75 percent of what it was prior to the cancer. The authors concluded that "obturation is an effective intervention for defects of the maxillary sinus and alveolar ridge on speech performance. Variations in effectiveness were noted based on site defect and patient satisfaction with the intervention" (p. 530).

For children born with clefts of the hard palate, the palate is typically repaired within the first 12 to 14 months of life. Scarring associated with the surgery has not been found to interfere with articulatory production in most cases.

Soft Palate

The relationship of the soft palate (velum) to speech sound production has been a topic of considerable research, much of it focusing on the sphincteral closure of the velopharyngeal port and the effect of velopharyngeal competence on articulation. *Velopharyngeal competence* refers to the valving that takes place to separate the nasal cavity from the oral cavity during nonnasal speech production. Inadequate velopharyngeal closure is frequently associated with (1) hypernasal (excessive nasal) resonance of vowels, vocalic consonants, and glides and liquids; (2) reduced or diminished intraoral breath pressure during production of pressure consonants (i.e., fricatives, stops, and affricates); (3) nasal air emission accompanying production of pressure consonants; and (4) unusual substitutions such as the use of glottal stops for stop consonants and pharyngeal fricatives for sibilants. These latter substitutions are sometimes referred to as *compensatory articulations*. Speakers unable to close off the airstream in the oral cavity may attempt to create closure at a location where it is possible for them to do so (i.e., below the level of the velum and other velopharyngeal muscles). Although velopharyngeal incompetence is often associated with individuals with clefts of the soft palate, some speakers without clefting also demonstrate such incompetence—for example, individuals with dysarthria related to neurogenic paresis or paralysis of the velopharyngeal muscles (Johns and Salyer, 1978).

When the oral cavity communicates with (is open to) the nasal cavity, for example, through palatal fistulae (openings) or following ablative surgery or velopharyngeal incompetence, varying degrees of hypernasality will usually result. On the other hand, hyponasality (denasality) may result when the nasopharynx or nasal cavity is obstructed during speech production. Inflammation of the mucous membranes of the nasal cavity or a deviated septum may also cause hyponasality.

In addition to immediate problems associated with speech production, children born with clefts of the soft palate also experience a higher frequency of middle ear infections (otitis media) (Sheahan et al., 2003) than children without clefts. The frequency of otitis media in children born with clefts appears to be the result of problems with either the structure or function of the Eustachian tube mechanism, which develops at about the same time in the embryo as the palate. Kemaloglou, Kobayashi, and Nakajima (1999) reported shorter and more horizontal Eustachian tubes in children with clefts of the palate compared to children without clefts. A higher incidence of otitis media may be important for speech because it may be associated with mild-moderate or moderate hearing loss (albeit temporary) and its potential impact on speech sound acquisition.

Nasopharynx

The nasopharyngeal tonsils (adenoids) are located at the upper or superior pharyngeal area. Hyperthrophied (enlarged) adenoids may compensate for a short or partially immobile velum by assisting in velopharyngeal closure. Thus, their removal may result in hypernasality. But the adenoids may become sufficiently enlarged as to constitute a major obstruction of the nasopharynx, resulting in hyponasal speech. Enlarged adenoids may also interfere with Eustachian tube function in some individuals. When adenoids constitute an obstruction of the Eustachian tube, they may be removed for medical reasons.

Summary

Although individuals with major oral structural deviations frequently experience articulation problems, the relationship between structural deficits and articulation skills is not highly predictable. The literature cites many instances of individuals with structural anomalies who have developed compensatory gestures to produce acoustically acceptable speech. Why some individuals are able to compensate for relatively gross abnormalities and others are unable to compensate for lesser deficits is not known. A speech-language clinician who evaluates or treats individuals with oral structural anomalies must work collaboratively with various medical and dental specialists during speech habilitation or rehabilitation. For an excellent review of the speech characteristics and treatment of individuals with glossectomy and other oral/oropharyngeal ablation, see Leonard (1994).

Genetic Disorders

A number of genetic disorders have been associated with problems related to speech sound acquisition and/or speech sound disorders. An excellent source of more detailed information about specific syndromes is Shprintzen (1997), and a recent review highlighting our growing knowledge of the influence of genetics on speech sound disorders is provided by Lewis (2009).

A classic example of a genetic condition with implications for speech sound production is *Down syndrome*, which is thought to occur once in about every 700 births. In most cases, DS results from an extra copy of chromosome 21 (hence, it is often called *Trisomy 21*). Several features associated with this syndrome likely contribute to difficulties with speech in this population. First, DS usually includes varying degrees of *cognitive* impairment that may lead to an overall delay in speech sound acquisition. Second, as mentioned previously, individuals with DS have *relative macroglossia*, or a normal sized tongue in a relatively small oral cavity resulting in less space for the tongue to maneuver during connected speech production. This might then explain why reduced intelligibility in conversation is such a common problem in this population (Kumin, 1994). Other problems for individuals with Down syndrome relative to speech include both generally *reduced muscle tone* and a *high frequency of otitis media* associated with Eustachian tube problems (Marder and Cholmain, 2006). Some controversy remains about whether the pattern of speech sound acquisition in DS is similar to what we see in typically developing children (but simply delayed) or actually follows a different course. An analysis by Roberts and colleagues (2005), which included 32 boys with DS and 33 typically developing boys matched for mental age, highlighted the difficulty in answering that question. Their findings showed an overall pattern of delayed speech sound development. However, these investigators also reported some examples of error patterns such as lateralization of sibilants and deletion of nasals, which are uncommon in even very young typically developing children. Additional discussion of speech sound problems in DS can also be found in Chapter 5 in the section "Language Development."

Another genetic disorder that has been shown to include difficulty with speech sounds (without clefting) is *Fragile X syndrome (FXS)*. Somewhat less common than Down syndrome, Fragile X is thought to occur once in about every 4,000 births. In this case, a mutation turns off a particular section of the X chromosome, resulting in failure to produce a particular protein. Males have only a single X chromosome and so are much more likely to be affected by FXS than females (for whom the mutation might be present on only one of their two X chromosomes). As with DS, FXS includes varying degrees of cognitive impairment that may delay speech sound acquisition. As in DS, the speech of individuals with FXS is frequently difficult to understand. The study by Roberts and colleagues (2005) also included 50 boys with FXS. In this case, error patterns were generally typical of much younger, typically developing children, suggesting a more straightforward diagnosis of delay (rather than deviance). A more recent study (Barnes et al., 2009) reported similar findings; boys with DS and FXS both exhibited reduced intelligibility, but the error patterns of boys with FXS more closely resembled those of younger typically developing children.

Recall also the previous discussion of true macroglossia and Beckwith-Wiedemann syndrome (BWS). In addition to speech concerns related to macroglossia, this genetic disorder may also include hemihyperplasia in which one side of the body (or just one side of some structures) is overdeveloped. This sometimes co-occurs with clefts of the palate. All of these issues may contribute to the difficulty these individuals have with anterior speech sounds, although macroglossia is likely the major factor (Stephens, 2011; Van Borsel, Morlion, Van Snick, and Leroy, 2000).

A final example of a genetic disorder that has been associated with speech sound disorders is galactosemia. This is an inherited disorder occurring once in about 53,000 live births; this condition manifests primarily as an enzyme deficiency that prevents the complete metabolism of the milk sugar lactose. Toxic by-products of incomplete metabolism accumulate and can lead to severe liver and neurological damage, and potentially death (Hoffman, Wendel, and Schweitzer-Krantz, 2011). Lactose-free diets reportedly halt any ongoing damage, but cognitive and speech deficits may remain. Hoffman, Wendel, and Schweitzer-Krantz studied 32 children and adults with this condition (age range 9–37 years). These authors reported that only 9/32 (28 percent) had full-scale IQ scores above 85 and only 5/32 (16 percent) produced no errors on a test of German speech production. Shriberg, Potter, and Strand (2011) reported that 8/33 (24 percent) of children with galactosemia presented speech characteristics that were consistent with a diagnosis of childhood apraxia of speech.

Hearing Loss

A third subgroup of organically based speech sound disorders includes individuals with significant hearing loss. One of the most important elements underlying the production and comprehension of speech, as well as the monitoring of one's own speech, is an auditory system that is sensitive to the frequency range where most speech sounds occur (500 to 4000 Hz). Individuals with more severe hearing loss will have difficulty decoding the incoming sound signal and will perceive words differently than individuals with normal hearing mechanisms.

The child who is hard of hearing or deaf faces the challenging task of learning how to produce speech without adequate auditory input. Learning to discriminate and produce speech must then be accomplished by watching how sounds look on the face, how they feel through vibrations, and what can be perceived from a distorted auditory signal. A certain level of hearing is required to learn and maintain normal speech production. Ling (1989) summarized this relationship by noting that the more normal a person's hearing, the more natural his or her speech is likely to be.

Several aspects of hearing loss have been shown to affect speech perception and production; these include the level of hearing sensitivity, speech recognition ability, and configuration of the hearing loss. Individual hearing losses can range from mild to severe or profound (more than 70 dB HL). Labels such as *hard of hearing* and *deaf* are frequently applied to persons with varying degrees of hearing impairment.

Hearing sensitivity typically varies somewhat from one frequency to another with speech and language differentially influenced by the frequency configuration and severity of the hearing loss. Although information recorded on an audiogram is a useful prognostic indicator of speech reception ability, children with similar audiograms may not perceive and process speech sounds in the same way. A pure-tone audiogram cannot measure a person's ability to distinguish one frequency from another or to track formant transitions (a skill critical to speech perception). Other factors (e.g., age of fitting and full-time use of amplification, concomitant factors, quality of early intervention programs) mean that individuals with similar pure-tone audiograms can differ greatly in their ability to understand and acquire speech.

A second hearing-related factor important to speech sound acquisition and maintenance is the age of onset and the age of detection of the hearing loss. If a severe loss has been present since birth, acquisition of language—including phonology, syntax, and semantics—is difficult, and specialized instruction and other interventions are necessary to develop speech and language. Such instruction may rely on visual, tactile, and kinesthetic cues and signing as well as whatever residual auditory sensation the person possesses or has been afforded via technology. For a discussion of the influence of hearing loss on infants' and toddlers' phonologic development, see Stoel-Gammon and Kehoe (1994). Children and adults who suffer a serious loss of hearing after language has been acquired usually retain their speech sound production patterns for a time, but frequently their articulatory skills deteriorate. Even those who are assisted with amplification may find it difficult to maintain their previous level of articulatory performance.

The most obvious characteristic of the speech of individuals with significant hearing loss is that it can often be very difficult to understand. Gold (1980) stated that for most listeners, it may be possible to understand only 20 percent of what speakers with congenitally severe or profound hearing loss are attempting to say without interventions such as cochlear implants. The difficulty with understanding the speech of these individuals appears to be problems at both the segmental and suprasegmental levels. At the segmental level, errors on both consonants and vowels can be observed (Levitt and Stromberg, 1983; Paterson, 1994).

At the suprasegmental level, persons who are deaf or hard of hearing generally speak at a slower rate than normal-hearing speakers because of longer duration of both consonants and vowels. They also use more frequent pauses and slower articulatory transitions. Stress patterns may also differ from those of normal-hearing speakers because many persons who are deaf or hearing impaired do not distinguish duration associated with stressed and unstressed syllables. Persons who are deaf or hearing impaired sometimes use too high or too low a pitch and nonstandard inflectional patterns. Harsh or breathy voice quality and hypo- or hypernasal speech are also commonly reported (Dunn and Newton, 1986).

As noted previously, even in cases of severe and profound hearing impairment, the specific types of perception problems and speech production errors are difficult to predict. There is a great deal of individual variability. Less information, however, is available for individuals with mild to moderate hearing losses than for those with more severe losses.

Calvert (1982) reported that errors of articulation common to children who are deaf are not confined to productions of individual phonemes; errors also occur because of the phonetic context in which the phones are embedded. Calvert documented specific examples of omission, substitution, distortion, and addition errors relative to particular target phonemes, classes of phonemes, and phonetic contexts. These are highlighted in Table 4.1.

The preceding discussion is most relevant for describing only those individuals with hearing loss who use hearing aids. The introduction of the cochlear implant has revolutionized the management of hearing loss, particularly for children who receive and are fitted with them early. Assuming there are no other handicaps present and recognizing that instruction/therapy is provided along with the implant, the speech, language, academic, and quality of life outcomes for individuals who receive these devices are generally much better than for those who rely on hearing aids. Cochlear implants include a series of tiny wires (called *electrodes*) that are surgically implanted into the inner ear. The electrodes are connected to an external microphone and a speech processor. Speech is received by the microphone and sent via the processor to the electrodes, which stimulate the auditory nerve via electrical pulses. A recent review of studies in this area (Flipsen, 2008) showed that the conversational speech produced by these children can be highly intelligible (up to 90 percent in some cases). However, other studies have shown types of errors and error patterns (albeit less frequent) similar to those found in individuals who are hearing impaired and use

TABLE 4.1   Common Speech Errors Seen in Deaf Speech

1. Errors of omission
   a. Omission of final consonants
   b. Omission of /s/ in all contexts
   c. Omission of initial consonants
2. Errors of substitution
   a. Voiced for voiceless consonants
   b. Nasal for oral consonants
   c. Low feedback substitutions (substitution of sounds with easily perceived tactile and kinesthetic feedback for those with less; for example, /w/ for /r/ substitution)
   d. Substitution of one vowel for another
3. Errors of distortion
   a. Degree of force (stop and fricative consonants are frequently made with either too much or too little force)
   b. Hypernasality associated with vowel productions
   c. Imprecision and indefiniteness in vowel articulation
   d. Duration of vowels (speakers who are deaf tend to produce vowels with undifferentiated duration, usually in the direction of excess duration)
   e. Temporal values in diphthongs (speakers who are deaf may not produce the first or the second vowel in a diphthong for the appropriate duration of time)
4. Errors of addition
   a. Insertion of a superfluous vowel between consonants (e.g., /sʌnoʊ/ for /snoʊ/)
   b. Unnecessary release of final stop consonants (e.g., [stop^h])
   c. Diphthongization of vowels (e.g., *mit* → [mɪʌt])
   d. Superfluous breath before vowels

Source: Calvert (1982).

hearing aids (Chin and Pisoni, 2000; Flipsen and Parker, 2008; Grogan, Barker, Dettmen, and Blamey, 1995). See Table 4.2 for a list of error patterns that have been observed in both children with hearing aids and cochlear implants.

In addition to errors on specific speech sounds or sound combinations, the supra-segmental aspects of speech may continue to be of concern for even the most successful cochlear implant recipients. Abnormal resonance and difficulty with the use of syllable and word-level stress may continue to be a problem for these children (Anderson, 2011; Lenden and Flipsen, 2007).

It should be noted, of course, that, as with children fitted with hearing aids, outcomes for children fitted with cochlear implants (although generally much closer to typical) can be quite variable (Geers, 2006). Age at implantation continues to be a crucial variable, with children receiving their implants at younger ages clearly evidencing better outcomes. Current criteria for implantation set by the U.S. Food and Drug Administration permit implantation in children as young as age 12 months, but there is ongoing debate about implantation at even younger ages. In some European countries, children are receiving implants as young as 4 months of age.

| TABLE 4.2 | Speech Sound Error Patterns Observed in Both Children Who Use Hearing Aids and Children Who Use Cochlear Implants |

Developmental Patterns*	Nondevelopmental Patterns†
Assimilation errors	Initial consonant deletion
Consonant cluster reduction	Glottal stop substitution
Final consonant deletion	Backing
Liquid simplification	Vowel substitution
Palatal fronting	Diphthong simplification
Stopping	
Unstressed (weak) syllable deletion	
Velar fronting	

*Error patterns seen in younger typically developing (normal hearing) children.
†Error patterns not usually seen in younger typically developing (normal hearing) children.
Source: Adapted from Parker (2005).

Regardless of the age limits for implants, not all children with hearing impairments are identified as early as they should be. Newborn infant hearing screening in the United States is widely conducted but is not yet universal. Other aspects of eligibility criteria for implantation are also changing. For example, more children with some degree of residual hearing in at least one ear are receiving implants. Preliminary data suggest that outcomes in such cases are better than for children with no residual hearing. Such children may especially benefit if a hearing aid is fitted in their nonimplanted ear. This arrangement (cochlear implant in one ear and hearing aid in the other) is referred to as *bimodal hearing*. In addition, many child implant candidates now receive cochlear implants in both ears (*bilateral implantation*). Some recent studies have shown that bimodal hearing (Ching, Incerti, Hill, and van Wanrooy, 2006; Madell, Sislian, and Hoffman, 2004) and bilateral implantation (Biever and Kelsall, 2007; Galvin, Mok, and Dowell, 2007) both result in significant improvements in speech perception outcomes over a single implant alone. Data still appear to be lacking, however, on long-range speech production outcomes for these groups.

Neuromotor Disorders

A fourth group of children with organically based speech sound disorders are those with identifiable impairments of speech movement control (i.e., those with neuromotor impairments). Speech production at a motor level requires muscle strength, speed of movement, appropriate range of excursion, accuracy of movement, coordination of multiple movements, motor steadiness, and muscle tone (Darley, Aronson, and Brown, 1975; Duffy, 2005). Damage that impairs one or more of these neuromuscular functions may affect motor speech production, including phonation, respiration, or velopharyngeal function. Neuromotor speech disorders more typically occur in adults than children because they are often associated with strokes or other forms of brain injury. When these disorders are present at birth or shortly thereafter, they are often described as being one of various forms of *cerebral palsy*.

Neurologists and speech-language pathologists have sought to understand the possible relationship between the clinical (behavioral) responses associated with neurologically impaired individuals and the site and extent of the neurological lesions (brain damage). The reason for such inquiry is to identify potential commonalities across patients between the nature and site of brain damage and the concomitant cognitive language impairment.

Although as noted earlier, entire books are devoted to motor speech disorders, the following offers a brief introduction to this topic.

Dysarthrias

The *dysarthrias* are neurologic motor speech impairments characterized by slow, weak, imprecise, and/or uncoordinated movements of the speech musculature. Yorkston, Beukelman, Strand, and Hakel (2010) stated that "dysarthrias form a group of disorders marked by impaired execution of the movements of speech production" (p. 4). Because dysarthrias are caused by different types of lesions, trauma, or disease that cause central or peripheral nervous system damage, dysarthrias cannot be described by a single set of specific characteristics.

Dysarthrias are characterized by a paralysis, weakness, or incoordination of the speech musculature, which may result from localized injuries to the nervous system, various inflammatory processes, toxic metabolic disorders, vascular lesions or trauma of the brain, and lesion, disease, or trauma to the nervous system. The most significant characteristic of dysarthric speech is reduced intelligibility. Dysarthric speech can involve disturbances in respiration, phonation, articulation, resonance, and prosody. Phonemes misarticulated in spontaneous speech are also likely to be misarticulated in other situations, such as reading and imitation tasks.

Apraxia

Apraxia is a motor speech disorder also caused by brain damage, but it is differentiated from the dysarthrias and described as a separate clinical entity. Apraxia of speech is characterized by an impairment of motor speech programming with little or no weakness, paralysis, or incoordination of the speech musculature. Whereas dysarthrias frequently affect all motor speech processes—respiration, phonation, articulation, resonance, and prosody—apraxia primarily affects articulatory abilities with secondary prosodic alterations.

A description of some of the clinical characteristics of apraxia has been provided by Duffy (2005):

> Deviant speech characteristics . . . include a number of abnormalities of articulation, rate, prosody, and fluency. The characteristics that best distinguish it from other motor speech disorders (the dysarthrias) are distorted sound substitutions and additions, decreased phonemic accuracy with increased rate, attempts to correct articulatory errors that cross phonemic boundaries, groping for articulatory postures, greater difficulty on volitional than automatic speech tasks, and greater difficulty on SMR [sequential motion rate] and multisyllabic word tasks than AMR (alternate motion rate] and single syllable tasks. . . . Articulatory distortions, reduced rate, and various prosodic abnormalities help distinguish AOS from aphasic phonologic errors. (p. 330)

Some clients who demonstrate apraxia of speech (verbal apraxia) also demonstrate similar difficulty in volitional oral nonspeech tasks, a behavior described as oral apraxia (Duffy, 2005). For example, an individual may protrude his or her tongue during eating but may be unable to perform this act voluntarily. Although oral apraxia often coexists with verbal apraxia, this is not always the case.

Duffy (2005) notes the following differences between AOS and dysarthria: (1) muscle strength, tone, range, and steadiness of movement are clearly affected in dysarthria but do not account for the deficits seen in apraxia of speech; (2) respiration, phonation, articulation, resonance, and prosody may all be affected in dysarthria, while AOS is limited to problems with articulation and prosody; (3) language difficulties (called *aphasia* in adults) are rarely seen in dysarthria but often co-occur with AOS; (4) speech errors are typically quite consistent in dysarthria while inconsistency is more typical of AOS; (5) distortions and substitution of simpler sounds are most common in dysarthria, but AOS may also include omissions, substitutions of more complex sounds, repetitions or prolongations; and (6) trial and error groping and self-corrections are common in AOS but uncommon in dysarthria. Lapointe and Wertz (1974) described patients who demonstrated a "mixed" articulation disorder consisting of a combination of apraxic and dysarthric speech characteristics.

CHILDHOOD APRAXIA OF SPEECH

One of the least understood speech sound disorder categories is *childhood apraxia of speech (CAS);* this condition has also been known by several other names, including *developmental apraxia of speech* and *developmental verbal dyspraxia*. Two reasons appear to have spawned a difficulty with this diagnosis. First, there have been disagreements about the specific distinguishing characteristics of this condition, or, in the past, even whether such characteristics exist. One of the more complete attempts to summarize the work was presented by Davis, Jakielski, and Marquardt (1998). Their review highlighted the fact that many of the characteristics that have been suggested as indicating CAS are not necessarily unique to it. Investigators who have tried to identify such unique characteristics do not always agree with one another. For example, Yoss and Darley (1974) reported that 16 children with delayed speech who also met their definition of CAS performed significantly poorer on "non-speech praxis abilities" compared to 14 children with delayed speech who did not meet their definition of CAS. On the other hand, Aram and Horwitz (1983) reported no such difference. Some have argued that such conflicts may simply reflect co-existing *oral apraxia* in some children with CAS. This is a similar issue in adult apraxia of speech. The failure to identify the unique features of CAS led some in the past to suggest that this disorder may not exist as a unique "diagnostic entity"; those taking this position argued that it simply represented the most severe form of speech delay of unknown origin (to be discussed later). However, others argue that CAS itself can be manifested along the entire continuum from mild to severe.

The second reason for the previous controversy surrounding CAS stems from concerns about applying the label *apraxia* because, unlike the adult form of apraxia, it is often not possible to document specific neurological damage that might have led to the problem. This latter question is another reason that CAS is often included with speech sound disorders of unknown origin (see next section). However, in some cases, a potential causal agent can be identified. Thus, CAS may not clearly fit into either the organic or unknown group. As such, it seems appropriate to discuss it separately here.

In 2002 in an effort to resolve the issue, the American Speech-Language-Hearing Association (ASHA) established an ad hoc committee on CAS. The committee reviewed the extensive and somewhat confusing literature in this area and in 2007 presented its findings. After considerable feedback, ASHA's legislative council adopted a position statement and the committee's technical report (ASHA, 2007a, 2007b). You may refer to the ASHA website where both documents can be obtained for more detailed study. The ASHA position statement defines CAS as follows:

> *Childhood apraxia of speech (CAS)* is a neurological childhood (pediatric) speech sound disorder in which the precision and consistency of movements underlying speech are impaired in the absence of neuromuscular deficits (e.g., abnormal reflexes, abnormal tone). CAS may occur as a result of known neurological impairment, in association with complex neurobehavioral disorders of known or unknown origin, or as an idiopathic neurogenic speech sound disorder. The core impairment in planning and/or programming spatiotemporal parameters of movement sequences results in errors in speech sound production and prosody. (2007a, pp. 1–2)

Note that the definition limits CAS to problems with speech; the possible co-existing but separate difficulties that children with CAS may demonstrate with nonspeech oral movements are thought to indicate the comorbidity of either an underlying neuromuscular problem (i.e., dysarthria) or oral apraxia.

The ASHA definition also emphasizes that although CAS is seen as a neurological problem, it may arise in more than one way. It may be a reflection of a known neurological condition such as cerebral palsy. It may also be comorbid with "known neurobehavioral disorders" such as autism, Fragile X syndrome, or Rett syndrome. In many cases, however, the origin of CAS is unknown (idiopathic).

Although the position statement has not solved all of the issues with CAS, this designation is generally accepted within the profession as a defined subpopulation of those with speech sound disorders of unknown etiology. In spite of this, it must be said that there is not yet a definitive list of diagnostic features for CAS. That is, we still do not fully know all of the characteristics that make CAS distinct from other disorders. However, as the definition indicates, the primary problem appears to be one of " . . . planning and/or programming . . . " for speech. The position statement then mentions an emerging consensus about three specific speech production features that may be unique to CAS. The first feature is inconsistent error on vowels and consonants; in this case, the term *inconsistent* specifically refers to multiple attempts at the same word resulting in different productions. Thus, a child with CAS who attempts the word *music* several times might produce them as /muzu/, /ugɪ/, and /mɪzu/. A second feature of CAS is difficulty with prosody, particularly as it relates to the use of phrasal or lexical stress. Shriberg, Aram, and Kwiatkowski (1997b), for example, noted a tendency toward excessive and equal stress in two-syllable words. To continue with our example, production of the word *music* by a child with CAS may be perceived as MUSIC instead of the normal MUsic (equal stress on both syllables rather than just the first). One study suggested that the difference between the syllables may be present but it may not be perceptible to listeners (Munson, Bjorum, and Windsor, 2003).

The third emerging feature of CAS cited in the position statement (which may be difficult to see in most clinical situations) is lengthened and disrupted transitions between syllables and sounds. A study by Maassen, Nijland, and van der Meulen (2001), for example, showed stronger "anticipatory coarticulation" in children with CAS compared to typically speaking children. These emerging characteristics raise the question of whether childhood apraxia of speech should be described as a purely motor speech disorder. Marquardt, Jacks, and Davis (2004) note that the inconsistency observed in CAS may just as easily be a product of an imprecise underlying phonological representation rather than a pure speech motor programming problem. As well, problems with the prosody of speech (i.e., excessive and equal stress) may indicate some lack of detail in the underlying representation about the hierarchical organization of speech. When combined with reports that children with CAS exhibit difficulty with reading and spelling (Gillon and Moriarty, 2007; McNeill, Gillon, and Dodd, 2009), it points to CAS being the result of a combination of representational and motor speech difficulties (McNeill, 2007). Such a conclusion remains speculative at this point.

Given the widespread use of the CAS label, it should be noted that the prevalence of this subcategory has not yet been established. Unfortunately, there have been no systematic population studies (ASHA, 2007b), but one estimate, based on clinical referral data, suggests an overall prevalence of one to two cases per 1,000 children (Shriberg, Aram, and Kwiatkowski, 1997a). It has also been suggested that the exact prevalence may vary depending on the specific origin of CAS. For example, findings reported by Shriberg, Potter, and Strand (2011) suggested a prevalence of CAS as high as 18 percent in individuals with galactosemia (i.e., 180 times the overall figure).

Chapter 9 presents some suggestions for assessment and treatment of CAS.

SPEECH SOUND DISORDERS OF UNKNOWN ORIGIN

The second and largest group of children with speech sound disorders is one that has puzzled investigators for many years. It includes those for whom there is no obvious cause. This has long raised the question: If we do not know how the problem arose in the first place, how do we help these children? Lacking clear answers, speech-language pathologists have for many years tended to do two things. First, we have often assumed that this is a single group, and second, we have tended to treat them all the same way. Until about the 1970s, most SLPs referred to these children as having *functional articulation disorders* (a term still used by some today). The word *functional* implies that these children have some sort of learning difficulty. And in this context, the word *articulation* implies that the problem is with learning to physically produce individual speech sounds. So, for many years, these children received what is now called *traditional articulation therapy* (sometimes also called *phonetic therapy*), which is a motor skill and perception-oriented approach to therapy. This approach will be described in Chapter 9.

In the 1970s, speech-language pathology began to be influenced by developments in the field of linguistics, particularly those brought forth by the publication of *The Sound Pattern of English* (Chomsky and Hallé, 1968), *A Dissertation on Natural Phonology* (Stampe, 1979), and *Phonological Disability in Children* (Ingram, 1976). These publications, combined with a growing interest in disorders of language (independent of difficulties with speech), forced SLPs to consider that in addition to learning how to physically produce speech sounds, children also have to learn how the sounds of their language are organized (i.e., they had to learn the phonology of the language). These publications and the subsequent research they spawned also made SLPs realize that there were patterns among what had always seemed like unrelated collections of individual errors. Previously, if a child said [wit] for *with,* [pan] for *fan,* and [too] for *Sue,* the diagnosis would have been simply that they had not learned to physically produce /θ/, /f/, and /s/. Therapy would focus on teaching the child to perceive and produce each of those sounds one by one. However, insights from linguistics made SLPs consider that these three errors might be related in some way. All of the intended sounds represent fricative targets being replaced by stop consonants. In this case, the child may be having troubling learning the *continuant* feature, which all fricatives share. Stampe took a different perspective and suggested that the child might have an immature speech production or perception system, and thus was temporarily unable to either perceive or produce fricatives. To get around this temporary limitation, Stampe suggested that the child was simplifying all fricatives to stops (a pattern known as *stopping*). As the child's perception or production systems matured, he or she would no longer find it necessary to simplify and would suppress the pattern (i.e., the child would, in this case, "stop stopping"). Ingram's book was perhaps the first to attempt to translate these developments in linguistic theory for the practicing clinician by speaking of "explicitly principled therapy." The net result was that the field suddenly began referring to these children as having *developmental phonological disorders* or simply *phonological disorders.* The emphasis had changed from articulation to phonology.

This change in labels was accompanied by changes in the approach to assessment and treatment. Many clinicians began to switch from teaching about the physical aspects of production to teaching children how using different sounds results in changes in meaning and proposed that one examine the error patterns in children with SSD. Instruction (therapy) focused on instruction on a pattern that might generalize to a number of speech sounds errors related to the same sound error pattern. This approach (also to be described in a later chapter) is called variously *contrast therapy, phonological therapy,* or *phonemic therapy.* Whatever it was called, many SLPs began to report that these children were progressing through therapy much more quickly than before with a sound-by-sound approach. Researchers began to validate this observation empirically. Klein (1996), for example, retrospectively compared 19 children who had received traditional articulation therapy with 17 children who had received phonological therapy. The two groups had been treated at different times by different clinicians, but within each group the therapy had been relatively controlled within a single university clinic. Klein reported that the children in the phonological therapy group spent significantly fewer months in therapy (13.5 vs. 22.3 months), were significantly less severely involved at their last treatment session, and were significantly more likely to have been dismissed from therapy with normal speech (17/17 vs. 2/19).

Unfortunately, this change in treatment approach was not universally successful. Even though outcomes tend to be better for many of these children, they do not all benefit equally. Some actually respond better to traditional articulation therapy, and some do not respond well to either approach. It is still not completely clear how to determine which child will respond best to which form of intervention.

In an attempt to more fully understand this group, researchers have examined a whole variety of variables to see whether these children differ in some more specific way from children who were developing speech normally or from those with organically based problems. To date, no consensus has emerged. As quickly as one study reports some unique difference, another study asks the same question and reveals contradictory results. For example, Dworkin (1978) reported that children with "functional articulation disorders" had lower tongue strength and slower diadochokinetic rates than typically speaking children. However, a follow-up study by Dworkin and Culatta (1985) revealed no such differences. Despite the lack of a consensus on the problem these children have, researchers have identified a whole range of factors that appear to be at least related to speech sound disorders. In Chapter 5, we discuss some of those factors. In terms of overall classification (i.e., organic; functional), the failure to identify any single factor that is unique to this group has led many to conclude that this may not be a single group. Perhaps there are subgroups. Several groups of investigators have tried to sort out what the subgroups might be.

One approach is to subdivide the group based on severity. Perhaps children with milder problems will respond better to particular treatments and those with more severe problems will respond better to other treatments. There are at least three problems with such an approach. First, although it is certainly true that children with speech sound disorders can be found anywhere along the continuum of severity (e.g., mild, moderate, or severe), there are no gold standards for determining severity of involvement in this population (Flipsen, Hammer, and Yost, 2005). Drawing the lines between the groups is therefore problematic. Second, if subgroups actually exist based on some other dimension, creating subgroups based on severity would result in only somewhat smaller but still heterogeneous groups. Third, and perhaps most important, "there seems to be no evidence that severity measures discriminate between subgroups of children with speech disorder in terms of the type of intervention indicated, or outcome" (Dodd, 2005, p. 5).

At least three other perspectives (etiological, psycholinguistic, symptomological) have begun to show potential for defining subgroups of children with speech sound disorders of unknown origin. The following sections describe these perspectives. It is important to note that, despite considerable efforts, no strong consensus has yet been reached about the best way to subdivide this population. What follows continue to very much be three "works in progress."

Classification by Possible Etiology

As we noted with each of the organically based subgroups, the cause was obvious. Shriberg (1982) argued that, in the case of speech sound disorders of unknown origin, the cause may simply be much more difficult to find. Despite the added difficulty, however, isolating the specific causes offers the possibility of both a better understanding of the nature of the problem and a better match between the child's problem and the chosen treatment approach.

The search for not so obvious causes is complicated by the fact that in many cases, what originally caused the problem (a *distal cause*) may have led to other problems (a *proximal cause*) that may now be maintaining the disorder (the distal cause may or may not still be operating). To illustrate, consider the child born with a significant hearing loss. The hearing loss results in an inability to hear all of the fine details of speech. This distal cause may lead to poorly developed or distorted long-term storage of the sound system (what linguists call a poorly developed or distorted *underlying representation*). This may contribute to inaccurate production; it would be difficult to accurately produce something if you do not have an accurate sense or perception of what the target is supposed to sound like. The hearing loss led to the problem originally and thus is the *distal cause* of the problem, but the poorly developed or distorted underlying representations may be the maintaining or *proximal cause* of the problem.

An early component of the search for etiological subgroups involved the identification of *causal correlates,* or factors that appeared very often in the case histories of these children (Shriberg and Kwiatkowski, 1994). This analysis yielded several candidates for possible subgroups. However, this approach proved to be insufficient because detailed case history information is not always available. Parents, who are often the primary source of case history information, may also not have very reliable memories about their children's histories (Majnemer and Rosenblatt, 1994). Complicating matters even further is that many children present with more than one of the causal correlates. This led Shriberg and his team to also search for *diagnostic markers,* or speech characteristics that are unique to each of the possible subgroups. Such markers are thought to offer insight into the perceptual, cognitive, or speech-processing mechanisms involved. These processing mechanisms then serve as confirmatory evidence for the subgroups by suggesting theoretical pathways from a distal cause to a particular subgroup. The diagnostic markers may also be ultimately useful clinically. They may, for example, serve as potential treatment targets or at least help to identify such targets. An understanding of both the diagnostic markers and the processing mechanisms leading to those markers might also help identify the best approach to treating those particular targets (Flipsen, 2002b).

Shriberg and colleagues (2010) have presented a version of this classification system that currently includes eight "putative" (i.e., potential and somewhat supported) subgroups. Together these subgroups make up the core of what is called the *Speech Disorders Classification System or SDCS* and are summarized in Table 4.3. The first three of the subgroups are classed as forms of *speech delay*. In such cases, these children present speech that is significantly behind developmental expectations during the preschool years. The speech of these children appears quite likely to normalize with treatment. The next three subgroups represent forms of childhood *motor speech disorder,* which may be less likely to normalize with treatment. The children in all six of these first subgroups typically qualify for and receive therapy. The distal cause for at least five of these subgroups is currently thought to be some form of genetic difference (some may also include the influence of environmental factors). Several studies have identified gene loci that appear to be associated with speech sound disorders (e.g., Lewis et al., 2006; McDermot et al., 2005; Shriberg et al., 2006). Lewis (2009) published a coherent review of these and related studies. For each subgroup, however, the specific genetic difference (not definitively identified yet) is thought to lead to a different processing mechanism and thus to different diagnostic markers. The last two subgroups in the SDCS system represent variations of *speech errors* in which no early concern is raised about speech, but the child simply fails to fully master one or two speech sounds during the developmental period (i.e., by age 9 years).

Evidence supporting etiological subgroups continues to accumulate (see Shriberg, 2009). The largest subgroup, speech delay–genetic (SD–GEN), includes approximately

TABLE 4.3 Shriberg's Eight Putative Subtypes of Speech Sound Disorders of Unknown Origin

Subgroup	Abbreviation	Prevalence* (%)	Sex	Distal Cause	Proximal Cause (processing mechanism)	Diagnostic Markers
Speech delay– Genetic	SD–GEN	56%	M > F	Genetic (polygenic) / environmental	Cognitive-linguistic processing	> deletion errors
Speech delay– Otitis media with effusion	SD–OME	30	M = F	Genetic (polygenic) / environmental	Auditory-perceptual processing	> backing errors; I-S gap[†]
Speech delay– Developmental psychosocial involvement	SD–DPI	12	M > F	Genetic (polygenic) / environmental	Affective-temperamental deficit	> severity ??
Motor speech disorder–Apraxia of speech	MSD–AOS	???	M >>F	Genetic (monogenic? or oligogenic?)	Speech-motor control	Lexical stress ratio; > coefficient of variation ratio
Motor speech disorder– Dysarthria	MSD–DYS	???	???	Genetic (monogenic? or oligogenic?)	Speech-motor control	???
Motor speech disorder–Not otherwise specified	MSD–NOS	???	???	???	Speech-motor control	???
Speech errors– Sibilants	SE–/s/	???	M < F	Environmental	Phonological attunement	> first spectral moment for /s/
Speech errors– Rhotics	SE–/r/	???	M > F	Environmental	Phonological attunement	< F3- F2

*Percentage of those children in the population who have speech sound disorders of unknown origin.
[†]I-S = Intelligibility – Speech gap (intelligibility far lower than predicted by speech sound accuracy).

56 percent of these children who have one or more family members who have or have had speech or language problems. As shown in Table 4.3, this subgroup includes more males than females. A particularly high proportion of omission errors occurring especially on later developing consonants (Shriberg et al., 2005) is proposed as the diagnostic marker for this subgroup; this suggests that they may be having difficulty identifying the phonemic details of the language (a cognitive-linguistic problem). Lewis et al. (2007) reported findings that support a unique cognitive-linguistic proximal cause for this subgroup. In that study, parents of children with speech sound disorders who themselves had a history of therapy for speech sound disorders performed significantly less well compared to parents without such histories on standardized measures of spoken language and spelling.

Research conducted by Felsenfeld and colleagues (1995) offers similar evidence. In a long-term follow-up study of individuals tested between 1960 and 1972 by Templin and Glaman (1976), the children of those earlier identified as "disordered" performed significantly poorer on tests of articulation than the children of those who had earlier been classified as "normal."

A second subgroup, speech delay–otitis media with effusion (SD–OME), includes approximately 30 percent of these children who have histories of early and frequent episodes of OME. The proportion of males and females appears to be roughly equal in this subgroup (Shriberg, 2009). At least two specific diagnostic markers have been proposed. Shriberg et al. (2003) identified the *intelligibility-speech gap*. The conversational speech of these children was consistently less understandable than children without such histories. However, looking only at the portions of speech that could be understood, the accuracy of their consonant production was better than that seen in some of the other subgroups. In other words, their speech was less well understood than would be expected given the accuracy of their consonant production. Shriberg et al. (2003) proposed a second diagnostic marker involving a higher frequency of backing errors (a very atypical pattern of using posterior sounds such as velar or palatal sounds in place of more anterior sounds such as alveolars). Like the SD–GEN subgroup, these two markers suggest difficulty extracting relevant phonemic details from the input language. In the case of SD–OME, the mechanism is thought to be intermittent hearing loss (Shriberg, Friel-Patti, Flipsen, and Brown, 2000).

A third possible subgroup, speech delay–psychosocial involvement (SD–DPI), is thought to include up to 12 percent of this population. As with SD–GEN, males outnumber females in this subgroup. Although the speech of this group has been characterized as more severely delayed than some of the other subgroups, a more specific diagnostic marker has yet to be identified. Hauner, Shriberg, Kwiatkowski, and Allen (2005) suggested that these children present with either (1) "approach-related negative affect" (i.e., described as aggressive, angry, or manipulative/control seeking) or (2) "withdrawal-related negative affect" (socially withdrawn, shy/fearful, or extremely taciturn). Thus, it is thought that these children may have temperaments that make it more difficult for them to obtain the feedback they need to develop and/or normalize their speech skills. These children may also be easily frustrated by their inability to communicate effectively and/or less likely to persist in their communication attempts.

Three other subgroups proposed by Shriberg include those with motor speech involvement. As noted earlier in the discussion of CAS, there is some justification for including at least those children with an idiopathic form of CAS in the population of speech sound disorders of unknown origin (referred to in Table 4.3 as MSD–AOS). In this group (Childhood Apraxia of Speech or CAS), males are thought to greatly outnumber females (Shriberg, 2009). Additional details on CAS can be found in the previous section. The other two subgroups of the speech delay type include those children with subtle or less obvious forms of dysarthria (MSD–DYS) or those for whom the motor system is clearly involved but where CAS or dysarthria do not clearly apply (MSD–NOS (Shriberg, Potter, and Strand, 2011). As indicated in Table 4.3, sex ratios are not yet well understood in either of these subgroups, nor is it clear which task(s) or speech behavior(s) would qualify as viable diagnostic markers.

The last two subgroups proposed by Shriberg (2009; speech errors–sibilants and speech errors–rhotics) are currently thought to reflect an environmental distal cause. Unlike the other six subgroups, Shriberg and associates (2005) noted that these children are not typically identified as requiring treatment for speech sound problems as preschoolers. Rather, they may have a "disposition to respond to the environmental press for mastery of speech sounds in the ambient language" (p. 838). In other words, these children may be so motivated to communicate that they attempt to master some aspects of speech before they are fully ready to do so. Put another way, they may "tune up" for speech too soon; hence, the proximal cause column describes the issue as one of "phonological attunement." These children may adopt a production pattern that is less than optimal but that is retained into the school years. It is perhaps noteworthy that problems with sibilants appear to be more common in females, but problems with rhotics appear to be more common in males.

In the SDCS system, production problems that extend beyond the normal developmental period are now referred to as *persistent speech disorder (PSD)*. These problems were previously referred to as *residual errors* (a label still used by some other investigators). Errors still occurring after age 9 years therefore would be classified as either PSD–SD, PSD–MSD, or PSD–SE with each label describing the earlier nature of the problem (e.g., PSD–SD would represent errors left over from a history of one of the forms of speech delay). It is worth noting that in most cases of PSD–SD and PSD–SE, the errors are usually distortions (rather than omissions or substitutions). Although listeners cannot usually hear the difference between the distortions arising from PSD–SD versus PSD–SE (i.e., a distorted /s/ from either source would sound the same), significant acoustic differences have been documented with the use of instrumentation (Karlsson, Shriberg, Flipsen, and McSweeny, 2002; Shriberg, Flipsen, Karlsson, and McSweeny, 2001).

Classification by Psycholinguistic Deficit

A second possible perspective that might be used to subdivide children with speech sound disorders of unknown origin into subgroups is to focus on the current underlying difficulty these children might be having with processing speech in the brain. Stackhouse and Wells (1997) argue that an etiological (what they term a "medical") approach to identifying the problem a particular child is having is limited both because reasons are often not apparent and because existing etiological schemes do not always point directly to specific treatment options. On the other hand, they argue that a focus on error patterns (what they term a "linguistic" approach) provides a description only of the output behavior and fails to explain why certain speech behaviors are occurring (i.e., it fails to account for even what we have here called the *proximal cause*). The better solution, according to Stackhouse and Wells, is to apply a psycholinguistic model. Psycholinguistic models (discussed briefly in Chapter 3) have been used for many years in the field of speech-language pathology (see Baker, Croot, McLeod, and Paul, 2001, for a review). Stackhouse and Wells provide a specific model for examining psycholinguistic processing in children with speech sound disorders (see Figure 4.1).

Note the term *phonological* that is used in Figure 4.1. Stackhouse and Wells (1997) point out that it is "important to distinguish a *phonological problem*—a term used to

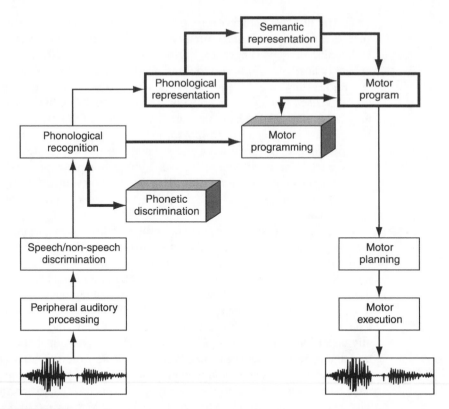

FIGURE 4.1   Speech-processing model by Stackhouse and Wells (1997).

Note: The broad arrows and shaded boxes represent processes hypothesized to occur offline.

Source: From *Children's Speech and Literacy Difficulties: A Psycholinguistic Framework* (p. 350) by J. Stackhouse and B. Wells, 1997. Copyright John Wiley & Sons Limited. Reproduced with permission.

describe children's speech output difficulties in a linguistic sense—from a *phonological processing problem*—a psycholinguistic term used to refer to the specific underlying cognitive deficits that may give rise to speech and/or literacy difficulties" (p. 8). Pascoe, Stackhouse, and Wells (2005) presented a detailed case study of the application of this model. "Katy" had difficulties with discriminating both real words and nonwords, which was interpreted as a problem with *phonological recognition.* In addition, she performed poorly on both real-word picture naming and nonword repetition, suggesting that she was having problems with her already stored *motor programs* as well as difficulty creating new motor programs (i.e., *motor programming*).

Stackhouse and Wells (1997) did not initially develop their model with the specific intention of identifying subgroups. However, Vance, Stackhouse, and Wells (2005) suggested that the use of profiles based on a particular pattern of problems might provide additional insight into the nature of a child's problem. Thus, using the model to identify subgroups seems at least plausible. One might, for example, evaluate large groups of children with speech sound disorders of unknown origin to determine whether certain profiles are more common than others. Stackhouse (2000) used this approach in a longitudinal study to suggest how different profiles might help differentiate children with speech sound disorders who have later literacy problems from those who learn to read normally.

Classification by Symptomatology

Barbara Dodd and her colleagues classify speech sound disorders of unknown origin in a different manner. Dodd, Holm, Crosbie, and McCormack (2005) note that "there is as yet no theoretically adequate or clinically relevant explanation of disordered speech . . . current models of the speech-processing chain . . . fail to disentangle causal, comorbid, and consequent difficulties" (p. 44). Dodd and her colleagues argue that "surface error patterns" (i.e., symptoms) provide the best perspective on classification and that such patterns do in fact explain the nature of the disorder. They have suggested four possible subgroups. The *Diagnostic Evaluation of Articulation and Phonology (DEAP)* (Dodd et al., 2006) was specifically developed for the classification of children using this system of subgroups.

The first subgroup proposed by Dodd is *articulation disorder* in which the child produces consistent substitution or distortion errors on a limited number of phonemes (often /s/ or /r/). Errors do not change whether the production is spontaneous or imitated. In a cohort study of 320 children with speech sound disorders, Broomfield and Dodd (2004) classified 40 (12.5 percent) children into this subgroup.

The second and largest of Dodd's subgroups, *phonological delay,* includes children whose errors can be described using phonological process labels that are also seen in much younger typically developing children (i.e., developmental patterns). Broomfield and Dodd (2004) classified 184/320 (57.5 percent) children into this subgroup.

Dodd's third subgroup, *consistent phonological disorder*, includes children who produce developmental patterns but also produce nondevelopmental patterns (i.e., those not usually produced by typically developing children). In this case, the nondevelopmental patterns are produced consistently. Broomfield and Dodd (2004) classified 66/320 (20.6 percent) children into this subgroup.

Dodd's final and smallest subgroup, *inconsistent phonological disorder*, includes children who produce nondevelopmental error patterns but do so inconsistently. In this case, *inconsistency* refers to variations in output on repeated productions of the same words. Broomfield and Dodd (2004) classified 30/320 (9.4 percent) children into this subgroup.

Dodd and her colleagues have attempted to empirically validate the categories. For example, Dodd (2011) compared 23 children classified as delayed (only producing errors seen in younger, typically developing children) against an age-matched group of 23 children classified as disordered (producing five or more instances of at least one atypical error pattern). The delayed group made significantly fewer consonant errors overall as well as fewer types of errors. Although the groups did not differ on general measures of language ability, the disordered group performed significantly less well on a nonlinguistic rule-learning task and showed less cognitive flexibility on two tests of executive function. Dodd interpreted the findings to mean that the disordered group was less able to sort out the sound system of the language. Validation of Dodd's categories is also being sought by demonstrating that the children in different groups respond differentially to different treatment approaches. For example, Dodd and Bradford (2000) presented case study data on three children: One child with a consistent phonological disorder received the most benefit from a phonological contrast approach, whereas two children with inconsistent phonological disorders initially responded most quickly to a core vocabulary approach. Once these latter children's errors became more consistent, one of them responded more quickly to phonological contrast therapy. These same associations between subgroup membership and response to therapy were also observed in a follow-up group study including a total of 18 children (Crosbie, Holm, and Dodd, 2005).

SUMMARY OF CLASSIFICATION

As comprehensive as the preceding discussion is, it represents only some current proposals as to how to classify children with speech sound disorders. Other perspectives are also possible. Clearly, considerable work remains. For the organically based disorders, clinicians know a great deal about how to assess and treat these children. As mentioned previously, specialized texts are available to provide the clinician detailed discussions regarding various organic categories. Considerable progress has also been made in understanding the nature of the problem where the origin is currently unknown, but clinicians do not yet have a clear consensus about the exact nature of this group. Lacking such a consensus, speech-language pathologists are left to choose from a number of available options for the assessment and intervention for these children. These options are outlined in subsequent chapters.

COMORBIDITY

The attempts at classification described above assume that the child's only communication problem is difficulty with speech sounds. However, practicing clinicians will tell you, such is not always the case. It is common for someone to have other communication problems in addition to SSD. For example, they may also a voice disorder, a language disorder, or a problem with fluency. The two (or occasionally more than two) disorders co-exist in the same individual. Put another way, we can say that the individual is *comorbid* for disorder X and disorder Y. The term *morbidity* arises from medicine and is just another term for illness. Physicians often talk about *morbidity rates* or rates of illness (as opposed to *mortality rates* or rates of death).

Understanding comorbidity of speech sound disorders with other disorders has important implications for clinical practice. First, it may be important to identifying the nature of the problem. For example, if a child leaves off plural –*s* endings, we would want to know whether this is because he or she cannot say /s/ (a speech sound problem) or does not understand the need for the plural marker (a morphological problem). Second, it may be important to understanding the relationship between the two disorders (i.e., which came first?). For example, if a child has unintelligible speech and a rough voice quality, is the roughness of the voice making it too hard for listeners to understand him or her? On the other hand, perhaps the speech sound disorder came first. The child may be quite unintelligible, which makes him or her work harder to be understood; this may lead to excess strain on the vocal mechanism, which then leads to the voice problem. A final reason for wanting to understand comorbidity is that it may have the implications for intervention. If two problems are present, do we treat them in a particular order (perhaps treating one first will cause the other problem to take care of itself?), or do we treat them simultaneously? But why might two disorders co-exist in the same individual? Several reasons are possible, and we have already alluded to one. Certain disorders may, by their very nature, lead to other disorders. Being unintelligible because of a speech sound disorder may lead to a voice disorder. Or when a child who is quite unintelligible attempts to communicate, others do not understand her or him. As a result, her or his conversations may end quickly because no communication is occurring. During such short conversations, such children miss out on opportunities to practice formulating and producing speech as well as language. They may also miss out on the valuable listener feedback that they normally would receive. Thus, being unintelligible may indirectly lead to delayed development of language skills. A second possible reason for comorbid disorders stems from the fact that communication is complex involving a number of components, all put into use at the same time. We do not normally produce speech sounds by themselves without some context. We are usually also producing morphemes (morphology), words (expressive vocabulary), as well as phrases and sentences (syntax). We are also modifying what we say based on our emotional state (prosody), the communicative situation (receptive language), and with whom we are communicating at that moment and in what setting (pragmatics). Two disorders of communication might therefore co-exist because the speech sound disorder results from some other disorder or problem (e.g., some genetic difference) that also affects other aspects of communication. A third possible reason for comorbid conditions may be that different aspects of language interact. Recall our earlier example of the child who leaves off the plural /s/ markers. Like many languages, English has *morphophonemic rules* in which a particular morpheme (e.g., plural markers) has several different phonetic forms (e.g., /s/, /z/. /ɪz/). Which particular form is used depends on the characteristics of the adjacent speech sound (i.e., is it voiceless, is it voiced, or is it another sibilant?). Producing these markers may be particularly difficult for some children because both the sound system and the morphology must be considered at the same time. Children need to learn all aspects of communication and how they work together. While attempting to master one, other aspects may lag behind at least temporarily. Finally, we cannot dismiss the possibility that comorbid disorders may be purely accidental and at least for some individuals may have nothing to do with each other.

How often do we see children with more than one disorder in the overall population? Data from the largest sample to date were reported in St. Louis, Ruscello, and Lundeen (1992), who reviewed records from the 1968–1969 National Speech and Hearing Survey (NSHS). That survey included testing of more than 38,000 school-age children (grades 1–12) from all over the United States. The NSHS reported individual prevalence values of 9.0 percent for "articulation disorders," 10.2 percent for voice disorders, and 0.8 percent for stuttering with an overall combined value of 5.7 percent. The NSHS also reported hearing impairments occurring in 2.6 percent of the sample. It should be noted that language was not a category included in this survey because at the time, language disorders in children were communication disorders just beginning to be recognized by speech-language pathologists.

In their review, St. Louis, Ruscello, and Lundeen (1992) reported that comorbidity appeared to be quite common. For example, only 41 percent of those children in the NSHS with articulation disorders had no other communication problem. "Nearly 57 percent had co-existing voice deviations. . . . Less than 1 percent of the articulation deviant group had associated stuttering . . ." (p. 8, St. Louis, Ruscello, and Lundeen) Interestingly, of those with voice disorders, only 38 percent had articulation disorders. Those who exhibited stuttering, 22 percent also had articulation disorders. These latter numbers highlight an important issue. The percentage values for comorbidity differ depending on which group you start with (sometimes called the *index disorder*). The reasons that the index disorder makes a difference probably reflect a combination of things. First, each disorder occurs at a different overall rate in the population. Second, some disorders (e.g., speech sound disorders) may be more likely to completely resolve than others (e.g., fluency disorders). St. Louis, Ruscello, and Lundeen reported that the percentage of children with articulation disorders declined steadily across grade levels, whereas the percentage who stuttered remained relatively consistent across grades. Third, the underlying nature of one disorder may differ from that of the other disorder, and thus each disorder may affect other aspects of communication differently. A good illustration of this is the finding that 41 percent of those with articulation disorders had no other problems. The same report said, however, that this was true for only 15 percent of those who stuttered.

Relying on the findings of the NSHS is not sufficient, of course. First, even in 1992, St. Louis, Ruscello, and Lundeen were concerned about the age of the data in that survey. Second, definitions of disorder have changed since 1968 as have the demographics of the population. Finally, as indicated previously, the NSHS failed to examine language disorders that have become a significant part of speech-language pathology practice. We now turn our attention to what we have since learned about several specific disorders known to be comorbid with speech sound disorders.

Speech Sound Disorders and Language Disorders

The speech sound system (i.e., the phonology) is one component of a child's developing linguistic system. As such, it is usually cited as a common link to language and is generally thought to account for comorbidity between speech sound disorders and (spoken) language disorders. In Chapter 5, we discuss this connection in more detail. In recent years, there has also been considerable interest in the extent to which speech sound disorders co-exist with problems with written language (i.e., difficulties with literacy). This is explored in Chapter 12.

The extent of the comorbidity between speech sound disorders and disorders of spoken language has been the subject of considerable study. Rather than do a detailed review of those studies, we can refer to one of the more extensive reviews of this literature conducted by Shriberg and Austin (1998). Their findings for studies with speech as the index disorder (our main focus here) are summarized in Table 4.4. Using findings from those studies and some of their own data, Shriberg and Austin concluded that up to approximately 60 percent of preschool children with speech sound disorders also have some type of language disorder. They also concluded that if we limit our discussion to co-existing *receptive language disorders* (i.e., problem understanding language spoken by others), the corresponding figure drops to 20 percent. Shriberg and Austin also suggested that there is some support for the idea that children who have more severe speech sound disorders may be more likely to have comorbid expressive language disorders. Although the comorbidity estimates in Table 4.4 vary from 20 to 60 percent, both are noticeably higher than the 7 percent prevalence figure now commonly cited for language disorders seen in the preschool population (Tomblin et al., 1997). Thus, having a speech sound disorder seems to increase the likelihood of having a language disorder, supporting a link between the two.

Speech Sound Disorders and Stuttering

Another area of comorbidity that has received considerable attention is the comorbidity of speech sound disorders and stuttering. Several connections have been suggested. Van Borsel and Tetnowski (2007), for example, reported that stuttering (just as we noted earlier for speech sound disorders) is more common in certain genetic disorders such as Down syndrome and Fragile X syndrome when compared to the general population. Genetic links are also suggested by the fact that both speech sound disorders and stuttering are more common in males than females. McKinnon, McLeod, and Reilly (2007), for example, collected data on 10,425 Australian elementary school children and reported male to female ratios of 2.85 to 1 for speech sound disorders and 7.5 to 1 for stuttering. More direct evidence for a link through genetics also comes from heritability studies; Van Beijsterveldt, Felsenfeld, and Boomsma (2010), for example, looked at data from more than 10,000 pairs of 5-year-old Dutch twins and concluded that stuttering is highly heritable (i.e., genetics play a large role). Although genetics may or may not be the distal

TABLE 4.4 Estimates of the Comorbidity of Language Disorders in Children with Speech Sound Disorders

Study	n	Mean Age*	Comorbidity Estimate (%)
Connell, Elbert, and Dinnsen (1991)	37	3	43%
Shriberg et al. (1986)	33	4	60
Shriberg and Kwiatkowski (1994)	64	4	66
Shriberg et al. (1986)	38	5	50
Paul and Shriberg (1982)	30	6	66
Shriberg and Kwiatkowski (1982c)	43	6	66
Schery (1985)	718	7	75[†]
St. Louis et al. (1994)	20	7	45[‡]
Ruscello et al. (1991)	24	12.5	54[§]
Ruscello et al. (1991)	24	12.5	21[#]

* Ages in years; rounded to nearest year
[†] No index disorder in this survey.
[‡] Estimated.
[§] Classified as having delayed articulation.
[#] Classified as having residual (persistent) errors.
Adapted from: Shriberg and Austin (1998).

(ultimate) connection, others have considered more proximal (immediate) connections between speech sound disorders and stuttering. The first of these is that both are motor-based problems (i.e., problems of speech production). Perhaps a common underlying motor problem accounts for both. An alternative perspective is that there may be a proximal connection through language (i.e., the phonology). Although we do not usually think of stuttering as a language problem, Bloodstein (2002) argued that stuttering is primarily a language problem. He notes that stuttering is most often evident at the beginning of syntactic units, it is largely absent in single word speech, and it is not usually elicited by single word tasks. Whether one considers the two disorders to be language or motor-based, both possibilities suggest that the comorbidity between speech sound disorders and stuttering may arise because of the child's limited capacity to manage several aspects of communication at the same time.

Whatever the link between speech sound disorders and stuttering, the search has been largely motivated by an interest in treatment. As previously noted, there may be some value in knowing whether we should treat one or the other first or treat them simultaneously. In the case of stuttering, however, a different issue has arisen. There has been a long-standing concern that working on speech sound production in an individual who also stutters will make the stuttering problem worse. The idea is that the stuttering may become worse in the short term because of the child's limited output capacity. Moreover, there is a greater fear that the stuttering may become worse because of the child's own negative reactions to being less fluent. Advocates of such a position would encourage an indirect approach to intervention for children who have both disorders. Nippold (2002) reviewed a series of studies related to this question and concluded that such a position may be unfounded. She found that (1) a higher frequency of stuttering is not associated with a higher number of speech sound errors, (2) stuttering severity has not been shown to be different in children with and without speech sound disorders, (3) type and frequency of speech sound errors does not appear to differentiate children who stutter from those who do not, (4) stuttering is no more common on complex versus simple words, and (5) speech sound errors do not seem to be any more common on stuttered vs. nonstuttered utterances. Nippold suggests therefore that there is little reason to expect a negative treatment interaction between stuttering and speech sound disorders when they are treated in the same individual.

Turning our attention to specific comorbidity values, the bulk of the work in the study of the co-occurrence of stuttering and SSD has used stuttering as the index disorder. This likely stems from the small number of individuals identified when speech sound disorders is the index. Recall our earlier discussion of the NSHS (St. Louis, Ruscello, and Lundeen, 1992) in which fewer than 1 percent of the children in that survey who had articulation problems also exhibited stuttering. On the other hand, the same survey reported that more than 20 percent of those who stuttered also had articulation problems. Blood and Seider (1981), who surveyed elementary school clinicians on this question, reported a similar value of 16 percent. Nippold (2002) cites more recent studies suggesting values in the 30–40 percent range as more common. This is consistent with Arndt and Healy (2001), who reported a figure of 32 percent. Whichever figures one accepts, all are higher than the 3.8 percent of 6-year-old children with speech sound disorders in the general population reported by Shriberg, Tomblin, and McSweeny (1999). A child who stutters appears to be at higher risk for a speech sound disorder than a child in the general population. Yaruss and Conture (1996) reached the same conclusion.

Speech Sound Disorders and Voice Disorders

Less commonly discussed comorbidities are speech sound disorders and voice disorders. As with stuttering, several different connections may account for the connection of SSD to voice disorders. Two have already been mentioned: (1) reduced intelligibility may lead to excess effort resulting in some type of damage to the laryngeal mechanism and (2) poor-quality sound associated with an underlying voice disorder may reduce intelligibility and lead to reduced practice and feedback. A third possible connection could be some common underlying problem that leads to both disorders. This is suggested by studies showing the co-existence of speech sound disorders and voice disorders (or at least voice quality differences) in two populations we have already discussed. Individuals with significant hearing loss lack the ability to adequately monitor their output. This is believed to explain the common reports of abnormal pitch, resonance, and poor control over speech sound accuracy (e.g., Leder & Spitzer, 1990). Another population is individuals with clefts of the palate with their inability to maintain adequate intraoral pressure. This is thought to lead to both speech sound errors and excess vocal effort, which may damage the vocal folds (e.g., Leder & Lerman, 1985).

Although frequently mentioned by clinicians, comorbidity values for speech sound disorders and voice disorders based on objective data are limited. As previously mentioned, the NSHS data suggest that almost 57 percent of school-age children with speech sound disorder may also have voice disorders. Another source is Shriberg and colleagues (1992), who reported on 137 children aged 3–19 years who had speech delay of unknown origin. Their data showed that 47 (34.3 percent) of the children failed the laryngeal quality portion of the *prosody-voice screening profile* (PVSP; Shriberg, Kwiatkowski, and Rasmussen, 1990). This means that fewer than 80 percent of their utterances in conversation were rated as having appropriate laryngeal (i.e., voice) quality. Values from both of these reports are again in stark contrast to the 10.2 percent of schoolchildren overall with voice disorders reported in the NSHS and 3.9 percent of the 2,445 preschool-age children studied by Duff, Proctor, and Yairi (2004). Having a speech sound disorder appears to increase the risk of also having a voice disorder.

Speech Sound Disorders and Emotional/Psychiatric Disorders

A final area of comorbidity has received somewhat less attention. Speech-language pathologists' caseloads often include children with other issues such as attention-deficit disorder (ADD), attention-deficit hyperactivity disorder (ADHD), or an anxiety disorder. Although not specific to speech sound disorders, studies such as that of Cantwell and Baker (1987) reported on 202 children referred for speech and/or language services. Overall, 46 percent also received some type of psychiatric diagnosis (*Note:* The word *psychiatric* here encompasses a spectrum of medically diagnosed disorders including ADD and ADHD); specifically Cantwell and Baker reported 17 percent of their participants had been diagnosed with ADD, 8 percent with conduct disorder, and 6 percent with anxiety disorder. A recent record review study by Pinborough-Zimmerman et al. (2007) identified 1667 children age 8 years in Utah with communication impairment (again not limited to speech sound disorders). Of these, 6.1 percent also had been diagnosed with ADD and 2.2 percent with anxiety disorder. More recently, a 2008 ASHA survey suggested that at least 60 percent of school clinicians provided some type of services to individuals with ADHD.

Might there be a connection between speech sound disorders and emotional or psychiatric problems? We can once again imagine a variety of possible accounts. As noted before, children with speech sound disorder may have considerable difficulty making themselves understood. This may lead to frustration and possibly considerable anxiety about communicating. Conversely, the child who is by nature overly anxious may not be the most desirable communication partner and may become somewhat ostracized. They may then miss out on opportunities to improve their speech sound accuracy. With ADHD, the child's difficulty staying on topic may also discourage conversational partners and limit practice time with speech. The connection may be in the other direction as well. The shortened conversations that unintelligible children often have may limit their opportunities to maintain their attention on a single topic for any length of time. Although specific evidence appears to be unavailable, one might also imagine a common underlying genetic problem leading to both disorders.

Our previous discussion of Shriberg's SD–DPI category is worth recalling at this point. A prevalence of 12 percent is shown in Table 4.3. Although Shriberg does not indicate that these children would necessarily qualify for a specific psychiatric diagnosis, his description of the nature of their problem implies it might be appropriate for at least some of them. Additional comorbidity data, particularly with speech as the index disorder, are somewhat limited. Keating, Turrel, and Ozanne (2001) used data from the 1995 Australian National Health Survey that included more than 12,300 children age 0–14 years. Results showed that about 8 percent of children with speech disorders were reported to also have "emotional problems." This contrasts with about 1 percent of children without speech disorders. That same study reported values of 5–7 percent and 1–2 percent, respectively, for "other mental disorders." This suggests once again an increased risk; if you have a speech sound disorder, you may be more likely to also have psychiatric or emotional problems, although as we know, this is not true for most of the speech disordered population.

CONCLUSION

For many children with speech sound disorders, the cause of the problem is known, and specific approaches to assessment and intervention have been and continue to be developed. In other cases, however, the origin of the problem is not known. This latter group of children does not consistently respond to the same intervention approaches, suggesting that there may be subgroups. Although many children in this population have historically been successfully provided intervention services, typically motor or linguistically oriented, several research teams continue efforts to unravel possible subgroups.

Children with speech sound disorders appear to be at increased risk for other kinds of problems including language impairments, stuttering, voice disorders, and psychological or emotional difficulties. Understanding the nature of these comorbidities may help us better understand the nature of the problem and how to treat them.

QUESTIONS FOR CHAPTER 4

1. What is meant by an "organically based" speech sound disorder? Cite some examples.

2. Briefly outline the three ways investigators have tried to identify subgroups of speech sound disorders of unknown origin.

3. Cite specific examples wherein knowledge of etiology is highly important, if not essential, to developing an effective and efficient intervention program.

4. What is *comorbidity*, and why is it important?

5. What are some possible ways to account for comorbid conditions in the same individual?

6. How common is it for an individual who stutters to also have a speech sound disorder?

CHAPTER 5

Factors Related to Speech Sound Disorders

PETER FLIPSEN JR.
Idaho State University

NICHOLAS W. BANKSON
James Madison University

JOHN E. BERNTHAL
University of Nebraska–Lincoln

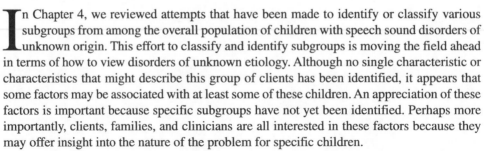

In Chapter 4, we reviewed attempts that have been made to identify or classify various subgroups from among the overall population of children with speech sound disorders of unknown origin. This effort to classify and identify subgroups is moving the field ahead in terms of how to view disorders of unknown etiology. Although no single characteristic or characteristics that might describe this group of clients has been identified, it appears that some factors may be associated with at least some of these children. An appreciation of these factors is important because specific subgroups have not yet been identified. Perhaps more importantly, clients, families, and clinicians are all interested in these factors because they may offer insight into the nature of the problem for specific children.

At the present time, the largest group of associated or causal factors that has been identified is in the area of structure and function of the speech and hearing mechanism. These are discussed first. Next, we discuss motor abilities followed by cognitive-linguistic factors, and in the final section, we discuss psychosocial factors.

STRUCTURE AND FUNCTION OF THE SPEECH AND HEARING MECHANISM

An obvious consideration when evaluating an individual's speech sound production skill relates to the potential for problems that may be manifested in the structure and function of the speech and hearing mechanisms. Problems of this nature may require medically related interventions. An example of this is surgical management for a child with cleft palate designed to facilitate velopharyngeal closure for production of stops, fricatives, and affricates. Lesser problems such as a mild case of macroglossia (enlarged tongue) in an individual with Down syndrome might suggest the need for teaching specific compensatory strategies such as controlling speaking rate (i.e., slowing down). Speech-language pathologists must draw on information from a number of professional disciplines in dealing with individuals who exhibit deficiencies in structure and/or function of the speech and hearing mechanisms.

Otitis Media with Effusion (OME)

It has long been supposed that frequent episodes of middle ear disease in children, which are accompanied by a buildup of liquid in the middle ear space (also called *otitis media with effusion*, or *OME*), may result in a delay in speech sound development. This is, of course, the basis for Shriberg's SD–OME subgroup of speech sound disorders of unknown origin discussed in Chapter 4. The assumption is that the accumulating liquid blocks the transmission of sound, resulting in a mild to moderate hearing loss, which may then impact speech sound acquisition. Although the condition invariably resolves and hearing usually returns to normal, frequent episodes may result in a history of inconsistent auditory input. However, research results to confirm these assumptions have been mixed. Shriberg, Flipsen, and colleagues (2000) identified 27 separate studies conducted on this question. Of the 27 studies, 17 (63 percent) suggested no impact, whereas 21 (78 percent) suggested some impact. (Some studies included comparisons using multiple measurement approaches; both impacts and no impacts were reported in some studies.)

Several reasons might account for this unclear picture. First, the majority of children experience at least one episode of OME during the preschool years (Adams and Benson, 1991). Assuming an average duration of 29 days per episode (Teele, Klein, Rosner, and the Greater Boston Otitis Media Study Group, 1984), a single episode would be unlikely to lead to a problem with the production of speech sounds. Some children, however, seem predisposed to multiple episodes of OME. Although comparisons were usually made between children with "frequent" OME and those with few or no episodes, the studies in this area differed widely as to their definition of the term *frequent*.

A second factor in the mixed findings for OME is that the studies differed as to the reliability of documenting actual episodes of OME. Some investigators relied solely on parent report; others evaluated available medical records. Even for studies using medical records, however, some physicians made their diagnosis by visualizing the tympanic membrane whereas others used tympanometry (even within the same study). Another complication to identifying OME is the reporting from longitudinal studies such as those by Marchant and associates (1984) of "silent otitis," or episodes in which the child displays no actual symptoms. Thus, in some studies, some children in the so-called control groups may have actually had OME that was not identified.

A third complication in the OME research is that few studies document or report the hearing status of the children during OME episodes. Although a temporary conductive hearing loss is often present during episodes of OME, the extent of the loss can vary widely across children. The timing of any hearing loss may also be crucial. Hearing loss occurring between 12 and 18 months of age may be especially troublesome for speech sound development (Shriberg, Friel-Patti, Flipsen, and Brown, 2000).

A fourth factor is access to medical care. Prompt medical treatment of OME may prevent significant accumulation of liquid in the middle ear space, and the resulting hearing loss may be of much shorter duration than without such treatment. If the children in the studies did not all have equal access to such treatment or if the treatment was not applied consistently, it should not be surprising that study outcomes varied widely.

A final factor that might account for some of the mixed findings in the OME studies is variation in socioeconomic status (SES) of the children both within and across studies. Socioeconomic status is discussed subsequently in more detail, but children from low SES backgrounds appear to be at higher risk for speech sound disorders because of either poorer-quality language stimulation and/or poorer access to health care.

Given the complexity associated with the mixed findings, it seems likely that they are the result of an interaction of several if not all of the factors cited. One proposal to deal with this complexity has been the use of longitudinal studies in which children are recruited in the first year of life and monitored for several years. Roberts, Rosenfeld, and Zeisel (2004) surveyed 14 such prospective studies using a statistical technique known as *meta-analysis* and concluded that there were "no to very small associations of OM to speech and language development in most children" (p. 247). Roberts and colleagues did note that such a conclusion assumes an optimal learning environment, which may not always be present. Thus, particular children may be at higher risk for delayed speech development from OME. Findings from a study by Shriberg, Flipsen, and colleagues (2000) support such a conclusion. Using two different groups, these authors reported that having frequent OME resulted in no increased risk of delayed speech in a group of children from a university-affiliated, general pediatric clinic group but a significantly increased risk of approximately 4.6 times for a group of Native American children living on a reservation. Children in the latter group were from a lower SES background and had poorer access to good-quality medical care.

Speech Sound Perception

Speech perception (often referred to as *speech discrimination*) skills likely play a role in several important aspects of speech sound acquisition: (1) making the association between the sounds of the native language and the meaning that can be expressed with those sounds, (2) making the association between the sounds the child her- or himself generates and the movements of the vocal tract, (3) making the association between the sounds the child produces and the meaningful units of the language, and (4) adapting the child's own productions to a changing vocal tract (i.e., adjusting what the child does to account for her or his own growth). Given its importance, it should not be surprising that speech-language pathologists have long been interested in the relationship between the perception and production of speech sounds in individuals with speech sound disorders who have normal auditory acuity (i.e., those who pass a standard hearing screening).

In the early days of the profession, many clinicians assumed that a major reason children produced sounds in error was because they didn't properly discriminate one sound from another (e.g., /s/ in *some* from /θ/ in *thumb*). The possibility of such a relationship was first investigated in the 1930s. This early perceptual research, referred to as *speech sound discrimination research*, relied primarily on general measures of speech sound discrimination (tests comparing sound contrasts), which required the participant to judge whether word or nonsense pairs verbally presented by the examiner were the same or different. In such tests, there was generally no attempt to compare the specific phoneme production errors with the specific perception errors the participant might have made. These early studies yielded mixed findings. Some (e.g., Clark, 1959; Kronvall and Diehl, 1954; Travis and Rasmus, 1931) found that normal speakers had significantly better discrimination skills, and several investigators found a positive correlation between performance on articulation tests and performance on tests of speech sound discrimination (Reid, 1947a; Carrell and Pendergast, 1954). Other studies, however, found no such relationship (Garrett, 1969; Hall, 1938; Mase, 1946; Prins, 1962b; Veatch, 1970).

Sherman and Geith (1967) suggested that one reason for the equivocal findings may have been that experimental groups were chosen on the basis of articulatory proficiency rather than speech sound discrimination performance, and consequently, etiologies associated with articulatory-impaired students may not have been limited to individuals with poor speech sound discrimination skills. To control for perceptual skill, Sherman and Geith studied 18 children with high discrimination scores and 18 with low scores. Based on a 176-item picture-articulation test, the children with high speech sound discrimination scores obtained significantly higher articulation scores than the group with lower discrimination scores. The authors concluded that poor speech sound discrimination skill may be causally related to poor articulation performance.

Schwartz and Goldman (1974) investigated the possible effects of the type of discrimination task required and found that their participants consistently made more errors when stimulus words were presented in a paired-comparison context (goat and coat; coat and boat) than when target words were included in carrier phrase and sentence contexts (as in "The man brought a coat"). They also found that when background noise was present during stimulus presentation, performance was poorer, particularly for the paired-comparison words.

General versus Phoneme-Specific Measures

In the late 1970s, a consensus that children with speech sound disorders did not have a general problem with speech perception emerged. Researchers such as Locke (1980a) pointed out that in children with speech sound disorders, the critical issue is their ability to discriminate the sound or segments that they misarticulate. Locke recommended going a step further, urging that measures of sound perception should be not only phoneme specific but also context specific. He argued that perceptual tasks should reflect the child's production errors and reflect those phonetic environments (words) in which error productions occur and include both the error productions and the target productions. Locke studied the ability of 131 children to perform a perceptual task in which the examiner produced imitations of the participant's error productions. The participants were then required to judge whether the examiner's productions were correct productions of the target word. Locke reported that 70 percent of the children correctly perceived the correct and incorrect forms of the target words, thus indicating that many children could correctly discriminate sounds made by an adult that they produced in error. About one-third of the contrasts misproduced were also misperceived.

More recently Rvachew and Grawburg (2006) tested 95 four- and five-year-old children with speech sound disorders and provided findings similar to that of Locke

(1980a). All scored within the normal range on a test of receptive vocabulary, which indirectly suggests no general problems with speech perception (i.e., a broader problem with speech perception might have meant poorer comprehension skills). However, only 62 percent achieved a passing score on a set of phoneme-specific speech perception measures.

In a study of 14 children 2 years of age, Eilers and Oller (1976) found some perceptual confusion in word and nonsense pairs when production of one segment was substituted for another. Yet other common production errors were discriminated by most of their participants. They concluded that some production errors may be related to perceptual difficulties and others to motor constraints.

External and Internal Monitoring

Recall the four aspects of speech sound acquisition mentioned earlier that are relevant to speech perception skills. The first of these (making the association between the sounds of the language in the environment and meaning) involves monitoring the speech of others. This is termed *external discrimination*, or monitoring. External discrimination can also include *external self-discrimination* of which listening to and making judgments of tape-recorded samples of one's own speech is an example. In both cases, the listener uses air conduction auditory cues.

The other three aspects of speech sound acquisition mentioned earlier involve evaluating one's own ongoing speech sound productions; this is called *internal discrimination* or *internal monitoring*. During internal discrimination, the speaker has available both air- and bone-conducted auditory cues. Testing the ability to internally discriminate typically involves asking the child to judge the accuracy of words or sounds immediately after they are produced.

Studies of speech sound discrimination skills of young children with delayed speech sound development have indicated that children frequently were able to make external judgments of sound contrasts involving their error sounds (Chaney and Menyuk, 1975; Locke and Kutz, 1975). A study by Aungst and Frick (1964) looked at the relationship between external and internal discrimination and /r/ production. Each participant was asked to (1) make an immediate right–wrong judgment of his or her /r/ production after speaking each word, (2) make right–wrong judgments of his or her /r/ productions after such productions had been audio recorded and played back, and (3) make same–different judgments of his or her /r/ productions as they followed the examiner's correct productions presented via audiotape recording. Moderate correlation coefficients of .69, .66, and .59 were obtained between each of the three phoneme-specific discrimination tasks and scores on the *Deep Test of Articulation* for /r/. In contrast, scores on a general test of auditory discrimination did not correlate well with the articulation measure. Lapko and Bankson (1975) conducted a similar study using a group of 25 kindergarten and first-grade children exhibiting misarticulations of /s/ and reported similar findings as did Wolfe and Irwin (1973) and Stelcik (1972).

But the results of other investigations (Woolf and Pilberg, 1971; Shelton, Johnson, and Arndt, 1977) have indicated that the findings in such studies may be influenced by factors such as the consistency of misarticulation, type of discrimination task used to test internal monitoring, and nature of the stimulus items.

Discrimination Training and Production Performance

Historically, clinicians routinely conducted some type of discrimination training, or "ear training," as a precursor to production training; however, that is no longer the case. This move away from such training appears to have followed on the heels of the mixed findings for studies of the relationship between general perceptual skills and production errors. However, if one assumes that at least some speech errors are perceptually based, a logical question is whether a functional relationship exists between speech sound production and discrimination and more specifically, whether discrimination training affects or perhaps enhances production of speech sounds.

Sonderman (1971) examined (1) the effect of speech sound discrimination training on articulation skills and (2) the effect of articulation training on speech sound discrimination skill. Sonderman administered Holland's speech sound discrimination program (1967) and the S-Pack (Mowrer, Baker, and Schutz, 1968) in alternate sequence to two matched groups of 10 children between 6 and 8 years old, all of whom produced frontal lisps. Improvement in both discrimination and articulation scores was obtained from both discrimination training and articulation training, regardless of the sequence in which the two types of training were conducted. Articulatory improvement did not necessarily mean that speech sound errors were corrected. Rather, shifts from one type of error to another (e.g., omission to substitution; substitution to distortion) were regarded as evidence of improvement.

Williams and McReynolds (1975) explored the same question. Two participants were first given production training followed by a discrimination probe and then discrimination training followed by a production probe. Two additional participants received the training in reverse order. The probe measures indicated that production training was effective in changing both production and discrimination; in contrast to Sonderman (1971), however, discrimination training did not generalize to production.

Shelton, Johnson, and Arndt (1977) explored the influence of articulation training on discrimination performance. One group of participants received production training on /r/ and a second group on /s/, and pre- and postdiscrimination probes, consisting of 40 items specifically related to the error sound, were administered. Results indicated that both groups of participants improved in articulation performance, but no improvement was noted in discrimination performance.

Rvachew (1994) studied the influence of various types of speech perception training that were administered concurrently with traditional speech sound therapy. Twenty-seven preschoolers with SSD who misarticulated /ʃ/ were randomly assigned to three groups, each of which received one of the following types of discrimination training: (1) listening to a variety of correctly and incorrectly produced versions of the word *shoe*, (2) listening to the words *shoe* and *moo*, and (3) listening to the words *cat* and *Pete*. Following six weekly treatment sessions, children who received types 1 and 2 training demonstrated superior ability to articulate the target sound in comparison to those who received type 3 training. Based on her data, Rvachew suggested that "speech perception training should probably be provided concurrently with speech production training" (p. 355). A later report of Rvachew, Rafaat, and Martin (1999) further supported this conclusion. Through two complementary studies, these researchers explored the relationship of stimulability, speech perception ability, and phonological learning. In the first study, participants were treated individually using a cycles approach as prescribed by Hodson (1989). They reported that children who were stimulable for a target sound and who demonstrated good pretreatment perceptual ability for that sound made more progress in therapy than those who were stimulable for the target sound but had poor speech sound perception for that sound. Children who were not stimulable did not make progress regardless of their perceptual skills. A second study included both individual and group instruction for the participants. Lessons involved phonetically based production activities and a computer-based program of perceptual training. Results from the second study indicated that all children, regardless of pretreatment stimulability and/or speech perception skills made progress in production. The authors concluded that "despite the independence of stimulability and speech perception ability before training, there is reason to believe that speech perception training may facilitate the acquisition of stimulability if both production and perception training are provided concurrently to children who demonstrate unstimulability and poor speech perception for the target sound" (Rvachew, Rafaat, and Martin, p. 40).

The findings reported by Rvachew and colleagues suggest that for children with poor speech sound perception of a target sound, including perceptual training along with production training, produces positive clinical outcomes in terms of speech sound acquisition. This conclusion is supported by findings of a third related study (Rvachew, Nowak, and Cloutier, 2004). In this case, the perception training program was combined with phonological awareness training (letter recognition, sound-symbol association, onset identification) and compared to a computer-based program for vocabulary development. The two approaches were used concurrently with speech production training for 34 preschool children. Findings again showed significantly superior outcomes for the children who received the perception training. Interestingly, the two groups did not differ on phonological awareness outcomes.

Self-Monitoring

The ability to identify errors in one's own speech (what we earlier called *internal discrimination*) during therapy has long been suggested as being important to therapy progress. Although formal study of internal discrimination has been limited, some investigators (Koegel, Koegel, and Ingham, 1986; Koegel, Koegel, Van Voy, and Ingham, 1988) have examined the relationship between self-monitoring skills and response generalization into the natural environment. School-age children were provided specific training in self-monitoring of the speech productions. These investigators reported that generalization of correct articulatory responses of the target sounds did not occur until a self-monitoring task was initiated in the treatment program. They concluded that such self-monitoring was required for generalization of the target sounds in the natural environment to occur. Using slightly different procedures, Gray and Shelton (1992) failed to replicate these findings. The authors indicated that different participant, treatment, and environmental variables may have accounted for different outcomes.

Kwiatkowski and Shriberg (1993; 1998) suggested that self-monitoring may actually result from the complex interaction of both (1) *capability* (linguistic and motor skills, physiological and cognitive limitations, and psychosocial factors) and (2) *focus* (attention, motivation, and effort). This might account for the mixed findings from studies of the role of self-monitoring in treatment outcomes. Reliable, objective measures of either self-monitoring or focus have not been developed. As such, the role of self-monitoring in speech sound disorders is still to be refined.

Summary

For many years, speech sound production errors were assumed to be based in large part on problems of speech perception. More recently clinicians have paid far less attention to perceptual skills in these children. A relationship between speech sound perception and production in some children with speech sound disorders appears to exist, although the precise nature of the relationship has not been determined. Available data suggest that this may be the case for perhaps as many as 30–40 percent of these children (Locke, 1980a; Rvachew and Grawburg, 2008) and that perceptual testing is justified in this population, particularly testing that is focused on speech sounds that the child misarticulates (Lof and Synan, 1997). Self-monitoring of error productions would appear to be an important skill for normalization of speech sounds in spontaneous speech, but instruments to assess such skill are lacking. More data are needed to better understand the relationship between discrimination errors and speech sound disorders. Although the efficacy of speech sound perception training as a predecessor to production training has often been questioned, when perceptual deficiencies are present, perceptual training prior to or concurrent with direct instruction would seem appropriate.

Minor Structural Variations of the Speech Mechanism

Speech clinicians, as part of an oral-mechanism examination, are required to make judgments about the structure and/or function of the lips, teeth, tongue, and palate. These oral structures can vary significantly, even among normal speakers. Investigators have attempted to identify relationships between speech sound disorders and structural variations of the oral mechanism.

Major variations were discussed in Chapter 4 regarding organically based disorders. The following sections highlight lesser variations and their potential impact on speech sound production. Although a strict cause–effect relationship has not been established, such variations may contribute to the difficulty that some children experience.

Lips

Approximation of the lips is required for the formation of the bilabial phonemes /b/, /p/, and /m/; lip rounding is required for various vowels and the consonants /w/ and /ʍ/. An impairment that would inhibit lip approximation or rounding might result in misarticulation of these sounds. Fairbanks and Green (1950) examined various dimensions of the lips in 30 adult speakers with superior consonant production and 30 with inferior consonant production and reported no differences on various lip measurements between the two groups.

Certain deformities of the lips such as the enlarged lips in Ackerman syndrome (Ackerman, Ackerman, and Ackerman, 1973) or congenital double lips (Eski, Nisanci, Aktas, and Sengezer, 2007) may interfere with speech production but not in every case. These findings suggest that only major deviations in lip structure or function are likely to impact speech sound production.

Teeth

Several English consonants require intact dentition for correct production. Labiodental phonemes (/f/ and /v/) require contact between the teeth and lower lip for their production, and linguadental phonemes require tongue placement just behind or between the teeth for /ð/ and /θ/ productions. The tongue tip alveolars (/s/, /z/) require that the airstream pass over the cutting edge of the incisors.

Researchers investigating the relationship between deviant dentition and consonant production have examined the presence or absence of teeth, position of teeth, and dental occlusion. *Occlusion* refers to the alignment of the first molar teeth when the jaws are closed, and *malocclusion* refers to the imperfect or irregular position of the teeth when jaws are closed. Lay terms to describe different types of occlusion include open bite and overbite. Refer to Figure 5.1 for examples of different types of occlusion.

A number of investigators have examined the relationship between different types of occlusion and speech sound disorders. Bernstein (1954) identified malocclusions in children with normal and defective speech but did not find a higher incidence of malocclusion in children with speech sound problems than in children with normal skills. Fairbanks and Lintner (1951) examined molar occlusion, occlusion of the anterior teeth, and anterior

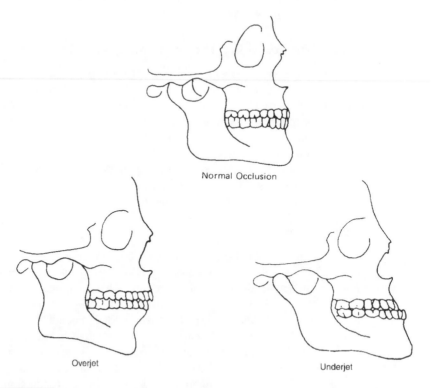

Normal Occlusion

Overjet

Underjet

FIGURE 5.1   Examples of types of occlusions.

spaces in 60 adults, 30 of whom were judged to have superior speech sound skills and 30 with inferior skills. When data from the participants were divided according to (1) no marked dental deviation and (2) one or more marked dental deviations, the authors found that marked dental deviations occurred significantly more frequently in the inferior speakers than in the superior ones. Laine, Jaroma, and Linnasalo (1987) conducted a study of speech errors and incisor teeth issues in 451 college-age students in Finland. They reported significantly higher amounts of horizontal overjet or vertical overbite in participants with "audibly clear" /s/ distortions compared to their peers with no speech errors. Subtelny, Mestre, and Subtelny (1964) found malocclusion to coexist with both normal and defective speech. They also noted that during /s/ production, normal speakers with malocclusion (distocclusion) tended to position the tongue tip slightly to the rear of the lower incisors (i.e., what some have called a *tongue-tip down /s/*) when compared to normal speakers with normal occlusion. In summary, although speakers with normal articulatory skills tend to have a lower incidence of malocclusion than speakers with articulatory errors, malocclusion itself does not preclude normal production.

The shape of the dental arch has also been examined. Starr (1972) reported that a speech sound problem is highly probable in individuals with a short or narrow maxillary (upper) arch and a normal mandibular (lower) arch. The consonants likely to be affected by such conditions are /s, z, ʃ, tʃ, f, v, t, and d/. He further noted that rotated teeth and supernumerary (extra) teeth do not generally present significant speech problems.

Another area of interest to investigators has been the influence of missing teeth on speech sound skill. Bankson and Byrne (1962) examined the influence of missing teeth in kindergarten and first-grade children. Initially, participants were identified as either children who had correct articulation with their teeth intact or children who had incorrect articulation with their teeth intact. After four months, articulation skills were reassessed and the number of missing central or lateral incisors tabulated. A significant relationship was found between presence or absence of teeth and correct production of /s/, but not of /f/, /ʃ/, or /z/. However, some children maintained correct production of /s/ despite the loss of incisors. Snow (1961) examined the influence of missing teeth on consonant production in first-grade children. Participants were divided into two groups: those with normal incisors and those with missing or grossly abnormal incisor teeth. Although Snow found that a significantly higher proportion of children with dental deviations misarticulated consonants, she also found that three-quarters of the children with defective dentition did not misarticulate these sounds. In contrast to Bankson and Byrne, who noted significant differences only for /s/, Snow found significant differences for all phonemes. Gable, Kummer, Lee, Creaghead, and Moore (1995) examined 26 children whose incisor teeth had to be extracted before age 5 years. At age 8 to 10 years, the speech sound production skills of these children were not significantly different from that of an age-matched group of children without the premature extractions. However, Pahkala, Laine, and Lammi (1991) reported that earlier appearance of the permanent teeth was associated with a decreased occurrence of speech sound disorders in a group of children acquiring Finnish.

Overall, although dental status may be a crucial factor in speech sound productions for some children, it does not appear to be significant for most. Many children appear to be able to adapt to abnormal dental relationships or atypical dental development.

Tongue

The tongue is generally considered the most important articulator for speech production. Tongue movements during speech production include tip elevation, grooving, and protrusion. The tongue is relatively short at birth, growing longer and thinner at the tip with age.

Ankyloglossia, or *tongue-tie,* is a term used to describe a restricted lingual frenum (sometimes called the *frenulum*). According to Hong, Lago, Seargeant, Pellman, Magit, and Pransky (2010), there is no consensus as to the precise definition of the term. Kummer (2009) noted that clinically it is usually defined as the inability to protrude the tip of the tongue past the front teeth. A review by Segal, Stephenson, Dawes, and Feldman (2007) indicated that prevalence estimates for ankyloglossia range from 4.2–10.7 percent of the population. The variability in these estimates is likely related to differences in definitions for tongue-tie.

At one time, it was commonly assumed that an infant or child with ankyloglossia should have his or her frenum clipped to allow greater freedom of tongue movement and better articulation of tongue tip sounds, and frenectomies (clipping of the frenum of the tongue) were performed relatively often. However, McEnery and Gaines (1941) examined 1,000 patients with speech disorders and identified only four individuals with abnormally short frenums. Their most extreme case of a short frenum was a 10-year-old boy whose only error was a /w/ for /r/ substitution, which was corrected following speech instruction. The authors recommended against surgery for ankyloglossia because of the possibility of hemorrhages, infections, and scar tissue. Fletcher and Meldrum (1968) examined two groups of sixth-grade students, 20 with limited lingual movement and 20 with greater lingual movement. These investigators reported that participants with restricted lingual movement scored within normal limits on a measure of articulation but tended to have more articulation errors than the group with greater lingual movement. The possibility of some relationship between frenum length and speech sound problems is supported by a more recent study that examined 200 children age 6 to 12 years. Ruffoli and colleagues (2005) classified the severity of ankyloglossia based on frenum length and reported "a relationship between the presence of speech anomalies and a decreased mobility of the tongue, but only for those subjects who frenulum length resulted in moderate or severe levels of ankyloglossia" (p. 174).

Clipping of the frenum does still occur, which raises the question as to whether it makes a difference. Messner and Lalakea (2002) reported results from a group of children age 1 to 12 years who underwent such procedures. Formal speech evaluations by speech-language pathologists indicated that 9 of 11 (82 percent) of the children with preoperative speech errors had improved their speech. A similar study by Heller, Gabbay, O'Hara, Heller, and Bradley (2005) reported improvement in 10 of 11 (91 percent) cases. These findings suggest that frenum clipping may make a difference for individuals for whom more severe ankyloglossia is affecting speech.

Another potential problem with the tongue relative to speech sound disorders is *macroglossia* (a tongue that is too large). This condition was discussed in Chapter 4. Whether it is true macroglossia or relative macroglossia (a normal size tongue in a small oral cavity), however, the relationship with speech sound production skills has still not been adequately investigated. The tongue is a muscular structure capable of considerable change in length and width and thus, regardless of size, is generally capable of the mobility necessary for correct sound productions. Put another way, many individuals with macroglossia appear to be able to compensate. The same appears to be true for individuals who have undergone partial glossectomy (removal of part of the tongue).

Hard Palate

The relationship between speech sound disorders and variations in hard palate dimensions has received limited attention. Fairbanks and Lintner (1951) measured the hard palates of a group of young adults with superior consonant articulation and a group with inferior consonant articulation. They reported no significant differences in cuspid width, molar width, palatal height, and maximum mouth opening. Removal of any part of the maxilla, whether or not restored surgically or prosthetically, may create a serious problem for the speaker.

Oral Sensory Function

Oral sensory and kinesthetic feedback plays a role in the development and ongoing monitoring of articulatory gestures, and thus the relationship between oral sensory function and speech sound productions has been of interest. Some treatment approaches include the practice of calling the client's attention to sensory cues. Bordon (1984) indicated the need for awareness of *kinesthesis* (sense of movement and position) during therapy. Almost any phonetic placement technique used to teach speech sounds (to be discussed in Chapter 9) typically includes a description of articulatory contacts and movements necessary for the production of the target speech sound.

The investigation of *somesthesis* (sense of movement, position, touch, and awareness of muscle tension) has focused on (1) overall oral sensitivity, (2) temporary sensory deprivation during oral sensory anesthetization (nerve block anesthesia) to determine the effect of sensory deprivation on speech production, and (3) assessment of oral sensory perception such as two-point discrimination or oral form discrimination to see whether such sensory perception was related to articulatory skill. Considerable research into oral sensory functioning has been conducted using a variety of methods.

Netsell (1986) has suggested that adults are likely not consciously aware of specific speech movements during running speech. He also speculated that children may not be aware of articulatory movements during the acquisition period. If Netsell is correct, the clinician who attempts to utilize somesthetic senses in monitoring running speech may be asking the client to respond to information that is not available at a conscious level without instruction.

Oral Tactile Sensitivity

Early investigators of oral sensory function attempted to explore the sensitivity or threshold of awareness of oral structures to various stimuli. Ringel and Ewanowski (1965) studied oral tactile sensitivity utilizing an esthesiometer, a device used in the measurement of two-point discrimination. They examined discrimination sensitivity of various structures in a normal population and found that the maximal to minimal awareness hierarchy for two-point stimulation (awareness of two points rather than one) was tongue tip, finger tip, lip, soft palate, and alveolar ridge and that the midline of structures tended to be more sensitive than the lateral edges.

Fucci and associates (Arnst and Fucci, 1975; Fucci, 1972) measured the threshold of vibrotactile stimulation of structures in the oral cavity in both normal and speech-disordered individuals. These investigators found that participants with misarticulations tended to have poorer oral sensory abilities than normal-speaking participants.

Oral Anesthetization

To study the role of oral sensation during speech, researchers have induced temporary states of oral sensory deprivation through the use of oral nerve-block and topical anesthetization (similar to what occurs prior to dental work). Then they examined a variety of variables, such as overall intelligibility, vowel and consonant articulation, rate, phoneme duration, and physiological and acoustic characteristics.

Gammon, Smith, Daniloff, and Kim (1971) examined the articulation skills of eight adult participants reading 30 sentences under four conditions: (1) normal, (2) with masking noise present, (3) nerve-block anesthesia, and (4) nerve-block anesthesia with masking noise. They noted few vowel distortions under any of the conditions and a 20 percent rate of consonant misarticulation (especially fricatives and affricates) under anesthesia and under anesthesia with noise. Scott and Ringel (1971) studied the articulation of two adult males producing lists of 24 bisyllabic words under normal and anesthetized conditions. They noted that articulatory changes caused by sensory deprivation were largely nonphonemic in nature and included loss of retroflexion and lip-rounding gestures, less tight fricative constrictions, and retracted points of articulation contacts.

Prosek and House (1975) studied four adult speakers reading 20 bisyllabic words in isolation and in sentences under normal and anesthetized conditions. Although intelligibility was maintained, speech rate was slowed, and minor imprecisions of articulation were noted. The authors reported that, when anesthetized, speakers produced consonants with slightly more intraoral air pressure and longer duration than under the normal nonanesthetized condition.

In summary, studies involving anesthetization have found that speech remained intelligible although participants did not speak as accurately as they did under normal conditions. However, the participants in these studies were adult speakers with normal articulation skills. It is unclear whether reduced oral sensory feedback might interfere with the acquisition of speech or affect remediation.

Oral Form Recognition

Oral sensory function has also been investigated extensively through form recognition tasks. Ringel, Burk, and Scott (1970) speculated that form identification (*oral stereognosis*) may provide information on nervous system integrity because the recognition of forms placed in the mouth was assumed to require integrity of peripheral receptors for touch and kinesthesis as well as central integrating processes. Most form recognition tasks require the participant to match forms placed in the oral cavity with drawings of the forms, or to make same-different judgments. Participants tend to improve on such tasks until adolescence when they ceiling out (i.e., achieve maximum performance possible). Stimuli for such testing are typically small, plastic, three-dimensional forms of varying degrees of similarity, such as triangles, rectangles, ovals, and circles.

Studies in this area have yielded inconsistent results. Arndt, Elbert, and Shelton (1970) did not find a significant relationship between oral form recognition and articulation performance in a third-grade population. But Ringel, House, Burk, Dolinsky, and Scott (1970) reported significant differences on an oral form-matching task between normal-speaking elementary school children and children with articulation errors. Speirs and Maktabi (1990) reported similar findings. Ringel and associates analyzed their data in more detail and noted that children with severe misarticulations made more form-recognition errors than children with mild articulation problems. However, a study by Hetrick and Sommers (1988) failed to find differences related to severity of articulation.

Some researchers have investigated the relationship between production of specific phonemes and oral sensory function. McNutt (1977) found that children who misarticulated /r/ did not perform as well as the normal speakers on oral form perception tasks; there were, however, no significant differences between the normal speakers and the children who misarticulated /s/.

Bishop, Ringel, and House (1973) compared oral form-recognition skills of deaf high school students who were orally trained (taught to use speech) with those who were taught to use sign language. The authors noted skill differences that favored the orally trained students and postulated that "while a failure in oroperceptual functioning may lead to [speech sound] disorders . . ., a failure to use the oral mechanism for speech activities, even in persons with normal orosensory capabilities, may result in poor performance on oroperceptual tasks" (p. 257).

Oral Sensory Function and Speech Sound Learning

Jordan, Hardy, and Morris (1978) studied the influence of tactile sensation as a feedback mechanism in speech sound learning. Their participants were first-grade boys, nine with good articulation skills and nine with poor articulation skills. Participants were fitted with palatal plates equipped with touch-sensitive electrodes and taught to replicate four positions of linguapalatal contact with and without topical anesthesia. Children with poor articulation performed less well on tasks of precise tongue placement than children with good articulation. Participants with poor articulation were able to improve their initially poor performance when given specific training on the tongue placement tasks.

Wilhelm (1971) and Shelton, Willis, Johnson, and Arndt (1973) used oral form-recognition materials to teach form recognition to misarticulating children and reported inconsistent results. Wilhelm reported articulation improved as oral form recognition improved. Shelton and colleagues reported results that did not support that finding. Ruscello (1972) reported that form-recognition scores improved in children undergoing treatment for articulation.

Summary

The role of normal oral sensory function or somesthetic feedback in the development and maintenance of speech production is complex. Despite efforts to identify the relationship between oral sensory status and articulatory performance, conclusive findings are lacking. A review of the literature, however, has revealed the following:

1. Oral form recognition improves with age through adolescence.
2. The role of oral sensory feedback in the acquisition of speech sounds is unclear.

3. During anesthesia, intelligibility is generally maintained but articulation tends to be less accurate.

4. Individuals with poor articulation tend to achieve slightly lower scores on form-perception tasks than their normal-speaking peers. However, some individuals with poor form-identification skills have good articulation.

5. Although some individuals with speech sound disorders may also have oral sensory deficits, the neurological mechanisms underlying the use of sensory information during experimental conditions may differ from those operating in normal running speech.

6. Information concerning oral sensory function has not been shown to have clinical applicability.

7. It is important to distinguish between the effects of sensory deprivation in individuals who have already developed good speech skills and the effects in individuals with speech sound disorders.

8. The effects of long-term sensory deprivation have yet to be explored.

MOTOR ABILITIES

Because speech is a motor act, researchers have explored the relationship between speech sound production and motor skills, investigating performance on gross motor tasks as well as oral and facial motor tasks.

General Motor Skills

Studies focusing on the relationship between general or gross motor skills and articulatory abilities have yielded inconsistent and inconclusive results. It may be concluded, however, that individuals with speech sound problems do not have significant retardation in general motor development.

Oral-Facial Motor Skills

Speech is a dynamic process that requires the precise coordination of the oral musculature. During ongoing speech production, fine muscle movements of the lips, tongue, palate, and jaw constantly alter the dimensions of the oral cavity. An assessment of the client's oral motor skills is typically a part of a speech mechanism examination. Tests of diadochokinetic (DDK) rate or maximum repetition rate (rapid repetition of syllables) have been used frequently to evaluate oral motor skills independent of phonological skills. This separation is made by using nonsense syllables to prevent the speaker from accessing their long-term word storage. These tasks also typically involve early developing sounds (stops and neutral vowels) that are assumed to be the simplest in terms of motor demands. The syllables most frequently used are /pʌ/, /tʌ/, and /kʌ/ in isolation, syllable repetition, and the sequences /pʌtʌ/, /tʌkʌ/, /pʌkʌ/, /pʌtʌkʌ/. These tasks are typically done at maximum rates (i.e., speakers are told to produce them "as fast as possible").

DDK rate is established either with a *count by time* procedure in which the examiner counts the number of syllables spoken in a given interval of time or a *time by count* measurement in which the examiner notes the time required to produce a designated number of syllables. The advantage of the time by count measurement is that fewer operations are required because the examiner needs to listen only to the syllable count and turn off the timing device when the requisite number of syllables has been produced. Performance is then sometimes compared to normative data. There is evidence that DDK rates improve with age. Fletcher (1972) reported that children increased the number of syllables produced in a given unit of time at each successive age from 7 to 13 years. Data reported by Canning and Rose (1974) indicated that adult values for maximum repetition rates were reached by 9- to 10-year-olds whereas Fletcher's data show a convergence after age 15.

McNutt (1977) and Dworkin (1978) examined DDK rates of children with specific misarticulations (errors on /r/ and /s/) and in their normal-speaking peers. Both investigators reported that the mean rate of utterances of the syllables tested was significantly lower in the participants with speech sound errors.

Some researchers have questioned the usefulness of rapid syllable repetition tasks such as DDK and their relationship to articulation skills because the movements of articulation are produced by the simultaneous contraction of different groups of muscles rather than the alternating contraction of opposed muscles (McDonald, 1964a). Findings from at least two studies of speech kinematics or movement patterns (Adams, Weismer, and Kent, 1993; Smith, Goffman, Zelaznik, Ying, and McGillem, 1995) also suggest a different organization of the movements at fast rates compared to normal rate. The two together suggest that fast rate productions are qualitatively different from normal rate productions. This makes it difficult to know how meaningful problems with DDK observed at fast rates really are.

Winitz (1969) also pointed out that because normal speakers have a history of success with speech sounds, they may have an advantage over speakers with misarticulations on DDK tasks. Tiffany (1980) pointed out that little is known about the significance of scores obtained on DDK tasks and thus "such measures appear to lack a substantial theoretical base" (p. 895). The one exception to this generality relates to those children that might be considered to evidence childhood apraxia of speech (discussed in Chapter 4). Poor performance in some DDK tasks often reflects syllable sequencing problems evident in this population. Another exception would be clients with a history of unusual or delayed oral-motor development, which may be evidenced in sucking, feeding, and swallowing in addition to delayed speech sound development. These children may evidence problems with muscle tone and movement of the oral structures, including independent movement of the tongue and/or lips from the jaw. It would appear that slow or weak oral-motor development may be a contributing factor to the presence of a speech sound disorder.

Although difficult to measure in most clinical settings, another perspective on possible motor deficits in speech sound disorders has involved the measurement of tongue strength. Dworkin and Culatta (1985) found no significant difference in the maximum amount of tongue force that could be exerted by children with speech sound disorders compared to children without any speech difficulties. Dworkin (1978) showed differences specific to children who were producing /s/ errors. A study by Bradford, Murdoch, Thompson, and Stokes (1997) revealed reduced tongue strength in children diagnosed with childhood apraxia of speech (CAS) compared to children with inconsistent phonological disorder and normal-speaking children. However, Robin, Somodi, and Luschei (1991) failed to find such a difference for the children with CAS in their study. The difference between the findings of these latter two studies, however, might be accounted for by differences in criteria for diagnosing CAS (see Chapter 4).

Like DDK rates, the value of measuring maximum tongue strength has been questioned. It has been suggested that people likely use only about 20 percent of their tongue strength capability during speech (Forrest, 2002; Kent, Kent, and Rosenbek, 1987). An alternative to measuring maximum tongue strength was conducted by Speirs and Maktabi (1990), who measured fine tongue control by asking their participants to maintain a low level of target pressure for short periods. The children with speech sound disorders showed significantly less stability (i.e., poorer fine control) than children without speech errors. In the previously mentioned study by Robin and colleagues (1991), although there was no difference in maximum strength, the children with CAS were significantly poorer at maintaining tongue pressure at 50 percent of maximum compared to normal-speaking children. Such findings lend some support to the idea that some children with speech sound disorders may have subtle motor deficiencies or delays.

Summary

Individuals with speech sound problems have not been shown to exhibit significantly depressed motor coordination on tasks of general motor performance. The relationship between oral-motor skills and articulation skills in speech sound disorders of unknown origin remains uncertain. Although such individuals have been found to perform more poorly on DDK tasks than their normal-speaking peers, these results cannot be accurately interpreted until the relationship between DDK tasks and the ability to articulate sounds in context is clarified.

Findings of tongue strength studies suggest that although overall strength may not be a problem for children with speech sound disorders, a more important issue may be fine tongue control or stability. It is not yet clear whether such findings represent children with speech sound disorders in general or are limited only to subgroups of this population such as those with abnormal tone or those with CAS.

Oral Myofunctional Disorders/Tongue Thrust

Speech-language pathologists observe oral myofunctional disorders (OMD), which include such phenomena as tongue thrusting, unusual oral movements, finger sucking, lip insufficiencies, and dental and oral structure deficiencies. The concern of speech-language pathologists relates to speech differences and disorders that may be related to such oral variations. Because tongue thrusting is the oral myofunctional disorder most commonly encountered by speech-language pathologists, in this section we focus on this phenomena.

Orthodontists and speech-language pathologists have been interested in tongue thrusting and a forward tongue-resting posture because of the perception that tongue function can cause certain types of (1) malocclusion problems, (2) altered patterns of facial development, and (3) speech sound problems. The type of speech sound disorder associated with tongue thrust and malocclusion is a frontal lisp characterized by anterior tongue placement for /s/ and /z/. The number of lisps is higher in children who evidence tongue thrusting than for children who do not evidence such behavior. Sometimes tongue thrust is also associated with anterior placement of /ʃ/, /tʃ/, /dʒ/, /ʒ/, /t/, /d/, /l/, and /n/.

Tongue thrust has been defined as frontal or lateral tongue thrust or strong contact of the tongue with the teeth during swallowing as well as inadequate lip closure or incorrect tongue rest posture (Neiva and Wertzner, 1996). Proffit (1986) pointed out that tongue thrust is something of a misnomer because it implies that the tongue is thrust forward forcefully when in reality such individuals do not seem to use more tongue force against the teeth than nonthrusters. Rather, *tongue thrust swallow* implies a directionality of tongue activity in swallowing. Hanson (1988a) suggested that a better description for these tongue position and movement behaviors would be "oral muscle pattern disorders." Other terms sometimes used to describe these behaviors include *reverse swallow, deviant swallow*, and *infantile swallow*. The latter terms should be avoided because of their inherent faulty implications (Mason, 1988).

The most salient features of a tongue thrust swallow pattern, according to Mason and Proffit (1974), include one or more of these conditions:

1. During the initiation of a swallow, a forward gesture of the tongue between the anterior teeth so that the tongue tip contacts the lower lip;
2. During speech activities, fronting of the tongue between or against the anterior teeth with the mandible hinged open (in phonetic contexts not intended for such placements); and
3. At rest, the tongue carried forward in the oral cavity with the mandible hinged slightly open and the tongue tip against or between the anterior teeth. (p. 116)

Everyone starts out life as a tongue thruster because at birth the tongue fills the oral cavity, making tongue fronting obligatory. Sometime later, the anterior tongue-gums/teeth seal during swallowing is replaced with a superior tongue-palate seal. There is some debate about when most children make this change. Hanson (1988b) suggested that this happens by age 5 years. A review of published studies by Lebrun (1985), however, concluded that "tongue thrust swallowing is the rule rather than the exception in children under 10 years of age" (p. 307). This is supported by a more recent study by Bertolini and Paschoal (2001) who examined a random sample of 100 Brazilian children age 7–9 years. These authors reported that only 24 percent of those children presented with a normal adultlike swallow.

Tongue thrust during swallow and/or tongue fronting at rest can usually be identified by visual inspection. Mason (1988) has pointed out that two types of tongue fronting should be differentiated. The first is described as a *habit* and is seen in the absence of any morphological structural delimiting factors. The second is *obligatory* and may involve factors such as airway obstruction or enlarged tonsils with tongue thrusting being a necessary adaptation to maintain the size of the airway to pass food during swallow. Shelton (1989) has questioned oral myofunctional therapy for obligatory tongue fronting because of the poor prognosis for change.

Wadsworth, Maul, and Stevens (1998) indicated that tongue thrust swallow frequently co-occurred with resting forward-tongue posture (63 percent), open bite (86 percent), overjet (57 percent), abnormal palatal contour (60 percent), and open mouth posture

(39 percent). Marshall (1992) indicated that some children who tongue thrust are described as having a tongue that is "too big." However, she stated that low muscle tone (flaccidity) of the tongue is often the real problem. She also attributes tongue thrusting to tongue instability, jaw instability, allergies, and poor sensory awareness.

Impact of Tongue Thrust on Dentition

The current view is that the resting posture of the tongue affects the position of the teeth and jaws more than the tongue function during swallowing (tongue thrust) or speaking does (Proffit, 1986). Tongue thrusting may play a role in maintaining or influencing an abnormal dental pattern when an anterior resting tongue position is present. If the position of the tongue is forward (forward resting position) and between the anterior teeth at rest, this condition can impede normal teeth eruption and can result in an anterior open bite. However, tongue-thrusting patients, in the absence of an anterior tongue-resting position, are not thought to develop malocclusions. The pressure or force on dentition associated with tongue thrust during speaking and swallowing are of short duration and do not exert enough force on the dentition to cause problems of dental occlusion. Mason (1988) pointed out that individuals who exhibit a tongue thrust pattern and forward tongue posture would be much more likely to develop a dental malocclusion than when only a tongue thrust is present.

Tongue Thrust and Presence of Speech Sound Errors

Investigators have reported that speech sound errors, primarily sibilant distortions, occur more frequently in children who evidence tongue thrust than in those who do not. Fletcher, Casteel, and Bradley (1961) studied 1,615 schoolchildren ages 6 to 18 and found that children who demonstrated a tongue thrust swallow pattern were more likely to have associated sibilant distortions than children who did not. They also reported that participants with normal swallow patterns demonstrated a significant decrease in sibilant distortion with age, whereas tongue thrusters did not. A similar relationship between tongue thrust patterns and sibilant distortions was reported by Palmer (1962), Jann, Ward, and Jann (1964), and Wadsworth, Maul, and Stevens (1998). Palmer also reported errors on /t/, /d/, and /n/, and Jann, Ward, and Jann noted additional problems with /l/.

Subtelny and colleagues (1964) used radiographic techniques to examine the relationship between normal and abnormal oral morphology and /s/ production. Their participants, 81 adolescents and adults, were divided into three groups: (1) normal speakers with normal occlusion, (2) normal speakers with severe malocclusion, and (3) abnormal speakers with severe malocclusion. In contrast to earlier investigators, these authors found that the incidence of tongue thrusting and malocclusion in normal speakers was comparable to that in abnormal speakers. This finding is consistent with the reported developmental decrease in the reverse swallow pattern. By contrast, Khinda and Grewal (1999) examined the relationship among tongue thrusting, anterior open bite, and speech sound disorders. In a group of children with tongue thrust and normal occlusion, 30 percent demonstrated speech sound disorders compared to 95 percent of children with tongue thrusting combined with an anterior open bite. Thus, significantly more speech sound disorders were associated with the combination of tongue thrust and anterior open bite.

Treatment Issues

In a review of the 15 studies that examined the effectiveness of tongue thrust therapy, Hanson (1994) reported that 14 of the investigators indicated that swallowing and resting patterns were altered successfully. Most studies reviewed patients at least one year following the completion of treatment. Only one of the studies that Hanson reviewed (Subtelny, 1970) found therapy to be ineffective in correcting the disorders.

Other support for tongue thrust intervention has often come from clinical reports by clinicians who conduct oral myofunctional therapy. For example, Hilton (1984) stated, "In my experience, many tongue-fronting children who begin speech articulation therapy without having had the early sensorimotor and stretching activities of myotherapy . . . begin with an unnecessary handicap. . . . I provide every tongue-fronting speech articulation case these initial oral awareness, control, and flexibility exercises prior to initiation of the place-feature oriented therapy" (p. 51). Umberger and Johnston (1997) agreed that combined speech therapy and oral myofunctional therapy provides the best opportunity for improved speech accompanying reduced tongue thrusting.

1991 Position Statement

Over the years there has been some question about the role of the speech-language pathologist in oromyofunctional disorders. In 1991, the American Speech-Language-Hearing Association (ASHA) adopted a position statement which notes that: "Investigation, assessment, and treatment of oral myofunctional disorders are within the purview of speech-language pathology" (p. 7).

In addition, the ASHA position statement includes the following:

1. Oral myofunctional phenomena, including abnormal fronting (tongue thrust) of the tongue at rest and during swallowing, lip incompetency, and sucking habits, can be identified reliably. These conditions co-occur with speech misarticulations in some patients.
2. Tongue fronting may reflect learned behaviors, physical variables, or both.
3. Published research indicates that oral myofunctional therapy is effective in modifying disorders of tongue and lip posture and movement.
4. Investigation, assessment, and treatment of oral myofunctional disorders are within the purview of speech-language pathology.
5. The speech-language pathologist who desires to perform oral myofunctional services must have the required knowledge and skills to provide a high quality of treatment. The provision of oral myofunctional therapy remains an option of individual speech-language pathologists whose interests and training qualify them.
6. Evaluation and treatment should be interdisciplinary and tailored to the individual. The speech-language pathologist performing oral myofunctional therapy should collaborate with an orthodontist, pediatric dentist, or other dentists, and with medical specialists such as an otolaryngologist, pediatrician, or allergist, as needed.
7. Appropriate goals of oral myofunctional therapy should include the retraining of labial and lingual resting and functional patterns (including speech). The speech-language

pathologist's statements of treatment goals should avoid predictions of treatment outcome based on tooth position or dental occlusal changes.

8. Basic and applied research is needed on the nature and evaluation of oral myofunctions and the treatment of oral myofunctional disorders. (p. 7)

Summary

The following can be said about oral myofunctional disorders:

1. Existing data support the idea that abnormal labial-lingual posturing function can be identified, including abnormal fronting (tongue thrust) of the tongue at rest and during swallowing, lip incompetency, and sucking habits.
2. A forward tongue-resting posture has the potential, with or without a tongue thrust swallow, to be associated with malocclusions.
3. There is some evidence that an anterior tongue-resting posture or a tongue thrust swallow and speech production errors co-exist in some persons.
4. Oral myofunctional therapy can be effective in modifying disorders of tongue and lip posture and movement.
5. Assessment and treatment of oral myofunctional disorders that may include some nonspeech remediation are within the purview of speech-language pathology but should involve interdisciplinary collaboration.
6. More research is needed on the nature and evaluation of oral myofunctions and the treatment of such disorders.

COGNITIVE-LINGUISTIC FACTORS

A second category of variables that have been studied relative to a possible relationship to speech sound disorders is that of cognitive-linguistic factors. Historically, the field of communication sciences and disorders has been interested in the relationship between intelligence and the presence of speech sound disorders. In more recent years, investigators have sought to describe the relationship between disordered phonology and various aspects of cognitive-linguistic functioning. This not only is useful in determining the type of instructional/intervention program that may be most efficacious for the child's overall language development but also helps to provide a better understanding of interrelationships of various components of language behavior.

Intelligence

The relationship between intelligence (as measured by IQ tests) and speech sound disorders has been a subject of many years of investigation. Early studies in this area (Reid, 1947a, 1947b; Winitz, 1959a, 1959b) reported low positive correlations between scores obtained on intelligence tests and scores on articulation tests. Thus, in terms of the relationship between intelligence and articulation in children of normal intelligence, data have indicated that one is not a good predictor of the other. A second perspective on the relationship between intelligence and phonology may be gleaned from studies of the phonological status of developmentally delayed individuals. Prior to 1970, a number of studies were conducted to explore the prevalence of speech sound disorders in developmentally delayed individuals. In a study of 777 children with cognitive impairments (what we used to call *mental retardation*) whose chronological ages ranged from 6 to 16 years, Wilson (1966) concluded that "there is a high incidence of articulatory deviation in an educable mentally retarded population, and the incidence and degree of severity is closely related to mental-age levels" (p. 432). Wilson's findings also indicated that articulatory skills, which continue to improve until approximately age 8 in the normal population, continue to show improvement well beyond that age in the cognitively impaired population. Schlanger (1953) and Schlanger and Gottsleben (1957) reported similar findings. Of note is that Schlanger and Gottsleben reported that individuals with Down syndrome (DS) or whose etiologies were based on central nervous system impairment demonstrated the most pronounced speech delay.

As noted previously in our discussion of classification and genetic disorders, the developmental pattern for speech sounds in persons with cognitive impairments is generally similar to that of younger typically developing children (Bleile, 1982; Smith and Stoel-Gammon, 1983; Sommers, Reinhart, and Sistrunk, 1988). However, Kumin, Council, and Goodman (1994) reported a great deal of variability in the age at which sounds emerge in the speech of children with DS. They also stated that these children do "not appear to follow the same order as the norms for acquisition for typically developing children" (p. 300) and that emergence of some sounds were as much as five years later than the age in which normally developing children acquire a sound.

Shriberg and Widder (1990) indicated that findings from nearly four decades of speech research in cognitive impairment can be summarized as follows:

1. Persons with cognitive impairments are likely to have speech sound errors.
2. The most frequent type of error is likely to be deletions of consonants.
3. Errors are likely to be inconsistent.
4. The pattern of errors is likely to be similar to that of very young children or children with speech sound disorders of unknown origin.

Several investigators have explored the speech patterns of individuals with DS, as discussed earlier, who represent a genetically controlled subset of individuals with cognitive impairment. Sommers and colleagues (1988) reported that among the speech sound errors evidenced by children with DS, ages 13 to 22 years, some were phonemes frequently seen in error in 5- and 6-year-olds of normal intelligence (i.e., /r/, /r/ clusters, /s/, /s/ clusters, /z/, /θ/, and /v/). The authors indicated that these errors would appear to support the assertion that the phonological development of children with DS follows the same general pattern as that of normal children. However, they also reported that DS children evidenced errors not typically seen in normal 5- and 6-year-olds (e.g., deletion of alveolar stops and nasals). They further reported that imitative and spontaneous single-word picture-naming responses of their participants failed to identify many of the omission errors found in connected speech samples of their participants.

Rosin, Swift, Bless, and Vetter (1988) studied the articulation of children with Down syndrome as part of a study of overall communication profiles in this population. They compared a group of 10 DS male participants (chronological age, or C.A. = 14;7 years) with a control group of individuals with other forms of cognitive impairment and two control groups of individuals with normal intelligence representing two age levels (C.A. = 6;1, 15;5). They reported that as mental age (M.A.) increased across participants, intelligibility on a language sample increased. The DS group was also significantly different from the group of individuals with other forms of cognitive impairment and the younger age normal group (the older group was not compared) in terms of the percent of consonants correctly articulated on the *Goldman-Fristoe Test of Articulation.*

In addition to the speech measures mentioned, Rosin and colleagues (1988) also included other language measures, an oral motor evaluation, and aerodynamic measures in their assessment. They reported that the DS group had difficulty with production measures as demands for sequencing increased (e.g., consonant-vowel repetitions, length of words). The DS group needed a significant amount of cueing in order to articulate the target /pataka/ and had more variable intraoral pressure when producing /papapapa/. The mean length of utterance of the DS group was also significantly shorter than the mentally retarded and normal groups. The authors indicated that these findings are in accord with observations of others and suggested that sequencing underlies both oral motor control and language problems evidenced in DS participants.

Summary

Investigators concur that there is a low positive correlation between intelligence and speech sound production skill within the range of normal intelligence. Thus, it can be inferred that intellectual functioning is of limited importance as a contributing factor to articulatory skill and can be viewed as a poor predictor of articulation. On the other hand, a much higher correlation has been found between intelligence and articulation in the cognitively impaired population. The articulatory skills in a subgroup of individuals with cognitive impairment (those with DS) reflect error patterns similar to those seen in young normally developing children; however, they also evidence errors that are considered different or unusual when compared to normal developing children.

Language Development

In our discussion of the comorbidity of speech sound disorders and language disorders in Chapter 4, we noted that the speech sound system (phonology) is part of the language system, so we might expect an interaction between the phonology and other aspects of language. Investigators have attempted to explain the interaction between phonology and other language disorders and delays. Understanding the nature of this interaction might help us understand the role of language development in speech sound disorders.

One aspect of language that has received considerable attention is syntax. A common perception is that language is organized "from the top down"—in other words, a speaker goes from pragmatic intent, to semantic coding, to syntactic structure, to speech sound productions. Thus, higher-level linguistic formulations may ultimately be reflected in a child's speech sound output. If this theory is accurate, it might be expected that the more complex the syntax, the more likely a child is to produce speech sound errors. Schmauch, Panagos, and Klich (1978) conducted a study in which 5-year-old children with both speech sound and language problems were required to produce certain nouns (drawn from phonologic inventories) in three syntactic contexts—that is, an isolated noun phrase (the simplest context), a declarative sentence, and a passive sentence (the most complex context). These investigators reported a 17 percent increase in speech sound errors between the noun phrase and each of the sentence contexts. They also reported that later developing consonants were those most influenced by syntactical complexity and that the errors reflected quantitative rather than qualitative changes.

Panagos, Quine, and Klich (1979) conducted a follow-up study. This study required 5-year-old children to produce 15 target consonants in noun phrases, declarative sentences, and passive sentences; the consonants appeared in the initial and final word positions of one- and two-syllable words. Syntax was again found to significantly influence speech sound accuracy as did number of syllables in target words, but word position did not. The authors reported that two sources of complexity—phonologic (including difficulty with later developing consonants as well as specific contexts) and syntactic—combined additively to increase the number of speech sound errors. From the easiest context (final word position of one-syllable words in noun phrases) to the hardest (final word position of two-syllable word in passive sentences), there was a 36 percent increase in speech sound errors. The effects of grammatical complexity were cumulative.

A second perspective on the language-phonology relationship suggests that linguistic influences operate "from the bottom up." In this view, language expression is regulated by feedback (internal and external) from speech output. The feedback is needed to maintain syntactic processing and accuracy, especially when errors occur and must be corrected.

Panagos and Prelock (1982) tested the hypothesis that phonologic structure influences children's syntactic processing. They required 10 children with language disorders to produce sentences containing words with varying syllable complexity—that is, *simple*: "The (CV) kid (CVC) pushed (CVCC) the (CV) car (CVC) in (VC) the (CV) room (CVC)," and *complex*: "The (CV) chocolate (CVCVCVC) is (VC) in (VC) the (CV) napkin (CVCCVC)." When participants repeated sentences containing words of more syllable complexity, they made 27 percent more syntactic errors and supported the hypothesis of a bottom-up influence. In addition, sentence complexity was varied from unembedded ("The girl washed the doll in the tub") to right embedded ("The cook washed the pot the boy dropped") to center embedded ("The lady the uncle liked sewed the coat") in this study, Panagos and Prelock also reported that syntactic complexity further compounded production difficulties. From the unembedded to the center embedded, there was a 57 percent increase in phonologic errors, which would suggest a top-down relationship.

These findings support the view that a simultaneous top-down bottom-up relationship exists between language and phonology. Another way of expressing this concept is to consider that children with disordered language-phonology have a limited encoding capacity; the more this capacity is strained at one level or another, the higher the probability of delay in one component or more of language. It should be pointed out that the investigators who have examined the effect of complexity on the language-phonology relationship have typically employed elicited imitation tasks; thus, the investigators controlled complexity of utterances. It can be argued that with this type of performance task, structural simplifications are the expected outcomes. Elicited imitation tasks do not reflect the conditions present when a child is engaged in conversation; thus, we cannot assume that constraints of the nature demonstrated by Panagos and Prelock (1982) can predict behavior in a conversational context (Paul and Shriberg, 1984). The complex demands of conversational speech may actually tax a child's capacity even more and may yield an even higher frequency of speech sound errors as a result. Additional formal study is needed to examine this issue.

Morphology is another aspect of language that has been investigated relative to speech sounds. Paul and Shriberg (1982) studied phonologic productions as they relate to particular morphophonemic structures. Continuous speech samples were obtained from 30 children with speech delays. In this case, certain of their participants were able to produce complex morphosyntactic contexts spontaneously without speech sound simplifications. In other words, some of their participants were able to maintain a similar level of speech sound production in spite of producing more complex syntactic targets. They (Paul and Shriberg, 1984) suggested that children may "do things other than phonologic simplification in an attempt to control complexity in spontaneous speech" (p. 319). They summarized by indicating that some children with speech delays are at times able to allocate their limited linguistic resources to realize phonologic targets consistent with their linguistic knowledge in the context of free speech, even though at other times they may use avoidance strategies or other means of reducing the encoding load.

The simultaneous top-down bottom-up relationship between phonology and other aspects of language is reflected in a synergistic view of language (Schwartz, Leonard, Folger, and Wilcox, 1980; Shriner, Holloway, and Daniloff, 1969). This perspective assumes a complex interaction and interdependency of various aspects of linguistic behaviors including language and phonology.

Several investigators have studied whether intervention focused on one aspect of the linguistic domain (e.g., morphosyntax) facilitates gains in an untreated domain (e.g., phonology). Matheny and Panagos (1978) looked at the effects of syntactic programming on phonologic improvement and the effects of phonologic programming on syntactic improvement in school-age children. Each group made the greatest gains in the treated domain as compared to a control group but also made improvements in the untreated domain. Wilcox and Morris (1995) reported similar findings. They noted that, based on comparison to a control group, children with speech sound and language impairments who participated in a preschool language-focused program made gains not only in language but also in phonology. In a study based on two siblings from a set of triplets, Hoffman, Norris, and Monjure (1990) also found that a narrative intervention program facilitated gains in both language and phonology for one brother while gains only in phonology were achieved by the brother who received only phonologic instruction.

Tyler and colleagues (2002) reported one of the more comprehensive studies of cross-domain improvement between language (morphosyntax) and phonology. They compared treatment outcomes for three groups of children, all of whom evidenced both speech sound and morphosyntactic disorders: (1) group 1 received morphosyntactic instruction for a 12-week block followed by 12 weeks in phonology, (2) group 2 reversed the order of the 12-week blocks, and (3) group 3 served as a control group. These investigators reported that in comparison to the control group, both interventions were effective; however, only morphosyntactic instruction led to cross-domain improvement (i.e., language therapy improved phonology but not the reverse). These findings have not been supported in all investigations of cross-domain improvements. Tyler and Watterson (1991) reported that participants with a severe overall language and phonological disorder made improvements in language when presented with language therapy; however, gains were not made in phonology (they actually reported a tendency for performance to become slightly worse). On the other hand, participants with mild-moderate but unequal impairments in phonology and language improved in both areas when presented with phonologic therapy. The authors suggested that a language-based intervention program may not result in improvement in phonologic as well as other language skills for children whose disorders are severe and comparable in each domain. However, children with less severe problems in one or both domains may benefit from therapy with either a language or phonology focus.

Fey and colleagues (1994) conducted an experimental treatment program with 26 participants, ages 44 to 70 months, with impairments in both grammar and phonology. Eighteen children received language intervention (grammar facilitation) in accord with one or the other of two designated teaching approaches; eight children served as controls. Results indicated that despite a strong effect for intervention on the children's grammatical output, there were no direct effects on the participants' speech sound productions. The authors indicated that trying to improve intelligibility by focusing on grammar is not defensible for children in the age and severity range of their participants. They further indicated that for most children who have impairments in both speech and language, intervention needs to focus on both areas. Although this study examined only one form of language intervention that anticipated phonologic effects, these data provide strong evidence that in children ages 4 to 6, treatment approaches should address phonologic problems directly if changes in phonologic performance are to be expected.

Tyler and colleagues (2002) have indicated that differences in findings between their study and that of the Fey and colleagues (1994) study may be due to differences in goal selection, intervention techniques, or measures used to determine changes in phonology. Further clinical studies are needed to clarify the synergistic relationship between language and phonology, including cross-domain improvements. The influence of age, nature and severity of both language and speech sound disorders, treatment approaches employed, and measures used to ascertain progress all need further study.

Summary

Language and phonology may be related in what has been termed a *synergistic relationship*. Investigators face the challenge of further defining the intricacies of the relationship between phonology and other linguistic behaviors in terms of both development and clinical management of disorders. It appears that for children with language impairment and moderate to severe speech sound disorders, direct phonologic intervention may be required to impact phonology. Further research in cross-domain generalization is needed to guide clinical practice in this area.

Academic Performance

The relationship between speech sound disorders and academic performance is of interest to clinicians working with school-age children because oral language skills are fundamental to the development of many literacy-related academic skills such as reading and spelling. Because the use of sounds in symbolic lexical units is a task common to learning to speak, read, and write, researchers for many years have studied the co-occurrence of reading and speech sound disorders and have discussed possible common factors underlying the acquisition of literacy and other language-related skills.

Hall (1938) compared 21 children with speech sound disorders of unknown origin with a normal control group on the *Gates Silent Reading Test* and the *Iowa Silent Reading Test* and reported no significant differences in silent reading achievement between the two groups. Everhart (1953) also used the *Gates Silent Reading Test* and reported no significant relationship between speech sound disorders and reading ability, although boys with normal articulation tended to obtain higher reading scores than the overall group of children with speech sound disorders.

Fitzsimons (1958) and Weaver, Furbee, and Everhart (1960) studied the relationship between reading readiness and speech sound disorders. Fitzsimons reported that below grade-level scores were more frequent among children with speech sound disorders than among those with normal speech development. Weaver and colleagues reported a significant relationship between articulatory performance and reading readiness as well as between articulatory performance and reading scores.

Flynn and Byrne (1970) took a different approach to this question. They compared articulatory performance of 52 advanced and 42 delayed third-grade readers on the *Templin-Darley Tests of Articulation*. Those who scored 4.2 or higher on the *Iowa Test of Basic Skills* were classified as advanced readers; those who scored 2.2 or lower were classified as delayed readers. The authors reported no significant difference between the two groups in articulation test scores.

Lewis and Freebairn-Farr (1991) examined the performance of individuals with a history of a preschool speech sound disorder on measures of phonology, reading, and spelling. Participant groups included at least 17 individuals from each of the following categories: preschool, school age, adolescence, and adulthood. Normal comparison groups at each age level were also tested. Significant differences between the disordered and normal groups were reported on the reading and spelling measures for the school-age group and on the reading measure for the adult group. Although the reading and spelling measures for the adolescent group and the spelling measure for the adult group did not reach significance, the trend was for the individuals with histories of disorders to perform more poorly than individuals who are normal. Data also indicated that participants who evidenced a speech sound disorder accompanied by additional language problems performed more poorly on measures of reading and spelling than participants with speech sound disorders only. This conclusion was also reached in a study by Raitano and colleagues (2004). The authors of these two latter studies indicated that children evidencing phonologic impairment are at risk for reading and spelling problems in school and may have special educational needs.

Felsenfeld, McGue, and Broen (1995) compared 24 adults with a documented history of a phonologic-language disorder that persisted from childhood until at least grade 11 (proband group), against 28 adults who were known to have had normal abilities as children (control group). These adults had originally been part of a large study in the 1960s (Templin and Glaman, 1976). Included among the comparison variables were several categorized under "educational performance." Results revealed that 28 percent of the children of the proband group repeated at least one grade compared to 0 percent from the control group. Likewise, 22 percent of the proband group had as children received academic tutoring compared to 4 percent of the control group. Speech treatment had been received by 33 percent of the proband group and 0 percent of the control group. Templin and Glaman also reported that half of the school-age children who were receiving speech treatment also either participated in remedial academic services and/or had repeated a grade. Recently, Overby, Trainin, Bosma Smit, Bernthal, and Nelson (2012) examined data from 272 individuals with a wide range of speech sound skills who were also part of the Templin and Glaman (1976) study; this dataset is now referred to as the *Templin archive* (2004) and is available to researchers interested in speech and language development. This archive offers a unique window on SSD because the data were collected prior to the time when school speech services were mandated by law. Given that few services were being provided, the impact of speech sound production skill on academic performance could be examined independent of speech intervention. Overby and colleagues looked at data on speech sound production skills as measured using the *Templin Prekindergarten Imitation Articulation Test (TPIAT),* which had been administered in the fall of their kindergarten year. Reading outcomes in first and second grade as well as spelling outcomes at third grade were examined. Findings indicated that the children with the poorest speech sound production skill in kindergarten had the poorest reading and spelling outcomes, and those with the highest speech sound production skill had the best reading and spelling outcomes.

Although interest has traditionally focused on the co-occurrence of reading-spelling and speech sound disorders in children, more recently there has also been interest in children's ability to process phonology as part of various reading tasks. More specifically, some students with reading disabilities may lack awareness of individual sounds, have difficulty dividing words into sounds and recalling sound-symbol relationships (phonologic awareness). Catts (1986) found that children with reading disabilities may have problems with these linguistically oriented tasks yet not reflect phonologic impairment.

Investigators have attempted to apply phonologic concepts to aid in the understanding of reading and spelling disorders. This is based on the assumption that acquisition of speaking, reading, and writing skills involves the analysis of sounds in lexical units, which may be related to underlying cognitive-linguistic processes. In particular, the concepts of phonologic processes and underlying internal knowledge of the sound system have been employed to aid in understanding the development of spelling and reading skills (Hoffman and Norris, 1989).

Liberman and Shankweiler (1985) indicated that reading success was related to the degree to which children were aware of "underlying phonologic structure" and that poor readers often were unable to segment words into their phonologic constituents. O'Conner and Jenkins (1999) reported that performance on phonological awareness tasks (e.g., initial sound identification, rhyme production, phoneme segmentation) in kindergarten predicted differences in reading achievement at the end of first grade and was reliable in identifying children who would later be diagnosed as having a reading disability.

Hoffman and Norris (1989) analyzed spelling errors of 45 elementary school children for evidence of phonologic process patterns. They reported that many of the spelling errors involved both syllable reduction and feature changes similar to the sound simplifications seen in the speech of young children with normal speech development. They further indicated that even though children had acquired normal speech, they exhibited spelling errors similar to those seen in the speech simplifications of younger children. A similar conclusion was reached by Clarke-Klein and Hodson (1995) who tested 29 third-grade children with a history of speech sound disorders; findings also indicated that the frequency of errors was significantly higher than that seen in a comparison group of 32 peers with normal speech sound development. Hoffman (1990) related specific types of developmental spelling patterns to stages of normal phonologic acquisition. For example, "precommunicative spellings" (seemingly random selection of letters of the alphabet to represent words) were described as parallel to the random sound productions of babbling. "Semiphonetic spellings" (letters used to represent sounds, but only some of the sounds are represented, for example, *E* for *eagle*) were described as parallel to the stage in which children delete syllables or segments and substitute sound classes for one another. Hoffman also indicated that because the speech-language pathologist is the school-based professional who has the most detailed knowledge of sound perception and production, phonologic organization, stages of acquisition, and methods of phonologic description, he or she is in a good position to serve as a resource to teachers regarding the application of phonologic concepts to the understanding of spelling errors. Chapter 12 focuses on phonological awareness and its relationship to literacy and the role of the speech-language pathologist in literacy.

Summary

Research investigations that have focused on the co-occurrence of speech sound disorders and literacy impairments indicate a relationship between these disorders in some children. Young children with severe speech sound and co-occurring language disorders may be at greater risk for academic problems. There may be a familial propensity for such difficulties. The role of "phonologic awareness" in the development of reading and spelling skills has been the focus of much study in the last decade. It appears that a relationship between phonological awareness and later literacy skills exists and that children with speech sound disorders are at risk for problems in both areas. Parallels have been made between the use of phonologic processes and stages in the acquisition of oral language and acquisition of reading and spelling skills. Speech-language pathologists are in a unique position to offer assistance to the classroom teacher in their efforts to assist children at risk for reading and/or spelling problems.

PSYCHOSOCIAL FACTORS

Psychosocial factors represent a third cluster of variables that have long fascinated clinicians in terms of their potential relationship to phonology. Age, gender, family history, and socioeconomic status have been studied in an effort to better understand factors that may precipitate or otherwise be associated with phonologic impairment.

Age

Investigations have revealed that children's articulatory and phonologic skills continue to improve until approximately 8 years of age, by which time the normal child has acquired most aspects of the adult sound system.

Speech-language pathologists have shown a particular interest in the effect of maturation on children identified as having speech sound disorders. Roe and Milisen (1942) sampled 1,989 children in grades 1 through 6 who had never received any formal speech therapy. They found that the mean number of articulation errors decreased between grades 1 and 2, grades 2 and 3, and grades 3 and 4. In contrast, the difference in the mean number of errors between grades 4 and 5 and grades 5 and 6 was not significant. The authors concluded that maturation was responsible for improvement in articulation performance between grades 1 and 4 but was not an appreciable factor in articulation improvement in grades 5 and 6.

Sayler (1949) assessed articulation in 1,998 students in grades 7 through 12 as they read sentences orally. His findings indicated a slight decrease in the mean number of articulation errors at each subsequent grade level, but because the improvement in speech sound productions was so small, he concluded that maturation does not appear to be an appreciable factor in improvement in the middle school and secondary grades.

The previously discussed National Speech and Hearing Survey (NSHS), as reported in St. Louis, Ruscello, and Lundeen (1992), sampled more than 38,000 school-age children prior to widespread availability of speech-language services. Findings indicated a gradual decline in the occurrence of speech sound disorders from kindergarten through twelfth grade. Thus, many speech problems appear to improve without formal treatment.

Finally, McKinnon, McLeod, and Reilly (2007) conducted a survey of teachers serving more than 10,000 Australian schoolchildren in kindergarten through grade 6. Findings indicated a decreasing proportion of speech sound disorders across grade levels.

Summary

A positive correlation between improvement in articulation skills and age in typically developing children appears to exist. Maturation generally is not a factor in speech sound acquisition after age 9 in typically developing children.

Gender

Child development specialists have long been interested in contrasts between males and females in speech sound acquisition, and, likewise, speech-language pathologists have investigated the relationship between gender and articulation status. Research in this area has focused on a comparison of (1) phoneme acquisition in males and females and (2) the incidence of speech sound disorders in males and females.

Dawson (1929) examined the articulatory skills of 200 children from grades 1 through 12 and reported that until approximately age 12, girls were slightly superior to boys. Templin (1963) reported similar findings: "In articulation development, girls consistently are found to be slightly accelerated . . . in all instances the differences are relatively small and often are not statistically significant" (p. 13).

Smit, Hand, Freilinger, Bernthal, and Bird (1990) conducted a large-scale normative study of speech sound development in children ages 3 through 9 from Iowa and Nebraska. They reported that the Iowa-Nebraska girls appeared to acquire sounds at somewhat earlier ages than boys through age 6. The differences reached statistical significance only at age 6 and younger and not in every preschool age group. Kenney and Prather (1986), who elicited multiple productions of frequent error sounds, reported significant differences favoring girls aged 3 through 5.

Speech surveys conducted by Hall (1938), Mills and Streit (1942), Morley (1952), Everhart (1960), and Hull, Mielke, Timmons, and Willeford (1971) indicated that the incidence of speech sound disorder was higher in males than females regardless of the age group studied. Smit and colleagues (1990) stated that "it is a well-known fact that boys are at much greater risk than girls for delayed speech, and this propensity continues to be reported" (p. 790).

Summary

The sex of a child appears to have some impact on speech sound acquisition. At very young ages, females tend to be slightly ahead of males, but the differences disappear as the children get older. As a consequence, many current tests of speech sound acquisition include separate normative data for males and females. Gender differences are reflected by the identification of significantly more male than female children as having speech sound disorders.

Family Background

Researchers have been interested in the influence of family background, both environmental and biological, and how it may affect a child's speech and language development. In the following paragraphs, we review literature related to family background and phonology organized around three topics: (1) socioeconomic status, (2) family tendencies, and (3) sibling influences.

Socioeconomic Status

The socioeconomic status (SES) of a child's family, as measured by parents' educational background, occupation, income, and/or location of family residence, is a significant part of the child's environment. Because some behavioral deficiencies occur more frequently in lower socioeconomic environments, SES has been of interest to speech-language clinicians as a possible factor in speech and language development.

Early studies of this question (Everhart, 1953, 1956; Prins, 1962a; Templin, 1957; Weaver et al., 1960) relied on parental occupation as the sole measure of SES and yielded conflicting findings. The studies by Everhart and that of Prins reported no significant association, but the studies by Templin and by Weaver and colleagues both indicated that the poorest articulation skills were exhibited by those from the lowest SES households.

Two more recent studies have measured SES differently. Smit and colleagues (1990) in the Iowa-Nebraska normative study used parental education level and reported no significant relationship to speech sound performance. A similar conclusion was reached by Keating, Turrell, and Ozanne (1995) with data from the Australian Health Survey, which used a combination of household income as well as parental occupation and education to index SES. Based on the study of more than 12,000 children age birth to 14 years, the authors also reported no significant association between SES and child speech disorders (which included both speech sound disorders and stuttering). These findings overall suggest that speech sound disorders are not that strongly associated with low SES (i.e., growing up in a low SES household does not suggest a problem with speech sounds). However, when combined with other factors, low SES may interact to result in a speech sound disorder. Recall our previous discussion in Chapter 4 of how children with frequent otitis media who also grow up in low SES households are at significantly increased risk of developing a speech sound problem.

Familial Tendencies

It is not uncommon for speech-language pathologists to observe a family history of speech and language disorders. Neils and Aram (1986) obtained reports from the parents of 74 preschool language-disordered children and indicated that 46 percent reported that other family members had histories of speech and language disorders. Of this group, 55 percent were reported to have speech sound disorders, the most prevalent familial disorder reported. Shriberg and Kwiatkowski (1994) reported data from 62 children, ages 3 to 6 years with developmental phonologic disorders. They found that 39 percent of the children had one member of the family with a similar speech problem, whereas an additional 17 percent (total = 56 percent) had more than one family member with a similar speech problem.

Two studies of twins have been reported that contribute to our understanding of familial influences, including genetic factors that may relate to speech sound disorders. Matheny and Bruggeman (1973) studied 101 same-sex twin sets, 22 opposite-sex twin sets, and 94 siblings between the ages of 3 and 8 years. An articulation screening test was administered to each child. Monozygotic twins' articulation screening correlated more closely with each other than did dizygotic twins' scores. The authors concluded that there is a strong hereditary influence on articulation status. In addition, sex differences were found to favor females. Locke and Mather (1987) examined speech sound productions in 13 monozygotic and 13 dizygotic twin sets. They reported more phonetic concordance in the monozygotic than the dizygotic twins (i.e., the identical twins were more similar in their errors patterns than the fraternal twins).

Lewis, Ekelman, and Aram (1989) compared sibling articulation status for a group of children identified as evidencing a severe speech sound disorder with a group who reflected normal speech development. Results revealed that the siblings of the children with communication disorders performed more poorly than control siblings on phonology and reading measures. Disordered participants' phonologic skills correlated positively with those of their siblings, whereas controls' scores did not. Families of children with disorders reported significantly more members with speech and language disorders and dyslexia than did families of controls. Sex differences were reflected in the incidence but not in the severity or type of disorder present. The authors concluded that their findings suggested a familial basis for at least some forms of severe speech sound disorders.

A familial basis of phonologic impairments is also supported by the findings from the previously mentioned study by Felsenfeld, McGue, and Broen (1995). Children of the 24 "disordered" participants performed significantly more poorly on all tests of articulation and expressive language functioning and were significantly more likely to have received articulation treatment than were the children of the 28 control participants.

A 2007 study by Lewis, Freebairn, Hansen, Miscimarra, Iyengar, and Taylor compared parents of children with speech sound disorders who themselves had histories of speech sound disorders with parents of similar children without such histories. The parents with histories of speech sound disorders themselves performed significantly more poorly on standardized tests of spoken language and spelling.

It may be inferred from these studies that genetic or biological inheritance factors may precipitate some speech sound disorders, yet it is often difficult to separate environmental from genetic/biological influences. Parlour and Broen (1991) reported on a study that examined environmental influences on speech sound disorders. Their research was predicated on the possibility that individuals who themselves experienced significant speech and language disorders as children are likely to provide a less than optimal cultural or linguistic milieu for their own families.

Using the same data set as that in the Felsenfeld and colleagues (1995) study mentioned above, Parlour and Broen (1991) employed two environmental measures, the *Preschool HOME Scale* and the *Modified Templin Child-Rearing Questionnaire.* These measures allowed them to ascertain qualitative aspects of a child's environment including physical, emotional, and cognitive support available to preschool children, and child-rearing practices based on direct observation of the examiner, parental reports, and parental responses to a written questionnaire.

The two groups performed in a comparable manner for all of the environmental domains sampled with one exception, acceptance, which assessed disciplinary practices. Parlour and Broen (1991) reported that families with a history of speech sound disorders relied more on physical punishment than did control families. In terms of future research efforts, the authors suggested that although differences were generally not significant between the groups, the disordered group received lower mean scores than controls on each of the *HOME* subscales, suggesting that some subtle differences may have been present, particularly for domains involving the use of punishment, learning, and language stimulation.

Recent advances in molecular genetics are allowing us to look more directly for genetic differences in individuals with speech sound disorders. Lewis (2009) reminds us of the complexity of the search because genes don't directly lead to the disorder but rather direct the production of proteins that then influence various aspects of development. She also points out that speech and language behaviors are likely related to a variety of neurological and biochemical processes, each of which may be active to differing degrees at different points in the developmental period. Those processes may also be involved with various speech and language behaviors (recall our discussion of comorbidity in Chapter 4). It is likely, therefore, that multiple genes are involved. Despite the complexity of the task, Lewis notes that candidate gene regions on several different chromosomes (e.g., 1, 3, 6, 7, 15) have been implicated as possible sources of speech sound production disorders by different investigator groups. Detailed discussion of this still very preliminary work is beyond the scope of the current text.

Sibling Influences

Another factor of interest to investigators of speech sound disorders has been sibling number and birth order. Because the amount of time that parents can spend with each child decreases with each child added to a family, some clinicians have questioned whether sibling order is related to articulatory development. Koch (1956) studied the relationships between certain speech and voice characteristics in young children and siblings in two-child families. In this study, 384 children between 5 and 6 years old were divided into 24 subgroups matched individual by individual on the basis of age, socioeconomic class, and residence. Data on speech and voice characteristics consisted of teachers' ratings. Koch reported that firstborn children had better articulation than secondborn, and the wider the age difference between a child and his or her sibling, the better the child's articulation. Likewise, Davis (1937) reported that children without siblings demonstrated superior artic-ulatory performance to children with siblings and to twins. On the other hand, Wellman, Case, Mengert, and Bradbury (1931) did not find a significant relationship between the number of siblings and level of articulation skill for 3-year-olds.

Twins have been reported to present unique patterns of speech sound acquisition (Perkins, 1977; Powers, 1957 Winitz, 1969). From birth, twins receive speech stimulation not only from others within their environment but also from each other. Powers indicated that the "emotional ties of twins, too, are likely to be closer than those of singled siblings, which further augments their interdependence in speech" (p. 868). It is not uncommon for twins to reflect common phonologic patterns and use similar phonologic patterns. Schwartz and colleagues (1980) reported, however, that in the very early stages of phonologic acqui-sition (the first 50 words), similarities in phonemes used, including phonologic patterns and lexical items, were not present. Unique patterns of speech are occasionally found in twins 2 years and older who have little resemblance to adult models and have meaning only to the twins; these are termed *idioglossia*.

Summary

Little relationship exists between socioeconomic status and speech sound disorders based on available reports. Although a higher number of misarticulating children tend to be found in lower socioeconomic groups (especially children under 4 years), socioeconomic status by itself does not appear to contribute significantly to the presence of a speech sound disorder.

Studies of phonologic development in twins as well as in families with a history of phonologic impairment suggest familial propensity toward the presence of such a disor-der. Investigations examining phonologic status and sibling relationships are limited, but findings have been fairly consistent. Firstborn and only children exhibit somewhat better articulation performance than children who have older siblings or twins during the preschool years. The age span between siblings also appears to affect phonologic proficiency with bet-ter articulation associated with wider age differences. One can speculate that the firstborn or only children receive better speech models and more stimulation than children who have older siblings. The possibility also exists that older siblings produce "normal" developmen-tal phonologic errors and, thus, at points in time present imperfect speech models to younger siblings. Unique patterns of sound productions have been reported in twins; reasons for these patterns are speculative and tend to focus on the stimulation each twin receives from the other. Unique speech patterns have, however, been reported, even in very young twins.

Genetic studies offer a tantalizing promise for tracking down the ultimate cause of at least some SSD. Preliminary work in this area suggests we may not be far from identifying specific genes involved.

The preceding discussion suggests a tension between the influence of the family environment (siblings, birth order, parenting style, SES) and genetic endowment on SSD.

Neither likely tells the whole story. It is probable that speech sound development and disorders reflect a complex interaction among many of these factors.

Personality

The relationship between personality characteristics and phonologic behavior has been investigated to determine whether particular personality patterns are likely to be associated with speech sound disorders. Researchers have examined not only the child's personality traits but also those of the child's parents, using various assessment tools.

Bloch and Goodstein (1971) concluded, in a review of the literature, that personality traits and emotional adjustment of individuals with speech sound disorders have shown contradictory findings and attributed this to two major problems with the investigations: (1) the criteria for defining articulatory impairment has varied from one study to the next and (2) the validity and reliability of tools or instruments used to assess personality and adjustment have varied.

In a causal-correlates profile based on 178 children with developmental phonologic disorders, Shriberg and Kwiatkowski (1994) presented data on psychosocial inputs (parental behaviors) and psychosocial behaviors (child characteristics) that were descriptive of this population. Of the parents, 27 percent were judged to be either somewhat or considerably ineffective in terms of behavioral management, and 17 percent were either somewhat or considerably overly concerned about their child's problem. An even smaller percentage of parents indicated that it was their perception that their child had difficulty with initial acceptance by peers. Over half of the children (51 percent) were described as somewhat too sensitive (easily hurt feelings), and an additional 14 percent were described as overly sensitive (very easily hurt feelings). Shriberg and Kwiatkowski reported that their descriptive data indicated that "a significant number of children with developmental phonologic disorders experience psychosocial difficulties" (p. 115). They indicated, however, that one cannot be completely certain that sampling biases did not inflate the magnitudes of the findings or whether the participants would differ significantly from data in a group without speech delay.

Summary

Although certain personality characteristics have been linked to some children with developmental phonologic impairments, no clear picture of personality variance from normals has emerged in this population. Likewise, certain parental/home variables have been associated with this population, but the strength of that association is not strong. Additional studies involving normal–disordered child comparisons are necessary before a definitive statement regarding this causal-correlate can be made.

Pacifier Use

A final topic is one frequently raised by parents and others. Is the use of a pacifier (also called a *dummy* in Australia and the United Kingdom) related to speech sound disorders in some children? Does the use of such devices interfere with speech sound acquisition in some way? An excellent review by Baker (2002) of the pros and cons of such devices suggested little direct evidence of their influence on speech development. Two more recent reports offer some insight into this question. Fox, Dodd, and Howard (2002) compared 65 German-speaking children age 2;7 to 7;2 with speech sound disorders against 48 age-matched typically developing children. Findings indicated that children with speech sound disorders were significantly more likely to have used a bottle as a pacifier (i.e., not just for feeding). The groups did not differ on use of pacifiers alone. A study in Chile by Barbosa and colleagues (2009) evaluated questionnaire data collected from parents of 128 children age 3 to 5 years. The authors concluded that for the 42 percent of the children who used pacifiers, there was a threefold increase in the odds of developing a speech sound disorder.

Although this limited group of reports suggests that children who use pacifiers may be at increased risk for speech sound disorders, definitive conclusions are premature. Additional study is clearly warranted.

CONCLUSION

A great deal has been discovered about factors related to speech sound disorders in children that can assist the speech-language pathologist in assessing phonologic status, planning remediation programs, and counseling clients and their parents. Yet many questions remain unanswered. One truth that emerges from the literature, however, is the absence of any one-to-one correspondence between the presence of a particular factor and the precise nature of most individuals' phonologic status. Prediction of cause-effect relationships represents a scientific ideal, but determination of such relationships in the realm of human behavior, including communication disorders, is often difficult. The likelihood of multiple factors being involved in cases of SSD complicates the search for such relationships. However, the progress being made suggests that they can ultimately be teased apart.

QUESTIONS FOR CHAPTER 5

1. What is the relationship of speech sound perception and speech sound errors?

2. What is the relationship between phonological disorders and morphosyntactic language impairments?

3. How is each of the following factors related to clinical phonology and speech production?

   a. Otitis media

   b. Tongue thrusting

   c. Missing teeth

   d. Cognitive impairment

   e. Lower socioeconomic status

   k. Family history of phonological difficulties

   i. Removal of part of the tongue

CHAPTER 6

Speech Sound Assessment Procedures

NICHOLAS W. BANKSON
James Madison University

JOHN E. BERNTHAL
University of Nebraska–Lincoln

PETER FLIPSEN JR.
Idaho State University

SPEECH SOUND SAMPLING

One of the unique contributions of the field of speech-language pathology to the assessment of verbal behavior is the development of speech sound *assessment* instruments. For several decades, the assessment of speech sounds, also referred to as *phonological* or *articulation assessments,* have remained almost the exclusive domain of speech-language pathologists, although linguists, child development specialists, psychologists, pediatricians, and special and regular educators also use such tools.

Evaluation of an individual's phonological status typically involves description of his or her speech sound productions and comparing them to that of the adult standard of the speaker's linguistic community. We call this type of analysis a *relational analysis,* a procedure that is designed to determine which sounds are produced correctly. For young children or speakers with limited phonological repertoires, the speech sound system is often described independently of the adult standard, in which case the examiner simply wants to know what speech sounds are produced regardless of whether they are used correctly or not. We call this an *independent analysis.*

Phonological assessment is often done in the context of a comprehensive communication evaluation that also includes assessment of voice quality, resonance, fluency, syntax, semantics, pragmatics, discourse, and prosodic aspects of language. Additional related measures such as hearing testing and an oral mechanism examination are usually included in a comprehensive communication evaluation/assessment. Although some clinicians have differentiated between phonological delay (children whose speech sound errors are similar to those found in younger normally developing children) and phonological disorders (children whose speech sound errors differ from normal developing children), we do not differentiate between the two here. In reality, most children with multiple misarticulations have errors that fall into both categories.

Phonological assessment is used to describe the phonological status of an individual and to

1. Determine whether his or her speech sound system is sufficiently different from normal development to warrant intervention.
2. Determine treatment direction, including target behaviors and strategies to be used in the management of the client.
3. Make prognostic statements relative to phonological change with or without intervention/therapy.
4. Monitor change in phonological performance across time.
5. Identify factors that might be related to the presence or maintenance of a phonological disability/delay.

In addition, the speech-language pathologist (SLP) might be called on to identify and describe dialectal variations of General American English. The need to describe such differences usually follows a request or inquiry for accent reduction by individuals who speak a regional or cultural dialect or for whom English is a second language. In the case of a client referred for a speech sound evaluation whose speech and language patterns reflect dialectal differences, the SLP must be able to differentiate which phonological characteristics can be attributed to dialect differences and which reflect a speech sound disorder.

The two primary purposes of a phonological assessment are to determine whether an individual needs instruction related to correct production and use of speech sounds, and if so, the direction of treatment. To make these determinations, the clinician engages in a multistep process that involves sampling the client's speech through a variety of procedures, analyzing the data gathered, interpreting the data that have been analyzed, and then making clinical recommendations. In this chapter, we discuss various sampling and testing procedures and discuss factors and issues that should be considered when analyzing and interpreting speech sound samples. This chapter focuses on impairments rather than accent/dialect reduction because the latter is discussed in detail in Chapter 11. In Chapter 7, you will find a case history of a child to whom procedures discussed in this chapter are applied.

SCREENING FOR SPEECH SOUND DISORDERS

A complete or comprehensive speech sound assessment, including analysis and interpretation of results, is not something that can be done quickly. Because of the time required for a complete speech sound assessment, clinicians often do a screening to determine whether a more comprehensive phonological assessment is warranted. Screening procedures are not designed to determine the need or direction of therapy but to identify individuals who merit further evaluation from those for whom further assessment is not indicated. Screening might be used for (1) children at a preschool or "kindergarten roundup" to determine whether they have age-appropriate speech sound production skills, (2) children in grade 3 (by which time maturation should have resolved most developmental errors), (3) individuals preparing for occupations, such as broadcast journalism, that require specific speech performance standards, and (4) clients referred for an undefined but suspected speech and language impairment to determine their phonological status.

Instruments used for screening consist of a limited sample of speech sound productions, which can usually be administered in 5 minutes or less. Screening measures can be categorized as informal or formal. *Informal measures* are often used when people wish to develop their own screening tools to meet their particular needs. *Formal* measures are often employed when users desire established norms or testing methodologies that are more uniform.

Informal Screening Measures

The examiner usually devises informal screening measures that are tailored to the population being screened. Although informal procedures can be easily and economically devised, they do not include standardized administration procedures or normative data, which are characteristics of formal screening measures. For example, in an informal screening procedure that could be used with a group of kindergarten children, the examiner asks each child to respond to the following:

1. Tell me your name. Where do you live?
2. Can you count to 10? Tell me the days of the week.
3. What do you like to watch on TV?

The focus of these questions is to engage a child in conversation so that one can obtain a sample of typical speech sound productions.

If the subjects are adults, the examiner might ask them to do one or all of the following:

1. Read sentences designed to elicit several productions of frequently misarticulated sounds, such as /s/, /r/, /l/, and /θ/. For example, "I saw Sally at her seaside house; Rob ran around the orange car."
2. Read a passage with a representative sample of English speech sounds, such as the "Grandfather Passage."

   Grandfather Passage. You wish to know all about my grandfather. Well, he is nearly 93 years old, yet he still thinks as swiftly as ever. He dresses himself in an old black frock coat, usually several buttons missing. A long beard clings to his chin, giving those who observe him a pronounced feeling of the utmost respect. When he speaks, his voice is just a bit cracked and quivers a bit. Twice each day he plays skillfully and with zest upon a small organ. Except in winter when the snow or ice prevents, he slowly takes a short walk in the open air each day. We have often urged him to walk more and smoke less, but he always answers, "Banana oil." Grandfather likes to be modern in his language.
3. Engage in an informal conversation about topics of interest such as a recent trip or a current event.

The examiner determines the criteria for the failure of an informal screening. An often-used rule of thumb is "If in doubt, refer for further testing." In other words, if an examiner is uncertain whether the client's speech sound system is not appropriate for his or her age and/or linguistic community, a referral should be made for a more complete assessment. The examiner can also choose to predetermine or establish ahead of time some performance standards on the screening instrument to help identify those to refer for further testing. Those individuals with the greatest need for additional testing and probable intervention are usually obvious to the examiner from even a small sample of their speech and language.

Formal Screening Measures

Formal screening measures include published elicitation procedures for which normative data and/or cutoff scores are often available. These formal measures are usually one of two types: tests that (1) are related to or are part of a more comprehensive speech sound assessment and (2) screen phonology as well as other aspects of speech and language. Tests designed explicitly for screening phonology are often used when screening speech sounds is a primary goal. Those instruments that combine phonological screening with other aspects of language screening are most commonly used for more general communication disorders screening in which information on phonology is just part of the communication assessment that is of interest.

The following is an example of a formal screening measure that is part of a more comprehensive assessment of phonology.

Diagnostic Screen (Dodd, Hua, Crosbie, Holm, and Ozanne, 2006)

The *Diagnostic Screen* is related to *The Diagnostic Evaluation of Articulation and Phonology (DEAP)* instrument. The screening portion includes 22 pictures that are imitated following examiner production (model), requires 5 minutes to administer, and provides an indication of whether further assessment could be appropriate. The authors indicate that the screening test is especially useful with children who are shy, immature, or have a short attention span.

The following tests include screening of phonology as part of an overall speech and language screening.

Fluharty Preschool Speech and Language Screening Test–Second Edition (Fluharty, 2001)

This test was designed for children ages 3 through 6 years. The speech sound assessment portion of the test includes 15 pictured objects to elicit 30 target speech sounds. Some stimulus items are designed to assess two sounds. Standard scores and percentiles for the articulation subtest are included.

Speech-Ease Screening Inventory (K–1) (Pigott and colleagues, 1985)

This test was designed for kindergartners and first-graders. The overall test takes 7 to 10 minutes to administer with the articulation section comprising 12 items. Through sentence completion items, 14 phonemes and three blends are assessed. Cutoff scores, which suggest the need for further testing, are provided.

Preschool Language Scale (Zimmerman, Steiner, and Pond, 2012)

This test was designed for children from birth through 6. The overall scale takes between 20 and 45 minutes to administer. Items used to assess speech sounds are only a portion of this test. Age-expected performance levels are provided.

Summary

Screening procedures are not designed to determine the need or direction of treatment. Rather, their purpose is to identify individuals who merit further testing. The criteria for failure on informal screening tests are often left up to the examiner. When available for formal screening tests, standard scores and percentile ranks can aid the examiner in establishing such criteria. It is common for scores one standard deviation or more below the mean to be used as a cutoff score. For some formal instruments, cutoff scores or age expectation scores are provided.

COMPREHENSIVE SPEECH SOUND ASSESSMENT: THE ASSESSMENT BATTERY

Sampling procedures involved in comprehensive speech sound assessments are more in-depth and detailed than those described for screening. When doing a phonological analysis, the clinician usually employs several assessment instruments and sampling procedures because no one sampling procedure or test provides all a clinician needs to know when making case selection decisions and/or for determining the direction that an intervention program should take. A phonological evaluation typically involves speech sound productions in speech samples of varying lengths and complexities (e.g., syllables, words, phrases), phonetic contexts, and response to various elicitation procedures (e.g., picture naming, imitation, conversation). This collection of samples is often referred to as an *assessment battery*.

As already stated, the two major purposes of a speech sound assessment are to determine the need for and direction of treatment. It is to these purposes that most of the writings, research, and testing materials on speech sound disorders have been addressed. The following pages present components of a phonological evaluation battery with an emphasis on procedures for obtaining speech sound samples. Following this, analysis and interpretation of data collected through sampling procedures are discussed. Throughout this chapter and the next, we attempt to synthesize the available literature and make suggestions based on the authors' clinical experience.

Speech Sound Samples Included in the Assessment Battery

Connected/Conversational Speech Sampling

Rationale.   All speech sound evaluations should include a sample of connected speech. Because the ultimate objective of phonological treatment is the correct production of sounds in spontaneous conversation, it is important that the examiner observe sound productions in as "natural" a speaking context as possible. Such samples allow one to transcribe phoneme productions in a variety of phonetic contexts, to observe error patterns, and to judge the severity of the problem and the intelligibility of the speaker in continuous discourse. Klein and Liu-Shea (2009) in a study of children with speech sound disorders, reported more and different types of errors in continuous productions than in single words productions. Sounds produced in connected speech can also be studied in relation to other factors such as speech rate, intonation, stress, and syllable structure. In addition, connected speech samples allow for multiple productions of sounds across lexical/vocabulary items.

Because spontaneous connected speech samples are the most valid or representative sample of phonological performance, some clinicians suggest that phonological analyses should be exclusively based on this type of sample (Morrison and Shriberg, 1992; Shriberg and Kwiatkowski, 1980; Stoel-Gammon and Dunn, 1985). Connected speech samples have the advantage of allowing the examiner to transcribe sound productions within the context of the child's own vocabulary and in running speech, which includes his or her natural prosodic patterns. In addition, these samples can be used for other purposes such as examining fluency, voice quality, and/or other aspects of language production. Following is a listing of practical problems associated with relying solely on such samples: (1) Many individuals with severe phonological problems can be unintelligible, and it can be impossible or very difficult to reliably determine and/or transcribe what they are attempting to say, (2) some children can be reluctant to engage in conversational dialogue with an adult they do not know, (3) it can also be very difficult to obtain a spontaneous speech corpus that contains a representative sample of English phonemes, and (4) as Ingram (1989a) has pointed out, sounds missing from a conversational sample can reflect a "selective avoidance" by the child; that is, the child chooses not to produce them. In summary, although connected speech samples are an essential part of an assessment battery, most clinicians do not rely on this type sample exclusively.

Elicitation Procedures.   The customary and preferred method for obtaining a sample of connected speech is to engage a client in spontaneous conversation. The clinician can talk with the client about such things as his or her family, television shows, or places the client has visited. The samples should be recorded so that the clinician can play them back as often as required to accurately transcribe the client's utterances. Clinicians should make notes about topics covered and errors noted to facilitate later transcription.

Some clinicians have the client read a passage orally as an alternative method for obtaining a connected sample of speech. Although this procedure provides a sample of connected speech, it has been demonstrated that fewer errors usually occur in a reading sample obtained in this manner than in a corpus of conversational speech (Wright, Shelton, and Arndt, 1969). Moreover, clinicians frequently test children who have not yet learned to read, in which case this procedure is obviously not a viable option.

Some speech sound tests specify procedures for obtaining a sample of connected speech. For example, in the "Sounds-in-Sentences" subtest of the *Goldman-Fristoe Test of Articulation–second edition* (Goldman and Fristoe, 2000), the client listens to a story while viewing accompanying pictures and is then asked to retell the story. Such a delayed imitation/repetition task (in contrast to immediate imitation in which the client repeats a designated stimulus immediately after it is presented) is designed to elicit particular sounds in specific words.

A more spontaneous method than the immediate or delayed imitation technique just described is for the client to tell a story about a series of pictures selected to elicit specific target words and sounds. Dubois and Bernthal (1978) compared productions in the same word stimuli elicited through a picture-naming task, a delayed imitation task, and a story-telling task. They reported that the highest number of errors was found on the storytelling task and the smallest number on the picture-naming task. These findings were not surprising because the task of naming single words requires different skills than the sequencing of words in phrases and sentences. Although the differences between the methods were statistically significant, the authors interpreted the differences as clinically nonsignificant. They did, however, report that some individuals varied from group trends in their production of certain sounds depending on the task; for example, some children made significantly more errors on the delayed imitation task than on the picture-naming task.

Summary.   A connected speech sample is a crucial part of any phonological assessment battery because it allows (1) assessment of overall intelligibility and severity, (2) determination of speech sound usage in its natural form, and (3) a database from which to judge the accuracy of individual sounds, patterns of errors, and consistency of misarticulations. The preferred method for obtaining connected speech samples is to engage the client in spontaneous conversation. If, for some reason, this cannot be accomplished, alternate procedures that can be used include (1) eliciting conversational responses via picture stimuli or toys, (2) utilizing a reading passage, and (3) telling a story following the clinician's model (delayed imitation).

Single-Word/Citation Form Sampling

Rationale.   From the standpoint of widespread usage, analyzing phoneme productions in a corpus of single-word productions (usually elicited by having an examinee name pictures) has been the most common method for assessing speech sounds. This is sometimes referred to as a *speech sound inventory*. Single words provide a discrete, identifiable unit of production that examiners can usually readily transcribe. Because transcribers often are interested in observing the production of only one or perhaps two segments (sounds) per word, they are able to transcribe and analyze single-word samples more quickly than multiple or connected word samples. Even though a test can prescribe the scoring of only one or two sounds in a word, we would suggest, particularly with children exhibiting multiple errors, that the tester consider transcribing the entire word, including the vowels. The efficiency of analyzing sound productions from single-word productions has resulted in widespread usage of such stimuli. As suggested earlier, this type of sampling provides data that are supplemental to information obtained from the connected speech sample.

When sampling single words, most inventories typically target only one or two consonants to be scored in a word. Sounds in words typically are assessed in the *initial* position (sound at the beginning of a word, for example, /b/ in /bot/), *final* position (sound at the end of a word such as /t/ in /ræbɪt/), and sometimes in the *medial* position (sounds between the initial and final sounds, for example, /ɔ/, /k/, and /I/ in /wɔkɪŋ/).

In some instances, each of the prefixes *pre-, inter-,* and *post-* is combined with the term *vocalic* to describe the location of a consonant sound within syllables. *Prevocalic* position refers to consonants that precede a vowel (CV) and therefore initiate the syllable (e.g., *s*oap, *c*at). *Postvocalic* position refers to consonants that follow the vowel (VC) and therefore terminate the syllable (e.g., soa*p*, ca*t*). *Intervocalic* position involves a consonant that is embedded (VCV) between two vowels (e.g., ca*m*el, ea*g*er). A singleton consonant in the initial position of a word is prevocalic. Likewise, a singleton sound in word-final position is postvocalic. A consonant in the intervocalic position often may serve the dual function of ending the preceding syllable and initiating the following syllable. A medial consonant can stand next to another consonant and serve to initiate (release) or terminate (arrest) a syllable and therefore is not necessarily intervocalic. More recently, the terms *onset* (elements of a syllable before a vowel) and *coda* (elements of a syllable after a vowel) have begun to be used. Thus, references to initial, medial, and final positions refer to location of consonants in a word, whereas the terms *prevocalic, intervocalic, postvocalic, releasor, arrestor, onset* and *coda* refer to consonant position relative to syllables.

Speech sound productions are influenced by the complexity of the syllables and words in which they are produced. We know that the number and juxtaposition of phonemes make some syllables more difficult to produce than others. For example, a syllable such as /*go*/ is easier to produce than /*grop*/. The first syllable shapes produced by children are generally CV, VC, and CVC, which constitute the simplest syllable shapes.

One of the key issues in assessment concerns the correlation between speech sound productions that occur in citation form (single words) and those that occur in connected speech. Research findings have shown a positive correlation between responses obtained from naming pictures and speech sound productions in spontaneous speaking situations. As noted earlier, differences in some clients are frequently observed between these two types of measures. Clinicians need to be aware that sound productions in single words may not accurately reflect the same sounds produced in a spontaneous speech context.

Morrison and Shriberg (1992) reviewed 40 years of studies that were designed to compare citation-form testing (single-word testing) with continuous-speech sampling. They reported that, in general, more errors occur in spontaneous connected speech as compared to production of single words, although there were instances and reports in which speech sound errors were more frequent in single words. However, in their own research, they reported that children produced sounds more accurately in connected speech when those sounds were well established but more accurately in citation-form testing when those sounds were just emerging.

Single-word testing does not provide the examiner an opportunity to evaluate the effect of context on speech sound productions (coarticulation). As discussed in Chapter 2, coarticulatory effects transcend phonetic, syllabic, and lexical (word) boundaries. Gallagher and Shriner (1975) reported that children's /s/ productions were affected by position in CCV consonant clusters. Curtis and Hardy (1959) reported that /r/ was more likely to be produced correctly in consonant clusters than in single phoneme productions. It is widely accepted that more variations occur in consonant productions when sounds are elicited in consonant-plus-vowel (CV) contexts rather than in consonant clusters (CCV).

Despite reservations about making inferences concerning conversational speech based on single-word samples, most clinicians value and include single-word productions in the assessment battery. Single-word tests, which can provide the clinician information concerning phonetic skills, typically include most consonants in a language and can provide useful phonological data in a relatively short time period. In addition, for unintelligible clients, the examiner has the advantage of knowing the productions the client has attempted to say. Because of frequent variations between productions of single words versus connected speech, we recommend that both types of samples should be included in the assessment battery.

Elicitation Procedures. Single-word citation tests involve having a client name single words in response to picture stimuli. Single words can also be obtained by having a child name toys or objects. For young children, the clinician may simply wish to transcribe single-word productions the child produced spontaneously. Because picture-naming tests are the typical method for sampling single words, the following discussion focuses on this type of sampling procedure.

Speech sound inventories typically sample consonants, consonant clusters, and occasionally vowels and diphthongs. Consonants are often assessed in the initial, medial, and final positions of words—for example, /s/ in *s*aw, pen*c*il, hou*s*e; /ʃ/ in *s*hoe, sta*t*ion, fi*s*h. Some instruments elicit sounds only in the initial and final positions. The specific sounds included in inventories vary from test to test but almost always include those sounds that have a high frequency of error in children's speech. Studies have shown the following as the most frequently misarticulated sounds: /s, z, θ, ð, ʃ, ʒ, tʃ, dʒ, v, r, ʍ/. With the exception of the /hw/ (a phoneme that is often collapsed with /w/ in English), these sounds are among those items usually included in single-word tests.

As stated previously, speech sound inventories have traditionally placed little emphasis on the assessment of vowels. Undoubtedly, this is a reflection of the fact that most preschool and school-age children with speech sound disorders have problems primarily with consonants and that vowels are typically mastered at a relatively early age. Because speech pathologists are increasingly involved in early intervention programs for children at risk for communication impairments, vowel productions have, however, been increasingly scrutinized. Although many speech sound tests do not target vowels, the examiner is encouraged to transcribe vowel productions even though a test is designed to examine only consonants.

When a clinician identifies the need for an in-depth analysis of vowel productions (typically this would be very young children), Pollock (1991) has suggested the following procedure for vowel sampling:

1. Clients should be provided multiple opportunities to produce each vowel.
2. Vowels should be assessed in a variety of different contexts, including (a) monosyllabic and multisyllabic words, (b) stressed and unstressed syllables, and (c) a variety of adjacent preceding and especially following consonants.

3. Limits for the range of responses considered correct or acceptable should be established because cultural or dialect influences can affect what is considered "correct." This will be discussed again in Chapter 11.

4. Recommended vowels and diphthongs to be assessed include the following:

Nonrhotic

/i/	/ou/
/ɪ/	/ɔ/
/ei/	/ɑ/
/ɛ/	/ʌ/ə/
/ae/	/aɪ/
/u/	/aʊ/
/ʊ/	/ɔi/

Rhotic

/ɝ, ɚ/	/ɔɚ/
/ɪɚ/	/ɑɚ/
/ɛɚ/	

To compensate for the lack of formal vowel assessment procedures, it is suggested that clinicians transcribe whole-word responses to the stimuli from commonly used phonological tests. To conduct a comprehensive review of vowels and diphthongs, it may be necessary, however, to supplement existing stimuli with additional vowels, diphthongs, and contexts not included in standard tests. For a comprehensive review of vowel disorders, refer to Ball and Gibbon (2001).

Another elicitation issue is the question of spontaneous versus imitated production. Studies comparing responses elicited via imitation with those elicited through spontaneous picture naming have produced inconsistent results. Investigators studying children between the ages of 5 and 8 years have reported that responses elicited via imitation tasks yield more correct responses than those elicited via spontaneous picture naming (Carter and Buck, 1958; Siegel, Winitz, and Conkey, 1963; Smith and Ainsworth, 1967; Snow and Milisen, 1954). Other investigators who studied children ranging in age from 2 to 6 years reported no significant differences in results from elicitation via picture naming and imitation (Paynter and Bumpas, 1977; Templin, 1947). It is best simply to assume that children, especially of school age, do better on imitation as compared to spontaneous picture-naming tasks.

Harrington, Lux, and Higgins (1984) reported that children produced fewer errors when items were elicited via photographs as compared to line drawings. These data again suggest that different response elicitation procedures frequently produce different findings; however, the clinical significance of such differences tends to be minimal. The clinician should be mindful that for a given client, the nature of the test stimuli could have a bearing on responses obtained.

In spite of their widespread use, single-word tests have a number of limitations. Such measures do not allow children to use their "own" words but a set of predetermined and sometimes complex syllable and word shapes. The use of multisyllabic test words can make more demands on a child's productions and elicit more errors than would monosyllabic words or the words used in a child's own spontaneous speech. Ingram (1976) reported that when initially occurring fricative and affricate word pairs were similar in stress pattern and syllable structure, phoneme productions tended to be similar, but when syllable structure and/or stress of the pairs differed, monosyllabic words were more likely to be produced correctly than were multisyllabic words. Clinicians should recognize that syllable shape and stress patterns of stimulus words could affect speech sound productions. The clinician should also keep in mind that citation tests primarily consist of nouns because they can be pictured; thus, citation tests do not reflect all the parts of speech used in connected conversational speech.

Another difficulty with tests designed to elicit a sample via picture naming is that they often elicit only a single production of a given sound in each of either two or three word positions. During phonological development, inconsistency in production is common, even in the same stimulus word. Because the production of a sound can fluctuate, the client's customary articulatory patterns can be difficult to determine with only one to three samples of a sound. The clinician can increase the number of sound samples obtained through a single-word test by transcribing all the sounds in each stimulus (lexical) item instead of focusing only on one or two sounds in each stimulus item. They can also add words that include particular phonemes in order to provide additional opportunities to produce sounds of interest.

Ingram and Ingram (2001) pointed out that during the acquisition process, children attempt to learn and say words, not phonemes/segments, and thus word-oriented measures can assist the clinician to better understand a child's phonological system and the child's learning. Ingram and Ingram suggest that the selection of target words for instruction should include an assessment of the complexity of the words to ensure that new sounds are introduced in word forms within the child's word system—that is, words within his or her vocabulary or those he or she can approximate. The goal of therapy is to expand not only the sound system and syllable shapes but also to increase the child's overall word complexity. It is of note that although Schmitt, Howard, and Schmitt (1983) reported a significant correlation between whole-word accuracy and articulation scores, Bankson and Bernthal (1990b) reported that many children's "whole-word correct" score varied from what would have been predicted from segmental and process scores, although no statistical analysis of the correlation was reported.

The most frequently used measures of speech sound productions are commercially produced tests. A number of phonological/articulation tests are commercially available. Despite the similarities between such tests, certain stimulus and response features differentiate one test from another. For example, one test can present items in the developmental sequence of sound mastery, whereas another can organize the analysis according to place and manner of articulation. Tests frequently employ colored drawings that are especially attractive to young children; however, they occasionally elicit responses with photographs or line drawings. Some tests elicit responses through imitation tasks rather than naming pictures, photographs, line drawings, or toys.

Summary.   Single-word samples, usually obtained via speech sound tests, provide an efficient and relatively easy method for obtaining a sample of speech sound productions. Although they can be a valuable part of the phonological assessment battery, they should not constitute the only sampling procedure. Among their limitations are the small number of phonetic contexts sampled, the failure to reflect the effects of conversational context, the questionable representativeness of single-word naming responses, and factors associated with variations of syllable shape, prosody, word familiarity, and parts of speech (e.g., nouns, verbs).

Stimulability Testing

Rationale.   Another sample of speech sound productions frequently included in a test battery is obtained through stimulability testing—that is, sampling the client's ability to imitate the correct form (adult standard) of error sounds when provided with "stimulation." Traditionally, this testing has examined how well an individual imitates, in one or more phonetic contexts (i.e., isolation, syllables, words, phrases), sounds that were produced in error during testing. Although descriptions of what constitutes stimulability testing have varied, a commonly used procedure is one in which the examiner asks an individual to imitate an auditory and visual model of a sound in one or more phonetic environments. A typical way of cueing the client is for the examiner to tell the client to "watch and listen to what I am going to say, and then you say it." In more recent years, investigators have gone beyond imitation to include additional cueing such as placement instruction and visual/tactile imagery. Glaspey and Stoel-Gammon (2005) have developed a detailed procedure for doing stimulability testing that includes systematically varying phonetic environments and cueing procedures. They have labeled their form of testing as a "scaffolding" procedure, including directions and scoring for this type of assessment. It should be recognized, however, that few standardized procedures for conducting stimulability testing are available. Some tests, such as the *Goldman-Fristoe Test of Articulation*, include a stimulability subtest. Adele Miccio (personal communication) suggested a measurement probe that would assess a child's stimulability for consonant errors by reviewing whether or not a client can imitate an error sound in isolation, and then in the initial, medial, and final positions when juxtaposed to the vowels /i/, /a/, and and /u/. For example, if /s/ is the target error sound, the client would be asked to imitate the sound in isolation, and then in the following syllable contexts—si, isi, is, sa, asa, as, su, usu, us. Thus, the child would be imitating the target sound in ten productions, for which a percentage of correct productions for each sound would then be obtained. Instruction prior to production is: "Look at me, listen, and say what I say." This stimulability probe is similar to that originally suggested by Carter and Buck (1958).

Stimulability testing has been used (1) to determine whether a sound is likely to be acquired without intervention, (2) to determine the level and/or type of production at which instruction might begin, and (3) to predict the occurrence and nature of generalization. In other words, these data are often used when making decisions regarding case selection and determining which speech sounds to target in treatment.

Investigators have reported that the ability of a child to imitate syllables or words is related to normal speech sound acquisition as well as to the probability of a child spontaneously correcting her or his misarticulations (Miccio, Elbert, and Forrest, 1999). Pretest and posttest comparisons with kindergarten and first-grade children have indicated that untreated children with high stimulability skills tended to perform better than children with low stimulability scores. For participants who were not stimulable, direct instruction on speech sounds was found to be necessary because most did not self-correct their errors. It has also been reported that good stimulability also suggests more rapid progress in treatment (Carter and Buck, 1958; Farquhar, 1961; Irwin, West, and Trombetta, 1966; Sommers et al., 1967). Carter and Buck reported, in a study of first-grade children, that stimulability testing can be used for such prognostic purposes. They reported that first-grade children who correctly imitated error sounds in nonsense syllables were more likely to correct those sounds without instruction than children who were not able to imitate their error sounds. Kisatsky (1967) compared the pre- to posttest gains in articulation accuracy over a 6-month period of two groups of kindergarten children, one identified as a high stimulability group and the other as a low stimulability group. Although neither group received articulation instruction, results indicated that significantly more speech sounds were self-corrected by the high stimulability group in the 6-month posttest when compared to the low stimulability group.

It can be inferred from these studies that individuals with poor stimulability skills should be seen for treatment because it is unlikely that such children will self-correct their speech sound errors. Children with good stimulability skills tend to show more self-correction on their speech sound errors, but this finding is not true for all children. As a result, stimulability is only one factor to be used in decisions about treatment and target selection. In summary, as one might expect, the prognosis for individuals who are stimulable or can imitate a sound is more favorable than that for individuals who are not stimulable or who cannot imitate their error sounds. Likewise, a child can be expected to make faster progress on sounds in which she or he is stimulable than on sounds that are not stimulable.

Stimulability has also been found to be an important factor in generalization. Elbert and McReynolds (1978) noted that generalization of correct /s/ production to a variety of contexts occurred as soon as the children learned to imitate the sound. In addition, Powell, Elbert, and Dinnsen (1991) reported that stimulability was the most decisive variable that they examined in explaining generalization patterns and could be used to explain and predict generalization patterns. They concluded that clinicians should target nonstimulable sounds first because nonstimulable sounds are unlikely to change, whereas many stimulable sounds can self-correct during treatment even without direct instruction on those stimulable sounds.

Elicitation Procedures.   As stated earlier, the examiner typically asks the client to look at the examiner's mouth or watch it in a mirror, listen to what is said, and then imitate the production. The examiner typically does not point out where teeth, tongue, or lips are positioned during production; the examinee is simply encouraged to listen and observe a production. If the client is unsuccessful at imitating the sound, some examiners engage in cueing or trial instruction, providing directions for how to make sounds. The latter information is also used in selecting targets and determining the direction of treatment.

Stimulability testing usually includes imitative testing of those sounds produced in error in word and/or conversational samples. Some articulation tests include a place on the scoring form to record stimulability results as well as sounds in isolation or in syllables. Clinicians usually want to assess imitation in isolation, nonsense syllables (usually in prevocalic, intervocalic, and postvocalic positions), and words (again across-word positions). The number of productions required at each level varies from one examiner to the next.

Cooperation of the child, number of sounds produced in error, and success with imitation are factors the clinician should consider when deciding how extensive the stimulability assessment should be.

For example, in the case of a client with a /θ/ for /s/ error or ([θʌn] for [sʌn]), the client could be asked to initiate /s/ as follows:

1. Isolation: /s/ 6 tries
2. Nonsense syllables:

*s*i	i*s*i	i*s*
*s*a	a*s*a	a*s*
*s*u	u*s*u	u*s*

3. Words:

sail	bicycle	ice
sun	baseball	horse
seal	missile	bus

Summary. Stimulability testing is useful in identifying those individuals most likely to need phonological intervention (those with poor stimulability scores), and for determining stimulus items for initiation of instruction. Stimulability scores have been found to have prognostic value for identifying those speech sound errors a child will likely self-correct, and/or that will generalize most quickly in therapy.

Contextual Testing

Rationale. As indicated earlier, speech sound errors, especially in children, can be variable and inconsistent. Sounds are often easier to produce in some contexts as opposed to others, thus accounting for some of the inconsistencies observed in sound productions, especially during the speech sound acquisition period.

Consistency of errors is a factor considered when deciding on the need for therapy. Contextual testing is most frequently used for making treatment decisions such as choosing sounds or sound patterns to work on in therapy or identifying a particular phonetic context that facilitates accurate sound production.

Contextual influences are based on the concept that sound productions influence each other in the ongoing stream of speech. McDonald (1964a) and others have suggested that valuable clinical information can be gained by systematically examining a sound as it is produced in varying contexts. McDonald coined the term *deep test* to refer to the practice of testing a sound in a variety of phonetic contexts. Coarticulatory effects consist of mechanical constraints associated with adjacent sounds and simultaneous preprogramming adjustments for segments later in the speech stream. This overlapping of movements (preprogramming) can extend as far as six phonetic segments away from a given sound (Kent and Minifie, 1977). Although the primary influence would appear to be sounds immediately preceding or following a target sound (Zehel and colleagues, 1972), we know that as a result of coarticulatory effects, segments can be produced correctly in one context but not in another. Such information is of value to the clinician who seeks to establish a particular sound segment in a client's repertoire.

Elicitation Procedures. The first published instrument for sampling contextual influences on sounds was the *Deep Test of Articulation* (McDonald, 1964b), a series of phoneme-specific tasks designed to assess individual speech sounds in approximately 50 phonetic contexts. This test is predicated on the hypothesis that when the consonants preceding or following the sound of interest are systematically varied, the client may produce the target sound correctly in at least one phonetic context.

More recent materials that have been developed to assess consistency-contextual influences include the *Secord Contextual Articulation Tests (S-CAT)* (Secord and Shine, 1997a) and the *Contextual Test of Articulation* (Aase and colleagues, 2000). The S-CAT consists of three components: (1) Contextual Probes of Articulation Competence (CPAC), (2) Storytelling Probes of Articulation Competence (SPAC), and (3) Target Words for Contextual Training (TWAC). The CPAC and SPAC are designed to assess 23 consonants and vocalic /ɝ/ in various phonetic contexts through word and connected speech samples and can be used with clients from preschool through adult. The *Contextual Test of Articulation* tests 5 consonant sounds and 15 consonant clusters through sentence completion items in several vowel contexts.

In addition to published contextual tests, an informal contextual analysis can be performed by reviewing a connected speech sample for contexts in which a target sound is produced correctly. Occasionally, facilitating contexts can be found in conversations that are not observed in single words or word-pairs. For example, the /s/ sound might be incorrect in production of /sʌn/ but be produced correctly when the /s/ sound is juxtaposed with /t/ as in /bæts/, /stɔp/. Phonemes can also be examined in various morphophonemic alterations to determine the effect of morpheme structure on phonological productions. Such alterations can be examined by having the client produce a sound in differing morphophonemic structures. For example, to determine whether word-final obstruent /g/ has been deleted in /dɔg/ (i.e., [dɔ]), the examiner might assess whether /g/ is produced in the diminutive /dɔgi/. Likewise, whether the child misarticulates /z/ in the word /roz/, the examiner might observe /z/ production in the morphophonemic context of /rozəz/. In this example, such testing can allow the clinician also to determine whether the error is a sound production problem or a problem marking plurality (a language-related difficulty).

Consonants can also be examined for correct phoneme productions in the context of consonant clusters. Although it is true that in most instances a consonant is more likely to be produced correctly as a singleton rather than in consonant clusters, it is not unusual for sounds to be produced correctly in the context of a cluster even when misarticulated in a singleton context. For example, one can find a correct /r/ or /s/ production in a cluster even though it can consistently be in error in a singleton context.

Summary. Contextual testing is conducted to determine phonetic contexts in which a sound error may be produced correctly. These contexts can then be used to identify a starting point for remediation. Contextual testing is also used as a measure of consistency of misarticulation.

Error Pattern Identification

For children with multiple errors, the assessment battery often includes a measure designed to identify sound error patterns or commonalities that occur across error productions.

Rationale. In an effort to obtain as broad an understanding of speech sound errors in a client with multiple errors as possible, clinicians need to identify error patterns that encompass several individual speech sound targets. A phonological *pattern* (the preferred term rather than *process,* which is also still used, however) is typically defined as "a systematic sound change or simplification that affects a class of sounds, a particular sequence of sounds, or the syllable structure of words." The identification of phonological patterns (phonological analysis) assumes that children's speech sound errors are not random but represent systematic variations from the adult standard.

One of the reasons pattern analysis procedures have appeal is that they provide a description of the child's overall phonological system. For example, if a child leaves /p, b, k, g, t, s, and z/ off the ends of words, the pattern can be described as "final consonant deletion." Khan (1985) furnished another illustration of a phonological process/pattern. A child who substitutes /wawa/ for *water* might be described in a traditional substitution analysis as substituting [w] for /t/ and substituting [a] for final /ɚ/. On the basis of what we know about speech sound acquisition, the [wawa] for *water* substitution is more accurately described as syllable reduplication, a common pattern seen in young children. The child in this instance is probably repeating the first syllable of the word *water* /wa/ rather than using sound substitutions for target sounds in the second syllable. In this example, the child is also demonstrating knowledge of syllable structure because *water* contains two syllables, as does /wawa/.

A second reason for doing a pattern analysis is the potential for facilitating treatment efficiency. When a pattern reflecting several sound errors is targeted for treatment, the potential exists for enhancing generalization across sounds related to that pattern by working on one or more sounds that reflect that pattern and looking for generalization to other sounds reflected in the same error pattern.

Systems of pattern analysis, whether based on a place-manner-voicing analysis or the more commonly employed phonological pattern procedures, are most appropriate for the client who has multiple errors. The intent of the analysis is to determine whether there are patterns or relationships among speech sound errors, and thus little would be gained with a child who made only a few speech sounds in error. For example, if a client is misarticulating only two consonants, /s/ and /r/, the clinician would develop a remediation plan that targets both consonants for direct instruction.

Phonological patterns identified in the child's speech can aid in treatment target selection. For example, if a child has eight speech sound substitutions reflecting three error patterns (e.g., stopping of fricatives, gliding of liquids, and fronting), remediation would likely focus on the reduction of one or more of these phonological patterns. The modification of one or more speech sounds (exemplars) reflecting a particular error pattern frequently results in generalization to other speech sounds reflecting the same error pattern. For example, establishment of /p/ and /f/ in word-final position for a child who deletes final consonants may generalize to other stops and fricatives deleted in word-final position. Another example of a pattern-oriented remediation strategy for instruction would be to target all speech sounds that appear to be simplified in a similar manner, such as fricatives being replaced with stops (i.e., stopping). In this instance, the clinician might focus on the contrast between stops and fricatives. By focusing on sounds that reflect a similar error pattern, treatment should be more efficient than if it focuses on individual sounds without regard to phonological patterns.

Elicitation Procedures.   Several analysis procedures that are based on identifying phonologic patterns have been published. Pattern analysis procedures have been published by Hodson (2004), Dawson and Tattersall (2001), Khan and Lewis (1986, 2002), Bankson and Bernthal (1990b), and Smit and Hand (1997). Through each of these single-word measures, phonologic patterns can be identified. In addition to these published analysis procedures, phonologic productions recorded during connected speech sampling and/or single-word testing can be analyzed for the presence of error patterns. It should also be pointed out that several computer-based programs can assist the clinician in analyzing error patterns (e.g., Hodson, 2003; Masterson and Bernhardt, 2001).

Summary.   Instruments designed to identify phonological patterns facilitate identification of commonalities among error productions. The unique aspect of these tests is the type of analysis they facilitate. A more detailed description of instruments developed to assess phonological patterns is presented in Chapter 7.

Criteria for Selecting Phonological Assessment Instruments

Formal test instruments selected by the clinician should be appropriate to the individual being tested and provide the information desired by the clinician. When selecting commercially available test instruments for phonological assessment, the clinician should consider the sample the instrument is designed to obtain, the nature of the stimulus materials (e.g., How easily recognized are the target pictures or objects?), the scoring system, and the type of analysis facilitated by the instrument. Practical considerations in test selection include the amount of time required to administer the instrument and analyze the sample obtained as well as the cost for purchasing the test and any test forms. The following is a discussion of some of these variables in more detail.

Sample Obtained

Test instruments will vary in the representativeness of the speech sample obtained. Variables to evaluate include the specific consonants, consonant clusters, vowels, and diphthongs tested as well as the units in which sounds are to be produced (i.e., syllables, words, sentences). In addition, stimulus presentation and type of sample elicited (e.g., picture naming, sentence completion, imitation, delayed imitation, conversation) should also be considered in selecting instruments.

Material Presentation

Another practical factor in selecting commercially available tests is the attractiveness, compactness, and manipulability of materials. Size, familiarity, and color of stimulus pictures and appropriateness to the age of the client can influence the ease with which the clinician obtains responses to test stimuli. In addition, the organization and format of the scoring sheet are important for information retrieval. Tests with familiar and attractive stimulus items and score sheets that facilitate analysis are desirable.

Scoring and Analysis

Because the scoring and analysis procedures that accompany a test determine the type of information obtained from the instrument, they are important considerations in test selection. Different assessment instruments currently available are designed to facilitate one or more of the following types of analysis: (1) phonetic and/or phoneme analysis of consonant and vowel sounds of the language, (2) sound productions in a variety of word positions and phonetic contexts, (3) place, manner, voice analysis, (4) phonological pattern/process analysis, (5) age appropriateness, and (6) speech sound stimulability. A practical consideration relates to how much time is required to complete an analysis versus the value of information obtained.

Transcription and Scoring Procedures

Methods for Recording Responses

The recording systems used by clinicians vary according to the purposes of testing, the transcription skills of the examiner, and personal preferences. The type of response recording the examiner employs will, however, determine the type of analysis the clinician is able to perform with the sample obtained. In turn, the type of analysis conducted can significantly influence instructional decisions, which frequently include a recommended treatment approach.

In the least sophisticated scoring procedure, phonological productions are simply scored as correct or incorrect based on the examiner's perception of whether the sound produced is within the acceptable adult phoneme boundary. This type of scoring is sometimes used to assess day-to-day progress but is not recommended when doing a speech sound assessment designed to determine the direction of treatment because more detailed description is required for this purpose.

The most common transcription system for recording sound errors is the *International Phonetic Alphabet (IPA)*, which includes a different symbol for each phoneme. As indicated in Chapter 2, more than 40 such symbols are utilized to identify the phonemes of the English language. This broad transcription system supplemented with a set of *diacritics* (narrow markers) usually provides sufficient detail for speech-language clinicians to adequately describe speech sound productions. For example, in a broad transcription of the word *key*, one would transcribe the initial segment with the symbol /k/. A more precise transcription of the initial /k/ would include the diacritic for aspiration [ʰ] following word initial [kʰ] because aspiration occurs in production of /k/ in word-initial contexts. The aspiration modifier [ʰ] in this transcription represents one example of a diacritic. Use of diacritics, sometimes called a *close* or *narrow transcription*, allows for recording specific topographical dimensions of individual segments and is recommended when broad transcription does not adequately describe an error. For example, if /s/ in the word /sʌn/ is lateralized (air emitted sideways rather than forward), the diacritic for lateralization is placed under the /s/, thus [ʂʌn]. See Table 6.1 for a list of common symbols and diacritics for clinical use.

TABLE 6.1   Symbols and Diacritics

[x]	voiceless velar fricative, as in *Bach*
[Φ]	voiceless bilabial fricative
[β]	voiced bilabial fricative
[ʔ]	glottal stop, as in [mʌʔi]
[ɹ̫]	r with [w] like quality

Stop Release Diacritics

[ʰ]	aspirated, as in [tʰap]
[⁼]	unaspirated, as in [p⁼un]

Diacritics for Nasality

[˜]	nasalized, as in [fæ̃n]
[˷̷]	denasalized
[˜̫]	produced with nasal emission

Diacritics for Length

[:]	lengthened

Diacritics for Voicing

[₀]	partially devoiced, as in [spun̥]

Diacritics for Tongue Position or Shape

[̪]	dentalized, as in [tɛn̪θ]
[̺]	lateralized, as in [s̺ op]

Diacritic markers are used to describe the speech of individuals whose speech sound productions cannot be adequately described by broad phonetic symbols. For example, in assessing the phonological status of an individual with a cleft condition who is unable to achieve velopharyngeal closure for certain speech sounds, diacritics indicating nasal emission (šnail) or nasalization (bæ̃n) can be useful in the description of the client's production of such segments. Similarly, when assessing the articulation of an individual with impaired hearing, symbols to indicate appropriate vowel duration (e.g., [si:] for lengthened), devoicing (e.g., [b̥]), and denasalization (e.g., ræ̃n) are recommended if these characteristics are present in productions. Likewise, with developmental articulation errors characterized by lateralization (e.g., [s̺]), dentalization (e.g., [s̪]), and devoicing (e.g., [n̥]), diacritics should be utilized.

Accuracy of Transcriptions

One of the major concerns regarding transcription of responses relates to accuracy. Clinicians must be concerned with whether their transcriptions are a valid representation of a client's productions. In making transcriptions, clinicians rely primarily on auditory perceptual judgments. These judgments are occasionally supplemented with physiological measures (such as aerodynamic measures) and acoustical measures (such as that obtained from spectrographic analysis), particularly in research investigations. These three types of data might not always be consistent with each other. For example, a glottal substitution for a stop in word-final position could be identified via a spectrographic analysis, yet a listener might not hear the glottal production and thus will transcribe it as a deletion (omission). It must be recognized, however, that even the more objective measures of speech segments (i.e., acoustical and physiological recordings) are not devoid of human interpretation and no one-to-one correspondence exists between a phoneme production, perception, and/or acoustical and physiological measurements. For most aspects of clinical phonology, auditory perceptual judgments by the examiner remain the primary basis of accuracy judgments and intervention decisions. Because of the dependence on perceptual judgments, it is important for clinicians to establish the reliability and validity of their perceptual judgments.

Interjudge Reliability. Traditionally, clinicians have used agreement between two independent transcribers as a means of establishing reliability of judgments. *Interjudge agreement* or *reliability* is determined by the comparison of one examiner's transcriptions with those of another and is essential for reporting the results of speech sound research. In addition, for students beginning to make judgments about accuracy of speech sound productions, establishing interjudge reliability with a more experienced person can assist in the development of accurate judgments. A commonly used method to determine interjudge reliability, called *point-to-point agreement*, compares the clinicians' judgments on each test item. The number of items judged the same is divided by the total number of items to determine a percentage of agreement between judges. As an example, if two judges were to agree on 17 of 20 items and disagree on 3, they would divide 17 by 20 and get 0.85, which would then be multiplied by 100 to obtain an interjudge reliability index of 85 percent agreement. Such point-to-point or item-by-item reliability is a typically employed method for establishing agreement between judges in phonological research.

Intrajudge Reliability. Along with knowing that his or her judgments agree with those of another examiner, the clinician also wants to know that his or her standards for judgments are consistent over time. Comparison of judgments made when scoring the same data on two separate occasions is referred to as *intrajudge reliability*. High reliability on such a measure indicates that the examiner is consistent in his or her judgments. Recordings of responses are used to determine this type of reliability because two judgments of the same responses are made.

In a study of point-to-point reliability of judgments of broad and narrow phonetic transcription, Shriberg and Lof (1991) reported that for interjudge and intrajudge reliability, average agreement for broad transcriptions exceeded 90 percent and for narrow transcriptions was 65 and 75 percent.

Phonologic Assessment in Young Children

Phonologic evaluation of young children (infants and toddlers) must be accomplished within the broader context of evaluating overall communicative behavior. Because phonologic development is integrally related to development of cognition, language, and motor skills, phonological development obviously is related to other aspects of a child's development. However, for purposes of this text, it is useful to isolate phonologic considerations from the overall communication process.

Much variability exists among young children in terms of the age at which specific speech sounds are acquired. Such variability makes it difficult to formulate strict developmental expectations and guidelines for the assessment of speech sound productions in infants and toddlers. Some guidelines, however, can be offered. One of the first assessments of phonologic development involves determining whether the infant is progressing normally through the stages of infant vocalization. Speech sound productions emerge within the context of infant vocalizations at the prelinguistic level. Information presented in Chapter 3 regarding the characteristics of these stages is helpful in knowing about sound productions that typically occur during this developmental period, including the gradual shift from prelinguistic to linguistic behavior that usually occurs during the first year.

The point in time and/or development of young children when clinicians frequently become involved in assessing phonology occurs after 18 to 24 months. By this age, children typically have acquired approximately 50 words and are stringing two words together. At this age, clinicians are usually interested in determining how a child is doing in comparison to age expectations. For younger children, or those with limited vocal repertoires, the clinician seeks to describe the sounds the child uses for communication regardless of correct usage. In normally developing children, first words typically occur at about 12 months of age, the transition stage occurs between 12 and 18 months, and two or three words are put together in sequence (strings) around 24 months. In children with speech delay, obviously these stages can occur at a later chronological age. Phonologic analysis in young children is inextricably bound to development of the child's vocabulary. Procedures for eliciting vocalizations from young children depend on the level of the child's development and can include a range of activities such as stimulating vocalizations during caregiving and feeding activities; informal play with a caregiver, sibling, or clinician; structured play; interactive storytelling; sentence repetition; retelling of a story told by the clinician (delayed imitation); narrative generation (about a favorite book); and spontaneous conversation.

Stoel-Gammon (1994) indicated that at age 24 months, children can be categorized into three groups: (1) those who are normal in terms of linguistic development (85 percent of children), (2) those who are slow developing (late talkers) but evidence no major deviations from patterns of normal acquisition, and (3) those whose developmental patterns deviate substantially from the broadest interpretation of norms in terms of order of acquisition or achievement of certain milestones. Stoel-Gammon indicated that the second and third groups together constitute 15 percent of the population. Children in the second group should be monitored to be certain that they "catch up" with the normal group. She indicated that children falling into this category would likely be those who, at 24 months, have a vocabulary of fewer than 50 words, have a phonetic inventory with only 4 to 5 consonants and a limited variety of vowels, and who, otherwise, are following the normal order of phoneme acquisition and do not have unusual error types. Children in the third group are those who should be considered for an early intervention program.

The type of phonological analysis usually employed during the early stages of speech sound acquisition is termed an *independent analysis of phonological behavior.* An independent analysis identifies the speech sounds produced by a child without reference to appropriateness of usage relative to the adult standard. This type of analysis is appropriate for the assessment of both normal and delayed phoneme acquisition. Morris (2009) has reported a study of test-retest reliability based on independent analyses of speech sound productions in toddler play sessions. She examined speech sounds in initial and final position, word shapes, syllable structure, and an index of phonetic complexity. She reported that the latter two elements had the highest degree of test-retest reliability. She suggested that larger samples could be necessary to improve reliability of independent analyses. For those children who have progressed to the point at which they have enough language that intelligibility is a concern (beyond 50 words in their vocabulary), a relational analysis can also be employed. As indicated earlier, relational analyses compare the child's phonological productions with the adult standard.

An independent description of phonology is typically based on a continuous speech sample and is designed to describe a child's productions without reference to adult usage. Analysis of a child's productions as a self-contained system (independent analyses) include the following (Stoel-Gammon and Dunn, 1985):

1. An inventory of sounds (consonants and vowels) classified by word position and articulatory features (e.g., place, manner, voicing)
2. An inventory of syllables and word shapes produced (e.g., CVC, CV, VC, CCV)
3. Sequential constraints on particular sound sequences (e.g., /ɛfʌnt/ for /ɛləfʌnt/)

As stated earlier, a relational analysis of phonological productions is typically used with children after age 2 as well as older children. Most of the assessment information presented elsewhere in this chapter pertains to relational analyses.

Summary.   Phonological evaluations with infants and toddlers are done within the context of an overall communication assessment because phonological development is integrally related to other aspects of development such as cognition, motor development, and other aspects of linguistic development. Informal assessment involving independent analyses is typically done with very young children and for those with limited verbal repertoires. Usually, these include an inventory of sounds, syllables, and word shapes produced and phonological contrasts employed. Once a child has a vocabulary of approximately 50 words, relational analysis typically is employed as part of the assessment battery.

RELATED ASSESSMENT PROCEDURES

The assessment of a child with a speech sound disorder includes testing and data-gathering procedures supplemental to those focusing directly on phonologic behavior. Information is gathered to provide a more comprehensive picture of an individual client and thereby contribute to a better understanding of her or his phonological status. It can also influence treatment recommendations that are made regarding a given client.

These additional assessment procedures often include a case history; an oral cavity examination; and hearing, language, fluency, and voice screenings. These procedures can aid the clinician in identifying factors that may contribute to or be related to the delay or impairment of phonology. Data gathered from these additional measures can lead to referral to other specialists and/or influence treatment decisions. If, for example, a child has a problem with closure of the velopharyngeal port, referral to a cleft palate team might result in pharyngeal flap surgery or the fitting of an intra-oral appliance such as a palatal lift prior to speech intervention.

Appropriate related personnel (e.g., audiological, medical) must corroborate the presence of suspected sensory, structural, or neurological deficiencies, and their recommendations must be considered part of the assessment. Any of these factors can be important in making decisions regarding the need for therapy, the point at which therapy should begin, and the treatment to be prescribed. Although language, fluency, and voice screening are part of overall communication evaluations, they are not reviewed here.

Case History

To facilitate an efficient and effective assessment, a case history is obtained from the client or a parent prior to the phonological assessment. This allows the clinician to identify (1) possible etiological factors, (2) the family's or client's perception of the problem, (3) the academic, work, home, and social environment of the client, and (4) medical, developmental, and social information about the client. Case history information is usually obtained in a written form completed by the client or parents. It is frequently supplemented by an oral interview. Specific questions on the phonological status of a young child might include the following: (1) Did your child babble? If so, can you describe it? (2) When did your child say his or her first words? What were they? When did he or she start putting words together? (3) Describe your child's communication problem and your concerns about it. (4) How easy is your child to understand by the family and by strangers? (5) What sounds and words does your child say? (6) What do you think caused your child's speech difficulty? (7) Is there a family history of speech difficulties, and if so, how would you describe them?

Although case histories obtained from the client or the client's family are products of memory and perception and thus might not reflect total accuracy (Majnemer and Rosenblatt, 1994), parents and clients in general are fairly reliable informants. In spite of shortcomings, the case history provides the clinician with important background information that frequently influences assessment decisions and subsequent management recommendations.

Oral Cavity Examination

Oral cavity (oral peripheral) examinations are administered to describe the structure and function of the oral mechanism for speech purposes. In particular, dentition is observed for bite and missing teeth; hard and soft palates are examined for clefts, submucous clefts, fistulas, and fissures. Size, symmetry, and movement of the lips; size and movement of the tongue; and symmetry, movement, and functional length of the soft palate are assessed.

To examine the intraoral structures, it is recommended that the client be seated immediately in front of the clinician with her or his head in a natural upright position and at a level that allows easy viewing. The examiner should wear surgical gloves. If the client is a child, the examiner might have the child sit on a table or the examiner can kneel on the floor. Although it might seem that the oral cavity would be viewed best when the client extends her or his head backward, such a position can distort normal relationships of the head and neck. The client's mouth usually should be at the examiner's eye level. A flashlight or other light source together with a tongue blade aids in the examination. Observations should start at the front of the oral cavity and progress to the back. Because the oral cavity examination is important in identifying possible structural abnormalities, a description of how an examination is conducted follows. For a more complete presentation of procedures for conducting an oral-mechanism examination, see St. Louis and Ruscello (2000).

Dentition

For the examiner to evaluate the occlusal relationship (i.e., alignment of upper and lower jaws), the client should have the first molars in contact with each other because the occlusal relationship of the upper and lower dental arch is made with reference to these molar contacts. The upper dental arch is normally longer and wider than the lower dental arch; therefore, the upper teeth normally extend horizontally around the lower dental arch; and the maxillary (upper) incisors protrude about one-quarter inch in front of the lower teeth and cover about one-third of the crown of the mandibular incisors. Such dental overjet is the normal relationship of the dental arches in occlusion.

The teeth are said to be in open bite when the upper teeth do not cover part of the lower teeth at any given point along the dental arch. Mason and Wickwire (1978) recommended that, when evaluating occlusal relationships, the clinician should instruct the client to bite on the back teeth and to separate the lips. They further stated that

> while in occlusion, the client should be asked to produce several speech sounds in isolation, especially /s/, /z/, /f/, and /v/. Although these sounds may not normally be produced by the client with teeth in occlusion, the standardization of airspace dimensions and increases in pressure in the oral cavity can unmask a variety of functional relationships. For example, the child who usually exhibits an interdental lisp may be able to articulate /s/ surprisingly well with teeth together. This occluded position can also unmask and/or counteract habit patterns related to the protrusion of tongue and mandible on selected sounds. (p. 15)

Mason and Wickwire (1978) also suggested that when an individual with excessive overjet has difficulty with /s/, he or she should be instructed to rotate the mandible forward as a means of adaptation to the excessive overjet. As pointed out in Chapter 5, however, dental abnormality and speech problems are frequently unrelated, and, thus, a cause-and-effect relationship between occlusion deviation and articulation problems should not be assumed.

Hard Palate

The hard palate (i.e., the bony portion of the oral cavity roof) is best viewed when the client extends his or her head backward. Normal midline coloration is pink and white. When a blue tint on the midline is observed, further investigation of the integrity of the bony framework is indicated. Such discoloration can be caused by a blood supply close to the surface of the palate and is sometimes associated with a submucous cleft (an opening in the bony palatal shelf). But a blue tint seen lateral to the midline of the hard palate usually suggests only an extra bony growth, which occurs in approximately 20 percent of the population.

When a submucous cleft of the hard palate is suspected, palpation (rubbing) of the mucous membrane at the midline of the most posterior portion of the hard palate (nasal spine) is recommended. Although many speech-language pathologists note the height of the hard palatal vault, it probably has little relationship to articulation deviations. The contour or height of the palatal vault could influence certain articulatory contacts, but most individuals with high palatal vaults use compensatory movements that allow for adequate speech sound production.

Soft Palate or Velum

The soft palate should be evaluated with the head in a natural upright position. When it is not in that position, changes in the structural relationships in the oral cavity area can prevent the viewing of velar function as it occurs during speech.

Mason and Wickwire (1978) cautioned that the assessment of velar function, especially velar elevation, should not be done with the tongue protruded or with the mandible positioned for maximum mouth opening. They recommended a mouth opening of about three quarters of the maximum opening because velar elevation might be less than maximum when the mouth is open maximally.

The coloration of the soft palate, like that of the hard palate, should be pink and white. A midline bluish tint should alert the clinician to the possibility of a submucous cleft of the velum in which case the surface of the velum is covered with mucous membrane, but the underlying layer of periosteum is absent.

The critical factor in velar function is the effective or functional length of the velum, not the velar length per se. Effective velar length is the portion of tissue that fills the space between the posterior border of the hard palate and the posterior wall of the pharynx. Effective velar length is only one factor in adequate velopharyngeal sphincter function and provides little or no information concerning the function of the sphincter's pharyngeal component (see the following description), another critical factor for adequate velopharyngeal valving.

The final velar observation typically made is velar symmetry and elevation. When asked to sustain a vowel such as "ahhh," the client's velum should rise vertically and not deviate to either side. If it does, it indicates normal movement, but because we cannot completely visualize velopharyngeal closure from the mouth, we cannot assume that velopharyngeal closure is normal. However, when the velum does not elevate, an inadequately functioning velopharyngeal sphincter should definitely be suspected. It should also be remembered that if the observation is made with the tongue protruded, velar elevation can be restricted.

The posterior-most appendage or extension of the velum is the uvula, which has little or no role in speech production in English. However, a bifid uvula should alert the clinician to other possible anatomical deviations. A bifid uvula appears as two appendages rather than one and is occasionally seen in the presence of submucous clefts and other abnormal anatomical findings.

Fauces

The next area to observe in the oral cavity is the faucial pillars and the tonsillar masses. Only in rare instances are these structures a factor in speech production. The presence or absence of tonsillar masses is noted and, if present, their size and coloration are observed.

Redness or inflammation could be evidence of tonsillitis, and large tonsillar masses could displace the faucial pillars and reduce the isthmus (or space between the pillars).

Pharynx

The oropharyngeal area is difficult to view in an intraoral examination. The pharyngeal contribution to velopharyngeal closure cannot be assessed through intraoral viewing because pharyngeal valving occurs at the level of the nasopharynx, a level superior to that which can be observed through the oral cavity. In some individuals, movement of tissue to form a prominence or ridge (Passavant's Pad) can be seen on the posterior wall of the pharynx; Passavant's Pad is not visible at rest but can usually be seen during sustained phonation. Passavant's Pad is present in approximately one-third of the individuals with cleft palates but is otherwise rare. Because its presence reflects a compensatory mechanism, the examiner should be alert to possible velopharyngeal valving problems. The presence of Passavant's Pad could suggest that adenoidal tissue is needed for velopharyngeal closure, and this factor should be considered in surgical decisions regarding adenoidectomies.

Considerable research has been conducted in the development of instrumental measures that can help in the assessment of velopharyngeal adequacy and function. Such measures are used to supplement clinical perceptions related to the adequacy of velopharyngeal function. Inadequate velopharyngeal function frequently is associated with hypernasal resonance, weak production of pressured consonants (i.e., stops, fricatives, and affricates), and nasal emission of air. A number of direct and indirect instrumental procedures can help to assess velopharyngeal function—for example, nasometer, videofluoroscopy, nasopharyngoscopy, and airflow (aerodynamic) measures. For more information about such techniques, see chapters in Bzoch (2004).

Tongue

As pointed out in Chapter 4, the tongue is a primary articulator, and individuals are able to modify tongue movements to compensate for many structural variations in the oral cavity. In terms of tongue size, two problematic conditions are occasionally found. The first, termed *macroglossia*, is an abnormally large tongue. Although the incidence of this condition is relatively low, historically some have associated it with Down syndrome. Research data, however, indicate normal tongue size in this population, but low muscle tone in the tongue and an undersized oral cavity may be present (the combination of a normal size tongue in a small oral cavity is what we previously termed *relative macroglossia*). The condition in which the tongue is abnormally small in relation to the oral cavity is termed *microglossia*, but this condition rarely, if ever, causes a speech problem.

It has been pointed out that tongue movements for speech activities show little relationship to tongue movements for nonspeech activities. Unless motor problems are suspected, little is gained by having the client perform a series of tongue movements used for nonspeech activities. Protrusion of the tongue or moving the tongue laterally from one corner of the mouth to the other can provide information about possible motor limitations or problems in control of the tongue.

The rapid speech movements observed in diadochokinetic tasks (syllabic repetition—e.g., pʌ pʌ pʌ, pʌ tʌ kʌ) provide some information with respect to speech function. The absolute number of syllables that an individual can produce in a given unit of time usually bears little relationship to articulatory proficiency except when gross motor problems are present. For a discussion of the relationship between diadochokinetic testing and articulation, see Chapter 4. Mason and Wickwire (1978) suggested that the clinician focus on the pattern of tongue movement and the consistency of contacts during diadochokinetic tasks.

A short lingual frenum can restrict movement of the tongue tip. As discussed in Chapter 5, most individuals, however, acquire normal speech in spite of a short lingual frenum. If the client can touch the alveolar ridge with the tongue tip, the length of the frenum is probably adequate for speech purposes. In the rare instance in which this is not possible, surgical intervention could be necessary.

Summary

In an oral cavity examination in which the clinician notes an inadequacy of structure or function that might contribute to speech sound errors, she or he has several options: (1) refer the client to other professionals (e.g., otolaryngologist, orthodontist, cleft palate team) for assessment and possible intervention, (2) engage in additional observation and testing to verify the earlier observation and note its impact on speaking skills, and (3) provide instruction related to compensatory or remedial behaviors.

Audiological Screening

The primary purpose of audiological screening is to determine whether a client exhibits a loss or reduction of auditory function, which could be an etiological factor associated with a phonological disorder. Audiological screening is usually conducted with pure tones and/or impedance audiometry prior to phonological assessment.

Pure tone screening typically involves the presentation of pure tone stimuli at 500, 1,000, 2,000, and 4,000 Hz at a predetermined intensity level. Usually, 20 dB HL is used for screening, but this level can be altered to compensate for ambient noise in the room. The pure tone frequencies used in screening are those considered most important for perceiving speech. The loudness of the pure tone stimuli reflects threshold levels needed to function adequately in the classroom and in the general environment.

Impedance screening measures eardrum compliance (movement of the eardrum) and middle-ear pressure as air pressure is altered in the external auditory canal. This screening test also yields basic information about the functioning of the tympanic membrane by eliciting the acoustic reflex. The acoustic reflex can be measured by presenting a relatively loud signal to the ear and observing the presence or absence of a change in the compliance of the eardrum. Screening of the acoustic reflex usually involves the presentation of a 1,000 Hz signal at 70 dB above a person's threshold. The acoustic reflex is a contraction of the stapedial muscle when the ear is stimulated by a loud sound and serves as a protective device for the inner ear. The client who fails a pure tone or impedance screening test should be referred to an audiologist for a complete audiological assessment.

Summary

As indicated in Chapter 5 in the discussion of hearing as it relates to an individual's speech sound productions, it is critical to know the status of a client's hearing. There is some indication that recurrent middle ear problems can contribute to phonological delay and speech sound disorders. In the case of more severe auditory impairments, a correlation between extent of hearing loss and level of speech and language development occurs frequently. Given this relationship, audiological screening must be a routine part of phonological assessment procedures.

Speech Sound Perception/Discrimination Testing

A review of the literature concerning the relationship between speech sound discrimination and articulation is presented in Chapter 5. The information presented there provides background for the assessment of speech sound perception, which is discussed here.

In the earlier years of the speech-language pathology profession (1920 to 1950), clinicians assumed that most children with articulation errors were unable to perceive the difference between the standard adult production and their own error production and then inferred that many phonological problems were the result of faulty perception. As a result of this assumption, speech sound discrimination testing that covered a wide variety of sound contrasts became a standard procedure in the assessment battery. These general discrimination tests did not examine contrasts relevant to a particular child's error productions (e.g., target sound vs. error sound—*rabbit* vs. *wabbit*) but sampled a wide variety of contrasts. An example of a general test of discrimination is the *Goldman-Fristoe-Woodcock Test of Auditory Discrimination* (Goldman, Fristoe, and Woodcock, 1970). Research findings have cast doubt on the relationship between general speech sound discrimination and phonological disorders. The result has been that today general speech sound discrimination tests are rarely used in clinical assessment. This testing is, however, recommended for those few clients suspected of having a generalized perceptual problem (e.g., inability to differentiate a wide variety of minimal pair sound contrasts). The type of testing recommended for clinical use is a phoneme task based on error production(s).

Locke's Speech Perception/Discrimination Testing

The *Speech Production Perception Task* (Locke, 1980b) is a perceptual measure designed to assess a child's perception of his or her articulatory errors and involves no preselected stimuli but stimuli based on the child's error productions. See Table 6.2 for the format for this task and Box 6.1 for instructions on how to administer the procedure.

Preliminary to the presentation of the *Speech Production Perception Task*, the child's speech sound errors must be identified. The child's error productions and the corresponding adult standard (correct) forms are then used to construct the perception task. In this procedure, the adult norm is identified as the stimulus phoneme (SP), the child's substitution or deletion as the response phoneme (RP), and a perceptually similar "control phoneme" is identified as CP. For example, if the client substitutes [wek] for /rek/, the

TABLE 6.2	Speech Production Perception Task

Speaker's Name _____**Sex** _____ **DOB** _____

Test Date:		**Test Date:**	
Usual Error Pattern / /[1] ....> / /[2]		**Usual Error Pattern** / /[1] ....> / /[2]	
Target Sound / / **Error** / / **Control** / /[3]		**Target Sound** / / **Error** / / **Control** / /[3]	
Stimulus - Category	**Response**[4]	**Stimulus - Category**	**Response**[4]
1. / / - Error	yes - NO	1. / / - Target	YES - no
2. / / - Control	yes - NO	2. / / - Control	yes - NO
3. / / - Target	YES - no	3. / / - Target	YES - no
4. / / - Target	YES - no	4. / / - Error	yes - NO
5. / / - Error	yes - NO	5. / / - Control	yes - NO
6. / / - Control	yes - NO	6. / / - Error	yes - NO
7. / / - Target	YES - no	7. / / - Target	YES - no
8. / / - Control	yes - NO	8. / / - Error	yes - NO
9. / / - Error	yes - NO	9. / / - Target	YES - no
10. / / - Target	YES - no	10. / / - Control	yes - NO
11. / / - Error	yes - NO	11. / / - Control	yes - NO
12. / / - Control	yes - NO	12. / / - Error	yes - NO
13. / / - Error	yes - NO	13. / / - Target	YES - no
14. / / - Target	YES - no	14. / / - Control	yes - NO
15. / / - Error	yes - NO	15. / / - Error	yes - NO
16. / / - Control	yes - NO	16. / / - Target	YES - no
17. / / - Target	YES - no	17. / / - Control	yes - NO
18. / / - Control	yes - NO	18. / / - Error	yes - NO
Mistakes: Error ____ Control ____ Target____		Mistakes: Error ____ Control ____ Target____	

Misperception = 3+ mistakes on "Error."
[1]Phonetic transcription of target word for this task.
[2]Phonetic transcription of what the speaker usually says in place of the target word.
[3]Control sound should be similar to both target sound and usual error but produced correctly.
[4]Correct responses are shown in UPPERCASE.
Source: Locke (1980b).

stimulus production (SP) would be *rake* /r/, the response production (RP) would be *wake* /w/, and an appropriate control production (CP) would be *lake* /l/ because /l/ is a liquid as is /r/.

    To administer the task, the examiner presents a picture or an object to the child and names it either correctly, using the target phoneme, using the client's incorrect response

BOX 6.1 Instructions for the Speech Perception—Production Task

Note that each form can accommodate testing for 2 different speech errors.

1. Identify the target sound and the child's usual error for that target. Also identify a control sound that is similar to both the target and the child's error but that the child produces correctly. For example, if the child says "fumb" for "thumb", the "th" would be the target sound, /f/ would be the child's error, and /s/ might serve as the control (assuming the child usually says /s/ correctly).

2. Under "production task," list the target word and the substitution. For example if he said "fumb" for "thumb":

$$thumb \rightarrow fumb$$

3. Indicate the target sound in the space marked Target ("th" in the above example), the substituted sound in the space marked Error ("f" in the above example), and a related sound as a control in the space marked Control (it should be similar to both the target and the error but one which the child produces correctly; "s" might be a good one for the above example).

4. In each of the 18 spots under "Stimulus—Class" fill in the appropriate sounds from #2 above depending on the item that is listed. For example if the item says Target, write "th," if it says Error write "f," and if it says Control write "s." This creates the stimuli for the test.

5. Using the target picture or an object as the visual cue, ask the speaker to judge whether or not you said the right word. For example:
   1. Is this "some"?
   2. Is this "fumb"?
   3. Is this "thumb"?
   4. Is this "thumb"?
   5. Is this "fumb"? etc.

If the speaker answers "yes," circle yes next to the item. If the speaker answers "no," circle no.

6. If the word "yes" or "no" appears in uppercase letters, that indicates the correct response. If it is in lowercase letters, that indicates it would be a mistake in perception.

7. Count the mistakes (the number of lower case responses) in each category (Target, Error, Control).

8. The speaker is said to have a problem with perception if 3 or more mistakes in perception are noted in response to the Error stimuli. Since there are 6 possible Error stimuli the child has then produced at least 50% incorrect responses and thus appears to be having trouble distinguishing what they usually say from what they should be saying.

9. If the child makes 3 or more mistakes on the Control sound, this suggests the child may not fully understand the task. Results of testing should be discarded and the test attempted at a later date.

(error) phoneme, or using a control phoneme. The control phoneme is one that the child produces correctly and is as similar as possible to both the target and the child's error. For each presentation, the child has to judge whether the word was produced correctly or not. The number of correct responses to the three types of stimulus items (target, error, control) are tabulated. A similar 18-item test is constructed for each sound substitution in which perception is to be examined in depth.

Phonological Contrast Testing

As can be ascertained from information presented in the preceding paragraphs, the type of perceptual testing recommended is the assessment of a client's perception of phonological contrasts related to her or his error productions. Perceptual testing usually involves the client's differentiating the adult standard production from her or his error production and/ or assessment of the child's perception of minimal pair phonological contrasts related to her or his error sound (e.g., *lake-rake*, where /r/ is the sound produced in error). In-depth perceptual testing of an error sound requires numerous phonemic pairings, all focusing on contrasts with the target sound.

Contrast testing is also useful with individuals learning English as a second language. Frequently, it is difficult for such people to hear sound differences that involve sounds not used in their native language. For example, native Japanese have trouble differentiating /r/ and /l/, and Spanish speakers sometimes have trouble differentiating /ɪ/ and /i/.

Assessment of a child's awareness of phonological contrasts provides the clinician data relative to the child's phonemic system at a perceptual level. Most clinicians improvise assessment tasks requiring the child to indicate awareness that certain contrasts are in her or his perceptual repertoire. For example, a child with sound substitutions of /t/ for /s/ could be shown pictures of the following pairs of words that contrast s/t, s/ʃ, and s/θ and be asked to pick up one picture from each pair as it is named.

sea	sea	some
tea	she	thumb

A child who cannot readily perceive these contrasts might be a candidate for perceptual training.

Summary

If it is suspected that a child's phonological errors are related to faulty perception, perceptual testing is appropriate. The primary concern relates to the child's ability to differentiate between the adult standard and his or her error productions. Perception tests should be based on the child's specific errors with assessment items based on phonemic contrasts the individual does not produce in his or her speech sound productions. Although our understanding of the relationship between phonological productions and perception is incomplete, it appears that improving perceptual skills may be useful in helping some children to improve their phonological productions. For individuals who are second language learners, perception testing is a very useful component to the assessment battery.

CONCLUSION

Speech sound assessment may consist of screening and/or comprehensive assessment. The former provides a quick evaluation to determine whether or not a problem may be present and whether more complete assessment is needed. A comprehensive assessment battery includes connected speech and single-word sampling, as well as stimulability and contextual testing. The battery also includes supplemental procedures such as the collection of a case history, an oral cavity examination, audiological screening and perceptual testing. All of these data are then compiled and interpreted. Such interpretation is the subject of Chapter 7.

QUESTIONS FOR CHAPTER 6

1. When is it appropriate to perform a comprehensive speech sound assessment versus a speech sound screening?

2. Describe the elements of a speech sound assessment battery and how each is accomplished.

3. What related assessments need to accompany the speech sound battery?

4. What are the strengths and limitations of citation testing and spontaneous speech assessment?

5. When is a pattern analysis appropriate, and how is it done?

6. What is the purpose of the case history?

7. Distinguish among target phonemes, error phonemes, and control phonemes used for speech perception testing.

CHAPTER 7

Determining the Need for Intervention and Target Selection

JOHN E. BERNTHAL
University of Nebraska–Lincoln

NICHOLAS W. BANKSON
James Madison University

PETER FLIPSEN JR.
Idaho State University

CASE SELECTION

After the clinician has collected various types of phonological samples, the data gathered during the assessment are analyzed and interpreted to determine (1) whether there is a phonological problem, (2) the nature of the problem if there is one, (3) whether the client should be seen for treatment, and (4) if treatment is indicated, a recommended plan of action. The primary goals of analyses are to score, sort, or otherwise organize data collected to describe phonological performance. The purpose of interpretation is to examine the results of the speech sound analyses and determine what course of action should be taken. Based on the interpretation of the analyses, the clinician must determine whether the client needs instruction, and, if so, select target behaviors for treatment and appropriate intervention strategies. In summary, the clinician reviews responses to the speech sound assessment tasks and interprets the analysis of these data to make appropriate and efficacious decisions.

In the case of children who receive therapy for speech sounds in the schools, services are often provided only for those children whose speech and language disorders interferes with their academic performance. In other school districts, social acceptability or parent request could also be used as factors in determining which children receive services. Qualifying children for phonological intervention requires the school-based speech-language pathologist to collaborate with a school-based diagnostic team to establish the need for services consistent with state and local eligibility criteria. In the paragraphs that follow, we review several factors or variables that the clinician should consider when reviewing assessment data and determining whether or not therapy is appropriate for a given child.

Intelligibility

Perhaps the first factor that is reviewed when making case selection decisions is the intelligibility or understandability of the client's spontaneous speech. The intelligibility of spontaneous speech in accord with a child's age reflects the client's verbal communication competence and is a most important factor when determining the need for intervention. Intelligibility of the speaker is the factor most frequently cited by both speech-language pathologists as well as other listeners when judging the severity of a phonological problem (Shriberg and Kwiatkowski, 1982a). It should be pointed out, however, that severity of a speech sound disorder and speech intelligibility are different although related concepts.

Speech intelligibility is a perceptual judgment made by a listener and is based, to a large extent, on the percentage of words in a speech sample that are understood. Intelligibility of speech reflects a continuum of judgments ranging from unintelligible (when the message is not understood by the listener) to totally intelligible (when the message is completely understood). Intermediate points along such a continuum might include the following: speech is usually unintelligible, speech is partially intelligible, speech is intelligible although noticeably in error, and speech sound errors are occasionally noticed in continuous speech. Furthermore, intelligibility may vary according to a number of variables, including level of communication (single words, conversation), topic under discussion, rate of speech, and familiarity of the listener with the speaker.

There is no standard procedure for quantifying the intelligibility of young children. Gordon-Brannan (1994) identified three general approaches for measuring intelligibility: (1) *open-set word identification* procedure in which the examiner transcribes a speech sample and determines the percentage of words identifiable, (2) *closed-set word identification* in which a listener identifies words repeated or read from prescribed word lists, and (3) *rating scale* procedures, which may take the form of either an interval scaling procedure in which a listener assigns a rating (number along a continuum of 5 to 9 points) or a direct magnitude scale from which a judgment of a speech sample is made relative to a standard stimulus. Although scaling procedures are often used because of their simplicity and efficiency, Schiavetti (1992) has pointed out that listeners have difficulty dividing interval scales evenly, and often it is difficult to establish reliability of listeners, particularly in the middle part of a scale.

Factors influencing speech sound intelligibility include the number and types of speech sound errors (e.g. sound omissions effect intelligibility more that sound distortions), consistency of sound errors, frequency of occurrence of error sounds, and phonological patterns used. In general, the higher the number of a speaker's productions that differ from the adult standard, the more intelligibility is reduced. However, a simple tally of the number of sounds in error is not an adequate index of intelligibility. As Shriberg and Kwiatkowski (1982a) reported, there is often a low correlation (they reported $r = .42$) between the percentage of consonants correct and the intelligibility of a speech sample.

As stated, factors in addition to the numbers of errors impact intelligibility. The nature of the clients' errors relative to the target is one such factor. For example, deleting a sound affects intelligibility more than a distortion of the same sound does. Intelligibility is also affected by the consistency of misarticulated sounds and the frequency with which an error sound occurs in the language. The more consistently a target sound is produced in error, and, likewise, the more frequently error sounds occur in the language, the more likely the listener is to have difficulty understanding the message.

Extraneous factors may influence intelligibility judgments. These factors include the listeners' familiarity with the speaker's speech pattern; prosodic factors such as speaker's rate, inflection, stress patterns, pauses, voice quality, loudness, and fluency; the linguistic experience of the listener; the social environment of the communication act; the message content; the communication cues available to the listener; and the characteristics of the transmission media. The complexity of these factors accounts for the finding that intelligibility ratings do not correlate highly with the percentage of speech sounds that are produced correctly.

In case selection, a general principle is that the poorer the intelligibility, the more likely the need for intervention is. According to parent reports, a stranger should understand typically developing 2-year-old children 50 percent of the time (Coplan and Gleason, 1988). Vihman (2004) reported a study of normal development in which her 3-year-old participants from well-educated families averaged more than 70 percent intelligibility in conversation (range of 50 to 80 percent). Gordon-Brannan (1994) reported a mean intelligibility of 93 percent (range of 73 to 100 percent) with normally developing 4-year-old children. Commonly accepted standards for intelligibility expectations are as follows: 3 years, 75 percent intelligible; 4 years, 85 percent intelligible; and 5 years, 95 percent intelligible. Bowen (2002) suggested the following expectations for intelligibility (percentage of words understood in conversation with an unfamiliar adult): 1 year, 25 percent intelligible; 2 years, 50 percent intelligible; 3 years, 75 percent intelligible; and 4 years, 100 percent intelligible. She arrived at this percentage by dividing a child's age in years by 4. It should be pointed out that these percentages are in keeping with commonly accepted standards of intelligibility, particularly for 3- and 4-year-old children. These percentages do not reflect the number of correct consonants but simply the ability of a listener to understand what a speaker intended to say. It is generally recognized that a client 3 years of age or older who is unintelligible to listeners is a candidate for treatment.

Following a review of the literature concerning the assessment of intelligibility of children, Gordon-Brannan (1994) suggested that calculating the actual percentage of words understood in a speech sample may be the most valid way to determine intelligibility. She suggested that the procedure could be enhanced by including orthographic transcription by a caregiver as a reliability check, and she pointed out that although rating scales for judging speech intelligibility are less time consuming than determining percentage of words understood, such intelligibility rating scales have not been validated or standardized for children with phonological deficits.

Shriberg and Kwiatkowski (1980) suggested another way to estimate intelligibility based on a conversational speech sample. The method is based on counting intelligible words. These researchers suggested that even when the speaker's word boundaries are difficult to determine, transcribers can reliably count and record the number of syllables that were produced and then group these syllables into words. They labeled their procedure an *intelligibility index (II)*. A study by Flipsen (2006b) compared Shriberg and Kwiatkowski's (1980) syllable identification and grouping procedures with several other methods. Flipsen reported that the differences among the methods were small enough to reflect measurement error and for clinical use, the original approach (counting intelligible words) had higher practical efficiency. Flipsen concluded that intelligibility of conversational speech of children can be reliably quantified and that clinicians and researchers need not limit themselves to less reliable and less valid scaling methods.

An example of one of the few published procedures for estimating speech sound intelligibility is the *Children's Speech Intelligibility Measure (CSIM)* developed by Wilcox and Morris (1999). This test involves a client imitating a list of words after the examiner's model with responses tape-recorded. Words are drawn from a pool of 600 that are grouped into 50 sets of 12 phonetically similar words. One word from each of the 50 sets is randomly chosen as a target item for each CSIM administration. Because of this large pool of items, intelligibility estimates may be repeated with a new set of similar words for each measure. Following the tape–recording, an independent judge listens to the tape and scores 50 words, selecting a response for each word from a list of 12 words that contain 11 phonetically similar foils. Although this test produces a quantitative index of intelligibility, it is based on single-word productions, and because the listener must identify one word or another from a list, he or she has the possibility of selecting the correct response even though he or she did not understand the word produced. It does provide, however, a quantitative index of single-word production intelligibility that does not rely on clinician transcription of productions.

Further research in the area of measuring speech intelligibility in children is anticipated to be conducted in the years ahead. For a more comprehensive review of procedures for evaluating the intelligibility of children's speech, see Kent, Miolo, and Bloedel (1994).

Severity

A second factor reviewed when determining the need for intervention is the severity of the speech sound disorder. *Severity* of a phonological disorder refers to the significance of a speech sound disorder and is associated with labels such as *mild, moderate*, and *severe*. Severity may also be looked at as representing the degree of impairment.

Historically, a frequently employed way to arrive at severity has been for the clinician to make an impressionistic judgment as to degree of impairment by using a scale (numerical, continuum of disability) that is designed to represent degree of severity (mild to severe). Such scales have been used because of their efficiency in terms of administration time and the lack of more definitive ways of determining severity. Despite the importance of severity estimations in terms of treatment decisions, there seems to be no clear consensus regarding the most valid way to arrive at level of severity of a speech sound disorder. In a study of clinicians' judgments of severity, Flipsen, Hammer, and Yost (2005) reported that clinicians tend to use judgments of both individual segments, including number, type, and consistency of errors, as well as whole-word accuracy in making such determinations. They also reported that there was such variability even among experienced clinicians in their perceptual ratings that they questioned the usefulness of such measures.

A more objective way of arriving at a determination of the degree of severity was developed by Shriberg and Kwiatkowski (1982a). These researchers developed a metric for quantifying the severity of involvement of children with speech sound disorders. They recommended the calculation of Percentage of Consonants Correct (PCC) as an index to quantify severity of involvement. Their research indicated that among several variables studied in relation to listeners' perceptions of severity, the PCC correlated most closely. The percentage of consonants correct requires the examiner to make correct–incorrect judgments based on a narrow phonetic transcription of a continuous speech sample. Such judgments were found to be a reasonable measure for the classification of many children's phonological disorders as mild, mild-moderate, moderate-severe, or severe.

Procedures outlined by Shriberg and Kwiatkowski (1982a, p. 267) for determining PCC are as follows:

> Tape record a continuous speech sample of a child following sampling procedures. Any means that yield continuous speech from the child are acceptable, provided that the clinician can tell the child that his exact words will be repeated onto the "tape machine" so that the clinician is sure to "get things right."

Sampling Rules

1. Consider only intended (target) consonants in words. Intended vowels are not considered.
   a. Addition of a consonant before a vowel, for example, *on* [hon], is not scored because the target sound /ɔ/ is a vowel.
   b. Postvocalic /r/ in fair [feir] is a consonant, but stressed and unstressed vocalics [ɝ] and [ɚ], as in *furrier* [fɝ·iɚ], are considered vowels.
2. Do not score target consonants in the second or successive repetitions of a syllable, for example, *ba-balloon* but score only the first /b/.
3. Do not score target consonants in words that are completely or partially unintelligible or where the transcriber is uncertain of the target.
4. Do not score target consonants in the third or successive repetitions of adjacent words unless articulation changes. For example, the consonants in only the first two words of the series [kæt], [kæt], [kæt] are counted. However, the consonants in all three words are counted as if the series were [kæt], [kæk], [kæt].

Scoring Rules

1. The following six types of consonant sound changes are scored as incorrect:
   a. Deletions of a target consonant.
   b. Substitutions of another sound for a target consonant, including replacement by a glottal stop or a cognate.
   c. Partial voicing of initial target consonants.
   d. Distortions of a target sound, no matter how subtle.
   e. Addition of a sound to a correct or incorrect target consonant, for example, *cars* said as [karks].
   f. Initial /h/ deletion (*he* [i]) and final n/ŋ substitutions (*ring* [rin]) are counted as errors only when they occur in stressed syllables; in unstressed syllables they are counted as correct, for example *feed her* [fidɚ]; *running* [rʌnin].

2. Observe the following:
   a. The response definition for children who obviously have speech errors is "score as incorrect unless heard as correct." This response definition assigns questionable speech behaviors to an "incorrect" category.
   b. Dialectal variants should be glossed as intended in the child's dialect, for example, *picture* "piture," *ask* "aks," and so on.
   c. Fast or casual speech sound changes should be glossed as the child intended, for example, *don't know* "dono," and "*n*," and the like.
   d. Allophones should be scored as correct, for example, *water* [warɚ], *tail* [teɪl̪].

   Calculation of percentage of consonants correct (PCC):

$$PCC = \frac{Number\ of\ Correct\ Consonants}{Number\ of\ Correct\ Plus\ Incorrect\ Consonants} \times 100$$

Based on research that related PCC values to listeners' perception of degree of handicap, Shriberg and Kwiatkowski (1982a) recommended the following scale of severity:

85–100%	Mild
65–85%	Mild/moderate
50–65%	Moderate/severe
<50%	Severe

Shriberg and colleagues (1997a, 1997b) have described extensions of this PCC metric developed to address concerns related to what some clinical phonologists perceived as limitations in the original procedure. Thus, the authors have presented additional formulas (e.g., percentage of vowels correct (PVC); percentage of phonemes correct (PPC); percentage of consonants correct adjusted (PPC-A)) that address such variables as frequency of occurrence of sounds; types of errors, including omissions and substitutions; the nature of distortions; and vowel and diphthong errors. Flipsen, Hammer, and Yost (2005) examined these measures along with several others as potentially more valid ways to determine severity. None of the alternatives appeared to be any better than the original PCC at capturing severity as judged by experienced clinicians.

Johnson, Weston, and Bain (2004) researched whether differences in PCC values would be obtained if the speech sample were based on sentence imitation rather than the conversational task recommended by Shriberg and colleagues. They compared scores of 21 children ages 4 to 6 years with speech delay that were derived from an imitative sentence task and a conversational task. Johnson and associates reported that PCC scores did not differ significantly with results indicating clinical equivalency. They cited advantages of sentence imitation samples that included providing opportunities to observe infrequently occurring speech sounds, reducing glossing problems, and providing for replicated samples in pre- and posttreatment assessment. Overall, the procedure made more efficient use of clinician and client time than conversational sampling and analysis. They cautioned, however, that clinicians should consider individual child characteristics when choosing an imitative approach.

Quantitative estimates of severity, such as the PCC, provide the clinician with an objective means for determining the relative priority of those who may need intervention and a way to monitor progress/change.

Phonological Error Patterns

In addition to the review of individual sound productions for age appropriateness, error patterns are also reviewed to determine whether a child is using such patterns at a level appropriate to the child's age. When conducting a phonological pattern analysis, the clinician reviews and categorizes errors according to commonalities among them. As discussed in Chapter 6, determination of a child's phonological patterns may be based on an assessment instrument designed specifically for that purpose. In addition, the clinician may use a connected speech sample as well as single words as the basis for the identification of patterns.

Types of Pattern Analysis

Place-Manner-Voicing.   The simplest type of pattern analysis involves classifying substitution errors according to place, manner, and voicing characteristics. A *place-manner-voicing analysis* facilitates the identification of patterns such as voiced for voiceless sound substitutions (e.g., voicing errors—/f/→[v] /t/→[d]), replacement of fricatives by stops (e.g., manner errors—/ð/→[d] /s/→[t/]), or substitution of lingua-alveolar sounds for lingua-velar sounds (e.g., place errors—/t/→[k] /d/→[g]). Another example is a child whose speech patterns reflect correct manner and voicing but produce errors in place of articulation, such as fronting of consonants, for example, /k/→[t] /g/→[d]. In this instance, the child is "fronting" consonants and substitutes sounds that are correctly produced in the front of the oral cavity for those in the back or posterior of the oral cavity.

Phonological Pattern/Process Analysis.   A second type of pattern analysis, sometimes called *phonological process analysis,* is the most frequently employed type of pattern analysis. As already discussed, phonological pattern analysis is a method for identifying commonalities among errors. Because speech sound productions are affected by such factors as position in words, phonetic context, and syllable structure of words, these factors are reviewed for patterns that occur across error sound productions. Before discussing interpretation of such analyses, we would like to review again some of the more common patterns (presented in Chapter 3 in terms of speech acquisition) observed in the speech of young children. Although there are differences in pattern terminology and listings of phonological patterns employed by various authors, most are similar to that which follows.

Whole Word (and Syllable) Patterns.   Whole word and syllable structure patterns are changes that affect the syllabic structures of the target word.

1. *Final consonant deletion.* Deletion of the final consonant in a word.

   e.g., *book*   [bu]
   cap   [ka]
   fish   [fɪ]

2. *Unstressed syllable deletion (weak syllable deletion).* An unstressed syllable is deleted, often at the beginning of a word, sometimes in the middle.

    e.g., *potato*   [teto]

    telephone   [tɛfon]

    pajamas   [dʒæmiz]

3. *Reduplication.* A syllable or a portion of a syllable is repeated or duplicated, usually becoming CVCV.

    e.g., *dad*   [dada]

    water   [wawa]

    cat   [kaka]

4. *Consonant cluster simplification.* A consonant cluster is simplified by a substitution for one member of the cluster.

    e.g., *brown*   [bwon]

    slide   [swʹɪd]

    ask   [æst]

5. *Consonant cluster reduction.* A consonant cluster is reduced to one member of the consonant cluster.

    e.g., *stop*   [tap]

    park   [pak]

    snow   [n̥ou]

6. *Epenthesis.* A segment, usually the unstressed vowel [ə], is inserted.

    e.g., *black*   [bəlæk]

    sweet   [səwit]

    sun   [sθʌn]

    long   [lɔŋg]

7. *Metathesis.* There is a transposition or reversal of two segments (sounds) in a word.

    e.g., *basket*   [bæksɪt]

    spaghetti   [pʌsgɛti]

    elephant   [ɛfəlʌnt]

8. *Coalescence.* Characteristics of features from two adjacent sounds are combined so that one sound replaces two other sounds.

    e.g., *swim*   [fɪm]   *tree*[fɪ]

Assimilatory (Harmony) Patterns.   In this type of error pattern, one sound is influenced by another sound in such a manner that one sound assumes features of a second sound. Thus, the two segments become more alike or similar (hence, the term *harmony*) or even identical. These sound changes are termed *progressive assimilation* if the sound that causes the sound change precedes the affected sound (*gate* [geɪk]) and regressive assimilation if the sound that causes the sound change follows the affected sound (*soup* [pup]). Types of assimilation include:

1. *Velar assimilation.* A nonvelar sound is assimilated (changed) to a velar sound because of the influence, or dominance, of a velar.

   e.g., *duck*   [gʌk]   (regressive assimilation)

   take   [kek]   (regressive assimilation)

   coat   [kok]   (progressive assimilation)

2. *Nasal assimilation.* A nonnasal sound is assimilated because of the influence, or dominance, of a nasal consonant.

   e.g., *candy*   [næni]   (regressive assimilation)

   lamb   [næm]   (regressive assimilation)

   fun   [nʌn]   (regressive assimilation)

3. *Labial assimilation.* A nonlabial sound is assimilated to a labial consonant because of the influence of a labial consonant.

   e.g., *bed*   [bɛb]   (progressive assimilation)

   table   [bebu]   (regressive assimilation)

   pit   [pip]   (progressive assimilation)

Segment Change (Substitution) Patterns.   In these patterns, one sound is substituted for another, with the replacement sound reflecting changes in place of articulation, manner of articulation, or some other change in the way a sound is produced in a standard production.

1. *Velar fronting.* Substitutions are produced anterior to or forward of the standard production.

   e.g., *key*   [ti]   (velar replaced by alveolar)

   monkey   [mʌnti]   (velar replaced by alveolar)

   go   [do]   (velar replaced by alveolar)

2. *Backing.* Sounds are substituted or replaced by segments produced posterior to, or further back in, the oral cavity than the standard production.

   e.g., *tan*   [kæn]

   do   [gu]

   sip   [ʃɪp]

3. *Stopping.* Fricatives or affricates are replaced by stops.

   e.g., *sun*   [tʌn]
   peach   [pit]
   that   [dæt]

4. *Gliding of liquids.* Prevocalic liquids are replaced by glides.

   e.g., *run*   [wʌn]
   yellow   [jɛwo]
   leaf   [wif]

5. *Affrication.* Fricatives are replaced by affricates.

   e.g., *saw*   [tʃau]
   shoe   [tʃu]
   sun   [tʃʌn]

6. *Vocalization.* Liquids or nasals are replaced by vowels.

   e.g., *car*   [kʌo]
   table   [tebo]
   tire   [talo]

7. *Denasalization.* Nasals are replaced by homorganic stops (place of articulation is similar to target sound).

   e.g., *moon*   [bud]
   nice   [deis]
   man   [bæn]

8. *Deaffrication.* Affricates are replaced by fricatives.

   e.g., *chop*   [sap]
   chip   [ʃɪp]
   page   [pez]

9. *Glottal replacement.* Glottal stops replace sounds usually in either intervocalic or final position.

   e.g., *cat*   [kæʔ]
   tooth   [tuʔ]
   bottle   [baʔl]

10. *Prevocalic voicing.* Voiceless consonants (obstruents) in the prevocalic position are voiced.

e.g., *paper* [bepɚ]
Tom   [dam]
table   [debi]

11. *Devoicing of final consonants.* Voiced obstruents are devoiced in final position.

e.g., *dog*   [dɔk]
nose   [nos]
bed   [bɛt]

The preceding list of phonological patterns is not exhaustive but represents most of the common patterns seen in normally developing children. These phonological patterns have also been used in analyzing the sound errors of phonologically delayed children.

Multiple Pattern Occurrence.   The examples of phonological patterns just presented included lexical items that reflected only a single pattern for each example. In reality, the child may produce forms that reflect more than one pattern operating, including some that are not reflected in the preceding definitions and descriptions. A single lexical item may have two or even more patterns interacting. When such productions occur, they are more complex and difficult to unravel than words that reflect a single pattern. For example, in the production of [du] for *shoe*, Edwards (1983) pointed out that the [d] for /ʃ/ replacement reflects the phonological pattern of (1) depalatalization, which changes the place of articulation, (2) stopping, which changes the manner of articulation, and (3) prevocalic voicing, which changes a voiceless consonant target to a voiced consonant. In the substitution of [dar] for *car*, the [d] for /k/ substitution is accounted for by the patterns of both velar fronting and prevocalic voicing. The identification of the sequence of steps describing how interacting patterns occur is called a *derivation* or *pattern ordering.*

Unusual Pattern Occurrence.   As indicated throughout this book, a great deal of individual variation exists in the phonological acquisition of children. Although most children use common developmental phonological patterns, the patterns observed across individuals vary. This is especially true in the speech of children with speech sound disorders. Unusual phonological patterns (e.g., use of a nasal sound for /s/ and /z/), called *idiosyncratic processes* or *patterns*, differ from the more common phonological patterns we have identified and are seen in children with both normal and delayed phonological development. The greatest variation in phonology occurs during the early stages of development and is probably influenced, in part, by the lexical items the child uses when acquiring his or her first words. When idiosyncratic patterns persist after age 3;0 to 3;5, they likely reflect a phonological disorder.

Sound Preferences.   Another type of sound pattern that some clinicians have reported is called *systematic sound preference.* In these situations, children seem to use a segment or two for a large number of sounds or sound classes. Sometimes a particular sound is substituted for several or even all phonemes in a particular sound class (e.g., fricatives). Other children substitute a single consonant for a variety of segments, such as [h] for /b, d, s, ʒ, z, dʒ, tʃ, ʃ, l, k, g, r/ (Weiner, 1981a). It has been postulated that some children avoid the use of certain sounds in their productions and instead simplify their sound productions.

Young children during the phonological acquisition stage simplify their productions as they learn the adult phonological system. The reasons that children simplify their productions likely include such factors as physiological and perceptual limitations/immaturities and a lack of linguistic knowledge. When such phonological simplifications (processes) persist in a child's speech sound productions, we identify these patterns as a way to describe the child's phonological system. It is difficult to determine the precise reason for the persistence of phonological patterns during speech sound acquisition.

Comments Regarding Phonological Patterns. A variety of efforts have been made to explain why some children have a propensity to produce error sounds in a pattern. As mentioned in Chapter 3, the theory of natural phonology assumes that the child has an adultlike underlying representation. As a consequence of a temporary limitation during the developmental period, however, the child is unable to translate those underlying sound representations into correct speech sound productions. Rather, they simplify their productions into something they are currently capable of producing. If a child attempts to say the word "dog" but produces [dɔ] instead, it could be hypothesized that adding a final consonant onto the end of an open syllable is difficult for this child. The way such a child produces the word is to leave off the final sound. Although this is a plausible explanation, it is not the only possible one. Hoffman and Schuckers (1984) suggested at least three other plausible explanations: (1) the child misperceives the adult word, for example, perceives [dɔg] as [dɔ], (2) the child's underlying representation for dog is [dɔ] so that is what she or he produces, (3) the child has a motor production problem (i.e., may have the appropriate perception but does not possess the necessary motor skill to make the articulation gesture to produce the sound). If the only evidence we have is that the child produced [dɔg] as [dɔ], there is no way to know the reason for the error production. Referring to the child's error as *final consonant deletion (FCD)* does not explain the reason for the error. The same might be said for the child who produces "tea" when intending to say "key." We can refer to this production as *velar fronting*, but we do not know why the child made that particular error. Thus, labels attached to phonological patterns do not explain why the child has made the error. Such labels only describe and identify error patterns and do not provide an explanation for the sound production.

That is not to say that labels for phonological patterns have no value. They can be a useful clinical tool for at least two reasons. First, we can use them to help determine whether a child is eligible for services by comparing their occurrence to developmental norms such as those discussed in Chapter 3 (see Table 3.9). Second, if we notice that a particular pattern such as final consonant deletion occurs frequently and includes a variety of different final consonants, we may be able to treat multiple targets simultaneously (see Chapter 10). Identification of phonological patterns can be useful clinical tools for both assessment and treatment (i.e., they can help us describe patterns of errors we observe), even though they do not explain the nature or reason for the child's problem.

Stimulability

In Chapter 6, procedures for conducting and interpreting stimulability testing were presented. As indicated, stimulability data are often used in making decisions regarding case selection and identifying target sounds for intervention. Investigators have reported that the ability of a child to imitate the correct form of an error sound in isolation, syllables, and/or words increases the probability that the child will spontaneously correct his or her misarticulations of that sound. The fact that a young child acquiring phonology can imitate error sounds suggests that the child may be in the process of acquiring those sounds.

The use of stimulability testing for predicting spontaneous improvement or the rate of improvement in remediation has not been documented sufficiently to make definitive prognostic statements. Stimulability testing is only a general guide for the identification of clients who may correct their phonological errors without intervention. False positives (i.e., clients identified as needing instruction but who ultimately will outgrow their problems) and false negatives (i.e., clients identified as not needing instruction but who ultimately will require intervention) have been identified in all investigations focusing on stimulability as a prognostic indicator. These findings must be considered when results from stimulability testing are used to make predictive statements regarding general clinical outcomes or outcomes for specific sounds that are stimulable.

Developmental Appropriateness

A final factor to consider in deciding whether a client is a candidate for intervention is the age appropriateness of his or her speech sound productions. We can evaluate this several different ways. For example, we can ask whether a child misarticulates sounds that are produced correctly by 75 or 90 percent of children at that age (depending on which criterion is selected), or we can ask whether a child's performance on a normed speech sound test is below the mean for his or her age (using whatever standard or cutoff is established), or whether a child evidences phonological patterns that typically are not used by other children of his or her age. No matter how we ask it, a yes answer would mean that the child would be identified as having a developmental delay or disorder.

Two methods traditionally have been employed to compare articulation performance and chronological age: (1) the number of correct responses on a speech sound articulation test are tabulated and then compared with normative data for a given age level on the same test (e.g., *Bankson-Bernthal Test of Phonology*; Bankson and Bernthal, 1990a) and (2) a comparison is made of the child's individual segmental productions with developmental norms for individual sounds (e.g., Prather, Hedrick, and Kern, 1975; Smit and colleagues, 1990).

Of the two methodologies just mentioned, probably the one most frequently used historically has been a comparison of a child's segmental (speech sound) productions with developmental norms for individual sounds. Although this appears to be a simple task, one must be cautious when assigning an age to a particular sound. Normative data for speech sound acquisition represent the point in time when a given percentage of children produce a sound correctly with 75 percent or 90 percent being the percentages most frequently reported in developmental studies of speech sound acquisition. One must remember, however, that children learn sounds at different rates and in different sequences. Thus, caution is required in the application of normative data for individual sounds produced by a given child. The normative data discussed in this chapter are primarily based on studies of children in the United States. Chapter 3 contains a more complete review of speech sound development in a variety of English speaking countries.

As stated, investigators have attached an age expectation to specific speech sounds by listing the age levels at which a given percentage of children in a normative group have mastered each sound tested. Table 3.3 in Chapter 3 provides a detailed summary of these investigations. Sander (1972) pointed out that such normative data are group standards that reflect upper age limits (i.e., 75 percent or 90 percent of children at a particular age produce the sound) rather than average performance or customary production (50 percent of children at a particular age produce the sound). Sander also argued that "variability among children in the ages at which they successfully produce specific sounds is so great as to discourage pinpoint statistics" (p. 58).

Prather, Hedrick, and Kern (1975) reported speech sound acquisition norms for children from age 2 through 4 years on a test designed to elicit consonants in the prevocalic and postvocalic positions. With respect to the age levels at which 75 percent of the children had mastered specific sounds, these investigators reported earlier age levels than Templin (1957), although the sequence of acquisition was similar in both studies. They pointed out that the differences in findings could be due to their use of two-position versus Templin's three-position testing.

Smit and colleagues (1990) gathered three-position data from children in two midwestern states. Using a 75 percent criterion level, they reported that children acquire sounds at ages similar to or younger than ages reported by Templin except for /ŋ/ and /r/, for which the 75 percent criterion was later than that reported by Templin. They also found that clusters of children tended to reach the 75 percent criterion at the same age or later than singletons contained in the clusters. It is interesting to note, however, the overall similarity between the data of Smit and colleagues and those of Templin gathered 33 years earlier.

Keep in mind that in using the data from any large group study, individual subject data are obscured. Although the precise sequence and nature of phonological development varies from one person to another, in general, certain speech sounds are mastered earlier than others, and this information is used in determining presence of phonological delay and the direction of treatment. For example, if 6-year-old Kirsten says all the sounds usually produced by 75 percent of 3-year-old children but is not yet using sounds commonly associated with 4-, 5-, and 6-year-olds, her phonological productions would be considered delayed. This developmental aspect of phonological acquisition makes age a useful factor in determining whether a child has a phonological delay.

A second commonly employed way of comparing phonology and chronological age is to compare a child's speech sound productions with norms for a specific phonological measure (as opposed to individual segmental norms). In this procedure, the number of speech sound productions produced correctly on a specific test is compared with normative data for that instrument. In other words, the number of sounds that the child produces correctly is compared with normative data to determine whether the child's articulatory performance is typical for her or his age. This analysis is appropriate for children 8 years old and younger because correct production of speech sound segments is usually expected by age 8 in typically developing children. This procedure is the basis by which many states and school districts determine whether children with phonological delay and disorders qualify for services. Tests such as the *Goldman-Fristoe Test of Articulation* (2000), the *Clinical Assessment of Articulation and Phonology* (Secord and Donahue, 2002), and the *Bankson-Bernthal Test of Phonology* (1990b) are examples of tests that report normative data.

An additional way to look at a child's individual speech sound productions from a developmental perspective is to review sound errors in terms of whether they tend to fall into one or another of the three developmental sounds classes (Shriberg, 1993) that were discussed in Chapter 3 (i.e., eight early developing sounds, eight middle developing sounds, eight late developing sounds). By reviewing a child's age and the nature of his or her errors, an additional perspective relative to developmental appropriateness can be obtained.

The age appropriateness of certain phonological processes/patterns that may be present in a young child's speech is an additional normative factor considered in case selection. Several investigators have provided data that are relevant to young children's use of phonological processes (see also Table 3.9 in Chapter 3). In a cross-sectional study, Preisser, Hodson, and Paden (1988) examined phonological patterns used by young children. Between 24 and 29 months, the most commonly observed patterns were cluster reduction, liquid deviation (which included deletions of a liquid in a consonant cluster, e.g., *black* → [bæk]), vowelization (e.g., *candle* → [kændo]), and gliding of liquids (e.g., red → [wɛd]). Next most common were patterns involving the strident feature.

Roberts, Burchinal, and Footo (1990) observed a group of children between 2;5 and 8 years in a quasi-longitudinal study—that is, children were tested a varying number of times over the course of the study. They reported a marked decrease in the use of patterns between the ages of 2;5 and 4. They also reported that at age 2;5, the percentage of occurrence for the following patterns was less than 20 percent: reduplication, assimilation, deletion of initial consonants, addition of a consonant, labialization shifts, methathesis, and backing. By age 4, only cluster reduction, liquid gliding, and deaffrication had a percentage of occurrence of 20 percent or more. Refer to Chapter 3 for a more complete summary of speech sound development.

Stoel-Gammon and Dunn (1985) reviewed studies of pattern occurrence and identified those patterns that typically are deleted by age 3 and those that persist after 3 years. Their summary is:

Patterns Disappearing by 3 Years	*Patterns Persisting after 3 Years*
Unstressed syllable deletion	Cluster reduction
Final consonant deletion	Epenthesis
Consonant assimilation	Gliding
Reduplication	Vocalization
Velar fronting	Stopping
Prevocalic voicing	Depalatalization
	Final devoicing

Bankson and Bernthal (1990b) reported data on the patterns most frequently observed in a sample of more than 1,000 children, 3 to 9 years of age, tested during the standardization of the *Bankson-Bernthal Test of Phonology (BBTOP)*. The *BBTOP* ultimately included the 10 patterns that appeared most frequently in children's productions during standardization testing. The patterns that persisted the longest in children's speech were gliding of liquids, stopping, cluster simplification, vocalization, and final consonant deletion. These data are almost identical to those reported by Khan and Lewis (1986) except they later (2000) found velar fronting also persisted longer in young children's speech.

Normative data on the use of phonological patterns can also be used in determining the need for intervention. In this case, one is looking for patterns or simplifications that are no longer typically used at a particular age. If patterns persist beyond the expected age level, or if a child uses unusual patterns, their presence is one of the factors that should be considered in case and target sound selection.

Comparison of children's performance age and phonological development (i.e., data for individual speech sounds) is widely practiced in making intervention decisions. Justifiable criticism has been made of using such data as the single criterion for case selection based on the following factors: (1) Speech sound developmental norms typically reflect upper age limits of customary consonant production (between 75 and 90 percent of children produce the sounds correctly) rather than average age of acquisition, (2) the norms are based on production in the initial, medial, and final positions of single words rather than spontaneous speech, (3) a great deal of variability exists across children in speech sound acquisition, (4) norms frequently are based on a single production of a particular sound in one to three contexts, (5) norms represent a statement of performance by age, but the sequence of acquisition may not be applicable to a given individual, (6) although sounds generally appear to be acquired in a sequence, prior acquisition of certain sounds is not necessarily required for the learning of other sounds, and (7) the nature of the error may be a critical factor in the determination of an age norm. For example, Stephens, Hoffman, and Daniloff (1986) reported that unlike most errors, lateralization of /s/ did not spontaneously improve with age. Our clinical experience is that lateralization of /s/ is a production that is not likely to self-correct with maturation. We would concur with the suggestion of Smit and colleagues (1990) that lateralized /s/ errors be treated earlier than other /s/ errors because unlike most speech sound errors, they do not generally spontaneously or self-correct with age.

Case Selection Guidelines and Summary

The first question that must be answered with data from phonological sampling is whether there is a phonological problem that warrants intervention. By reviewing the intelligibility of the speaker, the severity of the phonological problem, the developmental appropriateness of the productions, the error patterns that may be present, together with stimulability, a decision can be made regarding whether intervention is warranted.

As a general guideline for initiating intervention, a child typically would be one standard deviation or more (some state guidelines call for 1.5 to 2 standard deviations) below his or her age norm on a standardized measure of phonology. The clinician should recognize, however, that this is only a general guideline and that other considerations, such as nature of the errors and error patterns, consistency of errors, speaker's perception of his or her problem, and other speech-language characteristics, might also be important in intervention decisions.

Children between ages 2.5 and 3 who are unintelligible are usually recommended for early intervention programs, which typically include parental education and assistance. Children age 3 years or older who evidence pronounced intelligibility and/or severity problems or who evidence idiosyncratic phonological problems are also usually candidates for intervention. Children age 8 and below whose phonological performance is at least 1 standard deviation below the mean for their age could be candidates for intervention. Most children 9 years or older are recommended for intervention if they consistently produce speech sound errors—often called *residual or persistent errors.* Teenagers and adults who perceive that their phonological errors constitute a handicap should be considered for instruction. Likewise, children of any age should be considered for evaluation when they or their parents are overly concerned about their speech sound productions.

TARGET SPEECH SOUND SELECTION

Once the need for intervention is established, sampling data are further reviewed to determine goals or targets for intervention. The following paragraphs delineate how the various components of the assessment battery are utilized to establish target behaviors for remediation.

Stimulability

As you will recall, stimulability testing consists of assessing client performance when the client is asked to imitate the adult form of speech sound errors in isolation, syllables, and words. Many clinicians have postulated that error sounds that can be produced through imitation are more rapidly corrected through intervention than sounds that cannot be imitated. McReynolds and Elbert (1978) reported that once a child could imitate a sound, generalization occurred to other contexts. Thus, imitation served as a predictor of generalization. Powell, Elbert, and Dinnsen (1991) also reported that stimulability explained many of the generalization patterns observed during treatment. They found that sounds that were stimulable were most likely to be added to the phonetic repertoire regardless of the sounds selected for treatment. Miccio and Elbert (1996) suggested that "teaching stimulability" may be a way to facilitate phonological acquisition and generalization by increasing the client's phonetic repertoire.

Intervention is usually initiated at the level of the most complex linguistic unit the client can imitate (i.e., isolation, syllable, word, phrase). Sounds from different sound classes are often chosen as exemplars with stimulability data aiding in their selection. For example, if word-final stops, fricatives, and nasals are all deleted, the clinician might target one stimulable stop, one fricative, and one nasal as exemplars. Hodson (2007a) suggested selecting patterns on which the child is most stimulable to enhance the client's phonological repertoire.

Although there seems to be general agreement that more rapid generalization occurs for sounds on which the child is stimulable, some clinicians assign such sounds a lower priority for remediation. It has been reported that teaching sounds on which the child is not stimulable has the greatest potential to positively affect the child's overall phonological system although such sounds may be more difficult to teach (Powell et al., 1991). Thus, for children with multiple errors, greater gains in the overall phonological system can be made when intervention initially focuses on sounds not in the child's repertoire. This recommendation is in contrast to the notion that target selections should focus on sounds on which the client is stimulable because therapy will move rapidly and the child will enjoy faster success (Secord, 1989; Diedrich, 1983).

It has been postulated (Dinnsen and Elbert, 1984) that imitation of error sounds in words or syllables by the child may reflect correct underlying representations (storage of the adult form). One might speculate, then, that if a child is able to imitate a word, this performance could indicate that the child has acquired at a cognitive level the linguistic contrasts of the language necessary to produce a sound in at least some appropriate contrastive contexts. From this perspective, correct imitation is a reflection not only of phonetic or motor skill but also of the child's possession of the adult's (correct) underlying form of the error word. However, in a study of this issue, Lof (1994) concluded that one can only assume that stimulability testing reflects phonetic behavior.

As you have read, there is justification for choosing stimulable sounds as targets (e.g. faster progress in therapy), and justification for selecting nonstimulable sounds as targets (e.g. more overall gains in the child's system). Variables such as the client's age, severity of the disorder, and the need to experience immediate success are all related to how stimulability relates to target selection. Keep in mind that stimulability is only one of the variables to consider in selecting targets to work on initially. Other factors (to be delineated in the sections that follow) are also considered. General suggestions for target selection are presented after all the factors related to selection have been discussed.

Frequency of Occurrence

Another factor used in target sound selection is the frequency with which the sounds produced in error occur in the spoken language. Obviously, the higher the frequency of a sound in a language, the greater its potential effect on intelligibility. Thus, treatment will have the greatest impact on a client's overall intelligibility if frequently occurring segments produced in error are selected for treatment.

Shriberg and Kwiatkowski (1983) compiled data on the rank order and frequency of occurrence of the 24 most frequently used consonants in conversational American English from a variety of sources. Their compilation indicated that 11 consonants /n, t, s, r, l, d, ð, k, m, w, z/ occur very frequently in connected speech, so errors on these sounds are likely to have an adverse effect on intelligibility. The data reported by Shriberg and Kwiatkowski also show that almost two-thirds of the consonants used in conversational speech are voiced, 29 percent are stops, 19 percent are sonorants, and 18 percent are nasals. Dental and alveolar consonants accounted for 61 percent of the productions and labial and labiodental sounds for 21 percent. In other words, over four-fifths of consonant occurrences are produced at the anterior area of the mouth.

Developmental Appropriateness

Earlier in this chapter, we discussed the role of normative data in determining the need for therapy. That discussion is also relevant to target selection. Traditionally, clinicians have tended to select sounds for intervention that are earlier acquired and would be expected to be in a client's repertoire. Research by Gierut, Morrisette, Hughes, and Rowland (1996) has suggested, however, that for children with multiple errors, treatment of later as opposed to earlier developing sounds results in greater overall improvement in a client's phonological system than does targeting early developing sounds. This finding is in keeping with other research (Dinnsen, Chin, Elbert, and Powell, 1990; Tyler and Figurski, 1994), which suggests that targeting sounds evidencing greater as opposed to lesser complexity is a more efficient way to proceed with phonological intervention. Rvachew and Nowak (2001) reported data that do not support this assertion. In a study of children with moderate or severe phonological delays, these investigators found that children who received treatment for phonemes that are early developing and associated with some degree of correct productions (productive phonological knowledge) showed greater progress toward production of the target sounds than did children who received treatment for late-developing phonemes associated with little or no productive knowledge. Further research appears warranted before a definitive recommendation can be made regarding the efficacy of targeting early versus later developing sounds.

Some speech-language pathologists have suggested that target selection might be based on the concept of relating age and sound errors to the eight early, middle, and late developing sounds (Shriberg, 1993) that were discussed in Chapter 3. Bleile (2006) authored a book titled *The Late Eight*, which is a resource for teaching the late eight developing sounds (/θ, ð, s, z, ɝ, r, l, ʃ/). He indicated that these sounds are most likely to challenge school-age children and nonnative speakers, both children and adults.

Age appropriateness is one factor to consider in target selection; however, it should be pointed out that other variables discussed in this section should also be reviewed when selecting targets for phonological remediation. For older children in particular, other factors (e.g., frequency of occurrence, stimulability) usually weigh more heavily in terms of target selection.

Contextual Analysis

As stated earlier, contextual testing examines the influence of surrounding sounds on error sounds. Contextual testing may identify *facilitating phonetic contexts*, which are defined as surrounding sounds that have a positive influence on production of error sounds (Kent, 1982). Thus, contextual testing provides data on phonetic contexts in which an error sound can be produced correctly, which could be a helpful beginning point for treatment. Through the identification of such contexts, the clinician might find that a specific sound doesn't have to be taught but should instead be isolated and stabilized in a specific context because it is already in the client's repertoire. Both the client and clinician may save time and frustration that often accompany initial attempts to establish a speech sound by focusing first on contexts in which a sound is produced correctly and then gradually shifting to other contexts. For example, if a child lisps on /s/ but a correct /s/ is observed in the /sk/ cluster in [bɪskɪt] (biscuit), one could have the client say *biscuit* slowly, emphasizing the medial cluster (i.e., sk), and hopefully hear a good /s/. The client could then prolong the /s/ before saying the /k/ (i.e., [bɪs ss kɪt]) and ultimately say the /s/ independent of the word context (i.e., /sss/). This production could then be used to progress to other contexts using the stabilized /s/ production. In general, when contexts can be found where target sounds are produced correctly, such sound contexts can be used efficiently in remediation. The number of contexts in which a child can produce a sound correctly in a contextual test may provide some indication of the stability of the error. It seems logical that the less stable the error, the easier it might be to correct. However, some clinicians find that a stable error pattern is easier to focus on than is a more "elusive error." The clinician can utilize contexts in which a segment is produced correctly to reinforce correct production and facilitate generalization to other contexts. If a client's error tends to be inconsistent across different phonetic contexts, one might assume that the chances for improvement are better than if the error tends to persist across different phonetic contexts or situations.

Phonological Pattern Analysis

The comparison of a client's use of phonological patterns with normative data regarding the use of phonological patterns or simplifications can also be used in target selection. The patterns used by a phonologically delayed child can be compared with those that might be expected in the speech of normally developing children as shown, for example, in Table 7.1 (on page 237). Patterns that are not normally present in children of a particular age are those usually targeted for intervention. One caution, however, is that few data suggest that reduction in the use of phonological patterns occurs in a prescribed order although some patterns tend to persist in older children and others tend to occur only in younger children. Moreover, no data have been reported that suggest the elimination or reduction of one pattern in a child's speech should occur before another pattern is targeted for treatment. There are, however, general trends that could be helpful in targeting patterns for treatment, but a universally prescribed developmental order for pattern selection has not been established.

Hodson (2007a) suggested that clinicians focus on facilitating appropriate phonological patterns (rather than eliminating inappropriate patterns). For highly unintelligible children, she suggested focusing on the most stimulable pattern so that the child can experience immediate success. As a general guide, Hodson delineates the following potential primary targets for facilitation:

1. Syllableness (for omitted vowels, diphthongs, vocalic/syllabic consonants resulting in productions limited to monosyllables; using two-syllable compound words, such as *cowboy,* and then three-syllable word combinations, such as *cowboy hat*)
2. Singleton consonants in words (prevocalic /p, b, m, w/; postvocalic voiceless stops; pre- and postvocalic consonants, such as *pup, pop;* intervocalic consonants, such as *apple*)
3. /s/ clusters (word initial, word final)
4. Anterior/posterior contrasts (word-final /k/, word-initial /k/, /g/ for "fronters"; occasional /h/; alvolars/labials if "backers")
5. Liquids (word-initial /l/, word-initial /r/, word initial /kr/, /gr/—after the child readily produces singleton velars; word initial /l/ clusters—after child readily produces prevocalic /l/)

Target Behavior Selection Guidelines

Few Errors

For children evidencing a small number of sound errors, the clinician might wish to work simultaneously on all error productions. For example, if a child misarticulates /s/, /z/, /r/, and /l/, the clinician might target /s/ and /r/ (assuming that the client will generalize from /s/ to /z/).

If, however, a client is not able to handle multiple targets, one might wish to focus on a target that occurs most frequently in the language and/or that affects intelligibility the most. Age of the client, attention span, and length and/or frequency of treatment sessions are variables to consider in determining how many and which targets to focus on at any point in time.

Multiple Errors

For children with multiple speech sound errors, target selection has some similarity to selection for clients with a small number of errors; however, some additional considerations need to be made. The first step for determining targets in clients with multiple errors is to determine the patterns that are evident. In the preceding paragraphs, we presented the listing of Hodson's (2007a) suggested priorities for identifying target patterns for remediation.

When patterns have been identified for intervention, one is then faced with selecting specific sounds that need to be focused on to facilitate production of a particular pattern. The expectation is that a selected target(s) will generalize to other sounds within a given pattern. For example, if final consonant deletion is identified as the first target pattern, one must then choose a sound or sounds to work on to be established in the word-final position. Sound selection in this instance would be similar to the method identified earlier for choosing among sounds when there are a small number of errors (i.e., stimulability, frequency of occurrence of a target, developmental order).

Time-honored ways of selecting individual sound targets have been challenged because data have been provided (Gierut, 2001) that would suggest that other criteria for target sound selection might be more appropriate in terms of efficiency of treatment. More specifically, Gierut suggested that by targeting the following, a greater impact might be made on a child's overall sound system:

1. Later developing as contrasted with early developing sounds
2. Nonstimulable as contrasted with stimulable sounds
3. Clusters as contrasted with singletons
4. Difficult to produce as contrasted with easy to produce

Although many clinicians would suggest that these criteria for target selection should come into play after target patterns have first been identified, some suggest that one could employ these criteria without reference to overall patterns present in a child's errors. However, the nature of sound collapses might also influence target sound selection. For example, if /w/ is used for /r/, /l/, /s/, /z/, /θ/, /ð/, /h/, one might attempt to initially target /s/ and/or /h/ to establish a contrast between /w/ and a sound in another sound class.

OTHER FACTORS TO CONSIDER IN CASE SELECTION: INTERVENTION DECISIONS

Dialectal Considerations

As discussed in detail in Chapter 11, the linguistic culture of the speaker is a factor that must be considered when deciding on the need for speech-language intervention, particularly for those clients from ethnic or minority populations for whom one of the standard varieties of English might not be the norm. *Dialect*, as discussed in Chapter 11, refers to a consistent variation of a language, reflected in pronunciation, grammar, or vocabulary that a particular subgroup of the general population uses. Although many dialects are identified with a geographical area, those of greatest interest to clinicians are often dialects related to sociocultural or ethnic identification.

The phonological patterns of a particular dialect may differ from the general cultural norm, but these variations reflect only differences, not delays or deficiencies in comparison to the so-called standard version of the language. To view the phonological or syntactic patterns used by members of such subcultures as delayed, deviant, or substandard is totally inappropriate. As Williams (1972) put it years ago, "The relatively simple yet important point here is that language variation is a logical and expected phenomenon, hence, we should not look upon nonstandard dialects as deficient versions of a language" (p. 111). This perspective has obvious clinical implications: Persons whose speech and language patterns reflect a nonstandard cultural dialect should not be considered for remediation or instruction unless their phonological patterns are outside the cultural norm for their region or ethnic group, or the individual wishes to learn a standard dialect.

Phonological differences may also occur in the speech of individuals within subcultures. The language patterns of inner-city African Americans in New York City, for example, may be quite different from those in New Orleans. One cannot use normative data based on General American English (GAE) to judge the phonological status of individuals of some subcultures, nor should one assume that members of certain subcultures have homogeneous linguistic patterns, especially when geographic or ethnic factors are considered. Again, you are referred to Chapter 11 for additional information on this topic.

Clinicians need to know about a child's linguistic and cultural background in order to make appropriate assessment-related decisions, including the need for intervention and instructional goals. Peña-Brooks and Hegde (2000) suggest that clinicians need to know:

1. The language and phonologic characteristics, properties, and rules of the linguistically diverse child's primary language
2. How the primary language affects the learning of the second language
3. How to determine whether there are language or phonologic disorders in the child's first language, second language, or both

In the event that a speaker or the speaker's family wishes to modify the speaker's dialect or accent, the clinician may wish not only to use traditional sampling methods to describe the child's phonology but also to employ measures specifically designed to assess the dialect and nonnative speaker's use of English phonology. Instructional decisions are then based on samples obtained and the variations that exist between Standard English and the person's dialect or accent.

Social-Vocational Expectations

Another factor to consider in the analysis and interpretation of a phonological sample is the attitude of the client or the client's parents toward the individual's phonological status. In cases when a treatment recommendation is questionable, the attitude of a client or family may be a factor in decisions for or against intervention. This is particularly important for older children and adults. Extreme concern over an articulatory difference by the client or the client's parents may convince the clinician to enroll an individual for instruction. For example, the child who has a frontal lisp and has a name that begins with /s/ may feel very strongly that the error is a source of embarrassment. Crowe-Hall (1991) and Kleffner (1952) found that fourth- and sixth-grade children reacted unfavorably to children who had even mild articulation disorders. The literature contains many reports in which elementary children have recounted negative experiences in speaking or reading situations when they produced only a few speech sounds in error. Even "minor distortions" can influence how one is perceived. Silverman (1976) reported that when a female speaker simulated a lateral lisp, listeners judged her more negatively on a personality characteristics inventory than when she spoke without a lisp.

Overby, Carrell, and Bernthal (2007) reported that second-grade teachers had different expectations of children's academic, social, and behavioral performances when making judgments of children who were moderately intelligible and those with normal intelligibility. One-third of the teachers related children's school difficulty to their speech sound disorders and made expectations based on the speech intelligibility of the children.

The standard for acceptance of communication depends, to a large extent, on the speaking situation. People in public speaking situations could find that even minor distortions detract from their message. Some vocations—for example, radio and television broadcasters—may call for very precise articulation and pronunciations, and thus, some individuals may feel the need for intervention for what could be relatively minor phonetic distortions or even dialectal differences. We suggest that if an individual, regardless of age, feels handicapped or vocationally limited by speech errors or speech differences, treatment/instruction should usually be recommended or at least considered.

COMPUTER-ASSISTED PHONOLOGICAL ANALYSIS

Any discussion of phonological analysis and interpretation would be incomplete without calling attention to the fact that computer-based programs have been designed to assist with the analysis of phonological samples in clients who exhibit multiple errors. Masterson, Long, and Buder (1998) indicated that there are two primary reasons for using a computer-based analysis of a phonological sample: (1) it saves time and (2) it provides more detail of analysis than one typically produces with traditional paper and pencil (manual) analysis procedures. Computer phonological analysis (CPA) software involves inputting phonetic transcriptions from a computer keyboard and/or selecting from predetermined stimuli, displaying the data on the screen, and ultimately printing and/or reviewing the results of an analysis. Analyses often include both relational and independent analyses of consonants and vowels, word position analysis, syllable shapes used, patterns among errors, and calculation of percentage of consonants correct. Each CPA program has its own strengths and limitations, and undoubtedly future procedures will add new and helpful procedures for clinicians.

The Computerized Articulation and Phonology Evaluation System (CAPES) (Masterson and Bernhardt, 2001) is a good example of a computer system that was developed to elicit and analyze phonological productions. It elicits 47 single-word responses through digitized photographs presented on the computer. The clinician can tape-record responses or record them online. Following the initial 47-word productions, additional items of increasing word complexity are included based on the nature of the client's responses in the first items. These additional items are referred to as the Individual Phonological Evaluation (IPE). The end result of this assessment program is that the clinician has data that reflect the client's omission, substitution, and distortion errors for each consonant and consonant sequence in the initial, medial, and final positions of words as well as vowel productions. Analyses that describe the client's productions in terms of word length, syllable stress, word shape, place-manner-voice features, and phonological processes/patterns can also be generated. On the basis of these data, the program suggests treatment goals although, of course, the clinician must have a detailed enough speech sample to develop his or her own goals as well as intervention program.

In a study of time efficiency of procedures for phonological and grammatical analysis, comparing manual and computerized methods, Long (2001) reported that without exception for both phonology and language, computerized analyses were completed faster and with equal or better accuracy than were manual analyses. Phonological analyses included the evaluation of variability, homonymy, word shapes, phonetic inventory, accuracy of production, and correspondence between target and production forms. Long further indicated that time needed for analyses, both computer and manual, was affected by the type of analysis, the type of sample, and the efficiency of individual participants.

A listing of some of the current CPA software programs is as follows:

Hodson Computer Analysis of Phonological Patterns (HCAPP). Hodson, B. (2003). Wichita, KS: Phonocomp Software.

Computerized Profiling (Version CP941.exe). Long, S. H., M. E. Fey, and R. W Channell, (2002). Cleveland, OH: Case Western Reserve University.

Interactive System for Phonological Analysis (ISPA). Masterson, J., and F. Pagan (1993). San Antonio, TX: The Psychological Corporation.

Programs to Examine Phonetic and Phonological Evaluation Records (PEPPER). Shriberg, L. (1986). Hillsdale, NJ: Erlbaum.

Computerized Articulation and Phonology Evaluation System (CAPES). Masterson, J., and B. Bernhardt. (2001). San Antonio, TX: The Psychological Corporation.

CASE STUDY

Assessment: Phonological Samples Obtained

Client

Kirk

Age

3.0 years

Reason for Referral

Parental referral due to Kirk's poor intelligibility when speaking with familiar listeners and only slightly better (but still poor) when speaking with those who know him well.

Case History/Speech and Hearing Mechanisms Status

The case history submitted by the parents and supplemented with the examination interview revealed normal motor and language development; however, speech sound development was delayed. Hearing screening indicated that hearing was within normal limits. A speech mechanism examination indicated normal structure and function.

Language.   Vocabulary, syntax, and pragmatics appeared normal based on case history, language sample obtained, and social interaction between Kirk and the examiner. Language skills, as measured by the *Peabody Picture Vocabulary Test* and the *Preschool Language Scale*, indicated language within normal limits. Poor intelligibility made it difficult to assess expressive morphosyntactic structures; however, a spontaneous speech sample obtained through storytelling evidenced four 6-word utterances, a seemingly rich vocabulary, and appropriate concepts for a 3-year-old child. Based on these data, Kirk's language skills were determined to be within normal limits. This will, however, need to be confirmed later once his intelligibility improves.

Fluency and Voice.   Fluency was regarded as normal. However, a hoarse voice was noted. It was determined that vocal quality should be monitored over time by the parents and clinician to determine whether a problem was developing.

Phonological Samples Gathered

- *Conversation Connected speech sample* of 180 words was obtained, with Kirk telling the story of "The Three Little Pigs." This story was used because Kirk was familiar with it and words in the story were known to the examiner, thus facilitating phonological analysis.
- *Single-word productions*   were obtained through the *Bankson-Bernthal Test of Phonology (BBTOP)*. All consonants and vowels produced by Kirk in the stimulus words were transcribed.
- *Stimulability testing*   was done in isolation, syllables, and words for all target sounds produced in error.

Phonological Results and Analysis.   The transcription of the connected speech sample and the single words from BBTOP were analyzed with the Proph phonological analysis component of the Computerized Profiling (Long, Fey, and Channell, 2002) program. Individual sound transcriptions were entered into the program and served as the basis for the analysis.

Phonological Analysis Outcomes.   The percentage of consonants correct (PCC) was determined based on the connected speech sample. The PCC value was 34 percent, which translates to a rating of "severe" for connected speech.

Segmental Analysis. Segmental analysis revealed numerous sound substitutions, particularly the use of /d/ in place of fricatives, affricates, and some clusters. In addition, there were inconsistent initial and final consonant deletions, including deletion of the initial /h/, /r/, and /l/. Other substitutions included /f/ for /s/ and some prevocalic voicing. These errors were evidenced in both single-word productions and in running speech, although higher accuracy was reflected in single-word productions. Table 7.1 reflects consonant singleton transcriptions from single-word productions. Figures in the table indicate percent accuracy of production.

Stimulability Analysis. Kirk was instructed to "look at me, listen to what I say, and then you say it," followed by a model of the correct sound. Imitative testing (stimulability) was conducted for all sounds produced in error. Responses were solicited for sounds in isolation, syllables, and the initial position of words.

TABLE 7.1 Consonant Singleton Productions in Single-Word Productions Including Percent Accuracy of Production

| Target | Error Productions | | | |
	Error	Initial (%)	Error	Final (%)
p		100		100
b		100		100
m		100		100
w	ø	0		
f	/d/	0	/s/	0
v	/d/	0		100
θ	/d/	0	/t/	0
ð	/d/	0		
t		100		100
d		100		100
s	/d/	0	/f/	50
z	/d/	0	/v/	0
n		100		100
l	ø	0	/o/	0
ʃ	/d/	0	/f/	0
tʃ	/d/	0		100
dʒ	/d/	0		
j	ø	0		
r	ø	0		
k		100		100
g		100		100
h	ø	0		

Kirk was stimulable for most error sounds in isolation, syllables, and initial word position. He did not imitate clusters that were in error. The following sounds were not stimulable: /ʃ/, /tʃ/, /z/, /dʒ/, /r/, and /ɝ/. The /s/ was stimulable only in isolation even though it was observed in the word-final position of some words during testing.

Pattern Analysis.   A phonological process analysis was completed through the Proph program to determine error patterns that were evidenced in Kirk's single-word as well as connected speech sample. This analysis revealed that the most prevalent process was stopping with all fricatives and affricates impacted by this pattern (occurred in 85 percent of possible occasions in connected speech and with 44 percent occurrence in stimulus words from the BBTOP, particularly initial position). The most prevalent example of stopping was the use of /d/, which was substituted for initial /f/, /v/, /θ/, /ð/, /s/, /z/, /ʃ/, /tʃ/, /dʒ/, and the clusters /sl/, /sn/, and /fl/. Kirk used frication (e.g., /s/, /f/, although inappropriately) when producing some single words. A diagram of his sound collapses for /d/ is as follows:

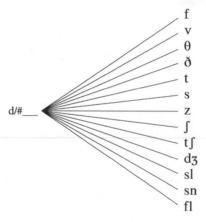

Clusters were simplified approximately 75 percent of the time in both isolated words and connected speech samples. Less frequently occurring patterns included *context-sensitive voicing* (prevocalic voicing), and *initial consonant deletions*. Prevocalic voicing occurred in less than 25 percent of possible instances and initial consonant deletions less than 12 percent. Process analysis scoring on the BBTOP revealed similar error patterns.

Vowel Analysis.   The Proph program assesses vowel accuracy, and, as might be expected for his age, Kirk's vowel productions were almost entirely accurate in both running speech and single-word productions. Inconsistent misarticulations were observed on the vowels /ɛ/ and /ʊ/ in running speech.

Summary

These data reflect a 3-year-old boy with a speech sound disorder that, according to his PCC, BBTOP norms, and examiner's subjective evaluation, is severe in nature. Although intelligibility was not formally measured, understanding his verbal productions was difficult even for family members. Most of Kirk's errors were sound substitutions with some deletions in both initial and final word positions. Substitution errors were predominately the /d/ being substituted for fricatives and affricates. The presence of initial consonant deletions is developmentally an unusual process, but it is present only for the aspirate /h/ and liquids. Final consonant deletion is a process usually eliminated by age 3 and was observed only occasionally in Kirk's speech. Inconsistencies in all types of error productions were noted.

Speech sound errors for which Kirk was not stimulable included the fricative /ʃ/, the affricates /tʃ/, and /dʒ/, the prevocalic /r/, and the vowelized /ɝ/. These error consonants will likely need to be stabilized in isolation and/or syllables and will require motor practice in single words before they are incorporated into word-pairs that reflect relevant sound contrasts. For /h/ and /k/, which were easily stimulated at the word level, it is likely that Kirk needs instruction in how these sounds are used contrastively in the language, or it might be necessary only to monitor these sounds to make sure they are acquired.

Assessment: Interpretation

Case Selection

Intervention is warranted for Kirk. Factors that influenced this recommendation are as follows:

1. Normative data indicate that most normally developing 3-year-old children are approximately 75 percent intelligible. Although Kirk has just turned 3, we would nonetheless expect him to be more intelligible than he is. Intelligibility was not formally determined in our assessment battery, but observational data as well as reports from his family indicate that much of Kirk's speech is unintelligible. This factor weighed heavily in our decision regarding Kirk's need for intervention.

2. With a PCC value in running speech of less than 40 percent, Kirk's impairment is regarded as severe in nature. This rating relates to level of handicap reflected in his speech.

3. Phonological analysis evidences numerous substitution errors, some deletions, and several phonological patterns that one would not expect in a child of his age. Positive indicators regarding Kirk's phonological status include the fact that he uses almost all vowels and some consonants correctly in his speech and is stimulable (with effort) for many of his error segments. His good vocabulary and the length of his utterances suggest that his linguistic deficits are confined to articulation and phonology, another positive indicator.

4. Intervention appears favorable because Kirk is stimulable for many of his error sounds, is highly verbal, and is not reluctant to speak.

Target Sound Selection

Because Kirk has numerous misarticulations, and because these errors fall into patterns, target selection should begin with a review of these patterns. The error pattern that occurred most frequently was that of stopping, with several initial sounds, predominately fricatives and glides, collapsed into /d/. He also evidenced voicing of voiceless consonants in the initial position, gliding of liquids, and cluster reductions.

Although stopping is a process that persists in children sometimes past the age of 3, it is unusual for a child of this age not to be using more fricatives in speech. Most children are expected to use /f/ correctly by this age, and many are using the /s/ as well. Because the fricative feature is diminished in Kirk's speech, reduction of stopping is the phonologic target of choice for initial therapy. The other two patterns evidenced in Kirk's speech (i.e., voicing, gliding) will be focused on later, largely because voicing does not have a great impact on intelligibility, and gliding occurred relatively infrequently and likely does not affect Kirk's intelligibility as much as stopping.

Intervention suggestions for Kirk are discussed in detail in Chapters 9 and 10. In terms of target selection, we would suggest approaches that allow for focusing on several error sounds in each lesson. Kirk's good attention span and good language skills will hopefully facilitate his handling multiple treatment goals. We would suggest addressing the sound collapses reflected in the /d/ replacement for numerous fricatives, other stops, and clusters.

Because Kirk is very young, one might choose to focus on only one or two sounds in the early sessions to avoid confusion among targets. As progress is made, additional targets can be identified and added to the sessions. If one chooses to focus on one or two target sounds at a time, our suggestion for a priority focus is /f/. This is a highly visible sound and one that develops early, would address Kirk's stopping pattern, and frequently develops in final position prior to initial position. Kirk already uses the sound as a substitution for other fricatives in the final position; for example, he says /tif/ for /tiθ/ but /lis/ for /lif/. A second treatment target, likely one to work on simultaneously, is the correct use of /s/. The /s/ is in Kirk's repertoire; however, it is used inappropriately. As stated already, length of attention span, including ability to focus on multiple sounds and/or sound contrasts simultaneously, will influence the choice of treatment approach. This issue is addressed in Chapters 9 and 10.

Summary

Kirk is a child who needs phonological intervention. Intelligibility, severity, and developmental level of his phonology support this decision. On the basis of his phonological samples, teaching frication to reduce stopping, producing sounds correctly in word-initial position, and further increasing Kirk's phonological repertoire would appear to be priority goals for initiating therapy.

CONCLUSION

Assessment data are interpreted for a variety of reasons including deciding if there is a problem, the nature of the problem, whether treatment is indicated, and what the treatment targets might be. Each decision requires the consideration of a number of different factors. In the next chapter we turn to a discussion of the basic considerations for treatment.

QUESTIONS FOR CHAPTER 7

1. Discuss how the following factors may be utilized in case selection:

   a. Intelligibility

   b. Severity

   c. Stimulability

   d. Error patterns

   e. Developmental appropriateness

2. Discuss how the following factors might influence target behavior selection:

   a. Stimulability

   b. Frequency of occurrence

   c. Developmental appropriateness

   d. Contextual analysis

   e. Phonological process analysis

3. Differentiate between intelligibility and severity.

4. How might treatment targets differ between a preschool child and a child age 12 years?

5. How do dialectal considerations influence intervention decisions?

CHAPTER 8

Remediation Procedures

NICHOLAS W. BANKSON
James Madison University

JOHN E. BERNTHAL
University of Nebraska–Lincoln

PETER FLIPSEN JR.
Idaho State University

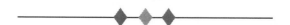

BASIC CONSIDERATIONS

Once a determination has been made that an individual's phonology is disordered or delayed and warrants intervention, the speech-language clinician uses assessment data in planning management strategies. As described in Chapter 6, phonological analyses are designed to assist the clinician in identifying appropriate target behaviors for instruction. After specific goals and objectives for intervention have been determined, the clinician is faced with the task of determining the type of treatment approach that is best suited for an individual client. Before discussing specifics of particular treatment approaches in the next two chapters, we focus in this chapter on some basic underlying concepts that should be considered when developing a treatment plan. Although the focus of the chapter is on disordered phonology, the concepts and principles described in this chapter may also be useful in terms of instruction related to other speech/language disorders as well as accent/dialect modification.

Framework for Conducting Therapy

Before clinical speech instruction is initiated, an organizational framework for the therapy sessions should be developed. In this section, we review several overarching components and strategies to be considered in treatment planning.

Once intervention objectives have been determined, the clinician formulates a treatment plan that spells out activities to be used in accord with the moment-to-moment temporal sequence of instructional components. The typical sequence of clinical speech instruction components is as follows:

Antecedent events (AE)	Delineation of stimulus events designed to elicit particular responses (e.g., auditory/visual modeling or pictures presented by the clinician, followed by a request for the client to imitate the model or name a picture)
Responses (R)	Production of a target behavior (e.g., often a particular sound in isolation or sound productions in a given linguistic and/or social context)
Consequent events (CE)	Reinforcement or feedback that follows the response (e.g., the clinician says "good" if a response is accurate or may say "try again" if inaccurate; tokens to reinforce correct responses)

Antecedent events are the stimulus events presented during or just prior to a response. Such events typically consist of a verbal model, a picture, printed material, or verbal instructions designed to elicit particular verbal responses. For example, if a client is working on /s/ at the word level, the clinician may show the child a picture of soap, and ask the child, "What do we wash with?" The child may be further asked to "say the word three times," or to "put it in a sentence." The type of antecedent events vary depending on whether the clinician is seeking to establish a motor behavior, teach a phonological rule or contrast, or help the client use a newly learned production.

Responses are the behaviors the clinician has targeted for the client. These may range from approximations of the desired behavior (e.g., movement of the tongue backward for production of /k/), to production of the correct behavior (e.g., /k/) in connected speech. The clinician is concerned with the functional relationship between an antecedent event and a response or, in other words, the likelihood that a given stimulus will elicit the desired response. Movement to the next level of instruction is often contingent on a certain number of correct responses. It is important in the establishment of a speech sound that clients have the opportunity to produce many productions in the course of a therapy session. A high rate of utterances provides the opportunity for both the clinician's external monitoring and the client's automatization of the response. It is usual that responses are stabilized at one level of complexity before proceeding to the next level (e.g., sounds are often easier to produce in syllables than in words; word production is easier than it is in phrases or sentences).

The third aspect of the temporal sequence for instruction is *consequent events* (CE). They occur following a particular response and usually are labeled reinforcement or punishment. Whether a response is learned (and how quickly it is learned) is closely related to what happens following the occurrence of a behavior or response. The most frequently used consequent event in clinical speech instruction is positive *reinforcement*. Tangible consequents such as tokens, points, chips, and informal reinforcers such as a smile or verbal feedback are typically used. Consequent events intended to reinforce should immediately follow the correct or desired behavior and should be used only when the desired or correct response is produced. Reinforcement is defined by an increase in a behavior following the presentation of consequent events. Providing a positive consequence after an incorrect production sends the "wrong message" to the speaker, possibly reinforcing an incorrect response, and does not facilitate learning of correct responses. The use of "punishment" as a consequence is seldom if ever used in treatment.

Instructional steps are organized so that a sequential series of antecedent events, responses, and consequent events are followed as one progresses through various levels of therapy (more on the levels in Chapter 9). See Table 8.1 for an example of a sequential series.

Goal Attack Strategies

An early intervention decision relates to determining the number of treatment goals targeted in a given session. Fey (1991) described three "goal attack strategies" applicable to children with speech sound disorders. The first strategy is called a *vertically structured treatment program* in which one or two goals or targets are trained to some performance criterion before proceeding to another target. Treatment sessions of this type involve a high response rate for a single target, involving lots of repetition of that target. The traditional approach to treatment of speech sound disorders, to be described in detail later in this book, is an example of a vertically structured program. In this approach, one or two phonemes are targeted for treatment and are worked on until they are produced in conversation before training is initiated on other target sounds. For a client who exhibits five different phonologic patterns, the clinician may target one process and focus treatment on one or two sounds related to that process/pattern until some criterion level is reached before proceeding to the next target process. Elbert and Gierut (1986) termed this vertical type of strategy *training deep*. The assumptions behind the vertical strategy are that (1) mass practice on a restricted number of target sounds with a limited number of training items facilitates generalization to other nontrained items and (2) some clients are best served by focusing on one or a few targets rather than many.

A second instructional strategy is a *horizontally structured treatment program* (Fey, 1991; Williams, 2000b), or what Elbert and Gierut (1986) have called *training broad*. Using this strategy, the clinician addresses multiple goals in each session. Thus, more than one goal may be incorporated into each session, and goals may change across sessions. By working on several sounds or patterns in the same session, the client will presumably

TABLE 8.1   Sequential Series of Antecedent Events, Responses, and Consequent Events

Step	Antecedent Event	Response	Consequent Event
1	Clinician: Put your tongue behind your teeth, have the tip of your tongue lightly touch the roof of your mouth as if you were saying /t/, and blow air. Say /s/.	/t/	Clinician: No, I heard /t/.
2	Clinician: Keep your tongue tip a little bit down from the roof of your mouth and blow air. Say /s/.	/s/	Clinician: Good! Perfect!
3	Now say /s/ 3 times.	/s/, /s/, /s/	Clinician: Great!
4	Now say /sa/.	/sa/	Clinician: Super!

learn commonalities or relationships among sound productions, and treatment will be more efficient. In contrast to the vertical approach, the client receives less intense training on specific targets, but the training presented is focused on a broader range of components of the sound system. The concept behind training broad is that limited practice with a range of exemplars and sound contrasts is an efficient way to modify a child's phonological system. The goal is to expose the child to a wide range of target sound productions so that this broad-based training facilitates simultaneous acquisition of several treatment targets.

A third strategy (Fey, 1986), which combines aspects of the vertical and horizontal approaches, is a *cyclically structured treatment program* (Hodson and Paden, 1991; Hodson, 2007a). In this approach, a single target (or pattern) is addressed for a single session or a week or more. After a fixed amount of therapy time (e.g., a total of 2 hours), another goal is addressed. The movement from goal to goal is essentially a horizontal approach to treatment whereas the focus on a single sound for a fixed time period may be viewed as vertical.

Historically, the most common strategy employed in speech sound remediation was the vertical approach, but many clinicians now favor the horizontal or cyclical approach, especially once clients have a sound in their repertoire (i.e., they can produce a sound at the motor level with some consistency). Our preference with children who produce multiple errors is the cyclical approach, although all three approaches have been shown to improve speech sound skill. For clients who evidence a small number of errors, such as misarticulating /r/, /s/, /l/, or /θ/ (persistent or residual errors), a vertical approach is preferable.

Scheduling of Instruction

Another consideration in planning for speech sound intervention relates to the scheduling of treatment sessions. Relatively little is known about the influence that scheduling of instruction has on remediation efficacy, and sufficient research has not been reported to determine which scheduling arrangements are most desirable. In addition, it is often not practical to schedule treatment sessions on an "ideal" basis. Treatment scheduling is usually determined by such factors as the client's age, attention span, and severity of the disorder and practical realities such as financial resources available, availability of instructional services, size of a clinician's caseload, and treatment models employed by a school system (e.g., pull-out versus classroom-based instruction). Investigators who have studied scheduling have generally focused on the efficacy of intermittent scheduling versus block scheduling of treatment sessions. *Intermittent scheduling* usually refers to two or three sessions each week over an extended period of time (such as eight months), whereas *block scheduling* refers to daily sessions for a shorter temporal span (such as an eight-week block). Several investigators have compared dismissal rates associated with intermittent and block scheduling, primarily for public school students with articulation disorders (Van Hattum, 1969). Based on these studies, Van Hattum reported that block scheduling was a more efficient way to achieve articulatory/phonological progress than was intermittent scheduling. Unfortunately, however, variables such as disorder severity, stimulability, and treatment methodology employed were not well enough controlled or described to make definitive clinical recommendations from these investigations.

Bowen and Cupples (1999) described a scheduling protocol in which children were seen once weekly for approximately 10-week blocks, followed by approximately 10 weeks without treatment. They reported positive results with this treatment schedule. It should be pointed out, however, that their treatment included multifaceted components including parent education. The specific influence of the break in treatment schedule on treatment outcome is unknown; however, this study reflects an approach that utilizes a form of block scheduling (Bowen, 2010).

Although controled experiments on scheduling are lacking, the following suggestions for scheduling of phonological intervention seem appropriate:

1. Scheduling of intervention four to five times per week for 8 to 10 weeks may result in slightly higher dismissal rates than intermittent scheduling for a longer period of time, the greater gains being made early in the treatment process. Some children, especially preschoolers, can generalize correct productions without a lot of instruction.
2. Intensive scheduling on only a short-term basis does not appear to be as appropriate with clients who have severe articulation/phonological disorders and need ongoing services.
3. Scheduling a child for three 20-minute sessions per week appears to yield better results than one 60-minute session.

Pull-Out versus Classroom-Based Instruction

A consideration related to treatment is the place and format of school-based service delivery. One decision relates to whether treatment is provided through a *pull-out model* (the client is instructed in a treatment room) or *inclusion model* (the client is instructed in a classroom setting), or a combination of the two. Historically, the pull-out model was the choice for articulation/phonological treatment. In recent years, an emphasis has been placed on integrating speech and language services within the classroom. The opportunity to incorporate a child's instruction with the academic curriculum and events associated with a child's daily school routine is the optimal way to enhance the efficiency and effectiveness of therapy. Furthermore, classroom inclusion capitalizes on the opportunity for collaboration among regular educators, special education educators, speech-language pathologists, and other professionals within a child's educational environment.

Masterson (1993) suggested that classroom-based approaches for school-age children allow the clinician to draw on textbooks, homework, and classroom discourse to establish instructional goals, target words, and instructional procedures. For preschoolers, classroom activities such as crafts, snacks, and toileting are similarly helpful activities for language and phonological instruction. In addition, for preschool and early primary-grade children, classroom-based phonological awareness activities may provide the clinicians the opportunity to extend services to all children in a classroom as they collaborate with teachers. Masterson further indicated that classroom-based approaches can be most useful for treating conceptual- or linguistic-based errors as opposed to errors that require motor-based habilitation. Instruction in the context of the classroom setting is typically less direct than that involved in a pull-out model and requires collaborative efforts between the clinician and the classroom teacher. The vocabulary used in the curriculum can be used by the speech clinician as the basis for target practice words. Classroom instruction is particularly appropriate when a client is in the generalization, or "carryover" phase of instruction, in which academic material and other classroom activities allow for an emphasis on communication skills. It is likely that both of these models (i.e., pull-out; classroom inclusion) are appropriate for a given client during the course of intervention depending on where they are on the treatment continuum, a concept that is discussed in the next chapter.

Clinicians must determine whether clients are treated individually or in a small group. Treatment is frequently conducted in small groups, which may be as effective as individual instruction in remediating speech sound disorders (Sommers et al., 1964; Sommers et al., 1966).

Sommers and colleagues (1964) reported that 50-minute group instruction based on the pull-out model resulted in as much articulatory change as 30-minute individual instruction when both group and individual sessions were conducted four times per week for 4 weeks. In a subsequent study (Sommers et al., 1966), similar results were obtained from group sessions held 45 minutes each week and individual instruction sessions held 30 minutes each week over a period of 8.5 months. These investigators concluded that group and individual sessions were equally effective and that the grade level (fourth to sixth grades versus second grade) or the severity of the speech sound disorder did not influence the results.

When children with speech sound disorders are grouped, such groups usually consist of three or four clients of about the same age who work on similar target behaviors. Unfortunately, such group sessions frequently have a tendency to become regimented so that all individuals work on the same target behavior and the same level of production.

Group instruction should be different from *individual instruction in a group* (the clinician works with each client individually while remaining group members observe). Group instruction can and should be structured so that individuals in the group can benefit from interaction with other members and from activities that involve the entire group. For example, individuals can monitor and reinforce each other's productions and can serve both as correct models for each other and as listeners to see whether the communication intent of the message is met or the productions correct.

It is our suggestion that a combination of group and individual sessions may be advantageous for most individuals with speech sound disorders. Furthermore, instructional groups should usually be limited to three or four individuals whose ages do not exceed a three-year range. Some suggest that when children are learning the motor skills involved in production of a given sound, individual instruction is perhaps the best format if only for a limited number of sessions or parts of sessions. Once a sound is in the child's production repertoire, group and classroom activities can easily be incorporated into the instructional plans.

Intervention Style

A final consideration before we begin our discussion of specific therapy approaches is intervention style. In addition to selecting target behaviors to be used in treatment, the clinician must also consider the management mode or style most appropriate for a given client. A key issue here is the amount of structure that may be prescribed for or tolerated by a given client.

Shriberg and Kwiatkowski (1982b) described the structure of treatment activities as ranging from drill (highly structured therapy) to play (little structure to therapy). These authors described the following four modes of intervention:

1. *Drill.* This type of therapy relies heavily on clinician presentation or some form of antecedent instructional events followed by client responses. The client has little control over the rate and presentation of training stimuli.
2. *Drill play.* This type of therapy is distinguished from drill by the inclusion of an antecedent motivational event (e.g., activity involving a spinner; card games).
3. *Structured play.* This type of instruction is structurally similar to drill play. However, training stimuli are presented as play activities. In this mode, the clinician moves from formal instruction to playlike activities, especially when the child becomes unresponsive to more formal instruction.
4. *Play.* The child perceives what he or she is doing as play. However, the clinician arranges activities so that target responses occur as a natural component of the activity. Clinicians may also use modeling, self-talk, and other techniques to elicit responses from a child.

These investigators conducted several studies with young children with phonological disorders to compare the relative effects of these four treatment modes. They reported that drill and drill play modes were more effective and efficient than structured play and play modes. In addition, drill play was as effective and efficient as drill.

Clinicians' evaluation of the four modes indicated that they felt drill play was most effective and efficient for their clients, and they personally preferred it. They also urged that three factors be considered when making a choice of management mode: (1) a general knowledge of the child's personality, (2) the intended target response, and (3) the stage of therapy (Shriberg and Kwiatkowski, 1982b).

Summary

Before deciding on a specific treatment methodology, the clinician must review the following:

1. What is the severity of the problem, and how many targets will be selected for treatment?
2. Which targets need to be focused on at a motor level and which can be approached from a rule or phonological basis?
3. How many targets will I work on in a given session, and how long will I stay with a target before I move on to another?
4. How frequently will therapy sessions be held, and how long will each session last?
5. Will instruction be individual or in a small group? If it is conducted in a school environment, will it be pull-out, classroom based, or a combination of the two? What is the best approach: drill and practice, play, or a combination of the two?
6. For children with both phonological and language impairments, how should intervention be structured (e.g., an integrated approach; target each area separately)?

MAKING PROGRESS IN THERAPY: MEASURING CLINICAL CHANGE

As discussed in Chapter 6, tools for measuring change can be employed to assist the clinician in determining whether intervention is successful and appropriate. Speech-language pathologists also need to assess progress (or lack of progress) in therapy. Evidence-based practice (ASHA, 2004b; 2005) requires that clinicians document treatment outcomes, which requires ongoing assessment.

Tools for Measuring Change

Norm-referenced tests such as the *Goldman-Fristoe Test of Articulation*, the *Clinical Assessment of Articulation and Phonology,* and the *Bankson-Bernthal Test of Phonology* can be used to determine eligibility for therapy and are designed for that purpose. It is tempting to simply readminister these tests on a regular basis and look for changes in test scores as a measure of progress. This is not a wise practice for several reasons. First, there is a statistical problem with such a practice known as *regression to the mean*, to be discussed later. Second, and from a more practical standpoint, such tests typically provide only a limited sample of the child's speech. They often include only a single word that tests performance on each sound in each word position (e.g., word-initial /s/). It is possible that when such a test is readministered, the child might remember having problems with that particular word during testing and may have practiced the word. The child may then appear to have mastered the sound, but is not necessarily able to produce that same sound in other words. On the other hand, the child may have become hypersensitive to that particular word because of her or his failure and might continue having difficulty with it even when she or he is perfectly capable of producing that sound in many other words.

To get around this limitation of norm-referenced tests, clinicians should and can create what is known as a *probe* (sometimes called a *generalization probe*) for each target sound being worked on in therapy (see Elbert, Shelton, and Arndt, 1967). Such probes include several words (typically 8 to 15) that contain the target sound. The S-CAT probes (Secord and Shine, 1997) discussed in Chapter 6 could easily be used or adapted for this purpose. Generalization probes are usually informal measures constructed by the clinician employing words that are not used in therapy. Using such words that are not practiced in therapy helps determine whether the child is really learning the sound and generalizing that sound into new/novel words in his or her sound system. Having a sound incorporated into the child's system allows the child to correctly produce any word containing the sound, even if that word has seldom been encountered before. Without such probes, clinicians can never be certain that the child isn't simply memorizing the set of speech movements for the particular words being practiced in therapy. Probes generally are not administered during each treatment session because clinicians don't want the child to become overly familiar with the probe items. A more typical practice is to administer a probe every 4 or 5 sessions, once a month, or at the point when the child reaches some predetermined production criterion on the practice words used in the instruction.

Determining What Caused the Change

Change either happens or it doesn't. Clinicians administer probes and determine whether the child is incorporating the sounds or other patterns being worked on to his or her sound system. If a client is not showing improvement, the speech-language pathologist has to decide whether to continue the intervention plan or modify it. On the other hand, an SLP who sees change is pleased because the goal is for the clients to make progress toward normal speech sound skills and produce intelligible speech. In an age of accountability and *evidence-based practice*, seeing change and positive outcomes may not be enough. Clinicians are increasingly being asked to demonstrate that the change occurred as a result of what they did, not as a result of something else.

What else might have caused the change in the individual's speech? If the clinician provided intervention and the child improved, did the treatment cause it? Perhaps, but there is a possibility that the change was unrelated to the treatment. Other influences could have resulted in the change. If something else besides the intervention caused the change, then the therapy might not have been necessary, and the SLP may have wasted his or her valuable time—time that could have been devoted to other clients on his or her ever-expanding caseload. Services cannot be provided for free. Someone has to pay for it, whether it's the taxpayers who fund the school district, an insurance company, or the client's family. The bottom line is that SLPs are being asked more and more often to demonstrate that intervention caused the change as well as to provide treatment in the most efficacious manner possible.

Other Sources of Clinical Change

If you enter a room and flip on a light switch and a light goes on, you generally assume that it was your action of moving the switch that caused the light to go on. But what if there was a motion sensor in the room that turns on the light? Your act of flipping the switch on may just have been coincidental. It was the movement of you coming into the room that actually turned on the light. Or what if the light was really turned on by sound activation? Your footsteps or the noise of turning the door handle as you entered the room was what turned on the light. Again, your flipping the switch on would have been just coincidental. Or what if a wireless device held by a friend who was with you controlled the light, and your friend actually turned on the light using that device just as you flipped the switch? Once again, your act of flipping on the switch may have been just a coincidence. The light just happened to come on right after you flipped the switch. Finally, what if there were a timer on the light and you just happened to flip on the switch exactly as the timer was turning the lights on? Again, it may just have been a coincidence.

Clearly, these are far-fetched examples. In clinical situations, things are not always so clear. A number of different things (sometimes called *extraneous effects*) might really have caused the change instead of or in addition to a clinician's intervention. Gruber, Lowery, Seung, and Deal (2003) identified several such effects that practicing clinicians need to be aware of. One of the first ones we think of when we work with children is normal development or maturation. With a child, it is always possible that her or his maturational development (e.g., fine-motor skills, auditory discrimination skills, grasp of a particular phonemic contrast) may have improved on its own so that the child is now capable of producing the sound on which the clinician and child have been working. The change may have had little or nothing to do with the intervention. This is part of what Gruber and colleagues call the *natural history effect* or the normal course of a condition over time. For children, the natural history effect includes factors such as normal development and the typical pattern of change seen in genetic disorders. For adults, the natural history effect includes things like normal recovery from neurological insult or the expected changes seen over time from a degenerative disease such as Parkinson's.

A second extraneous effect is the well-known *placebo effect* in which improvement results from the fact that any intervention is being applied. Gruber, Lowery, Seung, and Deal (2003) document a wide range of studies (in speech-language pathology and other disciplines) demonstrating this effect. Any attention being paid to the speech of young children has the potential to lead the child to focus on his or her speech and make changes that have nothing to do with the specific intervention that is being applied. Such changes may be temporary or even permanent. A variation on the placebo effect is the *Hawthorne effect* in which the client improves because he or she becomes convinced that the treatment he or she is receiving is working. A fourth extraneous effect discussed by Gruber and associates is the experimenter or *Pygmalion effect* in which the client responds positively to signals and/or interactions with the clinician so that change occurs. For all three of these effects (placebo, Hawthorne, Pygmalion), the client may put forth extra effort or extra focus on treatment targets. Or perhaps the client or his or her family reports improvement to the clinician when in fact there is none. Clinicians can't monitor clients' speech all the time, so they often rely on reports from the client or client's family to help determine therapy success and/or change in the speech of an individual.

Finally, there is also the extraneous effect known as *regression to the mean*. This is a statistical (but very real) phenomenon in which anyone who achieves an extremely low or extremely high score on some measurement will produce a subsequent score on that same measurement that is closer to the average (or the mean). People vary in their behavior from moment to moment, and that is certainly true of children with speech sound disorders. When the SLP measures a child's performance on a norm-referenced test, the SLP obtains a sample of the child's behavior. If at one point the child produces a very low score, part of the reason for that low score may be because he or she was not necessarily performing at his or her best on that particular day. Indeed, the child may have been performing at his or her worst. Statistically speaking, when the clinician measures the performance at a later time, the probability is very high that the child will have a better day and his or her score will go up (i.e., be closer to the mean). The higher score may have nothing to do with a change in the child's skill resulting from therapy.

In addition to the extraneous effects discussed by Gruber and colleagues (2003), there are also potential influences from outside "therapy" sources. Some children, for example, may be attending private therapy in addition to receiving services from clinicians in the public schools. Alternatively, parents or teachers who are often aware of the intervention goals may be emphasizing correct articulation in their interactions with the child, such as during book-reading activities. Such additional input is certainly a potentially positive influence, but it serves only to complicate the question of what caused the change.

As this discussion indicates, clinicians cannot assume that observed changes are always due to therapy. The dictates of evidence-based practice mean that it is the clinician's job to try to control for these effects so that treatment effectiveness can be demonstrated. Such demonstrations require proper data collection including the regular use of probes.

Controlling for Extraneous Effects

A variety of things might be done to control for extraneous effects. Researchers who are studying the effects of various treatments typically use a matched control group. This is a group of very similar children who either receive no treatment (usually hard to justify) or who receive an alternative treatment. The two groups are compared on how well they do. As a clinician, however, you usually will not have access to no-treatment groups of children with similar problems that you can compare. And ultimately, you will be interested in whether a particular child is making progress. An alternative solution is to have the child act as his or her own control, employing what is called a *single-subject design*. That means you measure change on several targets at the same time, but you provide treatment for only some of those targets (perhaps only one depending on your choice of goal attack strategy). You then compare progress on treated targets against progress on untreated targets. Ideally, the untreated target(s) would share few if any features with the target. Once the child achieves mastery on the target(s) being treated, additional (formerly untreated) targets are then introduced into the treatment sessions. This approach is sometimes called a *multiple baseline within-subjects design* and is illustrated in Figure 8.1 with a hypothetical example of a child who needed to improve his or her production of both /s/ and /r/. On the horizontal axis of each half of the figure is the number of the session in which the probes were presented and performance measured. On the vertical axis of the top half is the percentage correct for /s/ and on the vertical axis of the bottom half is the percentage correct for /r/. Sessions 1 through 3 are "baseline" sessions in which no treatment was provided and, as shown, no improvement was noted for either target. Such baseline measurements are important to establish that the behavior you are measuring is not beginning to change on its own. During sessions 4 through 7, treatment was provided for /s/ (Treatment I), but not for /r/. Notice an increase in the percentage correct for /s/ but no change in percentage correct for /r/. At that point, treatment changed to a focus on /r/, and an improvement is seen in the percentage correct for /r/ during sessions 8 through 11.

So, how does this approach account for extraneous effects? Well, we saw change when treatment was applied but no change when treatment was not applied. And when the focus of treatment changed to a new target, we saw change on the new target. It appears that the treatment was responsible for the change. If any extraneous effects were operating, we would expect improvement on at least some (if not all) of targets that were not receiving treatment.

Recently Lof (2010) described the collection of data to control for extraneous effects in a way that is consistent with evidence-based practice. He suggested that appropriate data collection by the clinician, including the use of treatment, generalization, and control probes, be referred to as the generation of *practice-based evidence* (or internal evidence). This would be integrated with available external evidence from published research (Baker and McLeod, 2011b).

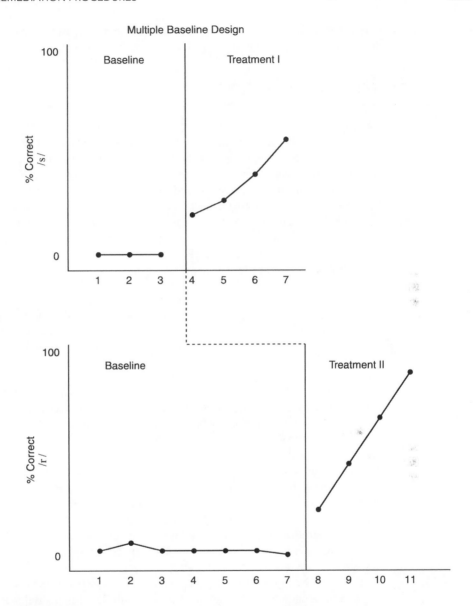

FIGURE 8.1 A multiple baseline design for investigating the effects of a phonological intervention procedure.

Is Significant and Important Change Occurring?

It is one thing to demonstrate that change is occurring as a result of treatment; it's quite another to say that the degree or quality of the change is significant or important. Olswang and Bain (1994) suggested that the clinician can answer yes to this question only if generalization is occurring. The nature of generalization and how to measure it are discussed in the next section.

FACILITATION OF GENERALIZATION

Once target behaviors are in a client's repertoire and can be produced on demand, the next task is to facilitate generalization to other linguistic contexts and nonclinical settings. *Generalization* is a process that is facilitated rather than taught, and it is relevant to correction of all speech sound errors whether they be viewed as motor and/or linguistic in nature. Generalization is a critical and all-important step in the learning process for all children who receive treatment for speech sound disorders. Our discussion of generalization includes an introduction to the concept, followed by a review of (1) across-position generalization, (2) across-context generalization, (3) across-linguistic unit generalization, (4) across-sound and feature generalization, and (5) across-situation generalization.

Stokes and Baer (1977) have defined *generalization* as

> The occurrence of relevant behavior under different non-training conditions (i.e., across subjects, settings, people, behavior, and/or time) without the scheduling of the same events in those conditions as had been scheduled in the training conditions. Thus, generalization may be claimed when no extra training manipulations are needed for extra training changes. (p. 350)

In other words, generalization (sometimes called *transfer*) is the principle that learning one behavior in a particular environment often carries over to other similar behaviors, environments, or untrained contexts. For example, if one learns to drive in a Ford Fusion, there is a high probability that one can also drive a Honda Accord. Generalization of training occurs from driving the Ford to driving the Honda. In terms of articulation remediation, if a client learns to produce /f/ in the word *fish*, [f] production will probably generalize to other words that contain /f/, such as *fun*. If generalization did not occur, it would be necessary to teach a sound in every word and context—an impossible task. The clinician must rely on a client's ability to generalize in order to effect a change in the use of speech sounds. Generalization, however, does not occur automatically, nor do all persons have the same aptitude for it. People vary in their ability to achieve generalization, but certain activities can increase the likelihood of generalization.

One type of generalization is *stimulus generalization*, which occurs when a learned response to a particular stimulus is evoked by similar stimuli. Behaviors that have been reinforced in the presence of a particular stimulus may be said to have generalized when they occur in the presence of novel but similar stimuli even though the response was not reinforced or taught. Consider this example: A client who utilizes the process of "velar fronting" (/t/ for /k/ substitution) has been taught to produce /k/ correctly at the word level in response to the auditory stimulus, "Say kangaroo." The client is later shown a picture of a kangaroo and asked to name it, but no model is provided. If the client says "kangaroo" with [k^h] produced correctly in response to the picture (i.e., the model is no longer necessary for a correct production), stimulus generalization has occurred.

Response generalization is another type of generalization that is especially relevant to speech sound remediation. This is the process in which responses that have been taught carry over to other behaviors that are not taught. An example of response generalization is as follows: A client with /s/ and /z/ errors is taught to say [s] in response to an auditory model of [s]. She or he is then presented an auditory model [z] and asked to imitate it. If the client emits a correct [z], response generalization has occurred. Such generalization is well documented in the literature, including an early study by Elbert, Shelton, and Arndt (1967) in which children with /s/, /z/, and /r/ errors were taught to say [s] correctly. Generalization was evident by correction of the untrained /z/, which has many features in common with /s/. However, no generalization to the untrained /r/ was noted. Obviously, sounds in the same sound class and having similar features with the target sound are those for which response generalization is most likely to occur.

Several other types of generalization can also occur during speech sound remediation, including generalization from one position to another, from one context to another, to increasingly complex linguistic levels, to nontrained words, to other sounds and features, and to various speaking environments and situations. Clinicians often attempt to facilitate generalization by sequencing instructional steps from simple to more complex behaviors. By proceeding in small, progressive steps, the clinician seeks to gradually extend the behavior developed during the establishment period to other contexts and situations.

The amount of training required for the different types of generalization has not been established and seems to vary considerably across subjects. Elbert and McReynolds (1978) have reported data from five children between 5 and 6 years of age indicating that between 5 and 26 sessions were required before across-word generalization occurred. They speculated that the error patterns exhibited by children affected both the time required and the extent of transfer that occurs.

For those clients who begin remediation with an established target behavior in their repertoire, generalization may be the primary task of instruction. Following is a discussion of the various types of generalization that are expected in the articulation remediation process.

Across-Word Position/Contextual Generalization

Generalization of correct sound productions across-word positions is well documented (Elbert and McReynolds, 1975, 1978; Powell and McReynolds, 1969). This term refers to generalization from a word position that is taught (initial, medial, or final) to a word position that is not taught. By teaching a sound in a particular position (e.g., initial position), generalization may occur to a second position (e.g., final position). Speech-language pathologists have traditionally taught target sounds first in the initial position of words followed by either the final or medial position. One rationale for beginning with the initial position is that, for most children, many sounds are first acquired in the prevocalic position (the most notable exception is certain fricatives, e.g., /f/ that appear first in word-final position).

Ruscello (1975) studied the influence of training on generalization across-word positions. Two groups, each containing three participants, were presented training programs that differed with respect to the number of word positions practiced in each session. Ruscello reported significantly more generalization across-training sessions for those subjects who practiced a target sound in the initial, medial, and final word-positions than the group who practiced a target sound only in the word-initial position. Weaver-Spurlock and Brasseur (1988) also reported that simultaneous training of /s/ in the initial, medial, and final positions of familiar words was an effective training strategy for across-position generalization to nontrained words.

It can be inferred from the available data that generalization from initial to final position is just as likely to occur as generalization from final to initial. A preferred word position that would maximally facilitate position generalization has not been established. Thus, the word position in which a target sound is trained does not seem to be a factor in position generalization. In terms of clinical management, unless the pattern of errors suggests a particular word position for initial training (such as final consonant deletion), it is recommended that the clinician train the word position that the client finds easiest to produce, check for generalization to other positions, and then proceed to train the other word positions if generalization has not already occurred. Except for selected fricative sounds (those that develop earliest in the final position), the easiest position to teach is the initial position. However, contextual testing could result in the identification of singleton or cluster contexts that are facilitating for an individual child. In the case of /s/, frequently it is taught in /s/-cluster contexts such as /sn/, /st/ or /ts/.

Technically, position generalization may be viewed as a type of contextual generalization. The term *contextual generalization*, however, also refers to phonetic context transfer—for example, generalization from /s/ in *ask* to /s/ in *biscuit* or to /s/ in *fist*. This type of generalization in which a production transfers to other words without direct treatment is an example of response generalization as previously described. When preliminary testing has indicated specific contexts in which an error sound may be produced correctly, clinicians frequently attempt to stabilize such productions—that is, see that a target sound can be consistently produced correctly in that context—and then provide instruction designed to facilitate generalization of the correct sound to other contexts. As with all types of generalization, the client must exhibit transfer to untrained contexts at some point for the remediation process to be complete. In a study of phoneme generalization, Elbert and McReynolds (1978) reported that although facilitative phonetic contexts have been posited as a factor in generalization, their data did not support the idea that certain contexts facilitate generalization across subjects. Instead, they found a great deal of variability in facilitative contexts across subjects. The authors also reported that once a child imitated the sound, generalization occurred to other contexts. They concluded that the status of the sound in the client's productive repertoire had more to do with generalization than did contextual factors.

Elbert, Powell, and Swartzlander (1991) examined the number of minimal word-pair exemplars necessary for phonologically impaired children to meet a generalization criterion. They reported that for their subjects (primarily preschool children), generalization occurred using a small number of word-pair exemplars (five or fewer for 80 percent of the children), but there was substantial variability across subjects. The occurrence of response generalization when teaching a small number of exemplars is consistent with findings from previous treatment reports (Elbert and McReynolds, 1978; Weiner, 1981b).

Across-Linguistic Unit Generalization

A second type of generalization involves shifting correct sound productions from one level of linguistic complexity to another (e.g., from syllables to words). For some clients, the first goal in this process is to transfer production of isolated sounds to syllables and words; others begin at the syllable or word level and generalize target sound productions to phrases and sentences.

Instruction begins at the highest level of linguistic complexity at which a client can produce a target behavior on demand. Instruction progresses from that point to the next level of complexity. When sounds are taught in isolation, the effects of coarticulation are absent, and therefore, the potential for generalization to syllables and words may be diminished. This notion received some support from a study reported by McReynolds (1972), in which the transfer of /s/ productions to words was probed after each of four sequential teaching steps: (1) /s/ in isolation, (2) /sa/, (3) /as/, and (4) /asa/. Although no transfer to words was observed following training on /s/ in isolation, more than 50 percent transfer to words was observed following training on /sa/. It should be recognized, however, that the training of /s/ in isolation prior to syllables might have had a learning effect and influenced the generalization observed following syllable instruction. Some clinicians prefer initially to teach sounds in isolation, syllables or nonsense words rather than in true words in order to decrease interference from previous learning.

Van Riper and Erickson (1996) and Winitz (1975) recommended that sounds be taught in nonsense syllables or nonsense (nonce) words before they are practiced in meaningful words, thereby reducing the interference of previously learned error productions of the target sound. This view is in contrast with the language-based perspective that phonologic contrasts should be established at the word level because *meaningful* contrasts are a key to acquisition. Powell and McReynolds (1969) studied generalization in four participants who misarticulated /s/. They reported that when two of the individuals were taught consonant productions in nonsense syllables, transfer of the target sound to words occurred without additional training. The other two individuals had to be provided instruction specifically at the word level for generalization from nonsense syllables to words to occur.

Elbert, Dinnsen, Swartzlander, and Chin (1990) reported that when preschool children were taught target sounds within a minimal pair contrast training paradigm, generalization occurred to other single-word productions as well as to conversational speech. Based on a 3-month posttreatment probe, they reported that participants continued to generalize to other nontrained productions.

In summary, it appears that some clients generalize from one linguistic unit to another without specific training; others require specific instructional activities for transfer from one linguistic unit to another. The process of generalization across linguistic units varies across individuals as do all types of generalization.

Across-Sound and Across-Feature Generalization

A third type of generalization is observed when correct production of a target sound generalizes from one sound to another. Generalization most often occurs within sound classes and/or between sounds that are phonetically similar (e.g., /k/ to /g/; /s/ to /z/ and /ʃ/).

Clinicians have long observed that training on one sound in a cognate pair frequently results in generalization to the second sound (e.g., Elbert, Shelton, and Arndt, 1967).

Generalization of correct production from one sound to another is expected when remediation targets are selected for linguistically based treatment approaches (see Chapter 10) based on pattern analysis. Often in these approaches, target behaviors that reflect patterns common to several error productions are selected. It is assumed that generalization will occur from exemplars to other error sounds within the same sound class or, in some instances, across sound classes.

A client can learn a feature and transfer the feature without necessarily correcting a sound. For example, a client who substitutes stops for fricatives may learn to produce /f/ and overgeneralize its use to several fricative sounds. Although the client no longer substitutes stops for fricatives, he or she now substitutes /f/ for other fricatives (e.g., [sʌn] → [fʌn]; [ʃou] → [fou]. Although the same number of phonemes is in error, the fact that the client has incorporated a new sound class into his or her repertoire represents enhancement of the child's phonological system (Williams, 1993).

Frequently, the establishment of feature contrasts is part of the effort to reduce and eliminate pattern usage and homonymy (in which one sound is substituted for several sounds in the language). The notion of feature and sound generalization, like other types of generalization, is critical to the remediation process. During the 1990s, several studies of children with multiple speech sound errors were conducted and data were collected regarding the impact on generalization of various types of treatment targets. Results of these studies are relevant to our discussion of across-sound and across-feature generalization.

In a study related to teaching stimulable versus nonstimulable sounds, Powell, Elbert, and Dinnsen (1991) reported that teaching a nonstimulable sound prompted change in the target sound and other stimulable sounds that were produced in error. However, teaching a stimulable sound did not necessarily lead to changes in untreated stimulable or nonstimulable sounds. The implication of this study is that treatment of nonstimulable sounds may lead to increased generalization and thus have a more widespread impact on the child's overall sound system than treating stimulable sounds.

Gierut, Morrisette, Hughes, and Rowland (1996) examined generalization associated with teaching early developing sounds versus later developing sounds. They reported that children taught later developing sounds evidenced change in the treated sound with generalization occurring both within and across sound classes. For those taught early developing sounds, improvements were noted on the target sound within class sounds, but not across class sounds.

Studies of generalization associated with teaching sounds evidencing "least" versus "most" knowledge of sounds in the sound system (Dinnsen and Elbert, 1984; Gierut, Elbert, and Dinnsen, 1987) have indicated that treatment focused on least knowledge resulted in extensive systemwide generalization in which treatment of most knowledge contributed to less change in a child's overall sound system. Studies comparing generalization associated with teaching phonetically more complex sounds to those less phonetically complex sounds (Dinnsen, Chin, Elbert, and Powell, 1990; Tyler and Figurski, 1994) have reported that more extensive changes were obtained when treatment was focused on more complex phonetic distinctions between error sounds as compared to simpler distinctions between sounds.

As a follow-up to the studies reported in the preceding paragraphs, Rvachew and Nowak (2001) studied the amount of phonological generalization associated with treatment targets that reflected early developing and more phonological knowledge (i.e., correct production in a larger number of contexts) as contrasted with later developing and little or no productive phonological knowledge. In contrast to previous findings, these investigators reported that greater treatment efficiency was associated with phoneme targets that reflected early developing and more productive phonological knowledge. Further investigation is necessary before definitive statements may be made with regard to the issue of targeting early versus later acquired sounds, and more versus less phonological knowledge.

Powell and Elbert (1984) investigated the generalization patterns of two groups of children with misarticulations. Specifically, they wanted to see whether the group receiving instruction on earlier developing consonant clusters (stop + liquid) would exhibit generalization patterns different from those of the group receiving instruction on later-developing consonant clusters (fricative + liquid). The authors reported that no clear overall pattern was observed; instead, the six participants exhibited individual generalization patterns. All participants evidenced some generalization to both the trained and untrained consonant clusters. The most interesting finding was that generalization to both cluster categories occurred on the final probe measure in five of six participants regardless of the treatment received. Powell and Elbert (1984) attributed generalization across sound and classes in part to the level of pre-treatment stimulability.

Across-Situations Generalization

The fourth and final type of generalization to be discussed in this chapter, called *situational generalization*, involves transfer of behaviors taught in the clinical setting to other situations and locations, such as school, work, or home. This type of generalization is critical to the remediation process because it represents the terminal objective of instruction (i.e., correct phonologic productions in conversational speech in nonclinical settings). Such generalization has also been called *carryover* in the speech-language pathology literature.

Most clinicians focus on activities to facilitate situational transfer during the final stages of remediation. Some, including the authors, have argued that clinicians should incorporate these activities into earlier stages of instruction. For example, once a client can produce single words correctly, efforts should be made to incorporate these words into nonclinical settings. A major advantage of providing phonological instruction in the classroom setting (inclusion model) is the opportunity to incorporate treatment targets into a child's natural communicative environment. For example, if a child's science lesson incorporates a word containing a target sound (such as /s/), the teacher or clinician can provide the opportunity for the child to utilize his or her new speech sound in words like *sun, solar, ice, estimate, season, summer*. Although much emphasis is placed on facilitating situational generalization, little experimental data are available to provide specific guidance to the clinician.

Studies by Costello and Bosler (1976), Olswang and Bain (1985), and Bankson and Byrne (1972) have shown that situational generalization is facilitated through treatment, but the extent of such transfer varies greatly from one individual to another. Costello and Bosler investigated whether certain clinical situations were more likely to evidence generalization than others. They recorded the transfer that occurred from training in the home environment to probes obtained in the following four settings:

1. A mother administered the probe while sitting across from her child at a table in a treatment room of the speech clinic.
2. An experimenter (who was only vaguely familiar to the child) administered the probe while sitting across from the child at the same table in the same room as setting 1.
3. The same experimenter administered the probe while she and the child were seated at separate desks facing each other in a large classroom outside the speech clinic.
4. A second experimenter (unknown to the child prior to the study) administered a probe while she and the child were alone and seated in comfortable chairs in the informal atmosphere of the clinic waiting room.

Although all three participants generalized from therapy to one or more of these testing settings, there was no evidence that generalization was more likely to occur in one environment than another. It may be that generalization variables differ so much from person to person that it is impossible to predict which environments are most likely to facilitate situational generalization.

Olswang and Bain (1985) monitored situational generalization for three 4-year-old children in two different settings during speech sound remediation. They examined connected speech samples recorded in conversational activities in a clinic treatment room and connected speech samples audio recorded by parents during conversational activities at home. They reported similar rates and amounts of generalization of target sounds for both settings.

One strategy that has been suggested to facilitate situational generalization is the use of self-monitoring. Self-monitoring techniques have included hand raising (Engel and Groth, 1976), charting (Diedrich, 1971; Koegel, Koegel, and Ingham, 1986), and counting of correct productions, both within and outside the clinic (Koegel, Koegel, Van Voy, and Ingham, 1988). Bennett, Bennett, and James (1996) suggested the following steps to facilitate self-monitoring:

1. External monitoring and verbal feedback
2. External monitoring with cues provided for revision (e.g., raise hand)
3. Self-revision by client when errors occur
4. Anticipating when errors may occur
5. Automatic usage of correct production

Koegel, Koegel, and Ingham (1988) examined generalization of /s/ and /z/ in seven children. They reported that when children self-monitored their conversational productions in the clinic, no generalization of the correct target production outside the clinic occurred. However, when children were required to monitor their conversational speech outside the clinic, "rapid and widespread generalization" occurred across subjects, although at slightly different rates. They reported high levels of generalization for all children. In contrast, when Gray and Shelton (1992) field-tested the self-monitoring strategy of Koegel, Koegel, and Ingham, the results did not replicate the positive generalization treatment effect reported by the Koegel, Koegel and Ingham.

In a retrospective study of efficacy of intervention strategies, Shriberg and Kwiatkowski (1987) identified self-monitoring procedures as a potentially effective component to facilitate generalization to continuous speech. In a subsequent experimental study, Shriberg and Kwiatkowski (1990) reported that seven of the eight preschool children generalized from self-monitoring to spontaneous speech. They concluded, however, that although self-monitoring facilitated generalization, it varied in terms of type, extent, and point of onset.

Despite a paucity of data on situational generalization, available evidence indicates that, as with other forms of generalization, the extent to which it occurs in different settings varies greatly among individuals. There is also the suggestion that situational generalization may be influenced by age and how well developed the child's phonologic system is (Elbert, Dinnsen, Swartzlander, and Chin, 1990).

Several investigators have suggested that productive phonologic knowledge (accuracy and consistency of sound production) influences children's generalization learning (Dinnsen and Elbert, 1984; Elbert and Gierut, 1986; Gierut, Elbert, and Dinnsen, 1987; Gierut, 1989). They have inferred that phonologic knowledge accounts for some of the individual differences that occur in generalization. Gierut, Elbert, and Dinnsen reported that more generalization occurred in sounds when children exhibited more knowledge (correct productions in a wide array of contexts) as opposed to less knowledge (correct productions in fewer contexts; more positional constraints), but the most generalization occurred on those sounds for which training was provided. They also reported that when intervention was directed toward sounds when the child evidenced the least phonologic knowledge, more generalization learning occurred across the child's phonologic system. These investigators recommended that clinicians choose sounds for treatment that reflect the least phonologic knowledge (inventory constraints). Even though training on sounds in which children showed most knowledge facilitated more generalization within a sound class, training on sounds for which children exhibited the least knowledge resulted in more broad-based generalization. Gierut, Elbert, and Dinnsen inferred from these findings that training on sounds in which children displayed the least knowledge (e.g., no correct production of a sound) resulted in more systemwide changes and reorganization of the child's phonologic system than did training on sounds in which children showed most knowledge (e.g., inconsistent productions).

Williams (1991) examined generalization of nine children on /s/ and /r/ sounds for which they exhibited the least phonologic knowledge as reflected by inventory constraints (i.e., the children did not produce /s/ and /r/ on a conversational sample or on a 306-item probe test). The misarticulated [s] and [r] were trained in consonant clusters. Williams reported three different generalization and learning patterns across the subjects and hypothesized that differences in generalization reflected different levels of phonological knowledge even though all error targets were classified in the least phonologic knowledge category (sound is not in child's repertoire). Williams questioned whether Gierut, Elbert, and Dinnsen's (1987) category of least knowledge was too broad to capture subtle differences in children's knowledge and recommended acoustical measurements to supplement transcription to further differentiate the amount of phonologic knowledge demonstrated for sounds in the least knowledge category of this system. This observation is consistent with recommendations from Weismer, Dinnsen, and Elbert (1981), Smit and Bernthal (1983), and Tyler, Edwards, and Saxman (1990).

Parental Assistance with Generalization

Clinicians have recognized that the generalization process in phonologic remediation might be facilitated if individuals from the client's environment could be drawn into the generalization phase of the treatment process. The assumption has been that persons significant to the client, including parents, teachers, and peers, could engage in activities designed to extend what the clinician was doing in the clinical setting. Several programs include instructional activities designed for parents to use with their children at home (Bowen and Cupples, 1999; Mowrer, Baker, and Schutz, 1968; Gray, 1974). Sommers (1962) and Sommers and colleagues (1964) studied several variables related to articulation instruction. More improvement between pre- and posttest scores was reported for children whose mothers were trained to assist with instruction than for a control group of children whose mothers had not received training. Carrier (1970) reported a study comparing a group of 10 children 4 to 7 years old who participated in an articulation training program administered by their mothers and a similar control group who received minimal assistance from their mothers. The experimental group obtained significantly higher scores on four phonologic measures than the control group. Other investigations in which parents provided directed articulation instruction for their children (Shelton, Johnson, and Arndt, 1972; Shelton, Johnson, Willis, and Arndt, 1975) reported that parents can be utilized to enhance phonological intervention.

The clinician must be sensitive to the role parents and other nonprofessionals can assume in the treatment process and must keep several things in mind. For example, parents can (1) provide good auditory models of target words, (2) have their child(ren) practice target words that the child(ren) can produce correctly, and (3) reinforce correct productions. Some things to keep in mind when utilizing parents include the following: First, if parents are to judge the accuracy of sound productions, they must be able to discriminate the sounds accurately. Second, the clinician should demonstrate to the parents the procedures to be used in the program; then the parents should demonstrate to the clinician the same procedures to ensure that they can carry them out. Third, the clinician must recognize that parents have only a limited amount of time; consequently, programs should be designed for short periods. Fourth, written instructions of the specific tasks should be provided to the caregivers/parents. Finally, clinicians should keep in mind that parents tend to function better as monitors of productions than as teachers. Often parents lack the patience and objectivity necessary to teach their own children. However, if parents or other individuals in the child's environment have the desire, skill, time, and patience to work with their children, the clinician may have a helpful facilitator of the generalization process.

Generalization Guidelines

1. For most rapid context and situational generalization, begin instruction with target behaviors (sounds) that are stimulable or in the client's repertoire.
2. For children with multiple errors, there are data to support each of the following as ways to facilitate generalization:
   a. Nonstimulable sounds are treated before stimulable sounds for system wide change.
   b. Sounds evidencing least knowledge are treated before those evidencing most knowledge for system wide change.

3. Because word productions form the basis of generalization, productions at the word level should be incorporated into the instructional sequence as soon as possible. When teaching a sound, utilize words and syllable shapes within the child's lexicon.

4. The more features that sounds have in common, the more likely that generalization will occur from one to another. For example, teaching /ɝ/ usually results in generalization to the unstressed /ɚ/ and the consonantal /r/; teaching one member of a cognate sound-pair, such as /s/, usually results in the client's correction of the cognate /z/.

5. Teaching a feature in the context of one sound, such as frication in /f/, may result in generalization of that feature to other untreated sounds (e.g., other fricatives such as /z/, or /v/).

6. Data to support a particular order for teaching sounds in various word positions to facilitate generalization are lacking. Beginning with the word position that is easiest for the client is an often used starting point.

7. When selecting sounds to target phonologic patterns, choose target sounds from across different sound classes in which the pattern occurs to increase the likelihood of generalization across the sound system (e.g., for final consonant deletion, one might select /d/, /f/, and /m/).

8. Nonsense syllables may facilitate production of sounds in syllable or nonword contexts during establishment of sound production because nonsense syllables pose less interference with previously learned behaviors than do words.

9. Activities to facilitate situational generalization are advised as soon as the client can say a sound in words.

10. In the case of preschool children, generalization frequently takes place without formal instruction to facilitate situational generalization in treatment.

11. Parents, teachers, and others in the child's environment can be used effectively to facilitate phonologic change in children.

DISMISSAL FROM INSTRUCTION

The final phase of phonologic instruction occurs when the client habituates new target behaviors and otherwise assumes responsibility for self-monitoring of target phonologic productions. This phase of therapy is an extension of the generalization phase.

During the final phase of therapy, sometimes referred to as the *maintenance phase*, clients decrease their contact with the clinician. Shelton (1978) labeled the terminal objective of articulation remediation as *automatization* and described it as the automatic usage of standard articulation patterns in spontaneous speech. The term *automatization* implies that phonologic productions can be viewed as motor behavior that develops into an automatic response. When phonologic errors are linguistic in nature, maintenance may be viewed as the mastery of phonologic rules or phonemic contrasts. In reality, both the motor production and phonologic rules become part of a person's everyday productive behavioral responses by this point in treatment. The maintenance phase may be considered complete once the client consistently uses target behaviors in spontaneous speech.

As mentioned in Chapter 5, self-monitoring appears to be important to consolidating the skills being learned. Clients should be expected to monitor their own productions during maintenance. Having the client keep track of target productions during specified periods of the day is a procedure that might facilitate self-monitoring of target productions.

Information from the learning literature offers insights into the maintenance or retention of newly acquired phonologic patterns. *Retention*, in the context of phonologic remediation, refers to the continued and persistent use of responses learned during instruction. Once an individual learns a new phonologic pattern or response, he or she must continue to use (retain) the response. In clinical literature, retention is sometimes discussed in terms of intersession retention and sometimes in terms of habitual retention. *Intersession retention* refers to the ability to produce recently taught responses correctly from one session to the next. Speech clinicians frequently observe "between-session forgetting" in many clients. In this instance, having parents monitor a child's productions of a selected group of words may be helpful. Short practice sessions between therapy appointments may improve intersession retention. *Habitual retention* is the persistent and continued use of the response after instruction has been terminated. The term *maintenance* is also used to refer to this phenomenon. Speech clinicians occasionally dismiss clients from instruction only to have them return for additional therapy some months later. Such individuals obviously did not habituate or retain their newly learned responses.

Sommers (1969) reported that articulation errors are susceptible to regression. In a follow-up study of 177 elementary school children who had been dismissed from articulation instruction during a six-month period, he found that approximately one-third had regressed. Based on conversational samples of target sound productions, 59 percent of those who had worked on /s/ and /z/ had regressed, but only 6 percent of those who had worked on /r/ had regressed.

In contrast, Elbert, Dinnsen, Swartzlander, and Chin, (1990) reported that for preschool children, learning continued to improve on both single-word and conversational speech samples obtained 3 months posttreatment. These data support the idea that young children are actively involved and continue to learn the phonologic system even after treatment has terminated. It appears that phonologic errors in preschool children are less habituated than in older school-age children and easier to correct.

Mowrer (1982) pointed out several factors that have been shown to influence the degree to which information will be retained in the child who is dismissed from therapy but then returns for lack of long-term maintenance or the child who has forgotten previous learning between sessions. First, the meaningfulness of the material used to teach the new responses may affect retention, although there is little empirical evidence in the articulation learning literature on this point. In general, as the meaningfulness of the material increases, the rate of forgetting tends to decrease, and, thus, the use of meaningful material is recommended during remediation. Thus, names of friends, family members, pets, familiar objects, and classroom vocabulary are appropriate choices. Although meaningfulness of material could be an important aid to long-term retention, the clinician might find, as stated earlier, that nonmeaningful material (e.g., nonsense syllables) may be useful during earlier phases of instruction (i.e., establishment). Leonard (1973) reported that when /s/ had been established in meaningful words, fewer training trials were required to transfer to other words than when nonsense items were utilized.

A second factor believed to affect retention is the degree or extent to which something has been learned. In general, the higher the number of trials during the learning process, the greater the retention. Retention improves when some overlearning of verbal material takes place. To avoid unnecessary practice, it is important to determine the minimum amount of learning needed to provide a satisfactory level of retention. The optimum point for stopping instruction occurs when additional training does not produce sufficient change in performance to merit additional practice; however, there are few data to guide the clinician about when this point might be.

A third factor affecting retention is the frequency of instruction or the distribution of practice. Retention is superior when tasks are practiced during several short sessions (distributed practice) than during fewer, longer sessions (massed practice). On the basis of this fact, frequent, short practice sessions are recommended. In his review of this topic, Mowrer (1982) concluded: "On the basis of controlled learning experiments in psychology alone, it could be recommended that clinicians could increase retention by providing frequent instruction; but bear in mind that no data are available from speech research that confirms this recommendation . . . the important factor in terms of frequency of instruction is not how much instruction . . . but the total number of instruction periods" (p. 259).

A fourth factor shown to affect retention is the individual's motivation. The more motivated a person, the greater the extent to which the retention of the material has been learned. Little, if any, experimental work reported in the phonologic literature has attempted to examine motivational state during speech instruction.

Baker (2010a) reviewed eight studies that reported on children whose speech was judged to be normal at the time of dismissal. She found that there was a wide range of sessions and hours required for normalization of children's speech and a wide range of dismissal criteria reported. The dismissal criteria for speech sounds ranged from 50 percent accuracy of targeted sounds during conversational speech (Williams, 2000a) to 75 percent accuracy on a single-word probe (McKercher, McFarlane, and Schneider, 1995).

Dismissal of children who have achieved intelligible speech usually occurs because treatment goals have been achieved. However, not all dismissals are the result of the child's having achieved treatment goals but can occur for other reasons. Dismissal might occur when services are restricted by policies for enrollment or caseload size. For example, Baker (2010a) points out that sometimes dismissals are the result of the need for a clinician to serve other children who are judged to have a greater need for intervention. In such instances, it may be disheartening for both the client and the clinician and it is best to prepare parents and children.

Dismissal Criteria

The maintenance phase provides a period for monitoring retention, and dismissal decisions are made during this period. Limited data on dismissal criteria have been reported, and thus evidence is lacking to support a single dismissal criterion. Elbert (1967) suggested dismissal might be based on two questions: (1) Has the maximum change in this individual's speech behavior been attained? (2) Can this individual maintain this level of speech behavior and continue to improve without additional speech instruction? No matter what criteria are used for dismissal, they should be based on periodic samples of phonologic behavior over time. The maintenance phase provides the final opportunity for the clinician to monitor, reinforce, and encourage the client to assume responsibility for habituation of the new speech patterns.

Diedrich and Bangert (1976) reported data on articulatory retention and dismissal from treatment. Some of the children studied were dismissed after reaching a 75 percent criterion level for correct /s/ and /r/ productions as measured on a 30-item probe word test plus a 3-minute sample of conversational speech. Four months later, 19 percent of the children had regressed below the 75 percent criterion level. No higher retention was found, however, among those children who remained in treatment until achieving higher than 75 percent criterion level on the probe measure. Diedrich and Bangert concluded that most speech clinicians tend to retain children with /s/ and /r/ errors in articulation instruction longer than necessary.

Maintenance and Dismissal Guidelines

1. The reinforcement schedule should continue to be intermittent during maintenance, as during the latter stages of generalization.
2. During the maintenance phase, clients assume increased responsibility for self-monitoring their production and maintaining accurate productions.
3. Dismissal criteria may vary depending on the nature of the client's problem and the client's age. Preschool children with multiple errors generally require less stringent dismissal criteria than older children because they have been reported to continue to improve phonological productions without instruction once they begin to incorporate a new sound(s) into their repertoire. School-age and older clients who evidence residual errors /r/, /s/, and /l/ and whose speech patterns are established and resistant to change might require more stringent dismissal criteria to retain the productions.
4. It has been suggested that clinicians may tend to keep many clients enrolled for phonologic remediation longer than is necessary. In other words, the cost-benefit ratio for intervention may significantly decline after a certain point is reached in treatment.

QUESTIONS FOR CHAPTER 8

1. When in the treatment process would it be appropriate to use continuous versus intermittent reinforcement?
2. What are critical considerations in selecting consequent events?
3. Describe vertical, horizontal, and cyclical structured treatment programs.
4. Describe and give examples of three types of phonological generalization.
5. Present five expectations relative to phonological generalization.

CHAPTER 9

Motor-Based Treatment Approaches

PETER FLIPSEN JR.
Idaho State University

JOHN E. BERNTHAL
University of Nebraska–Lincoln

NICHOLAS W. BANKSON
James Madison University

◆ ◆ ◆

APPROACHES TO INTERVENTION

In Chapter 8, we discussed concepts and principles that underlie remediation of speech sound disorders. These principles and considerations are applicable to all the treatment approaches that are discussed both in this chapter as well as those in Chapter 10.

As discussed in Chapter 4, speech-language pathologists historically approached the correction of speech sound errors from the standpoint of teaching a motor behavior. Most clinicians viewed speech sound errors as an individual's inability to produce the complex motor skills required for the articulation of speech sounds. Since the 1970s, clinicians have also viewed speech sound disorders from a more linguistic (phonological) perspective. The linguistic perspective is based on the recognition that some individuals produce speech sound errors because they have not learned to use certain phonologic rules, especially sound contrasts, in accord with the adult norm. In other words, many error productions reflect a client's lack of rules for appropriate sound usage rather than an inability to physically produce the sounds.

Before discussing specific intervention approaches, a few general comments are in order. First, although it is convenient to dichotomize approaches to intervention into *motor/articulation* (to be discussed in this chapter) and *linguistic/phonologic* (to be discussed in Chapter 10) aspects of phonology, it is important to remember that normal speech sound production involves both the production of sounds at a motor level and their use in accordance with the rules of the language. Thus, the two skills are intertwined and may be described as two sides of the same coin. At a clinical level, it is often difficult or impossible to determine whether a client's errors reflect a lack of motor skills to produce a sound, a lack of linguistic knowledge, or deficiencies in both. It may be that, in a given client, some errors relate to one factor, some to another, and some to both. By careful observation of a client and the nature of his or her problem and at times a bit of experimentation, the clinician usually is able to determine when one type of intervention should be emphasized. In cases of persistent (i.e., residual) errors such as the child who distorts or lateralizes [s], a motor approach is usually the treatment of choice, and the child's knowledge of the linguistic aspects of the sound is generally assumed.

A second point to be made is that even though a disorder may be perceived as relating primarily to either the motor or linguistic aspects of phonology, instructional programs typically involve elements of both. Some activities undoubtedly assist the client in the development of both linguistic knowledge and appropriate motor skills. That said, we have divided the intervention approaches we discuss primarily on the basis of the degree to which they emphasize either motor or linguistic aspects of speech sound learning.

A third point to keep in mind is that several of the treatment approaches presented in this chapter and the next were not developed from a particular theoretical perspective. Many have emerged from pragmatic origins and continue to be used simply because clinicians feel that "they work." Thus, some of the approaches we describe in this and the following chapter can be related to theory, some are atheoretical, and others lie somewhere between. In the summary of each approach, we provide a "Background Statement" that reflects our perception of the theoretical perspective from which the approach has emerged. A challenge for the future is to develop, refine, and revise theories that provide rationale, support, explanations, and direction for intervention procedures.

Lastly, as discussed in Chapter 1, we are now well into the era of evidence-based practice. That means clinicians must demonstrate that the treatment being applied can and is making a real difference over and above any extraneous effects (e.g., maturation) as described in Chapter 8. Baker and McLeod (2011b) noted that this includes using the best available published evidence. This will be highlighted under "Research Support" for the approaches to be presented. Baker and McLeod also note that the application of the evidence-based approach also requires the collection of our own clinical evidence (data) using appropriate control and generalization measures as described in Chapter 8. Clinician-gathered data to support treatment effectiveness is called *practice-based evidence* (Lof, 2010).

THE PUBLISHED EVIDENCE

The published evidence regarding whether treatment of speech sound disorders works has been slowly accumulating. A comprehensive narrative review by Baker and McLeod (2011a) identified 134 studies examining various treatments that were published between 1979 and 2009. This review did not include studies of treatments for childhood apraxia of speech, dysarthria, or persistent (residual) errors, nor did it include expert committee reports that relied primarily on opinion. Among the studies they reviewed, Baker and McLeod documented 46 different approaches with 23 different approaches having been studied more than once.

Having amassed all of this evidence, what factors do we need to consider when reviewing various studies? One thing to be aware of when comparing evidence for different approaches is that different treatment approaches may not have been compared in the same study. Only 40/134 studies (30 percent) reviewed by Baker and McLeod (2011a) made such direct comparisons. Another factor to be aware of when comparing multiple studies of the same approach is that different investigators may have reached different conclusions. In such cases, perhaps some studies examined the problem in a way that gives us more confidence in the results. Not all published research studies are equal. Different investigators choose different ways to answer the same research question (i.e., they use different research designs). As well, regardless of the research design, no study or investigation is perfect. For example, some participants may not have completed the study, sample data may have been lost, or participants may not have perfectly fit the selection criteria for the study. All studies have limitations, and some studies may have more limitations than others; put another way, some studies are of higher quality than others. Baker and McLeod (2011a) suggested at least two different ways to evaluate research evidence. We can examine the research designs that were used, and/or we can look at the quality of the studies. Unfortunately, there is not much agreement on how to compare the quality of studies. But we can compare research designs. Doing so is worthwhile because different designs offer different amounts of control over the influence of extraneous effects. A discussion of how they specifically do this is beyond the scope of the current text, but you will likely discuss research designs in a course on research methods, which is included in most speech-language pathology programs.

In 2004, in addition to a position statement, the American Speech-Language-Hearing Association (ASHA) also adopted a technical report on evidence-based practice that provides a set of *evidence levels,* which is similar to what is used by other professions to evaluate research evidence. The levels reflect the research designs that were used and are arranged so that higher-level studies (i.e., those with a lower numerical rating) provide greater degrees of control over extraneous effects than those with a higher number. The levels are:

Level Ia	Well-designed meta-analysis of >1 randomized controlled trial
Level Ib	Well-designed randomized controlled study
Level IIa	Well-designed controlled study without randomization
Level IIb	Well-designed quasi-experimental study
Level III	Well-designed nonexperimental studies (i.e., correlational and case studies)
Level IV	Expert committee report, consensus conference, clinical experience of respected authorities

Although at this stage of your education, you are not likely familiar with these different research designs, it is important for you to be aware that the lowest level (level IV) is *expert opinion*. Expert opinion can, however, be valuable because it is usually based on extensive experience and is often where we start if a new approach appears. We have to remember, however, that, despite their experience, experts may be biased (often unknowingly) toward a particular approach, which indicates that more objective evidence/documentation obtained through formal research studies should always take precedence.

In addition, different clinicians may have more success with one approach than another because they know it better and thus do a better job in administering it than one with which they are less familiar.

In their review of the research studies on speech sound disorders, Baker and McLeod (2011a) used the ASHA scheme to assign evidence levels to each of the studies they reviewed. Of the 134 studies, Baker and McLeod found that only 2 meta-analyses (level Ia) had been conducted. There were also 20 randomized control trials (level Ib), but 100 (74 percent) of the studies were either level IIb or level III (recall that level IV reports were not included). This suggests that much of our available evidence regarding treatment effectiveness related to speech sound disorders is at the lower evidence levels. Baker and McLeod did note a positive trend in the literature for higher evidence levels of studies conducted more recently. They also pointed out that the majority of the studies (63.6 percent) reviewed involved 10 or fewer participants, which seriously limits our ability to make broad conclusions or generalize from such studies. The bottom line appears to be that although we have a fairly large body of treatment literature concerning speech sound disorders, much work remains to be done.

Results of studies using specific approaches are discussed later, but it is possible to make a general conclusion about whether treatment for speech sound disorders works by examining the findings of the two meta-analyses (overall reviews of studies) that have been conducted. Both Law, Garrett, and Nye (2004) and Nelson, Nygren, Walker, and Panoscha (2006) looked broadly at outcomes for both speech and language interventions and reported specific findings for speech sound disorders. In each review, they examined findings from studies that spanned a number of years in which participants were randomly assigned to either an experimental group or a control group. Both sets of authors concluded after their reviews that, when comparing the groups receiving intervention to those receiving no treatment, the intervention group consistently performed better than the no treatment groups on outcome assessment measures. This positive treatment effect was seen when measuring the percentage of consonants correct in conversation as well as on single-word, speech sound articulation (criterion) measures. Thus, it would appear that intervention for speech sound disorders does make a difference; however, additional information is needed regarding the effectiveness of specific treatment methods.

TREATMENT CONTINUUM

Treatment has typically been viewed as a continuum of activities comprising three stages: establishment, facilitation of generalization, and maintenance. This continuum, which comes from the motor learning literature, is applicable to most types of speech and language disorders and constitutes a framework for a wide variety of specific teaching techniques and procedures. The goal of the first phase of instruction, called *establishment*, is to elicit target behaviors from a client and then stabilize such behaviors at a voluntary level. For motor-based approaches, this generally involves teaching the correct production of an individual sound, whereas for linguistically based approaches, it involves ensuring correct production of a target along with some contrasting sound such as the child's typical error for that sound. If the child's problem is judged to be primarily linguistically based, the establishment phase is likely to be much shorter than for motor-based problems because the physical skill to produce the target is often present.

Motor-based establishment procedures are often based on production tasks as in the example of a clinician teaching a child who does not produce /l/ where to place his or her tongue to say /l/. In addition, for a child who can say /l/ but deletes it in the final position (e.g., *bow* for *bowl*), the contrast between word-pairs, such as *bow* and *bowl* or *sew* and *soul*, may need to be taught during the establishment phase. Once the client is able to readily produce the correct form of the sound and is aware of how it is used contrastively, he or she is ready to move into the generalization phase of instruction.

The second phase of instruction is called *generalization*. As discussed in Chapter 8, it is designed to facilitate transfer or carryover of behavior at several generalization levels: positional, contextual, linguistic unit, sound, and situational. The treatment process includes instructional activities or strategies designed to facilitate generalization or carryover of correct sound productions to sound contrasts, words, and speaking situations that have not been specifically trained. An example of a context generalization activity would be practicing /s/ in a few key words (e.g., *see, sit, seek*) and then determining whether /s/ is produced correctly in other words. An example of a situational generalization activity would be practicing /l/ in sentences in the treatment setting and then observing whether the child uses /l/ in words, phrases, and sentences produced in his or her classroom or home.

During the generalization phase, clinicians usually follow a very predictable progression from smaller to larger linguistic units (e.g., sounds to syllables to words to sentences to conversation). Moving from one level to the next occurs once the client achieves some predetermined level of success (e.g., 80 percent correct across three consecutive treatment sessions). Some preliminary work by Skelton (Skelton, 2004; Skelton and Funk, 2004) has suggested that progress may be faster if, during generalization, different levels of practice are randomly presented within an activity. Additional investigation of this approach to generalization appears warranted.

The third and final phase of remediation, *maintenance*, is designed to stabilize and facilitate retention of those behaviors acquired during the establishment and generalization phases. Instructional activities related to the generalization and maintenance phases of treatment generally overlap. Frequency and duration of instruction are often reduced during maintenance, and the client assumes increased responsibility for "maintaining" and self-monitoring correct speech patterns. The client may also engage in specific activities designed to habituate or automatize particular speech patterns. A maintenance activity could consist of a client's keeping track of his or her /s/ productions at mealtime or use of r-clusters during 5-minute phone conversations every evening for a week. It should be pointed out that although establishment, generalization/carryover, and maintenance have been identified as discrete phases of treatment, in practice there might be considerable overlap among these phases.

Clients might enter the treatment continuum at different points, the exact point being determined by the individual's articulatory/phonological skills. Consider these two examples: Mark is able to produce a sound correctly in words and is able to perceive the target contrastively. Mark therefore begins instruction at the generalization stage and would likely focus on incorporating target words into phrases. Kristy is able to produce a sound imitatively in syllables, perceives the sound contrast in word-pairs, but fails to incorporate the target production of the sound into words. She also enters the treatment continuum at the generalization stage but at an earlier point than Mark. In her case, the clinician will seek to establish the target sound in a set of target words selected on the basis perhaps of facilitating context or even vocabulary items used in her classroom. For Mark, the clinician will facilitate generalization to phrases and sometimes other contexts. For Kristy, the clinician will facilitate generalization from syllables to words, including words not specifically focused on in a therapy session. The clinician must identify not only the appropriate phase of the treatment continuum but also the appropriate level within a phase at which to begin instruction.

MOTOR LEARNING PRINCIPLES

Motor-based approaches to treating speech sound disorders were designed to focus primarily on the motor skills involved in producing target sounds. They also frequently include perceptual tasks as part of the treatment procedures. Most motor-based approaches represent variations of what is often referred to as a *traditional approach* or *traditional articulation therapy*. Treatment based on an articulation/phonetic or motor perspective focuses on the placement and movement of the articulators in combination with auditory stimulation (e.g., ear training and focused auditory input). This remediation approach involves the selection of a target speech sound or sounds with instruction proceeding through the treatment continuum we described previously until the target sounds are used appropriately in spontaneous conversation. Thus, from the perspective of advocates of motor-based approaches, speech production is viewed as a learned motor skill with remediation requiring repetitive practice at increasingly complex motor and linguistic levels and situations until the targeted articulatory gesture becomes automatic.

It is somewhat surprising that, despite our long-standing use of motor-based approaches, we have limited research available about how speech motor learning occurs, particularly in children. Fortunately, research in other disciplines such as physical therapy as well as in adults with acquired speech disorders has begun to reveal a series of basic principles that may be applicable to children with speech sound disorders. Recently Maas and colleagues (2008) summarized much of this research indicating three areas of study in which progress has been made:

Prepractice Goals.   Prior to beginning practice, clinicians need to consider how to increase motivation for learning by including the child (or parent) in establishing goals to work on and making those goals functionally relevant. For very young children and/or those with cognitive impairments, we would likely rely more heavily on parental input. Also, we need to ensure that the child understands the tasks being asked of her or him; we do this by ensuring that we have both simple, easy-to-understand instructions and good models of both the goal behavior and what would be unacceptable output. We may need to either practice or record examples of both correct productions and errors so we can reliably present these models to the child so she or he understands what is and is not acceptable. As we know, prior to any sort of remediation planning, we need to be sure of the child's perceptual abilities (i.e., hearing acuity) to avoid frustration during the learning process.

Principles of Practice. As Ruscello (1984) pointed out, practice is the key variable for mastery of any skilled motor behavior. We must therefore arrange therapy so that there are lots of opportunities to practice the desired behavior. In addition, Maas and colleagues (2008) also point out that:

1. If we have the option, many shorter treatment sessions are probably more productive than fewer but longer sessions.
2. Practice under a variety of conditions (e.g., different rates with different intonation patterns) is preferable to repeating the targets many times under the same conditions.
3. Random presentation of targets is better than multiple repetitions of the same target.
4. Having the child focus on the output (target) is preferable to having her or him focus on the details of the individual articulator movements.
5. Practicing the entire speech target (even if it is only the sound in isolation) is better than breaking that target down into tiny pieces and repeating those pieces multiple times.

Principles of Feedback. Maas et al. (2008) note that the way we provide feedback to the child may be crucial to his or her learning. Early on in therapy, it appears best to provide the child with *knowledge of performance* or feedback about what specifically he or she is doing correctly or incorrectly. But once the target begins to be established, feedback should quickly change to *knowledge of results,* or a focus on whether the target was produced correctly. Interestingly the research Maas et al. cite also suggests that less feedback is better than more because it gives the child the opportunity to reflect internally on what he or she has done. Therapy may need to begin with a lot of feedback, but it appears best to quickly fade the feedback out so that it becomes relatively infrequent. Finally, when feedback is delivered, there should be a slight delay (i.e., a few seconds) to give the child the opportunity to reflect on his or her own (auditory, tactile, kinesthetic, and proprioceptive) feedback. However, the clinician must take care that some extraneous event doesn't occur prior to the feedback lest the event be reinforced rather than the desired behavior.

It bears repeating that these principles are drawn largely from research outside of speech learning or from a small number of studies of adult speech motor learning. Thus, extending them to children learning speech (and more particularly to children with speech sound disorders) is still somewhat speculative at the moment. However, these principles have been shown to be valid for many types of motor learning outside of speech. In addition, many of them are consistent with what clinicians report they have been doing for years and with our discussion of shaping and positive reinforcement of behaviors discussed in Chapter 8. We await further validation of these principles with children.

TEACHING SOUNDS/ESTABLISHMENT

For clients who do not produce target behaviors on demand or who have perceptual and/or production difficulty with particular adult phonologic contrasts, the first step usually involves teaching sounds, which may include perceptual training. Clients who enter the treatment continuum at this point often include those who (1) do not have a specific sound in their repertoire and are not stimulable, (2) produce a sound in their repertoire but only in a limited number of phonetic contexts and are unable to readily produce the segment on demand, (3) do not perceive the sound in minimal pairs, and (4) produce a sound on demand but do not easily incorporate the sound into syllabic or word units, particularly combining the consonant with a following or preceding vowel.

Two basic teaching strategies are used to establish sound productions. The first involves discrimination/perceptual training prior to or along with direct production training. The second involves initiating treatment with a production focus and makes the assumption that the client learns to discriminate and perceive the sound as an indirect benefit of production training. Perceptual training might include a number of different tasks such as (1) minimal contrast training (e.g., sorting word-pairs such as *two* and *tooth* into two categories that reflect the presence of the final consonant and the deletion of the final consonant), (2) traditional discrimination tasks (e.g., discrimination of [s] from [θ]), and (3) auditory stimulation—that is, the child listens only (does not produce) to 5–10 words with the target sound produced correctly.

Perceptual Training

Traditional Ear Training

The type of perceptual training that historically was used most commonly is called *ear training* or *speech sound discrimination training*. Instructional tasks designed to teach discrimination stem from the traditional motor approach to articulation treatment and typically involve making same-different judgments about what is heard (e.g., "Tell me if these are the same or different: *rake-wake*").

Van Riper and Emerick (1984), Winitz (1975, 1984), Powers (1971), and Weber (1970) recommended that discrimination training occur prior to production training during the establishment phase of the treatment continuum. As discussed in Chapter 5, however, routine perceptual training may be of little value. It would appear to be more appropriate to use discrimination (or perceptual) training only in cases in which perceptual difficulties have been documented and then targeted only to sounds in which both a perceptual and a production problem are present. Such an approach is supported by a study conducted by Overby (2007) who reported that a group of second-grade children with speech sound disorders had lower overall scores on a speech perception task than typically developing children. She did not find, though, a consistent pattern or relationship of the specific speech sound errors children made and performance on the speech perception task for the specific speech sound error.

Traditionally, speech sound discrimination training has focused on judgments of external (clinician-produced) speech sound stimuli. Speech sound discrimination training procedures are often sequenced so that the client goes from judgments of another speaker's productions to judgments of one's own sound productions.

It should be noted that perceptual instruction is frequently an inherent aspect of production training. For example, when a client is asked to say *house* but says *hout*, the clinician may say, "No, not *hout* but *house*." In this instance, although instruction is production oriented, perceptual training is inherent to the task. Some clinicians may therefore choose not to do perceptual training as a separate step.

Winitz (1984) suggested that auditory discrimination training precede articulation production training and be concurrent with production training at each stage of production (e.g., isolation, syllable, word, sentence, conversation) until the client can make the appropriate speech sound discrimination easily at that level. The idea that perceptual training should precede production training is based on the assumption that certain perceptual distinctions are prerequisites for establishing the production of a speech sound in the child's phonologic system, although this assumption is not universally accepted. As noted in Chapter 5, there is some evidence that using concurrent perceptual training with production training may improve production skill and possibly perceptual skill as well.

Methodology for Traditional Ear Training (Van Riper and Erickson, 1996)

1. *Identification.* Call the client's attention to the target sound—what it sounds like, what it looks like as you observe the lips and mouth—and, as best you can, help her or him be aware of kinesthetic sensations or what it feels like inside the mouth. For some children, it may help to label the sound and have an appropriate picture or object to go with it (e.g., /f/ is the angry cat sound; /t/ is the ticking sound; /k/ is the throaty sound).

   After auditorily stimulating the child with repeated productions of the target sound, then ask the child to raise her or his hand, ring a bell, or otherwise indicate when she or he hears the target sound in isolation. Intermingle the target with other sounds. Initially, the other sounds should have several feature differences from the target in terms of voicing, manner, and place of production (e.g., /s/ and /m/). However, as instruction progresses, the number of feature contrasts between the target and the other sounds should be fewer (e.g., /s/ and /θ/).

2. *Isolation.* Have the client again listen for the target sound by identifying it in increasingly complex environments. Begin by having the child raise her or his hand, show a happy face, or otherwise indicate when she or he hears the sound in a word (begin with the initial position). We can then progress to having the child listen for the sound in phrases and sentences. This step might also include practice identifying the presence of a sound at the middle or end of the word. Note that this step is very difficult for young children before they have learned to read and is not usually included unless the child has a good grasp of the concept's beginning and end.

3. *Stimulation.* Provide the client an appropriate auditory model of the target sound in both isolation and words. This activity might include limited amplification and varying stress and duration of the target sound. Hodson and Paden (1991) advocate this type of activity as part of the cycles approach to remediation and in the treatment program is referred to as *auditory bombardment* or *amplified auditory stimulation.*

4. *Discrimination.* Ask the client to make judgments of correct and incorrect productions you produce in increasingly complex contexts (i.e., words, phrases, sentences). In this activity, the client is comparing someone else's production with his or her own internal image of the correct form of a sound. For example, if a child substitutes /θ/ for /s/, the clinician might say: "Here is a picture of a thun. Did I say that word right? Did you see my tongue peeking out at the beginning of the word? Did you hear /θ/ instead of /s/? See if I am right when I name this picture (picture of school): *thcool, thcool.* Did I say that correctly?"

Perceptual Training of Sound Contrasts

One aspect of the influence of linguistics on clinical phonology has been its impact on the nature of perceptual training that should either precede or be a part of phonological treatment. Rather than focus on discrimination between sounds, the phonological perspective suggests that perceptual training should focus on minimal pair-contrast training. The particular minimal pair would reflect the child's error pattern. LaRiviere, Winitz, Reeds, and Herriman (1974) first proposed this training, which focuses on the client's differentiation of minimally contrasting word-pairs. For example, when consonant clusters are reduced, the child would be taught to sort contrasting word-pairs (e.g., led-sled) into categories that reflect simplification of a consonant cluster and those that reflect appropriate production of the target consonant cluster (e.g., sick versus stick). Another example is a task for final consonant deletion in which the client picks up pictures of "tea" and "teeth" as the clinician randomly names them. The intent of this training is to develop a perceptual awareness of differences between minimal pairs (in this case, the presence or absence of a final consonant in the word), and the training serves to establish the appropriate phonologic contrasts. Such training might also be used for single errors (i.e., those that don't necessarily reflect a wider pattern). For example, with the child who substitutes /t/ for /k/, the focus might be on discriminating pairs such as "tea" and "key." Many clinicians employ perceptual training of this type, and a method for using it is presented here. The topic is further described in Chapter 10 when minimal pair intervention strategies are discussed.

Methodology for Perceptual Training of Sound Contrasts

1. *Introduction of a minimal pair.* Present to the client a word that contains the target sound. For example, if the child is substituting /t/ for the fricative /ʃ/, the word *shoe* might be used in a perceptual training activity. The child listens as the clinician points to five identical pictures of a shoe and names each one.

   Next, present to the client a second word also with associated pictures of the word, which contain a contrasting sound that is very different from the target sound (i.e., has several different features from the target sound.) For example, *shoe* might be contrasted with *boo* (ghost picture). The phonemes /ʃ/ and /b/ differ in voicing, manner, and place of articulation. For this step, the clinician identifies the original five pictures of a shoe plus the five pictures of "boo."

2. *Contrast training.* Practice differentiating the two contrasting words at a perceptual level. Line up the 10 pictures, 5 of which are of a shoe, and 5 of boo. Ask the client to hand you the picture you name. Make random requests for either *boo* or *shoe*. If the child can readily do this, he or she has established at a perceptual level the contrast between /ʃ/ and /b/. If the child has difficulty with this task, it should be repeated, possibly with different words. Once the child can do this task, contrast training should be repeated with a minimal pair involving the target and error sound (e.g., *shoe-two; shop-top*).

   When the clinician is satisfied that the client can discriminate the target sound from other sounds and that he or she can perceive the target in minimal pairs involving the target sound and error sound, the client is ready for production training. It should be pointed out that in our experience, many children readily discriminate accurately through external monitoring tasks—that is, discriminate the clinician's productions although they may not produce the contrast.

Perceptual Training Software

An alternative to the classic perceptual training described above is the use of commercially developed programs such as the *Speech Assessment and Interactive Learning System* (SAILS; AVAAZ Innovations, 1994). This is a software program specifically intended to improve speech perception skills in children with speech sound disorders. The child is presented a variety of correct and incorrect real-speech examples of the target phoneme and is asked to make judgments about whether the production was correct or not. The software provides visual feedback about the accuracy of the child's judgment. According to Rvachew and Brosseau-Lapré (2010), the child usually works with an adult who also provides specific feedback about the child's judgments (e.g., *"Yes, that was a good /s/ sound"* or *"That /s/ didn't sound right, did it?"*). The software also tracks the child's success rate to assist the clinician in monitoring progress. Administration of the SAILS program can be done either prior to beginning production training or concurrently (e.g., for 5–10 minutes at the beginning of each therapy session).

There is published evidence that the SAILS program can be effective. At least three randomized control trials (Level Ib) have been conducted using it. One of these (Rvachew, 1994) was discussed in Chapter 5. More recently, Wolfe, Presley, and Mesaris (2003) conducted a study with nine preschool children who had speech sound disorders. Five of the children received production training only, and 4 received a combination of production and SAILS training. The two groups performed equally well overall, but performance was better with the SAILS training on targets when perceptual skills were poor at pretreatment testing. Rvachew, Nowak, and Cloutier (2004) conducted the third randomized control trial involving SAILS. A group of 34 preschool children with speech sound disorders received weekly treatment sessions for a variety of targets with whatever production approach their clinician thought was appropriate. In addition, half the children underwent SAILS training sessions while the other half (controls) listened to computerized stories and answered questions about the stories. The children who received the SAILS training demonstrated better speech production skills at the end of 16 weeks of therapy; in addition, prior to entering first grade, 50 percent of those who received SAILS training had fully normal speech compared to only 19 percent from the control group.

Amplified Auditory Stimulation

Hodson and Paden (1991) developed this approach to perceptual training as an integral part of their *cycles training,* which is discussed in Chapter 10. Clinicians have also used it in conjunction with other treatment approaches including motor-based treatments. This method is sometimes referred to as *auditory bombardment* (a term actually coined by Charles Van Riper). It is intended to be used concurrently with speech production training and involves presentation of lists of up to 20 words containing the target sound or sound pattern at the beginning and end of each treatment session. A mild gain amplification device is used to ensure that the input is loud enough but not distorted (*Note:* There is a natural tendency to distort speech when speaking louder than normal). The child merely listens; no production or judgment is required of the child.

Hodson and Paden (1991) described a variation on this perceptual training (referred to as *focused auditory input*) for a client who "... either has not been willing or was unable to produce a target at the time of initial contact (e.g., children functioning below the 3-year-old level)" (p. 107). In this case, initial treatment sessions are conducted in which no production is required of the child. A series of play activities is used in which the child is exposed to many models of specific target sounds or patterns (one or two specific targets per session) produced by the clinician or the parent during the natural course of the play activities.

With either version of this form of perceptual training, Hodson and Paden (1991) also suggested that word lists containing the target sounds be sent home for additional listening practice.

Summary of Perceptual Training

Many speech clinicians teach their clients to perceive the distinction between the target and error sounds or to identify phonemic contrasts as part of the establishment process. Such activities may precede and/or accompany production training. As stated earlier, routine discrimination/perceptual training in treatment has been questioned because many individuals with phonologic disorders do not reflect discrimination problems. In addition, production training unaccompanied by direct perceptual training has been shown to modify phonologic errors. Perceptual training in cases when a perceptual problem accompanies a production problem may be justified.

Production Training

Motor-based intervention typically begins with a focus on helping a client learn to produce a target sound. Whether perceptual training is included or whether it precedes or is interwoven with production training, the goal during this phase of training is to elicit a target sound from a client and stabilize it at a voluntary level. These procedures may also be used occasionally with linguistically based interventions (Chapter 10).

When a sound is not in a person's repertoire, it is sometimes taught in isolation or syllables rather than words. It should be remembered that some speech sounds, such as stops, are difficult to teach in isolation because stops by their physical nature are produced in combination with vowels or vowel approximations. Glides, likewise, involve production of more than the glide when they are produced. Fricatives can be taught in isolation because they are sounds that can be sustained (e.g., s-s-s-s-s-s). Stops and glides are usually taught in CV contexts (e.g., stop + schwa = /gə/).

Whether sounds should be taught initially in isolation, syllables, or words is a matter of some controversy. McDonald (1964a) urged that syllables be used in production training because the syllable is the basic unit of motor speech production. Some clinicians (e.g., Van Riper and Emerick, 1984) argued that because isolated sounds are the least complex units of production and afford the least interference between the client's habitual speech sound error and the learning of a correct (adult) production, they should be taught first. Words sometimes elicit interference from old error patterns and in such cases may not be a good place to initiate instruction. Others advocate words (lexical items) as the best place to begin instruction because the client can benefit from contextual influences in meaningful productions and because of the communicative benefits that accrue from the use of "real words." The clinician can determine the level of production that is most facilitative for correct production and then determine whether interference from previous learning (i.e., long-established habits) is a problem.

Speech-language clinicians commonly employ four methods to establish the production of a target sound: imitation, phonetic placement, successive approximation, and contextual utilization. Each of these approaches is discussed here:

1. *Imitation.* We recommend that the clinician attempt to elicit responses through imitation as an initial instructional method for production training. Usually, the clinician presents several auditory models of the desired behavior (typically a sound in isolation, syllables, or words), instructs the client to watch his or her mouth and listen to the sound that is being said, and then asks the client to repeat the target behavior. Sometimes, the clinician may amplify the model through some type of mild gain amplification device.

Procedures for Eliciting a Sound (θ) through Imitation

CLINICIAN: Watch my mouth and listen while I say this sound—/θ/ (repeat it several times). Now you say it.

CLINICIAN: That's right, I heard the /θ/ sound. Now say this—/θa/ (repeat it several times).

CLINICIAN: Good, now say /θi/. (Proceed to have the client combine /θ/ and a couple of other vowels.)

CLINICIAN: Now say *thumb* (repeat it several times).

Sometimes the clinician tape-records productions to play them back for the client's self-evaluation. Clients may also be asked to focus on how a sound feels during correct production and to modify their productions to maintain this kinesthetic awareness.

When an individual can imitate a target sound, the goal during establishment is simply to stabilize target productions. Subsequent instruction usually begins at the most complex linguistic level at which the client is able to imitate, whether it be isolation, syllables, or words. The level at which a client can imitate may already have been determined during stimulability testing, but it should be rechecked at the initiation of instruction. Even if the client was not stimulable on a sound during assessment, it is recommended that the clinician begin remediation by asking the client to imitate target productions using auditory, visual, and tactile cues.

2. *Phonetic placement.* When the client is unable to imitate a target sound, the clinician typically begins to cue or instruct the client regarding where to place his or her articulators. This type of instruction is called *phonetic placement.*

Procedures for Using the Phonetic Placement Technique to Teach Sounds

a. Instruct the client where to place the articulators to produce a specific speech sound (e.g., for /f/, tell the client to place his or her upper teeth on his or her lower lip and blow air over the lip; for /ʃ/, tell the client to pull the tongue back from the upper teeth past the rough part of the palate, make a groove in the tongue, round the lips, and blow air).

b. Provide visual and tactile cues to supplement verbal description (e.g., model the correct sound and provide verbal cueing as the client attempts the sounds: "Remember to lightly touch the lower lip as you blow air for /f/; remember the groove as you blow air for the /ʃ/.").

c. It may be helpful, depending on the client's maturity level, to analyze and describe differences between the error production and the target production. Sometimes clinicians like to use pictures or drawings reflecting placement of the articulators as part of the instruction.

The phonetic placement method has probably been used as long as anyone has attempted to modify speech patterns. Over three-fourths of a century ago, Scripture and Jackson (1927) published *A Manual of Exercises for the Correction of Speech Disorders,* which included phonetic placement techniques for speech instruction. These authors suggested:

a. Mirror work

b. Drawings designed to show the position of the articulators for the production of specific sounds

c. "Mouth gymnastics"; that is, movements of the articulators (lips and tongue) in response to models and verbal cues and instructions

d. The use of tongue blades to teach placement of sounds and straws to help direct the airstream

The phonetic placement approach involves explanations and descriptions of idealized phoneme productions. The verbal explanations provided to the client include descriptions of motor gestures or movements and the appropriate points of articulatory contact (tongue, jaw, lip, and velum) involved in producing the target segments. This approach to teaching sounds frequently is used alone or in combination with imitation plus successive approximation and context utilization (described in the following discussion). Appendix A describes techniques for teaching various consonants, some of which utilize phonetic placement cues.

Application of the Phonetic Placement Procedure for Teaching /s/

a. Raise the tongue so that its sides are firmly in contact with the inner surface of the upper back teeth.

b. Slightly groove the tongue along the midline. Insert a straw along the midline of the tongue to provide the client a tactile cue as to the place to form the groove.

    c. Place the tip of the tongue immediately behind the upper or lower teeth. Show the client in a mirror where to place the tongue tip.

    d. Bring the front teeth (central incisors) into alignment (as much as possible) so that a narrow small space between the rows of teeth is formed.

    e. Direct the airstream along the groove of the tongue toward the cutting edges of the teeth.

3. *Successive approximation.* Another procedure for teaching sounds that is, in some respects, an extension of using phonetic placement cues involves shaping a new sound from one that is already in a client's repertoire or even a behavior the client can perform, such as elevating the tongue. Complex behavioral responses such as speech sound productions often need to be broken down into a series of successive steps or approximations that lead to the production of the target behavior(s). A teaching method that utilizes successive approximation is termed *shaping*. The first step in shaping is to identify an initial response that the client can produce and one that is related to the terminal goal. Instruction moves through a series of graded steps or approximations, each progressively closer to the target behavior. Shaping has been found to be an efficient method for teaching complex behavioral tasks but requires careful planning in the sequencing of events to be used for treatment.

Shaping Procedure for Teaching /s/

    a. Make [t] (the alveolar place of constriction is similar for both /t/ and /s/).

    b. Make [t] with a strong aspiration on the release, prior to the onset of the vowel.

    c. Prolong the strongly aspirated release.

    d. Remove the tip of the tongue slowly during the release from the alveolar ridge to make a [ts] cluster.

    e. Prolong the [s] portion of the [ts] cluster in a word such as *oats.*

    f. Practice prolonging the last portion of the [ts] production.

    g. Practice "sneaking up quietly" on the /s/ (delete /t/).

    h. Produce /s/.

Shaping Procedure for Teaching /ɝ/ (Shriberg, 1975)

    a. Stick your tongue out (model provided).

    b. Stick your tongue out and touch the tip of your finger (model provided).

    c. Put your finger on the bumpy place right behind your top teeth (model provided).

    d. Now put the tip of your tongue "lightly" on that bumpy place (model provided).

    e. Now put your tongue tip there again and say [l] (model provided).

    f. Say [l] each time I hold up my finger (clinician holds up finger).

    g. Now say [l] for as long as I hold my finger up like this: (model provided for 5 seconds). Ready. Go.

    h. Say a long [l] but this time as you are saying it, drag the tip of your tongue slowly back along the roof of your mouth—so far back that you have to drop it. (Accompany instructions with hand gestures of moving fingertips back slowly, palm up.) (p. 104)

These examples for /s/ and /ɝ/ reflect ways that clinicians capitalize on successive approximations: by shaping behavior from a sound in the client's repertoire (e.g., /t/) and by shaping from a nonphonetic behavior in the client's repertoire (e.g., protruded tongue). Once the client produces a sound that is close to the target, the clinician can use other techniques, such as auditory stimulation, imitation, and phonetic placement cues, to reach the target production. Descriptions of selected ways to elicit various sounds are provided in Appendix A and are frequently discussed on the Internet phonology listserve (www.phonologicaltherapy@yahoogroups.com). A more complete list of various ways to elicit sounds can be found in Secord and colleagues (2007).

4. *Contextual utilization.* Another procedure used to establish a sound involves isolating a target sound from a particular phonetic context in which a client may happen to produce a sound correctly even though he or she typically produces the sound in error. As indicated in Chapter 6, correct sound productions can sometimes be elicited through contextual testing because sounds are affected by phonetic and positional context, and some contexts may facilitate the correct production of a particular sound. In Chapter 6, contextual testing was recommended for some clients selected for remediation.

Correct consonant productions can occasionally be observed in clusters even when absent in singletons. Therefore, clusters should be included in contextual testing. Curtis and Hardy (1959) reported that more correct responses of /r/ were elicited in consonant clusters than in consonant singletons. Williams (1991) reported that when teaching /s/ in clusters, the sound generalized to /s/ in singletons, which is consistent with the notion that teaching sounds in more complex contexts will generalize to less complex contexts. Hodson (2007b) supports this idea by suggesting that targeting /s/ in clusters during treatment has the potential to facilitate widespread change within a child's phonological system. If a context in which the target behavior is produced correctly can be found, it can be used to facilitate correct production in other contexts.

Procedures for Teaching Sounds through Context Utilization

If /s/ is produced correctly in the context of the word-pair "bright sun," the /t/ preceding the /s/ may be viewed as a facilitating context.

a. Ask the client to say *bright sun* slowly and prolong the /s/. Demonstrate what you mean by saying the two words and extending the duration of /s/ (e.g., *bright—sssssssssun*).
b. Next ask the client to repeat *bright—sssssink*, then *hot—ssssssea*. Other facilitating pairs may be used to extend and stabilize the /s/ production.
c. Ask the client to only say /s/ without the "lead-in."

Using phonetic/linguistic context as a method to establish a sound allows the clinician to capitalize on a behavior that could already be in the client's repertoire. This procedure also represents a form of shaping because one is using context to help the client isolate and stabilize production of an individual phoneme.

Establishment Guidelines

Individual variations among clients preclude a detailed set of specific instructions applicable to all clients; however, the following are general guidelines for establishment:

1. Perceptual training, particularly contrast training employing minimal pairs, is suggested as part of establishment when there is evidence that the client's production errors are due to problems perceiving appropriate phonologic contrasts.
2. When teaching production of a target sound, look for the target sound in the client's response repertoire through stimulability (imitation) testing, contextual testing (including consonant clusters, other word positions, and phonetic contexts), and observation of a connected speech sample. Our recommended hierarchy for eliciting sounds that cannot be produced on demand is (a) imitation (verbal stimulation), (b) phonetic placement, (c) successive approximation (shaping), and (d) contextual utilization. Stabilize correct productions and use them as a starting point for more complex linguistic units and contexts.

BEYOND INDIVIDUAL SOUNDS

Teaching a sound (establishment) is typically the first step in motor-based intervention, and it may be used in linguistically based interventions as well. But correction of phonologic errors involves stages of the treatment continuum that go beyond establishment. Several motor-based treatment approaches include procedures designed to move a client through a multistep process from establishment through correct production of target sounds in conversational speech.

Traditional Approach

The *traditional approach* to articulation therapy was formulated during the early decades of the 1900s by pioneering clinicians of the field. By the late 1930s, Charles Van Riper had assimilated these treatment techniques into an overall plan for treating articulation disorders and published them in his text titled *Speech Correction: Principles and Methods* (originally published in 1939 and modified in subsequent editions). As an outgrowth of his writings, the traditional approach is sometimes referred to as the *Van Riper method*.

The traditional approach is motor oriented and was developed at a time when those receiving treatment were typically school-age clients, often with persistent (residual) errors. At that time, clinicians were seeing few children with language disorders, and caseloads included more children with mild disorders than at present. However, the traditional approach was successfully used with clients representing a range of severity. The traditional approach to articulation therapy is still widely used and is particularly appropriate for individuals with errors considered to be articulatory or motor in nature.

The traditional approach progresses from the speaker's identification of error productions to the establishment of correct productions and then moves on to generalization and finally to maintenance. As Van Riper and Emerick (1984) stated:

> The hallmark of traditional articulation therapy lies in its sequencing of activities for (1) sensory-perceptual training, which concentrates on identifying the standard sound and discriminating it from its error through scanning and comparing; (2) varying and correcting the various productions of the sound until it is produced correctly; (3) strengthening and stabilizing the correct production; and finally (4) transferring the new speech skill to everyday communication situations. This process is usually carried out first for the standard sound in isolation, then in the syllable, then in a word, and finally in sentences. (p. 206)

A characteristic of this approach is its emphasis on perceptual training. During this part of therapy, the client is not required to produce the sound, but instead, instruction is designed to provide a perceptual standard by which the client can contrast his or her own productions. Thus, perceptual training becomes a precursor to production training. Procedures for doing perceptual training were presented earlier in this chapter in our discussion of methods for teaching sounds and is not repeated here.

The primary ingredient of traditional instruction is production training with the focus on helping a client learn to produce a sound on demand. Production training usually includes four sequential instructional phases wherein a target sound is (1) produced in isolation (the target sound is elicited in isolation or, in the case of stops and certain glides (in a CV context such as /pa/), (2) produced in syllables (the sound is produced in CV, VC, and VCV syllables), (3) produced in words (the target sound is produced in a word or lexical context in initial, final, and medial positions), and (4) produced in increasingly complex syntactic utterances (i.e., phrases, sentences, conversational speech).

Instructional Steps for Traditional Production Training
(Secord, 1989; Van Riper and Erickson, 1996)

1. *Isolation.* The first step in the traditional method is to teach a client to produce a sound in isolation. An explanation for beginning with production of the target sound in isolation is the assumption that the articulatory gestures of a sound are most easily learned when the sound is highly identifiable and in the least complex context. The goal at this level is to develop a consistently correct response. Specific techniques for teaching sounds were discussed earlier and are included in Appendix A. It should be pointed out that training should begin at whatever level of sound complexity a child can produce—isolation, sound clusters, syllables, or words.
2. *Nonsense syllables.* The second step involves teaching the client to produce a sound in a syllable. The goal at this step is consistently correct productions in a variety of nonsense syllable contexts. A suggested sequence for syllable practice is CV, VC, VCV, and CVC. It is also suggested that the transition from the consonant to the vowel should be accomplished with sounds that are similar in place of articulation.

For example, an alveolar consonant such as /s/ should be facilitated in a high front vowel context, as in [si]. The clinician might also wish to use the target sound in nonsense clusters.

3. *Words.* The third step involves having a client produce a sound in meaningful units—that is, words. This step begins once the client can consistently produce the target sound in nonsense syllables. Instructions at this level should begin with monosyllabic words with the target consonant (assuming instruction is focusing on consonants as opposed to vowels) in the prevocalic position (CV). Instruction then moves to VC, CVC, CVCV, monosyllabic words with clusters, followed by more complex word forms. Table 9.1 reflects a hierarchy of phoneme production complexity at the word level as presented by Secord (1989).

    Once a core group of words in which the client is readily able to produce the target sound is established, the clinician seeks to expand the small set of core words to a somewhat larger set of training words. Usually target words are selected on the basis of meaningfulness to the client (e.g., family names, places, social expressions, words from the academic curriculum), but other factors such as phonetic context and syllable complexity should also be considered just as they were for the initial set of core words.

4. *Phrases.* Once the client can easily produce a target sound in words, instruction shifts from single-word productions to practicing a target sound in two- to four-word phrases. This level of production represents a complexity level between single words and sentence-level productions. This is especially true if carrier phrases are employed. *Carrier phrases* are phrases in which only a single word is changed with each repetition (e.g., I see the *car*; I see the *cup*; I see the *cane.*). In phrase-level productions, one should begin with phrases in which only one word contains the target sound. As the client produces a target sound in a single word, the clinician might wish to add a second word in the phrase that contains the target sound.

5. *Sentences.* An extension of phrase-level productions is sentence-level practice. Just as practice at other levels has involved careful sequencing of task complexity, this

TABLE 9.1 Substages of Word Level Stabilization Training for /s/

Substage	Syllables	Examples for /s/
1. Initial prevocalic words	1	*sun, sign, say*
2. Final postvocalic words	1	*glass, miss, pass*
3. Medial intervocalic words	2	*kissing, lassie, racer*
4. Initial blends/clusters	1	*star, spoon, skate*
5. Final blends/clusters	1	*lost, lips, rocks*
6. Medial blends/clusters	2	*whisper, outside, ice-skate*
7. All word positions	1–2	(any of the above)
8. All word positions	any	*signaling, eraser, therapist*
9. All word positions; multiple targets	any	*necessary, successful*

Source: Secord (1989).

principle also holds at this level. Consideration should be given to factors such as phonetic context, syllable structure of words, and number of words in the sentence. The following sequence of sentence levels is suggested:

a. Simple short sentence with one instance of the target sound
b. Sentences of various lengths with one instance of the target sound
c. Simple short sentences with two or more instances of the target sound
d. Sentences of various lengths with two or more instances of the target sound

6. *Conversation.* The final step in production training involves using a target sound in everyday speech. At this point, the clinician is seeking to facilitate generalization of productions that have already proceeded through more structured production tasks. Initially, generalization situations are structured so that the client produces her or his sound correctly in situations in which the speech is monitored. Activities such as role-playing, talking about future plans, attempting to get information, interviewing, and oral reading can be used at this level. Following structured conversations, subsequent activities are more spontaneous and free and sometimes characterized as "off-guard" type conversations. The intent is to provide activities to facilitate transfer that approximates real-life situations. Activities should include speaking situations in which the client focuses not on self-monitoring but on what she or he says. Telling personal experiences, talking about topics that evoke strong feelings, and taking part in group discussions are used at this stage of instruction. Some clinicians include "negative practice" to help to stabilize a new response. In negative practice, a client deliberately produces a target sound incorrectly and then contrasts it to a correct production; Van Riper and Erickson (1996) stated that such deliberate productions of error sounds increased the rate of learning.

At this point, the clinician also seeks to facilitate the carryover of conversation to situations beyond the therapy environment. It is suggested that such situational generalization be encouraged once the client can produce a target sound at the word level. By encouraging transfer in earlier stages of instruction, it is assumed that generalization beyond the word level will be significantly enhanced and will perhaps decrease the amount of time needed at the phrase, sentence, and conversational levels.

Summary of the Traditional Approach

Background Statement.   The underlying assumptions of the traditional approach to remediation include the following: (1) Faulty perception of speech sounds may be related to speech sound errors and (2) speech sound errors may be viewed as an inadequate motor production of speech sounds. Thus, the traditional approach relies heavily on motor production practice combined with activities related to perceptual training.

Unique Features.   Until the 1980s, the traditional approach to speech sound remediation constituted the basic methodology employed by most clinicians for instruction and treatment of speech sound errors and is still widely used today. The traditional method focuses on motor learning of individual speech sounds. The approach provides a complete instructional sequence for correcting articulatory errors. It can be modified to fit the needs of clients of all ages. Perceptual training is recommended as a precursor to or an accompaniment of direct work on sounds.

Strengths and Limitations. This approach has been widely used over time and forms the basis of several current treatment approaches. Its widespread usage is likely related to the logical sequence of training tasks, the success that accrues through motor practice, and the adaptability and applicability of the approach. The value of perceptual training has been questioned and studied with the suggestion that it not be used routinely. There is, however, some evidence for its use when there is a documented perceptual problem. In addition, the traditional approach may not be the most efficacious approach for clients with multiple errors including those whose errors are linguistic rather than motor based (recall the study by Klein, 1996, which was mentioned in Chapter 4 in which children who received a traditional approach spent more time in therapy and were less likely to be dismissed with normal speech than were children who received a more linguistically based approach).

Research Support. This approach has stood the test of time because it has "worked" for many clinicians with many clients. Many investigators have reported phonological change in association with intervention that has been based on this approach. Two relatively high-level published studies illustrate this. Note that in both cases, prerecorded stimuli were used for perceptual training rather than live voice presentations. A randomized control trial (level Ib) by Rvachew (1994) used concurrent perceptual training and traditional therapy with three groups of children. Groups 1 and 2 (with 10 and 9 children, respectively) did discrimination tasks with minimal pairs (either correct versus distorted versions of /ʃ/ in "shoe" or correct versus another phoneme—"shoe" versus "moo"), while group 3 (with 8 children) did discrimination tasks with a nonminimal word-pair ("shoe" versus "Pete"). Across 8 weeks of therapy, group 3 made on average no gains on either production or perception of /ʃ/ while groups 1 and 2 made significant improvement on both production and perception. None of the children had been stimulable for /ʃ/ at the beginning of the study. Another level Ib study by Wolfe, Presley, and Mesaris (2003) compared traditional therapy with concurrent perceptual training (4 children) to traditional therapy without perceptual training (5 children). Treatment targets were specific to each child. All targets were stimulable prior to treatment. Overall, after an average of 11 treatment sessions, both groups made similar amounts of improvement in production skill. There was also no difference between the groups for progress on target sounds that had been well perceived prior to therapy. However, the children who received the concurrent perceptual training achieved significantly better production outcomes on those target sounds that were not well perceived prior to therapy.

The emphasis on external discrimination training as part of the treatment process with the traditional approach for all children has been questioned. The findings from Wolfe, Presley, and Mesaris (2003) support the notion that the addition of perceptual training may be appropriate only for those targets wherein the child is also having difficulty with perception.

Context Utilization Approaches

Some clinical phonologists (McDonald, 1964a; Hoffman, Schuckers, and Daniloff, 1989) have advocated contextual or sensory-motor-based approaches to intervention. Treatment suggestions related to these approaches are based on the recognition that speech sounds are not produced in isolation but rather in syllable-based contexts and that certain phonetic contexts could be facilitative of correct sound usage. McDonald suggested that instruction for articulatory errors be initiated in a context(s) in which the error sound can be produced correctly. He provided an example of a child with a /s/ distortion who produced [s] correctly in the context of *watchsun*. He suggested the following sequence of instructions after *watchsun* was identified as a context when /s/ was correctly produced: (1) Say *watchsun* with "slow-motion" speed, (2) say *watchsun* with equal stress on both syllables, then with primary stress on the first syllable, and then with primary stress on the second syllable, (3) say *watchs* and prolong [s] until a signal is given to complete the bisyllable with [ʌn], and (4) say short sentences with the same facilitating context such as "Watch, sun will burn you." The sequence is repeated with other sentences and stress patterns. The meaningfulness of the sentence is not important because the primary focus of the activity is the movement sequences.

Following these steps, the client is instructed to alter the movement patterns associated with the correct /s/ by changing the vowel following the segment in a suggested sequence such as:

watch-sun	*watch-sat*
watch-sea	*watch-soon*
watch-sit	*watch-sew*
watch-send	*watch-saw*

The next step is to practice words that include a second context using words such as *teach, reach, pitch, catch,* and *beach* that would be used in combination with one-syllable words beginning with /s/ and followed by a variety of vowels (such as *sand, sun, said,* and *soon*). Various sound combinations are practiced with different rates and stress patterns and should eventually be practiced in sentence contexts.

Hoffman, Schuckers, and Daniloff (1989) described another variation of the contextual approach that involves a sequenced set of production-based training tasks designed to facilitate the automatization of articulator performance. The basic assumption behind their suggestions is that "revision of over learned, highly automatic behavior is possible through carefully planned and executed performance rehearsal" (p. 248). Intervention is seen as involving instruction and practice of motor articulatory adjustments to replace previously learned (incorrect) productions. The paragraphs that follow present the sequence of tasks and instructional activities these authors suggest.

Prior to working directly on error targets, the clinician elicits, via imitation, sound segments that the client can produce correctly. Such "stimulability tasks" provide the client an opportunity to experience success in a speech task as well as the opportunity to observe and imitate the clinician's productions. It is suggested that the clinician not only model the correct form of sounds in the child's repertoire but also distort such productions through excessive movements (e.g., lip rounding for /m, p, f/) for the purpose of giving the client the opportunity to practice manipulation of the articulators in response to the clinician's model. It is hoped that such activity will facilitate the client's skill at identifying, comparing, and discriminating the clinician's and his or her own sound productions.

Following stimulability tasks, the client needs to learn the articulatory adjustments necessary for correct target sound production. It is suggested that the clinician be able to repeat sentences using error productions similar to those of the client in order to be aware of the motoric acts involved in the client's misarticulations. The emphasis at this point is on doing interesting things with the speech mechanism (e.g., view their productions in the mirror or listen to recordings of themselves).

Rehearsal involves four levels of complexity: nonsymbolic units, words and word-pairs, rehearsal sentences, and narratives. Once the narrative level has been reached, rehearsal can include a mixture of the four levels.

Practice with *nonsense syllables* provides practice with articulatory gestures that were begun during pretraining. Nonsymbolic instruction focuses on target productions in VC, CV, VCV, and VCCV syllables. It is asserted that production of nonsymbolic units imposes minimal constraints on the speaker by allowing her or him to focus on the speech task rather than morphology, syntax, and semantics. The emphasis on nonsense words is also supported by recent findings from Gierut, Morrisette, and Ziemer (2010), who reported greater and more rapid generalization compared to the use of real words.

Word and word-pair practice is the next step in the program. Initial targets should reflect a transition from nonsymbolic units to meaningful units that encompass the non-symbolic syllables already practiced. Practice activities at this level are designed to encourage the client to assume responsibility for recognizing and judging the adequacy of her or his performance. Table 9.2 reflects a list of words and word-pairs by word position that might be used at this level.

The next step in the program involves *rehearsal sentences*. At this stage, the client repeats the clinician's model of sentences that includes words practiced at the word level followed by practice on a word containing the target segment and then embedding it in a

TABLE 9.2 Word and Word-Pair List for [s]

Prevocalic		Intervocalic		Postvocalic
Initial	**Cluster**	**Medial**	**Final**	**Word-Pair**
Sam	scat	passing	pass	Jack sat
seed	ski	receive	niece	jeep seat
soup	scooter	loosen	loose	room soon
saw	scar	bossy	toss	cop saw
sit	skit	kissing	miss	lip sip
sign	sky	nicer	mice	right side

spontaneously generated sentence. For example, using key words from Table 9.2, sentences such as the following could be practiced:

> *Jerry was very sad today.*
>
> *The sky was very cloudy on Tuesday.*
>
> *His leg muscle was sore.*
>
> *Bison is another word for buffalo.*
>
> *Don't drink all the juice.*
>
> *The ace is the highest card.*

The final step in this program involves using a target sound in *narratives* that can be illustrated, acted out, or read. A series of clinician-generated narratives are employed—for example, for a preschool client, "This is Poky the turtle. Today is his birthday. He is 6 years old. He says, 'It's my birthday.' What does he say?" This is followed by the client saying, "It's my birthday." Through such narratives, practice of the target sound is embedded in communicative tasks. The clinician may have a client practice individual sentences from these narratives for additional practice at the sentence level.

Although this program has been presented as a series of steps or levels, the authors point out that these steps should overlap. Throughout the program, the client is the primary judge of adequacy of productions, describing the movement patterns and articulatory contacts.

Sacks and Shine (2004) suggested another variation on the context utilization approach. As with the preceding two approaches, the *Systematic Articulation Training Program Accessing Computers (SATPAC)* approach uses both facilitating contexts and systematic progression through the treatment continuum. The SATPAC approach also puts a heavy emphasis on the use of nonsense words as a means to overcome strongly ingrained error habits. The systematically organized lists of stimuli containing the nonsense words are generated with the SATPAC software program.

Summary of Contextually Based Approaches

Background Statement.   The theoretical concept underlying contextual approaches is that articulatory (i.e., motor-based) errors can be corrected by extensive motor practice of articulatory behaviors with syllabic units as a basic building block for later motor practice at more complex levels. To employ this approach, a sound must be in the client's repertoire.

Unique Features.   The emphasis on imitated, repetitive productions is a unique aspect of this approach. The systematic variation of phonetic contexts in productions of both sounds produced correctly and error sounds targeted for remediation sets this approach apart from others. A major value of context testing is to identify contexts that may be useful in therapy.

Strengths and Limitations.   A major strength of this approach is that it builds on behaviors (segmental productions in particular phonetic contexts) that are in a client's repertoire and capitalizes on syllables plus auditory, tactile, and kinesthetic awareness of motor movements. It may be particularly useful for clients who use a sound inconsistently and need methodology to facilitate consistent production in other contexts. The concept of syllable practice and systematic variation of phonetic contexts and stress may be useful to any training method that includes syllable productions. An often-cited limitation of this approach is the difficulty in motivating many children to engage in the extensive imitation and drill that this approach requires.

Research Support.   Contextual testing designed to locate facilitating contexts can be used with clients who are not stimulable in their attempts to produce the target. Published clinical investigations that provide support for the efficacy of using a context facilitation approach to intervention are very limited and relatively low level. One report by Stringfellow and McLeod (1991) involved a case study (evidence level III) in which a facilitating context was used successfully to teach a child to produce distinctive versions of /l/ and /j/. Dunn and Barron (1982) also reported moderate improvement in another case study (level III) when word-final /z/ was targeted. One phase of the mixed approach (i.e., it was not purely a context utilization approach) involved the use of two word sequences for which the context was systematically modified by changing the word immediately following the target. Finally, Masterson and Daniels (1991) reported a case study (level III evidence) of a child age 3;8 who exhibited both dentalized distortions of sibilants and /w/ for /r/ substitutions. Three semesters of therapy using a linguistically based approach resulted in complete correction of the /r/ errors. The sibilant errors were corrected in therapy sessions but did not generalize to conversational speech. Within one month of introducing the Hoffman, Schuckers, and Daniloff (1989) context-based approach described previously, generalization of correct production of the sibilants occurred and was maintained at the 100 percent correct level at a 3-month follow-up visit.

Alternate Feedback Approaches

As discussed in Chapter 2, speakers receive various kinds of feedback including internal feedback (tactile, proprioceptive, kinesthetic, auditory) while they are speaking and external feedback from others about whether they understood the intended message. Speakers might also get negative external feedback about specific errors they produce. In therapy, clients also receive external feedback from the clinician regarding the accuracy of production, what they might be doing wrong, and/or what they might do to produce the target correctly. But what if this feedback is not sufficient to help the child improve her or his speech? Over the years, a number of instrumentation/appliance-assisted approaches in which the client receives supplemental feedback from such instruments have been suggested. These approaches are usually recommended for older children and/or adults with persistent (residual) errors on the assumption that conventional feedback has not been sufficient. Some of these approaches involve considerable expense on the part of the clinician or the family (and occasionally specialized training for the clinician) that is difficult to justify before more conventional approaches have been exhausted.

Tactile Feedback Approaches

To enhance tactile feedback, a removable appliance similar to an orthodontic retainer, was developed by Blakeley and Louis in 1975 (as reported in Clark, Schwarz, and Blakely, 1993) to assist with correction of /r/ and /ɝ/ errors. A small acrylic block is built into the posterior portion of the device to provide a landmark for correct tongue placement. The device is custom fit to each child's maxillary arch and attached to the back teeth during therapy and practice sessions.

Visual Feedback Approaches

For some children, putting a device into the mouth may be unacceptable. Also, in some cases, additional tactile feedback may be insufficient. Shuster, Ruscello, and Toth (1995), for example, have argued that tactile feedback is quite minimal during normal production of /r/ or /ɝ/. Several alternative approaches have been developed to provide the child visual feedback.

Sounds involving the bilabial, labio-dental, and interdental places of articulation are naturally visible. However, that is not the case for most other consonants and vowels. One fairly direct visual feedback approach is the use of ultrasound imaging. Similar to its use to visualize the heartbeat patterns of an unborn child during a pregnancy, it is possible to visualize the tongue during the act of speaking.

Other types of visual feedback approaches offer somewhat less direct visual feedback. The most widely known of these is palatography, which involves creating images of how the tongue contacts the palate during speech. According to Fletcher (1992), this has been of interest since at least 1803. Work by Samuel Fletcher and others in the 1970s and 1980s led to the development of the modern version of this approach, which is known as electropalatography (EPG). This procedure involves creating a custom mouthpiece that covers the palate. The *artificial palate or pseudopalate*, as it is sometimes called, has a series of small pressure sensors embedded within and connected to small wires. The wires extend out one corner of the mouth and are connected to a computer. When the child speaks, his or her tongue contacts the sensors and there is an image created on the computer screen showing the pattern of contact along the palate. The clinician can have an artificial palate created for themselves that can then be used to generate a model of what the pattern of contact should look like for particular speech sounds. The child is instructed to move his or her tongue around to create the right pattern of contact, which will be shown on the computer screen. At the same time, the client can get feedback on how her or his productions sound.

Even less direct feedback is possible through the use of microphones connected to computers with software that generates *spectrograms,* which show how the acoustic signal changes over time. Like EPG, the clinician can use spectrograms of his or her own productions to model what the correct version should look like on the display.

Summary of Alternate Feedback Approaches

Background Statement.   The basic premise behind each of these approaches is that typical internal and external feedback is insufficient to help some children learn to produce some sounds. Each takes a slightly different approach but offers a different form of feedback that the child may be able to use to modify what they do during speech sound production.

Unique Features. In addition to the novel feedback, the use of some sort of instrumentation for feedback is a unique aspect of these approaches, which may offer additional motivation for the older child or adult who has been unsuccessful with more conventional treatment.

Strengths and Limitations. A notable strength of these approaches is that the presence of the novel feedback and/or the use of instrumentation could assist some clients to get past their long-established incorrect productions. As mentioned earlier, the major limitation with these approaches is often cost. In addition, many clinicians have limited experience with using and/or interpreting the information provided with approaches such as ultrasound or spectrograms. Another limitation is that many of these approaches require the presence of something unnatural in the oral cavity and may require the child to produce speech in an unnatural way. This may limit the child's ability to transfer the placement or movement being learned to more natural speaking situations. These approaches have generally been applied to older children with persistent (residual) errors.

Research Support. Relative to tactile feedback, Ruscello (1995) noted that much of the evidence for the /r/ appliance has been anecdotal. The highest level study available appears to be that of Clark, Schwarz, and Blakeley (1993), who randomly assigned 36 children ages 8–12 years to one of four treatment groups (random assignment and the use of control groups made this a level Ib study). Two groups used the appliance (one with and one without auditory models of correct /r/) and two other groups were given traditional therapy (again one group with and one group without auditory models). All four groups showed some improvement over 6 weeks of therapy, but the two groups who used the appliance improved to a significantly greater degree than the other groups. Limited generalization to conversational speech was noted, however. These findings suggested improved performance *might* be possible with the appliance.

Relative to visual feedback approaches, research overall has been limited mostly to case studies (level III), but the vast majority of studies have reported positive outcomes. Ultrasound has received very limited research attention. Adler-Bock, Bernhardt, Gick, and Bacsfalvi (2007) used ultrasound imaging with two adolescents who had long-standing difficulty with /r/. Ultrasound provided documentation and visual feedback of tongue position and shape during pretreatment and posttreatment. Results of this level III study showed significant improvement in the percentage of /r/ productions judged as accurate by uninvolved SLP listeners. Subjective judgments of the ultrasound images also suggested more accurate tongue shapes during /r/ production posttreatment.

Outcomes of studies using spectrograms have also been very limited. In a level III study, Shuster, Ruscello, and Toth (1995) used this approach with two children (age 10 and 14 years) to target production of /r/. After 3–6 hours of treatment, both were consistently producing correct versions of /r/ as judged by both listeners and via acoustic analysis.

Of all the visual feedback approaches, EPG (which requires the use of a custom dental appliance) appears to have been the most frequently studied. Gibbon and Wood (2010) suggest at least 150 reports of EPG being applied to a variety of different speech-disordered populations are available. They note, however, that none was above level III (i.e., all involved case studies). A few examples of EPG studies for children with speech sound disorders are presented here to illustrate the findings with this approach. Carter and Edwards (2004) conducted a post hoc review of 10 cases of children with speech sound disorders of unknown origin ages 7 to 14 years who had been treated with EPG for a variety of speech sound targets. After 10 weeks of treatment, a significant improvement in overall conso-nant accuracy as well as in specific target sounds in a single word probe task was found. McAuliffe and Cornwell (2008) reported findings for an 11-year-old girl treated with EPG for lateralized /s, z/. After four weeks of direct therapy with an SLP and six weeks of home practice (using a portable EPG unit), she was producing normal versions of the targets (without the artificial palate in place) as determined by listener ratings and acoustic analy-sis. Despite the positive result, analysis of EPG displays suggested only minimal change in the pattern of tongue contact with the artificial palate in place. Dagenais, Critz-Crosby, and Adams (1994) also reported a similar outcome of normal production of /s/ (previously lat-eralized) but abnormal tongue contact for an 8-year-old girl. This latter study also reported no noticeable improvement with EPG for a second child despite 28 treatment sessions. Thus, outcomes with EPG, while promising, are not universally positive.

Summary of Motor Approaches to Remediation

The treatment approaches described on the previous pages focus on the development and habituation of the motor skills necessary for target sound productions. An underlying assumption is that motor practice leads to generalization of correct productions to untrained contexts and to automatization of behaviors. Motor approaches to remediation are espe-cially appropriate for phonetically based errors but are frequently employed in combination with procedures described in Chapter 10 under linguistic-based approaches. Approaches that use alternate forms of feedback are available and have shown some promise for treat-ing older children and adults with persistent (residual) errors.

REMEDIATION GUIDELINES FOR MOTOR APPROACHES

1. A motor approach to remediation is recommended as a teaching procedure for cli-ents who evidence motor production problems. One group of individuals who fre-quently are candidates for motor approaches includes those with persistent (residual) errors. A motor approach can also be incorporated into treatment programs for clients reflecting linguistically based errors. Instruction should be initiated at the linguistic unit level (isolation, syllable, word) at which a client can produce target sounds.
2. Perceptual training for those clients who evidence perceptual problems related to their error sounds is recommended as part of a motor remediation program.

CORE VOCABULARY APPROACH

One approach that does not fit neatly into either the motor-based or linguistically based category is the core vocabulary approach. It targets children with severe but inconsistent speech sound productions (i.e., different sound substitutions across productions and ≥ 40 percent variable productions) (Dodd, Crosbie, and Holm, 2004). "Children with incon-sistent speech disorders" are one of the four symptomatology subgroups described in

Chapter 4. Their speech is characterized by variable productions of words or variable phonological features across contexts and also within the same context. Dodd and colleagues hypothesize that the reason for such children's unstable phonological system reflects a deficit in phonological planning (i.e., phoneme selection and sequencing). The authors differentiate this subgroup of children with inconsistent speech sound disorders from childhood apraxia of speech (CAS), although similar forms of inconsistency are present in both types of disorders. Dodd, Crosbie, and Holm state that the core vocabulary approach is "the treatment of choice" for children with inconsistent speech sound productions who may be resistant to contrast treatment or traditional therapy. They suggest that this treatment results in a systemwide change by improving the consistency of whole-word production and addressing speech processing deficits.

The core vocabulary procedure includes the following steps:

1. The child, parents, and teacher select a list of approximately 50 words that are "functionally powerful" for the child and that includes names (family, friends, teachers, pets), places (*school, library, shops, toilet*), function words (*please, sorry, thank you*), foods (*drinks, soda, hamburger, cereal*), and the child's favorite things (*games, Batman, sports*). Words are chosen because they are used frequently in the child's functional communication.

2. Each week 10 of the functional 50 words are selected for treatment. The clinician teaches the child his or her best production using cues or teaching the word sound-by-sound. If the child is unable to produce a correct production of the word, developmental errors are permissible. The child is required to practice the 10 words during the week and at the therapy sessions with a high number of responses per session. Teachers and parents are to reinforce and praise the child for "best" word production in communication situations. The intent is to make sure that the 10 words are said the same way each time rather than to target correct productions. If a child produces a word differently from his or her best production, the clinician would imitate the word and explain that the word was said differently and how it differed from the best production. However, the clinician does not ask the child to imitate the target word but provides information about the best production because when a child imitates they can produce it "without having to assemble/generate their own plan for the word" (p. 228; Dodd, Holm, Crosbie, and McIntosh, 2006)

3. At the end of the weekly sessions (twice weekly), the child is asked to produce the words three times. Words produced consistently are then removed from the list of 50 words. Inconsistently produced words remain on the list, and the next week's words are randomly chosen from the 50-word list. Once every two weeks, untreated words from the 50-word list are selected as probe words. The probe words are elicited three times each to monitor generalization.

Background Statement.   The core vocabulary procedure focuses on functional outcomes in which a consistent (even if not fully correct) output is targeted. An underlying assumption of this approach appears to be that, if the child changes what she or he does to make the outcomes more consistent, listeners will be better able to understand the intended message. She or he will then be able to provide consistent feedback, which will allow the child to either make systemwide changes to her or his sound system or modify her or his speech motor programs.

Unique Features.   This approach does not dictate any specific teaching approach but rather assumes that with the assistance of the clinician, the child will do whatever she or he needs to do to modify the output. Likewise, the focus is on making the child more consistent and thus more understandable without any emphasis on a particular linguistic level of production.

Strengths and Limitations.   Because intelligibility is the overriding goal of all communication, a clear strength of this approach is that, unlike most other approaches, it focuses on that important goal. An apparent limitation is that the approach is intended for only those with inconsistent speech who constitute a small percentage of children with speech sound disorders. Finally, the lack of detail on how to achieve consistency may be frustrating for some clinicians.

Research Support.   Dodd and her colleagues have conducted a number of studies to validate this approach. The highest level of treatment study available (level IIb) appears to be that of Crosbie, Holm, and Dodd (2005). These authors compared treatment using a phonological contrast approach (auditory discrimination with either minimal pairs or multiple oppositions; the specific approach depended on the child) with a core vocabulary treatment approach. Eighteen children ages 4;8 to 6;5 with severe speech disorders received two 8-week blocks of both of the intervention treatments. All of the children increased their accuracy of production of consonants (PCC) as well as their consistency of the production. They reported that core vocabulary intervention resulted in more change in children with "inconsistent" speech sound disorders and that "contrast therapy" resulted in improved changes in children with "consistent" speech disorders.

THE USE OF NONSPEECH ORAL-MOTOR ACTIVITIES

Some clinicians continue to use *nonspeech oral-motor* training as a precursor to teaching sounds or to supplement speech sound instruction (Lof and Watson, 2008). Such activities include horn or whistle blowing, sucking through straws, and tongue wagging for which no speech sounds are produced. This contrasts with any activity that includes the production of speech sounds (even if just a single phoneme), which would be better described as *speech motor* training.

Despite their widespread use, nonspeech oral–motor activities have long been questioned. Until recently, the case against them was largely made philosophically (i.e., using indirect logic rather than direct evidence). Forrest (2002) argued the logical point of view in addressing the four justifications that clinicians have historically used in support of nonspeech oral-motor activities in therapy:

1. They simplify the task? Forrest pointed out that evidence from studies of complex motor skills other than speech suggests that mastery of such skills requires performance of the entire task rather than what are perceived as the individual components

of the task. Brief discussion of components used in speaking for production of an individual sound may be helpful, but extensive practice of individual components is not sufficient to learn the overall skill.

2. They strengthen the articulators? Forrest noted that (a) most of the nonspeech oral-motor activities used are not practiced with sufficient frequency or against enough resistance to actually enhance strength, and (b) studies indicate that we usually need only 15–20 percent of our strength capacity for speech.

3. They enhance the sensitivity of the articulators? Forrest noted (as we did in Chapter 5) that there is no clear relationship between oral motor sensitivity and speech sound disorders.

4. They replicate normal development? Although it seems counterintuitive, Forrest cited considerable evidence that suggests that speech does not normally develop from nonspeech behaviors; the latter just happens to emerge earlier in development. Nonspeech activities such as sucking, blowing, chewing, and swallowing are quite different from speech in terms of the types of movements, level of muscle activity, and coordination among the muscles. This is true even in very young children in whom speech is just emerging (Moore and Ruark, 1996; Ruark and Moore 1997). Put another way, speech and nonspeech activities may share structure, but they differ greatly in how those structures are used, and they appear to develop independently.

Recently, a small body of direct evidence regarding the value of nonspeech oral-motor activities has begun to accumulate. Lass and Pannbacker (2008) identified 11 studies that examined speech outcomes following nonspeech oral-motor treatments. Only 2 of the 11 studies showed significant change that might be attributed to the use of nonspeech oral-motor activities. One of these (Fields and Polmanteer, 2002) was a level Ib study, but it has been criticized on methodological grounds (e.g., inappropriate statistical analysis) and has never been published in a peer-reviewed journal. The other was a level III study by McAllister (2003) that examined only voice quality and did not report outcomes for speech sounds. Thus, the vast majority of the direct evidence does not support the use of nonspeech oral-motor activities to improve speech sound production.

In summary, the logical arguments and the research evidence both point to the same conclusion. They support the long-held dictum that "if you want to improve speech, you should focus on speech." We recommend against the use of nonspeech oral-motor activities for speech sound intervention and treatment.

INTERVENTION FOR CHILDHOOD APRAXIA OF SPEECH

The topic of childhood apraxia of speech (CAS) was introduced in Chapter 4 in our discussion of classification of speech sound disorders. In this section, we address issues relevant to clinical assessment and intervention with this subpopulation.

As noted in Chapter 4, we do not have a clear sense of how CAS differs from other speech sound disorders. The 2007 ASHA position statement, however, provides a starting point for such differentiation. From that perspective, CAS is generally viewed as primarily a problem of planning and programming speech sound production that manifests itself in errors of both precision and consistency of production. Children with CAS have difficulty reaching precise speech sound targets and may produce the same word in different ways on multiple attempts. Children with CAS could also have associated (comorbid) neuromuscular problems (i.e., dysarthria) and/or other types of apraxia such as oral or limb apraxia (i.e., problems with nonspeech movements). The position statement also indicates that CAS is likely a problem that is neurological in nature and might result from known neurological impairments such as cerebral palsy, or it might be associated with complex neurobehavioral disorders such as autism, Fragile X syndrome, or Rett syndrome. However, the origin of any neurological limitations is in many cases unknown (idiopathic).

Consistent with the idea of problems with planning and programming of speech output, Velleman and Strand (1994) have stated that children with CAS may be capable of producing the individual aspects of speech production (i.e., articulatory postures, phonemes, words), but have great difficulty "bridging among the various elements that constitute language performance" (p. 120). Put another way, CAS likely includes difficulty not only with phonology but also with other aspects of language.

In regard to higher levels of language, Velleman (2003) noted that many of these children often demonstrate receptive language skills that are superior to their expressive abilities. Lacking such a gap, another diagnosis such as specific language impairment might be appropriate (although CAS could coexist in some cases). Gillon and Moriarty (2007) also supported the possibility of a higher level of language problems in children with CAS; the authors reported an increased risk for reading and spelling difficulty in this population. It should also be noted that many children with CAS also manifest social and behavioral problems (Ball, 1999). This may be a consequence of the significant difficulty that many of these children appear to have in making themselves understood (i.e., having greatly reduced intelligibility).

Assessment

Assessment of this population is not unlike that used with any child with a speech sound disorder and, in addition to a standard articulation/phonological battery, typically includes a case history, hearing screening, and screening for other areas of communication (language, voice, fluency). However, specific aspects of evaluation of the CAS population warrant elaboration.

The oral mechanism examination should be particularly thorough to determine whether comorbid dysarthria or oral apraxia is present. It should include an assessment of strength, tone, and stability of the oral structures (e.g., can the child move the tongue independently of the mandible? Does the child do anything special to stabilize the mandible, such as thrust it forward?). A review of the child's feeding history may be of interest in this regard. Young children, in particular, might exhibit uncoordinated feeding patterns without dysphagia (swallowing problems). Overall motor skills, both automatic and volitional, including the ability to perform imitative and rapidly alternating tongue movements, in addition to diadochokinetic (DDK) tasks should be part of the assessment. As noted previously, one feature that is emerging as potentially unique to CAS is difficulty with transitions between sounds. Although static articulatory positions (sounds in isolation) might be produced correctly, rapid combinations of movements frequently are difficult for this population. DDK tasks involving changing place of articulation might be especially problematic in cases of CAS. In addition, the rapid successive movements (e.g., syllable to syllable) of connected speech entail constant approximations of specific articulatory targets because no absolute or static positions are associated with speech sounds. For children with CAS, the inherent dynamic overlapping movement involved in producing sequential motor speech elements is a problem. Velleman and Strand (1994) indicated that sequencing difficulties may not manifest themselves in phonemic sequencing errors per se but are more evident at the articulatory level, affecting the relative timing of glottal and articulatory gestures. These latter factors result in perceived errors of voicing and vowels, especially diphthongs.

Strand and McCauley (1999) proposed using an utterance hierarchy for assessment. In their procedure, evaluation includes speech sound productions in a variety of utterance types, for example, assessing connected speech through conversation, picture description, and narrative; employing DDK tasks; using imitative utterances that include vowels (V), consonant-vowels (CV), and vowel-consonant (VC) combinations; assessing CVC productions when the first and last phoneme are the same and when they are different; and repetition of single words of increasing length, multisyllabic words, plus words in phrases, and sentences of increasing length.

In analyzing speech performance, the clinician must keep in mind the nature of CAS as a disorder involving the hierarchical levels of speech and language, including motor planning for syllable sequencing. Movements, transitions, and timing should be observed as speech is produced at a variety of linguistic levels from simple to complex. For children with a limited verbal repertoire, an independent phonological analysis of a speech/language sample is recommended by assessing the child's individual speech sound productions without comparison to the standard use of these productions in the general population. For those with more normal verbal skills, a traditional phonologic assessment battery (relational analysis) is recommended with particular attention to the analysis of speech sounds within syllabic units. In this instance, a connected speech sample is critical because it allows the examiner to review syllable and word shapes produced by the child. To evaluate consistency of productions, particular attention should be paid to words that occur multiple times in the sample.

Phonologic assessment should also include imitation of words that increase in number of syllables (e.g., *please, pleasing, pleasingly*). Because children with CAS evidence problems with the dynamic organization of communication efforts, it is not unusual for problems to be present with the suprasegmental (e.g., phrasal stress) aspects of speech. Coordinating the laryngeal and respiratory systems with the oral mechanism is often very difficult. This problem may result in difficulty with varying intonation contours, modulation of loudness, and maintaining proper resonance. Vowels may be prolonged because the child needs time to organize coordination for the next series of speech sound movements. Recall also that the 2007 ASHA position statement cited excessive and equal stress as another emerging feature of CAS.

It may be prudent to refer more seriously impaired children with suspected dysarthria and/or CAS to a pediatric neurologist to determine the status of current neurological functioning. Seizure history, associated limb apraxia, presence of oral apraxia, and general knowledge of neurological functioning could influence the overall management program for a given child and thus warrant such a neurological referral.

Recommended Assessment Battery for CAS

1. Case history (including review of feeding history)
2. Hearing screening/testing
3. Screening of voice and fluency characteristics
4. Speech mechanism examination
   a. Structure and function
   b. Strength, tone, stability
   c. DDK tasks
5. Connected speech sample
   a. Segmental productions
   b. Syllable and word shape productions
   c. Phonologic patterns present
   d. Intonation, vocal loudness, resonance
   e. Analysis of consistency (words occurring more than once)
6. Segmental productions (citation form testing; independent analysis for those with a limited phonological repertoire)
   a. Consonants, vowels, and diphthongs
   b. Syllable shapes used
7. Intelligibility—how well the acoustic signal is understood with and without context
8. Stimulability testing (include multiple opportunities)
   a. Segments
   b. Syllables
   c. Words with increasing number of syllables
9. Phonological awareness assessment
10. Interpersonal skills
    a. Social interaction
    b. Behavioral interactions
    c. Academic/community interactions
11. Language evaluation
    a. Comprehension and production
    b. Sound productions at various semantic and syntactic levels

A number of published tests specifically designed for use in the assessment of children with suspected CAS are available. These include the *Screening Test for Developmental Apraxia of Speech-Second Edition* (STDAS-2; Blakely, 2001), the *Apraxia Profile* (AP; Hickman, 1997), and the *Kaufman Speech Praxis Test for Children* (KSPT; Kaufman, 1995). It should be noted that all of these tests were developed prior to the publication of the ASHA position statement on CAS. Each includes the authors' own sense of what tasks to include. None of them examines all three of the emerging features of CAS (consistency across multiple attempts, difficulty with transitions, prosodic disturbances), and in particular, none of them examines consistency. A possible supplement to the above assessment battery might therefore be the *Diagnostic Evaluation of Articulation and Phonology* (DEAP; Dodd and colleagues, 2006), which includes a consistency subtest.

Treatment

Velleman (2003) noted that relatively little empirical research supports the use of any particular treatment program with children who have CAS. Evaluating what research is available remains a challenge, however, because much of what is available was published prior to the adoption of the ASHA position statement. Therefore, most treatment studies would not necessarily have defined CAS the same way, and the children being treated might have been quite different across studies.

Assuming that the core problem in CAS is difficulty with programming or planning for speech, neither traditional motor approaches nor linguistic approaches would likely work well for these children. Indeed, some clinicians have suggested a slow response to these typical interventions as a diagnostic marker for CAS; that is, perhaps very slow progress in therapy is a characteristic of children with CAS. Velleman (2003) noted a diagnosis of CAS on the basis of slow progress in therapy would be unwise because slow progress may simply reflect poorly applied therapy and may not necessarily mean that there was a mistake in the original diagnosis.

Because of what we know about CAS, two aspects of therapy would appear to require particular attention: short-term goals and production units. Rather than focusing on individual speech sounds, a major short-term therapy goal is to build a functional vocabulary for the child with CAS. Often these children have significant intelligibility problems, and efforts need to be directed toward building a core of intelligible words to facilitate the communication process. To the extent possible, production activities should include attention to syllabic structures and combinations of these syllables so that the child gains verbal building blocks for words. Some elements of the previously discussed core vocabulary approach may be appropriate for children with CAS. Recall that in Chapter 4, we noted that some children with speech sound disorders of unknown origin share the pattern of inconsistency seen in children who might be classified as having CAS. Frequent drill and practice on a variety of target syllables and words are the focus of treatment.

Another perspective on short-term goals in CAS is to use other approaches to communication in general. Cumley and Swanson (1999) suggested the use of some type of augmentative or alternative system such as a voice output communication aid or sign language or both. The goal in this case is to provide a short-term bridge to encourage communication as well as better feedback from conversational partners; those same partners would be more likely to understand the message and less likely end communication exchanges prematurely. Using three cases studies (i.e., a level III study), Cumley and Swanson showed that multimodal AAC intervention (i.e., using a combination of speech, sign, and voice output device device):

> ... provided them with greater opportunities for communicative success and flexibility for initiating, participating in, and repairing their communication breakdowns ... [and] afforded greater opportunities for supporting and facilitating the language development, communicative interaction, and academic success of these children. (p. 121)

Relative to production units, a focus of instructional activities should be the motor-planning component of the disorder. Rather than using drill activities that focus on repetition of the same sounds or syllables, a variety of speech and language motor planning activities should be provided to practice transitions and timing movements required in the dynamic process of ongoing speech. Emphasis is placed on shifting the stimulus materials to incorporate a wider variety of syllable sequences. For example, one could start by having a child name a succession of animals with one-syllable names (e.g., *bat, bear, bird, bug*), then shift to animals with two-syllable names (e.g., *baboon, beaver, camel*), and then increase to three-syllable names (e.g., *buffalo, butterfly, bandanna*). Names could then be combined, emphasizing being able to do the motor planning necessary to accommodate shifts and variations in syllable sequencing that represent increasing linguistic complexity. Rosenbeck, Kent, and LaPointe (1984) also recommended continually shifting the segmental targets in a succession of syllables beginning with CV or VC, repeating the patterns, and then systematically varying the CV pattern and moving into word combinations.

Strand and Skindner (1999) recommended integral stimulation methods that included tactile and proprioceptive monitoring of articulatory configurations, movement paths, and practice with movements to provide knowledge of results to the child. They suggested that more frequent distribution of sessions (always a good idea when scheduling therapy sessions) might result in better motor learning (e.g., 2 hours of therapy per week is better distributed in four half-hour sessions than in two 1-hour sessions). They also suggested choosing stimuli for treatment that are useful and meaningful to the child to allow him or her to experience successful communication. They emphasized the importance of stimulus selection, including length and phonetic context of the target words. Some positive outcomes have been reported using variations of this approach with case study or level III research designs (Edeal and Gildersleeve-Neumann, 2011; Strand and Debertine, 2000; Strand, Stoekel, and Baas, 2006). Strand, Stoekel, and Baas refer to the child-specific form of integral stimulation as *Dynamic Temporal and Tactile Cueing (DTTC)*.

Square (1999) outlined three additional types of interventions, including tactile-kinesthetic, rhythmic and melodic facilitation, and gestural cueing. In "touch-cueing" (Bashir, Grahamjones, and Bostwick, 1984), the clinician touches a particular area of the face or neck as each sound in a sequence is produced. Children learn the sound associated with each touching cue. Thus, children can be presented simultaneous touch, auditory, and sometimes visual cues as they produce sounds in various movement patterns. The "touch-cue" method is an example of a tactile-kinesthetic approach. Another tactile-kinesthetic approach is *Prompts for Restructuring Oral Muscular Phonetic Targets (PROMPT)* developed by Chumpelik (1984). This approach specifies jaw height, facial-labial contraction, tongue height and advancement, muscular tension, duration of contractions, and airstream management for phoneme production. An example of a rhythmic and melodic facilitation approach is known as *Melodic Intonation Therapy* (Helfrich-Miller, 1984). This program uses stimuli that progress over a hierarchy of difficulty while being intoned with Signed English use as a pacer.

A set of suggestions for working with clients with CAS is presented in Table 9.3. This is based on a combination of the recommendations and/or findings from Velleman and Strand (1994), McNeill (2007), and Edeal and Gildersleeve-Neumann (2011). For children who are very young or severely impaired, gestures and pantomime may be encouraged. An augmentative communication system assessment may be desired, particularly for children who are unintelligible. Such assessment should target the various systems that

TABLE 9.3	Suggestions for Speech Production Treatment for CAS

1. Include an emphasis on expanding both phonetic and syllable shapes inventories.
2. Avoid repetitive drill of the same target except when initially teaching a new sound. When doing so, quickly move beyond single sounds and focus on teaching motor planning by gradually moving to longer and more complex sound sequences (i.e., syllable shapes).
3. Use both visual and auditory clues for modeling correct production.
4. Frequent, short sessions with breaks are likely to be more successful than longer, less frequent sessions.
5. Consider randomly ordered presentation of stimuli across different linguistic levels (e.g., mix word, phrase, and sentence-level stimuli in random order within the same activity).
6. Activities incorporating music may assist with possible prosodic problems.
7. Include phonological awareness activities.

may be appropriate for facilitating language development, reading, spelling, and written language. Facilitating communication through these techniques is often viewed as a means to develop verbal communication as well as other aspects of language. Perhaps the most comprehensive set of instructional materials for treating clients with motor planning difficulties is the *Nuffield Centre Dyspraxia Programme* (1994), which was developed at the Royal National Throat Nose and Ear Hospital in London, England. Velleman (2003) has also presented treatment suggestions for children with CAS. Programs commercially available might provide assistance in organizing treatment strategies; however, such programs currently lack formal empirical support. It is important to remember that individualized programs designed specifically for a child based on his or her assessment performance is likely to result in the most effective interventions and progress.

CASE STUDY REVISITED: MOTOR PERSPECTIVE

Intervention Recommendations

In Chapter 7, we discussed the speech samples obtained from Kirk with an analysis and interpretation of his test data. We now discuss how one might proceed in developing an intervention plan based on that interpretation. In this chapter, we take a motor-based perspective. In Chapter 10, we assume a linguistic perspective.

As you recall, Kirk is a 3-year-old child with multiple errors who needs intervention because of poor speech intelligibility. You might wish to review the case study report at the end of Chapter 7 at this time. As you move through the discussion that follows, bear in mind that the steps involved and the variables considered are applicable to many clients with speech sound impairments.

Kirk is stimulable for most error sounds, but there are exceptions: /ʃ/, /tʃ/, /θ/, /r/, and /ɝ/. Intervention for these exceptions could readily be seen as needing a motor-based approach. Likewise, some of the stimulable sounds were more easily imitated than others, so instruction must also include teaching or stabilization of the motor production of sounds that he cannot consistently imitate on demand.

First Consideration: How Many Targets Should I Address in a Session?

As we noted in Chapter 7, Kirk has multiple error sounds suggesting that a focus on several targets is more appropriate either within a single lesson or across lessons within a 3- or 4-week time frame (cycles or horizontal approach). This could include targets in which a motor-based approach is appropriate as well as targets in which a linguistically based approach makes more sense (i.e., those sounds that are readily stimulable).

Second Consideration: How Should I Conceptualize the Overall Treatment Program?

Because Kirk has so many sounds in error and some of those sounds are not stabilized at an imitative level, it is suggested that the clinician begin a session by spending about 5 minutes engaged in what has been identified as "sound stimulation/practice," an activity designed to enhance Kirk's stimulability for all error sounds. Kirk is young and still acquiring phonemes, so it seems advisable to provide him the opportunity to produce a variety of sounds that are not produced correctly in his conversational speech. Sound stimulation can include practice not only on error sounds (e.g., /ɝ/, /s/, /f/) but also sounds that he does say correctly (/p/, /h/, /f/). Successful production of such sounds might facilitate his willingness to try other sounds he has made in error.

Kirk should make five attempts to produce each sound target during sound stimulation, using a cueing hierarchy for those in error, based on the level of support necessary to produce a sound (e.g., modeling, phonetic placement, or selected contexts). After five attempts, another sound is practiced. With only five attempts, the client is not overwhelmed with repeated failures if he or she cannot produce a sound. It is hoped that by briefly focusing in each session on production of a variety of sounds and levels of complexity (i.e., isolation, syllables, words), a child will acquire the skill to imitate the sound when given an auditory and/or visual model. Production in this type of activity is a building block for focusing on phonological contrasts and for facilitating generalization when a child is stimulable. Following sound stimulation/production practice, the treatment program focuses on those errors for which more linguistically based interventions are more applicable.

Third Consideration: How Do Instructional Goals Relate to the Treatment Continuum and Specific Instructional Steps?

The treatment continuum, including establishment, generalization, and maintenance which provides the focus for much of what we do in therapy, was discussed earlier. In the case of Kirk, the /ɝ/ or other nonstimulable sounds require an establishment activity such as sound stimulation mentioned previously. His other error patterns (i.e., initial consonant deletion; stopping; final consonant deletion) fit into the generalization phase of the continuum because he is stimulable on many of the sounds required to eliminate these patterns. Earlier we discussed that in each stage of the treatment, the continuum of therapy comprises a sequence of steps and activities that include antecedent events from the clinician, responses from the client, and consequent events from the clinician based on client responses. One of the initial planning tasks is to determine how one is going to sequence antecedent events (e.g., verbal instruction, pictures, printed symbols, game activity) and consequent events (e.g., verbal reinforcement, tokens, back-up reinforcers).

A more complete outline of the overall treatment plan for Kirk is presented at the end of Chapter 10.

QUESTIONS FOR CHAPTER 9

1. How would one assess auditory perception in a child who is suspected of having difficulty with sound contrasts?

2. Outline a traditional approach to articulation therapy and specify for whom it is appropriate.

3. What characteristics distinguish children with CAS from other phonologically delayed children, and what distinguishes their treatment?

4. What is meant by *nonspeech oral motor activities?* Why are these often regarded as not worthwhile?

5. Outline a shaping procedure for teaching /tʃ/.

6. What is meant by evidence-based practice? What is meant when we talk about varying levels of support for treatment procedures?

CHAPTER 10

Linguistically Based Treatment Approaches

PETER FLIPSEN JR.
Idaho State University

NICHOLAS W. BANKSON
James Madison University

JOHN E. BERNTHAL
University of Nebraska–Lincoln

◆ ◆ ◆

We now turn our attention to a second category of treatment approaches for speech sound disorders, linguistically or phonologically based instruction. Whereas the motor approaches we discussed in Chapter 9 may be described as phonetically based and focus on teaching the physical aspects of producing speech sounds, linguistic approaches are focused more on teaching sound contrasts and appropriate phonological patterns. As such, linguistically based intervention focuses on strategies for reorganizing a child's phonological system. Although a linguistic based approach is most suitable for a child with multiple speech sound errors, elements of the approach can and continue to be used in combination with more traditional, or motor-based, approaches.

As we did in Chapter 9, for each approach discussed, we provide sections on "Background Statement," "Unique Features, Strengths and Limitations," and "Research Support." The latter will be framed based on the levels of evidence that American Speech-Language-Hearing Association (ASHA) has adopted and that were outlined near the beginning of Chapter 9. As in the earlier chapter, the emphasis is on the best available evidence.

The primary focus of linguistic approaches to remediation is the establishment of the adult phonological system, including the inventory of phonemes (i.e., sounds used to contrast meaning), allophonic rules (i.e., use of different allophones in different contexts), and phonotactic rules (i.e., how sounds are combined to form syllables and words). Treatment programs designed to facilitate acquisition of the phonological system are not associated with a single unified method; however, they share two primary characteristics. The first characteristic relates to the behaviors targeted for treatment and the second to the instructional procedures themselves.

As discussed in Chapter 7, selection of target behaviors is usually based on patterns that describe the errors. Following pattern or phonological process identification, individual sound(s), called *exemplars*, are chosen that are likely to facilitate generalization from the exemplar to other sounds related to a particular error pattern. Treatment is then designed to facilitate the acquisition of appropriate sound contrasts and/or sequences with the expectation that generalization will occur to other sounds that are part of the same pattern (e.g., in targeting final consonant deletion, teaching several final consonants is assumed to generalize to other final consonants that are also deleted).

Many treatment protocols that are based on a linguistic model employ minimal contrast word-pairs, which involve minimal or maximal feature contrasts (Weiner, 1981b; Gierut, 1989; Fey, 1992). For example, minimal pairs such as bu*s*-buc*k* and bu*s*-bu*t* represent minimal pairs with greater and lesser contrasts, respectively, because of the differences in both place and manner of articulation between /s/ and /k/ and only a manner difference between /s/ and /t/.

The primary focus of linguistic approaches has been to (1) establish sound and feature contrasts and (2) replace error patterns with appropriate phonological patterns. Linguistic approaches have targeted elimination of homonyms (one word used for two referents—for example, *shoe* used for both *chew* and *shoe*) and establishment of new syllable and word shapes and of new sounds or sound classes.

MINIMAL PAIR CONTRAST THERAPY

A signature approach of linguistic based remediation is *minimal pair contrast therapy*. Contrast therapy employs pairs of words that differ only by a single phoneme (e.g., *b*at-*p*at, *m*ove-*m*oo*d*, *s*un-*t*on). The underlying concept of this type of therapy is that focusing on word-pairs that typically differ by a single phonemic contrast will teach the client that different sounds signal different meanings in words. The phonemic contrasts are related either to feature differences between sounds (e.g., *pat-bat* differ by the voicing feature; *pat-fat* differ by the manner feature), or syllable shape (e.g., *bow-boat* differ by the presence or absence of the final sound; *key-ski* differ by the presence or absence of the initial sound[s] in the syllable initiation—cluster versus noncluster or cluster reduction). Investigators have reported changes in children's phonological systems (Weiner, 1981; Elbert and Gierut, 1986; Gierut, 1989, 1990; Williams, 1991) following training with word-pair contrasts. Contrast therapy focuses on the establishment of sound contrasts necessary to differentiate one word from another. Although this communication-oriented therapy emerged from a linguistic orientation, it is also occasionally used in traditional treatment approaches.

An example of a contrast approach to treatment can be observed in remediation strategies employed with a client who deletes final consonants. Such a client might produce stops correctly in word-initial position but delete them in word-final position (the syllables lacks closure also called open syllables). In such a circumstance, the clinician can assume that the final consonant deletions are probably not a production (phonetic) problem but in this case likely reflect a conceptual rule related to syllable structure (use of the open syllable). Treatment would focus on helping the client to recognize that the presence of a consonant in word-final position is a necessary contrast to distinguish certain word-pairs in the language (e.g., *two-tooth*; *bee-beet*). Because the client is able to produce the target correctly in initial position, the motoric production of a target consonant is assumed to be within a client's productive repertoire, and thus motor production of the sound is not the focus of instruction. Rather, the focus is on the development of cognitive awareness of final consonant contrasts/syllable closure.

The most common type of contrast training typically focuses a substituted or deleted sound with a target sound. For example, if a client substitutes /t/ for /k/ in word-initial position, contrast training words might include *tea-key* and *top-cop*. Similarly, if a child deletes the final /t/, contrast pairs might include *bow-boat* and *see-seat*. Minimal contrast instruction is appropriate when two or more contrasting sounds in the adult language are collapsed into a single sound unit with the result that sound contrasts are not produced (e.g., both /t/ and /k/ are realized as /t/), or segments are deleted, such as in final consonant deletions. Training is designed to establish sound contrasts that mark a difference in meaning.

Minimal contrast instruction typically focuses first on perception of contrasts and then on the production of contrasts. La Riviere and colleagues (1974) first proposed a training task that focused on perceptual training utilizing contrast pairs. In this procedure, the child was taught to identify words where the target sounds and errors were presented in word-pairs. For example, if a child deletes /s/ in /s/ clusters (cluster reduction), the clinician names several pictures representing minimal pair words such as *spool-pool* or *spill-pill* to the client. The clinician names items to be picked up and then requires the client to pick them up or perhaps sort the words into one or two categories (/p/ singletons or /sp/ clusters).

A production-based minimal pair task requires the client to produce both words as truly different words. For example, a client who deletes final consonants might ask the clinician to give him or her the picture of either a *bee* or a *beet* and then be reinforced by the clinician for the appropriate production. In this task, the client must be able to produce the distinction between *bee* and *beet*. As stated earlier, the reverse of this procedure (i.e., the clinician asks the client to give him or her certain pictures) can be used to establish perceptual contrasts (i.e., recognizing the distinction between *bee* and *beet*).

Weiner (1981b) reported a study in which minimal contrast training was used to reduce the frequency of selected phonological patterns. He used minimal pairs in activities that required accurate word productions for the child to communicate successfully. For example, Weiner used a game to teach final /t/ in a minimal contrast format. He placed such words as *bow* and *boat* into minimal pairs. Sample stimuli consisted of several pictures of *bow* and several pictures of *boat*. The instructions for the game were as follows:

> We are going to play a game. The object of the game is to get me to pick up all the pictures of the *boat*. Every time you say boat, I will pick one up. When I have all five, you may paste a star on your paper." If the child said *bow*, the clinician picked up the *bow* picture. At times he would provide an instruction, e.g., "You keep saying *bow*. If you want me to pick up the *boat* picture, you must say the [t] sound at the end. Listen, *boat, boat, boat*. You try it. Okay. Let's begin again" (p. 98)

Weiner (1981b) reported that such training established additional phonological contrasts in the child's repertoire and then generalization to nontrained words. A variety of word lists (e.g., Bleile, 1995) and treatment materials (e.g., Bird and Higgins, 1990; Palin,

1992; Price and Scarry-Larkin, 1999) are available commercially to assist clinicians in finding contrasting word-pairs and pictures for treatment. The software program *Sound Contrasts in Phonology* (SCIP; Williams, 2006) also serves this purpose.

Protocol for Employing a Minimal Pair Training Procedure

1. Select a sound contrast to be trained based on the client's error patterns. For example, if the child substitutes /t/ for /ʃ/ (stopping), one might select *tea-she, toe-show*, and *tape-shape* as contrasting words when targeting the stopping pattern. Select five pictures for each of the contrast words.
2. Engage the client in minimal contrast training at a perceptual level (e.g., "I want you to pick up the pictures that I name. Pick up _____.").
3. Pretest the client's motor production of each of the target words containing the error sound, and, if necessary, instruct him or her in production of the target phoneme. Such instruction usually needs to be only brief in duration; when more intensive instruction becomes necessary, treatment with a more motor-based approach (see Chapter 9) might need to be carried out before linguistic instruction proceeds.
4. Have the client imitatively produce each target word.
5. Engage the client in minimal contrast training at a production level (e.g., "I want you to tell me which picture to pick up. Every time you say *show*, I will pick up this picture").
6. Engage the client in a task that requires him or her to incorporate each of the contrast words in a carrier phrase (e.g., "I want you to point to a picture and name it by saying 'I found a _____.'").
7. Continue the carrier phrase task, incorporating each of the contrasting words into the phrase (e.g., "I found a *tea* and a *she*").

Clinicians can use their creativity and clinical knowledge to modify a protocol such as that just presented. Descriptions in the literature of minimal pair treatment approaches as well as several commercially available sets of materials are designed to facilitate this treatment approach. It should be mentioned that for those instances when meaningful minimal pairs cannot be found to reflect a particular contrast, "near minimal pairs," in which one word might not have meaning, are sometimes used (e.g., *van-shan*). In this instance, the clinician may point to an abstract drawing and, as in the preceding example, say, "This is a *shan*." Thus, the child is taught a nonsensical but contrasting word to use in the minimal pair activity.

Different Kinds of Minimal Pairs

Thus far we have assumed that all minimal pairs are the same. This is not necessarily the case. If we compare the contrasting sounds in the pairs, sometimes the sounds differ on only a single feature. For example, in the pair sun-ton the /s/ and /t/ are contrasted, and they differ only on a single feature; in this case it is manner of articulation. Likewise in the pair tea-key the /t/ and /k/ only differ on place of articulation. Sound contrasts in minimal pairs that include a single feature difference are referred to as minimal opposition contrasts. On the other hand, some contrasts in minimal pairs may differ on more than one feature. For example, in the pair tea-she the contrasting sounds differ on both place and manner of articulation. Or in the pair sew-go the difference is three features (place, manner, and voicing). Contrasts that differ on more than a single feature are sometimes called maximal opposition contrasts. Therapy based on both minimal and maximal oppositions has been proposed. Advocates of the maximal oppositions approach note that phonological oppositions of more disparity may facilitate more change in the client's acquisition of feature contrasts; they also suggest that the contrasts between the word-pairs are more salient and thus easier for the client to perceive. Examples of minimal and maximal opposition pairs are as follows:

Minimal Oppositions	*Feature Differences*
*s*un—*t*on	manner of production
*th*umb—*s*um	place of production
*ch*ew—*sh*oe	manner of production

Maximal Oppositions	*Feature Differences*
*ch*ain—*m*ain	manner of production, nasality, place of production
*c*an—*m*an	manner of production, nasality, place of production
*g*ear—*f*ear	manner of production, voicing, place of production

The treatment methodologies outlined earlier for minimal contrast therapy are also applicable to maximal contrast training.

The use of maximal oppositions is supported by data from Gierut (1989, 1990). Her research indicated that for children with multiple errors, maximal contrast training facilitated a greater overall change in the phonological system than did minimal contrast training. In her research, the sound contrasted to the target sound was a phoneme that was already in the subject's phonological repertoire, not one that had to be taught before being used in the minimal pair. Nonetheless, by focusing on maximal oppositions, more generalization to other sounds occurred than with minimal opposition minimal pairs. In other studies in which two new target sounds were paired and introduced at the same time (Gierut, 1991, 1992; Gierut and Neumann, 1992), this strategy resulted in more generalization to other sounds than did pairs in which the target sound was paired with substitute sound or the target sound with a known sound.

Multiple Oppositions Therapy

A treatment methodology that represents another variation of the minimal contrast approach is the multiple oppositions approach (Williams, 1993, 2000a, 2000b, 2003). The *multiple oppositions* approach simultaneously contrasts several target sounds with a comparison sound. This approach is counter to the singular contrastive approach (i.e., including either minimal or maximal oppositions), which addresses sound errors or collapses one at a time. The multiple oppositions approach is designed for children who have multiple sound errors characterized by severe to profound phonological impairments.

The underlying premise behind this approach is that multiple errors produced by children evidencing numerous phoneme collapses into a single sound (i.e., one sound is used in place of two or more other sounds) are best treated with a "systematic" view as opposed to individual sound focus. The goal is to help a child reorganize his or her sound system by focusing on numerous minimal contrast pairs at the same time and help the child recognize the nature of his or her phoneme collapses. For example, if a child substitutes /t/ in the final word position for each of the following sounds—/k/, /tʃ/, /s/—treatment might focus on contrasting the word *bat* with *back* and *batch* with *bass*. In these examples, instead of focusing on a single contrast (e.g., *bat-back*), the procedure uses three minimal pair contrasts in the same activity (i.e., *bat-back; bat-batch; bat-bass*). A treatment session might also include instructional activities related to additional phoneme collapses. Lessons are centered on words evidencing "multiple oppositions" related to error targets. Eventually, instruction moves from focusing only on contrastive word-pairs to using sounds in increasingly complex linguistic structures.

A list of a child's phoneme collapses followed by sets of contrasting training items focusing on multiple oppositions (Williams, 2000a, 2000b) can be found in Figure 10.1.

Data reported by Williams (1993, 2000a, 2000b) indicated that by using the enlarged treatment sets included in the multiple oppositions approach with severely impaired children, clinicians were able to expand the number of phonemic contrasts. She hypothesized that through such an approach, the greatest change occurs in the smallest amount of time with the least effort. Williams (2006) has developed a software program, *Sound Contrasts in Phonology (SCIP)*, that includes contrasting vocabulary items available for multiple oppositions therapy.

Metaphon Therapy

Howell and Dean (1991) indicated that children with phonological disorders who fail to respond well to minimal pair therapy need to be taught the characteristics of sounds as a way to facilitate development of sound contrasts in their phonological repertoire. Instruction in this approach is designed to teach the awareness and skills necessary to succeed with minimal pair therapy. It structures treatment to facilitate children's development of metaphonological skills, that is, the ability to pay attention to the detailed aspects of the phonological system of the language followed by a broader perspective of the overall system. The detailed portion is part of what is described as *phonological awareness.* Investigators have reported that children with phonological disorders do not perform as well as their normally developing peers on metaphonological tasks (Kamhi, Friemoth-Lee, and Nelson, 1985). Metaphon therapy focuses on feature differences between sounds in order to develop an awareness that sounds can be classified by characteristics such as duration (*long-short*), manner (*noisy-whisper, stopping-flowing*), and place (*front-back*). The goal is to use this new awareness to assist with speech sound production. Direct instruction of phonological awareness is sometimes a goal in itself, because it is a skill needed for reading and spelling and is discussed in Chapter 12.

Therapy begins by teaching awareness of sound differences followed by the way that these concepts apply to sounds in general. Treatment then moves to identifying features across target speech sounds and then focuses on word-pairs, which incorporate targeted sound contrasts. An example activity might be sorting picture cards into groups containing

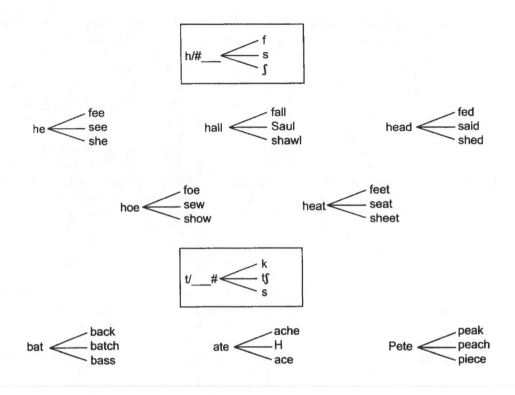

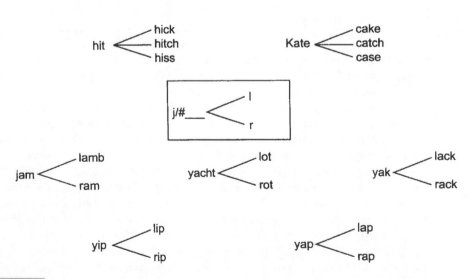

FIGURE 10.1 Phoneme collapses with related minimal pair treatment sets focusing on multiple oppositions.

Source: Williams (1999). Used with permission.

one target versus the contrasting target. The second phase of therapy is designed to transfer the metaphonological knowledge gained in the first phase to communication situations in which the client must convey his or her intended message through appropriate use of sound contrasts. These would be essentially the same as production tasks used in conventional minimal contrast training.

Summary of Minimal Pair Contrast Training

Background Statement. The establishment of sound contrasts (contrast training) is a linguistic approach to phonological remediation. Instruction typically involves perceptual and production tasks of word-pairs that reflect phonemic contrasts described as minimal, maximal, or multiple oppositions within the context of minimal pairs. Contrast training procedures facilitate the reorganization of the phonological system to reduce the use of phonemic collapses and to establish additional phonemic contrasts and syllable shapes.

Unique Features. Contrast training is primarily communication oriented by requiring the listener-speaker to select the appropriate word of the word-pair for communication intent to occur. That is, the listener-speaker must perceive and produce a particular phonemic contrast to communicate (act or get someone else to act appropriately) with the listener. It focuses on the ways that sounds are used in the language (i.e., to signal contrasts in meaning).

Strengths and Limitations. The approach is designed for clients who collapse sounds and do not contrast sounds consistent with the rules of the language. It is particularly useful with children who evidence numerous misarticulations or phonological patterns that are not consistent with the adult standard. It also is recommended for use with any client who needs to establish phonemic contrasts regardless of whether errors have a motor component. Clinicians need to have a plan for fitting contrast training with other treatment activities, including motor instruction and practice with increasingly complex linguistic utterances.

Research Support. More than 40 treatment studies to date have included the use of minimal pair contrasts (Baker & McLeod, 2011a). However, the vast majority of the studies represent lower levels of evidence (levels IIb and III). At least two randomized control trials (level Ib studies) have been conducted with minimal pair approaches. Dodd and colleagues (2008) randomly assigned 19 children to either a minimal contrast group or a nonminimal contrast group in which the contrasts appeared to be maximal (e.g., *key* versus *me; mop* versus *stop*). They reported significant progress for both groups but no significant differences between the groups. A study by Ruscello, Cartwright, Haines, and Shuster (1993) compared a minimal pair approach administered by clinicians with the same approach that included parents administering half of the therapy sessions at home. Once again, both groups made significant progress, but neither achieved more gains than the other. In a recent review, Baker (2010) reported that despite being lower level, the majority of the evidence suggests that the minimal contrast approach works. However, Baker also reported that the studies varied widely in what was included as part of the treatment. For example, many studies began with imitation training, but many did not. Some studies included some type of perceptual component, but many did not. Some studies specifically targeted the phrase and sentence level, whereas many were limited to the word level. This makes direct comparisons across studies and determination of what the critical components might be for optimum effectiveness very difficult.

CYCLES APPROACH

The cycles approach (Hodson and Paden, 1991) represents another linguistic approach designed for children with multiple sound errors. This approach targets deficient phonological patterns for instruction, uses sounds to teach appropriate phonological patterns, and moves through these targets in a sequential manner that is not based on a criterion level of performance before moving onto another sound and/or pattern. The cycles approach helps children to acquire appropriate phonological patterns rather than focusing on helping children eliminate inappropriate patterns or deviations. The procedures followed in a cycles approach treatment session typically include (1) auditory stimulation of a target sound with amplification (the client focuses attention on auditory characteristics on the target sound), (2) production practice (to help the child develop new kinesthetic images), and (3) participation in experiential play activities involving picture and object naming tasks that incorporate the target pattern into word productions.

The remediation plan is organized around treatment cycles that range from 5 to 16 weeks, depending on the client's number of deficient patterns and the number of stimulable phonemes within each pattern. Hodson's (2007a) suggestions for treating behaviors through a cycles approach include the following:

> Each phoneme (or consonant cluster) within a pattern is targeted for approximately 60 minutes per cycle (i.e., one 60-minute, two 30-minute, or three 20-minute sessions) before progressing to the next phoneme in that pattern and then on to other deficient phonological patterns. Furthermore, it is desirable to provide stimulation for two or more target *phonemes* (in successive weeks) within a pattern before changing to the next target *pattern* (i.e., each deficient phonological pattern is stimulated for two hours or more within each cycle). Only one phonological pattern is targeted during a beginning cycles session allowing the child to focus on a specific pattern. Patterns are not intermingled (e.g., final /k/ in the same session as initial /st/) until the third or fourth cycle. (pp. 90–91)

A cycle is complete when all phonological patterns selected for remediation at a given point in time have been treated. Following completion of one cycle, a second cycle that will again cover those patterns not yet emerging and that need further instruction is initiated. Phonological patterns are recycled until the targeted patterns emerge in spontaneous utterances. Hodson (1989) indicated that three to six cycles of phonological remediation, involving 30 to 40 hours of instruction (40 to 60 minutes per week) are usually required for a client with a disordered phonological system to become intelligible.

In the *Hodson Assessment of Phonological Patterns* (Hodson, 2003), the author recommended that patterns (deviations or processes) targeted for remediation should include those in which at least 40 percent of the opportunities for their occurrence is present. Phonological patterns targeted for remediation are also those patterns on which the client is stimulable.

An example of target selection and implementation of the cycles approach is the following. If fronting of velars occurs at least 40 percent of the time and if velars are stimulable, the appropriate use of velars could be selected as a target pattern for remediation. Initially, a target velar (e.g., final /k/) is selected as an instructional target and, following the instructional sequence delineated next, activities related to this sound would be focused on for approximately 1 hour. Following work on this sound, a second velar (e.g., initial /g/) could be targeted. Following work on this pattern, a second pattern would be selected as part of this cycle (e.g., /s/ clusters).

Hodson (2007b) has identified "optimal primary target patterns for beginning cycles" and "potential secondary target patterns." The potential primary targets are (1) syllableness (omission of the syllabi nuclei: vowels, diphthongs, vocalic/syllabic consonants), (2) singleton consonants when consistently omitted in a word position (i.e., in CV, VC, CVC, or VCV, (3) /s/ clusters either in word-initial or word-final position, (4) anterior/posterior contrasts where the child lacks either velars or alveolars/labials and either fronts or backs sounds, and (5) liquids /l/, /r/, /kr/, /gr/, and /l/ clusters all in word-initial positions.

Potential secondary target patterns are not targeted until the child has acquired the following patterns in spontaneous speech: (1) syllableness, (2) basic word structure, (3) anterior/posterior contrasts, and (4) some evidence of stridency, suppression of gliding, and substitution for liquids in spontaneous utterances.

Secondary target patterns are (1) palatals (i.e., /j/, /t/, /ʒ/, /tʃ/, /dʒ/), /ɚ/, /ɝ/, and word-medial /r/, (2) other consonant sequences (some which may be primary targets), such as /s/ cluster in word-final position, /s/ plus stop in word-medial position (basket), glide clusters (tw, kj), liquid clusters /tr/, and CCC /skw, skr/, and (3) singleton stridents, such as /f, s/, voicing contrasts (prevocalic, vowel contrasts, assimilations, and any other deviations).

Hodson (2007b) also recommends against targeting the following in preschool children: voiced-final obstruents /b, d, g, v, z, ð, ʒ, dʒ/, postvocalic /l/, word-final /n/, unstressed syllables, and /θ, ð/.

The instructional sequence for each session is as follows:

1. *Review.* At the beginning of each session, the prior week's production practice word cards are reviewed.
2. *Listening activity.* This step requires listening for about 30 seconds while the clinician reads approximately 20 words containing the target pattern. This auditory stimulation is done at the beginning and end of each session using two different word lists and includes the use of amplification (i.e., a mild gain assistive listening device). The clinician may also demonstrate the error and contrast it with the target.
3. *Target word cards.* The client draws, colors, or pastes pictures of three to five carefully selected target words based on phonetic environment of the words on 5" × 8" index cards. The name of the picture is written on each card, and the child says each word prior to its selection as a target word to evaluate it for difficulty.
4. *Production practice.* The client participates in experiential play production practice activities. The client is expected to have a very high success rate in terms of correct productions. Shifting activities every 5 to 7 minutes helps to maintain a child's interest in production practice. The client is also given the opportunity to use target

words in conversation. Production practice incorporates auditory, tactual, and visual stimulation and cues as needed for correct production at the word level. Usually, five words per target sound are used in a single session. The client must produce the target pattern in words in order to get his or her turn in the activity.

5. *Stimulability probing.* The target phoneme in the next session for a given pattern is selected based on stimulability probing (checking to see what words a child can imitate), which occurs at this point in the treatment session.

6. *Listening activity.* Amplified auditory input with amplification is repeated using the word list from the beginning of the session.

7. *Phonological awareness activities.* Activities such as rhyming and syllable segmentation are incorporated for a few minutes each session because many children with speech sound disorders are "at risk" for later problems with literacy skills. See Chapter 12 for a review of the relationship among children with speech sound disorders, phonological awareness skills, and literacy skills.

8. *Home program.* Parents are instructed to read a word list (5–10 words) to the child at least once a day, and then have the child name the words on the picture cards used in the listening activity. The five cards used during the session for production practice are also sent home for the child to practice daily. This activity should take only about 2 minutes each day.

The client is not required to meet a criterion level prior to moving to treatment of other patterns within a cycle. When patterns persist, they are recycled for treatment at a later time.

Summary of Cycles Approach

Background Statement.   The cycles approach is based on the phenomenon of gradualness (moving ahead and recycling) with mastery eventually occurring as sessions progress as observed in normal phonological acquisition. The emphasis on the acquisition of phonological patterns stems from a linguistic perspective of phonological behavior. Production practice of target sounds along with auditory stimulation (listening tasks) reflects aspects of a more traditional approach to intervention.

Unique Features.   The most distinctive feature of this approach is its focus on shifting and cycling of remediation targets and the fact that a phoneme related to a particular pattern is focused on for a given length of time rather than a set criterion level of performance, with a new target being worked on after an hour of instructional time. Focusing on pattern acquisition rather than on elimination of inappropriate patterns is a developmentally sound way to conceptualize intervention.

Strengths and Limitations.   The attributes just identified are all strengths of this approach. Although it was designed for unintelligible children, aspects of this approach can be used with less severely impaired clients. The cycles approach has been adapted for use with children with cleft palate (Hodson, Chin, Redmond, and Simpson, 1983), developmental dyspraxia (Hodson and Paden, 1991), and recurrent otitis media and hearing impairments (Gordon-Brannan, Hodson, and Wynne, 1992) as well as developmental delay.

Research Support. The authors have a wealth of clinical experience to support this approach to intervention and report good success with unintelligible children. This approach, like many others, represents a composite or "package" of various instructional components and has been widely adopted by clinicians for unintelligible and phonologically delayed children. The available evidence supporting this approach has tended to be lower level (III or IV) with at least two exceptions. Almost and Rosenbaum (1998) conducted a randomized control trial (level Ib evidence) involving 26 preschool children. Half of the group was randomly assigned to a 4-month block of immediate treatment, but treatment for the other half was delayed. Treatment involved a modified version of the cycles approach; one significant modification involved the use of minimal pairs (not a necessary component of cycles) to teach the contrast between the child's error and the adult pattern. At the end of 4 months, the groups were reversed (the first group received no treatment while the second entered treatment). Speech production accuracy improved for both groups with significantly more change occurring during the treatment periods (and significantly less change during the periods of no treatment). Both groups improved equally well on a control measure (mean length of utterance) over the 8-month period. The second study was a level IIa investigation by Tyler, Edwards, and Saxman (1987) involving four preschool children. Two children received a minimal pairs treatment approach while two received the cycles approach. After 2 months of treatment, all four children showed significant reduction in the use of the treated phonological patterns and little or no change in untreated (control) patterns. The two treatments were judged to be equally effective.

BROADER-BASED LANGUAGE APPROACHES

The approaches discussed so far assume a bottom-up orientation in which individual sounds or error patterns are the initial focus with therapy progressing through longer and longer linguistic units. At least two approaches take a top-down approach and begin with a focus on higher-level language to improve speech sound skill.

Whole-Language Intervention

As discussed in Chapter 4, children with severe phonologic disorders frequently have difficulty with other aspects of language (Camarata and Schwartz, 1985; Panagos and Prelock, 1982; Hoffman, Schuckers, and Daniloff, 1989; Paul and Shriberg, 1982; Fey and colleagues, 1994; Tyler, Lewis, Haskill, and Tolbert, 2002; and Tyler and Watterson, 1991). And as we discussed in Chapter 5, the relationship between phonology and other language impairments has been shown to be strong, and this relationship impacts clinical practice. Such coexisting impairments suggest that many children have a generalized difficulty with the language learning process. Although the precise nature of the relationship between phonology and other aspects of language is unknown, it has been suggested that phonologic delay, especially when it coincides with other language impairments, can be at least partially remediated by employing a language-based intervention approach (Gray and Ryan, 1973; Matheny and Panagos, 1978; Hoffman, Norris, and Monjure, 1990; Tyler, Lewis, Haskill, and Tolbert). Because higher-level language organization likely has an effect on speech sound production (recall the discussion in both Chapter 2 and Chapter 5), Hoffman, Norris, and Monjure (1990) suggest that remediation of speech sound disorders outside the broader context of overall language development may not be the most efficacious way to treat children with speech sound disorders

Others have indicated that the efficacy of a language-based approach to treating phonological disorders may be related to the degree of severity of the impairment (Fey et al., 1994; Tyler and Watterson, 1991), although results reported by Tyler, Lewis, Haskill, and Tolbert (2002) did not support this view. However, many clinicians use a language-based approach to remediation for children with mild phonological problems and language delay/disorders. For those with more severe phonological disorders, instruction may need to be focused specifically on phonology as well as the language problem. It may be that as children with severe speech sound disorders progress in treatment, instruction may need to become more language based. The following paragraphs delineate possible ways to use language-based therapy to ameliorate a speech sound disorder.

Norris and Hoffman (1990) described a storytelling language-based approach to phonologic intervention based on client generation of narratives. Preschool children constructed verbal stories in response to pictures from action-oriented children's stories and shared them with a listener. The clinician's primary role was to engage the children in constructing and talking about the pictures. The goal for each child was to produce meaningful linguistic units, syllable shapes, phonemes, and gestures that are shared with a listener. The clinician seeks to expand each child's language-processing ability by asking the child to produce utterances that exceed their current level of functioning.

Norris and Hoffman (1990, 2005) believe that language-oriented intervention should be naturalistic and interactive as the clinician seeks to simultaneously improve semantics, syntax, morphology, pragmatics, and phonology because all are components of language. Such an approach puts all the perceptual and motor cues of speech sound production into a broader communication context; in so doing it integrates all aspects of communication which all speakers must ultimately do. In terms of treatment priorities, phonology is the last component emphasized, because intelligibility is a concern only after children have expressive language. Such child–clinician interactions should be based on spontaneous events or utterances and communicative situations that arise in the context of daily play routines and instructional activities. They outline three steps for intervention:

1. Provide appropriate organization of the environment/stimulus materials for the child to attend to, which enables the clinician to alter language complexity systematically throughout the course of therapy.
2. Provide a communicative opportunity, including scaffolding strategies that consist of various types of prompts, questions, information, and restatements that provide support to the child who is actively engaging in the process of communicating a message.
3. Provide consequences or feedback directly related to the effectiveness of the child's communication.

Norris and Hoffman (1990) described an "interactive storytelling" technique in which the clinician points to a picture and models language for the client and then gives the child an opportunity to talk about the event. If the child miscommunicates the idea, the adult provides feedback designed to assist her or him in reformulating the message. The clinician can use three primary responses with the child:

1. *Clarification.* When the child's explanation is unclear, inaccurate, or poorly stated, the clinician asks for a clarification. The clinician then supplies relevant information to be incorporated in the child's response, restates the event using a variety of language forms, and asks the child to recommunicate the event. Hoffman, Norris, and Monjure (1990) presented the following example of this type of response: If a child described a picture of a man cooking at a grill by saying, "Him eating," the clinician might say:

   "No, that's not what I see happening. The man isn't eating yet, he's cooking the food. See his fork, he is using it to turn the food. I see him—he is cooking the food. He will eat when he's done cooking, but right now the food is cooking on the grill. He is cooking the food so that they can eat." (p. 105)

   Then the clinician provides an opportunity for the child to restate the information (e.g., ". . . so tell that part of the story again"). Thus, feedback is based on meaning rather than structure.

2. *Adding events.* If the child adequately reports an event, the clinician points out another event to incorporate in the story using a variety of language models. The child is then given the opportunity to retell the story. In an example from Hoffman, Norris, and Monjure (1990), the clinician points to specific features in the picture and says something like:

   That's right, the man is cooking. He is the dad and he is cooking the hamburgers for lunch. Mom is putting plates on the table. Dad will put the hamburgers on the plates. So you explain the story to the puppet. (p. 105)

3. *Increasing complexity.* If the child adequately describes a series of events, the clinician seeks to increase the complexity of the child's story by pointing out relationships among events such as motives of the characters, cause-effect relationships among the individual events, time and space relationships, and predictions. The child is given the opportunity again to reformulate his or her own version of the story. Another example from these authors is, "If the child said, 'The daddy is cooking hamburgers and the mommy is setting the table,'" the clinician might prompt the child to link these two events in time and space by saying:

   That's right, mommy and daddy are making lunch for the family. When daddy finishes cooking the hamburgers he will put them on the plates, so tell that part of the story to the puppet. (p. 105)

Although such interactive storytelling focuses on syntax, semantics, and narrative language skills, correct phonological models and feedback are also being provided the child. More recently, Hoffman and Norris (2010) have begun to include a significant emphasis on written language in their approach. They have developed three visual tools to assist in this regard. Phonic Faces includes alphabet letters overlaid on a face drawing to help make the association between the speech sound and the letter usually associated with it. MorphoPhonic Faces presents a Phonic Face for the first letter of a word along with drawings to illustrate the meaning of the intended word. Phonic Faces storybooks incorporate Phonic Faces and other images along with text to help solidify the association among speech sounds, letters, words, and meanings.

Naturalistic Intervention

A second top-down approach to improving speech sound skill is more directly intended to improve speech sounds by initially targeting improvement of overall speech intelligibility. It is based on two ideas: (1) the primary presenting symptom for many children with speech sound disorders is reduced intelligibility (problems making themselves understood by others) and (2) accuracy of production of speech sounds is not the only factor influencing how well speech is understood. Camarata (2010) proposed that the initial step for these children should be to increase the proportion of messages that are being understood. This would allow conversations with these children to move beyond what are often brief, unproductive encounters. By focusing on intelligibility first, the child obtains feedback about her or his messages. This feedback may enhance learning by encouraging both more speech attempts and more practice. Speech and language development are then seen as highly interactive processes that are stimulated in natural interactions. Once intelligibility has improved, attention can turn to accuracy of production of individual speech sounds.

Naturalistic intervention is a highly child-centered approach in which the clinician arranges the therapy environment in ways that encourage communication attempts. Toys and activities of interest to the child are made available and the clinician (or a parent or other caregiver). These activities can include requiring the child to ask for assistance and can involve more than one participant. The clinician and child interact in whatever natural ways arise with the clinician providing facilitating feedback referred to as *recasts*. The environment is to be organized so most of the target words the child attempts are known and the clinician provides both confirmation of the communicative attempt and a correct model of the target (e.g., Child: "*a wion*"; Clinician: "*yes, it's a lion.*"). The conversation can continue, and the child can learn to improve his or her speech from the feedback received. Providing good speech and language models and ensuring that the conversation between the child and the clinician continues are both critical to the process (Camarata, 1993). Once the majority of utterances are intelligible, the focus of therapy can switch to speech sound accuracy by including toys, games, and pictures geared to specific speech sound targets. As with the whole-language approach described earlier, this approach can also be used for children with comorbid language impairments; in such cases, once intelligibility improves, specific language targets may also be incorporated.

Summary of Broader-Based Language Approaches

Background Statement.   Language-based approaches are generally founded on two basic premises: (1) phonology is a part of the overall language system and should be treated in a language/communication context and (2) improvement in phonologic behaviors also occurs when instruction is focused on higher levels of language (morphosyntax, semantics).

Unique Features.   These approaches emphasize a top-down communication-oriented therapy that focuses on the interactive nature of communication. They assume that such emphasis facilitates phonological development/remediation and may also help facilitate higher-level language learning.

Strengths and Limitations. From a theoretical perspective, the rationale behind these approaches is attractive (i.e., teaching higher-level language communication context will result in phonological improvement). It appears that at least for some phonology clients, this concept is useful, although it is not entirely clear which ones it might be best suited for. Data suggest that these approaches may be the most useful for those who have severe impairments of both speech and language. In addition, they may be useful when a client is at the point in treatment at which carryover to connected speech is the goal.

Research Support. The highest-level direct evidence in support of the whole-language approach for improving speech sound production appears to be a level IIa (quasi-experimental) study by Nettleton and Hoffman (2005). Four children (age 4 years) with specific expressive language disorders and difficulty with speech sounds received intervention with Phonic Faces storybooks. For the first half of the treatment period, the target was /f/, and /ʃ/ served as a nontreated control sound. For the second half of the treatment period, the targets were reversed, and /ʃ/ became the treated sound. Production of /f/ improved immediately for all four participants and production of /ʃ/ improved only in the second half (for three participants; no change was seen with the other participant who was the only one who had not been stimulable for /ʃ/). As discussed in Chapter 8, observing change only when treatment was applied suggested that the storybook treatment was likely responsible for improving speech sound production.

More recently, some higher-level but indirect evidence in support of the whole-language approach has begun to accumulate. The evidence is indirect because the studies involved typically developing children rather than children with speech sound difficulties. This evidence is in the form of two unpublished doctoral dissertations involving randomized control trials (level Ib evidence) with typically developing 2-year-old children. Terrel (2007) demonstrated that Phonic Faces led to better letter name knowledge, letter-sound association, and speech sound production accuracy compared to those for a no-treatment control group. McInnis (2008) compared the use of MorphoPhonic Face cards to cards containing plain text and reported that the former led to significantly better word recognition, phonological awareness, and early literacy skills.

Relative to naturalistic intervention, Camarata (2010) reported findings from a randomized control study (level Ib), which indicated that this approach was equally as effective as imitation and drill at increasing spontaneous output compared to a no-treatment control group. A second randomized control trial by Yoder, Camarata, and Gardner (2005) included 52 preschool children with both speech and language impairments. Half of the children received the naturalistic intervention, and the other half (control group) was free to seek out whatever other treatment to which they might have access; parents of the control group participants documented how much treatment they received. Data indicated that the children in the control group actually received more treatment than those in the naturalistic intervention group. Intelligibility gains were seen with both groups, but no overall difference in the amount of gain between the two groups was observed. However, the naturalistic treatment resulted in signficantly more gains for the children with the poorest pretreatment accuracy, suggesting that a focus on overall intelligibility might be particularly helpful for children with the most severe speech sound disorders and possibly those with coexisting language disorders.

REMEDIATION GUIDELINES FOR LINGUISTICALLY BASED APPROACHES

1. A linguistic approach is recommended when there are multiple sound errors that reflect one or more phonologic error patterns. These approaches are particularly useful with young children who are unintelligible.

2. Once error patterns have been identified, a review of the child's phonetic inventory assists in the identification of target sounds (exemplars) to facilitate correct pattern usage. This review usually includes examination for stimulability and may include phonetic contexts that facilitate correct production of a target, frequency of occurrence of potential target sounds, and the developmental appropriateness of targets.

3. Selection of training words should reflect the syllabic word shapes the child uses. For example, if the child uses only CV and CVCV syllable shapes, multisyllabic target words would not be targeted. This guideline is obviously inappropriate if the focus on remediation is on syllable structure simplifications and/or word structure complexity.

4. Selecting target words that facilitate the reduction of two or more patterns simultaneously could increase treatment efficiency. For example, if a child uses stopping and deletes final fricatives, the selection of a final fricative for training could aid in the simultaneous reduction of the processes of stopping and final consonant deletion.

5. When errors cross several sound classes (e.g., final consonant deletion affecting stops, fricatives, and nasals), select exemplars that reflect different sound classes or possibly the most complex sound class.

6. Instruction related to phonologic patterns may focus on the broader pattern and less on the phonetic accuracy of individual sounds used in treatment. For example, if a child deletes final consonants but learns to say [dɔd] for [dɔg], the /d/ for /g/ replacement might be overlooked during the *initial* stage of instruction because the child has begun to change his or her phonologic system to incorporate final consonant productions.

7. Linguistic-based approaches have been shown to effective in treating children with multiple errors.

8. Minimal contrast therapy usually focuses on both perception and production. When using contrast therapy, minimal pairs with maximal feature differences between contrasting sounds (maximal oppositions) and contrasting two target sounds might be the most efficient way to establish contrasts and impact the child's entire sound system than are word-pairs that reflect few feature differences (minimal oppositions).

9. For children with many sound collapses, a multiple oppositions approach might be an efficient way to impact the child's overall sound system.

10. For children with co-existing language impairments, a broader-based language (top-down) approach might be appropriate.

CASE STUDY REVISITED: LINGUISTIC PERSPECTIVE

Intervention Recommendations

Again we visit the case of Kirk, whom we introduced in Chapter 7 and have also discussed in Chapters 8 and 9. Kirk was stimulable for many of his errors, suggesting that motor-based treatment would be unnecessary for those errors. Some of the stimulable sounds were more easily imitated than others. Because he could imitate most of his error sounds, a major goal of instruction was to help Kirk learn to use sounds contrastively, or in other words, diminish his sound collapses by using sounds appropriately to ensure word contrasts.

First Consideration: How Many Targets Should I Address in a Session?

Because Kirk has multiple error sounds, a focus on several targets is suggested, either within a single lesson or across lessons within a 3- or 4-week time frame (cycles or horizontal approach). It is suggested that treatment sessions for Kirk should address error patterns, beginning with stopping and the sound collapses reflected in that pattern (i.e., /d/ replacing several other sounds and clusters such as /s, z, tʃ, θ/ and clusters /sl, sn, fl/).

Second Consideration: How Should I Conceptualize the Treatment Program?

One treatment option for addressing Kirk's errors is to use a cycling approach in which one or more sounds are targeted in a given lesson to help him learn to use a particular phonological pattern (e.g., frication because he currently substitutes stops for most fricatives). In a subsequent lesson within the same cycle, other fricatives related to that pattern would be the focus, continuing until most of the fricatives have been practiced. At that point, another pattern would be targeted, including one or more sounds in a given lesson (e.g., use of final consonants). This cycling approach might employ amplified auditory input, perceptual training of minimal pairs, and sound production of minimal pairs, including drill and play activities. The linguistic complexity of activities increases as progress is made (e.g., going from words to phrases to sentences to conversation).

An alternative treatment approach that specifically addresses sound contrasts is to teach multiple oppositions that simultaneously address the collapse of numerous sounds to /d/. Instruction might initially focus on sound collapses that include sounds in Kirk's repertoire and then, as other sounds are established, expand to other sound collapses. In the following example, solid lines indicate initial collapses to focus on because the sounds are in Kirk's repertoire; broken lines reflect targets that can be addressed as additional sounds are added to Kirk's repertoire.

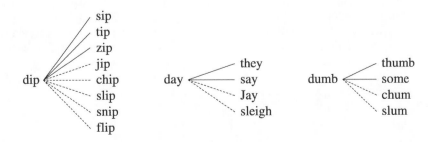

Another way to approach Kirk's stopping pattern is the use of focused minimal pairs rather than the multiple-oppositions approach. This method is a more traditional approach to using minimal pairs to establish sound contrasts; that is, it focuses on a single pair and then progresses to other minimal pairs to establish other contrasts in his system. Instruction would begin with a minimal pair evidencing maximal opposition between a target sound and a contrasting sound. For example, instruction might first focus on the word-pair *seal-meal*, and once Kirk can produce that pair, go to *seal-veal*, and finally *deal-seal*. The hope is that by initially contrasting /s/ with /m/ (sounds that evidence several feature differences from /d/), such practice will facilitate more rapid acquisition of other sound contrasts.

Overall Treatment Plan

As indicated by our preceding discussion and that in Chapter 9, the nature of Kirk's errors suggests an overall mixed approach with some targets being treated with a more motor-based approach but the remainder with a more linguistic approach. For either group of targets several different options have been outlined. One possible general plan for his overall treatment is presented in Table 10.1.

TABLE 10.1   Possible Intervention Sequencing for Kirk

Component	Procedure	Rationale
Sound stimulation/ practice	Ask the client to produce a variety of sounds five times each (both incorrect and correct sounds). Provide auditory models and cueing as necessary.	Child's stimulability has been shown to highly influence generalization. Therefore, we must help children acquire all the sounds at a motor level. Brief practice periods serve to encourage continued attempts at sounds that may be difficult for Kirk to produce.
Production activities	Focus on teaching frication and final consonant usage. Focus on one or two sounds per session, moving from /f/ to /m/ to /s/ and other stimulable sounds. Use minimal pairs at a perceptual level before practice on pairs at a production level. Drilling/playing games and activities are recommended. Use a listening task to introduce each sound. Consider using multiple opposition contrasts for the /d/ collapses.	Cycling across patterns and sounds is helpful for children with multiple errors. Kirk is young and still developing his sound system, and he has a good attention span. Therefore, he could benefit from shifting focus from week to week. Multiple oppositions can be helpful for phoneme collapses and are recommended because Kirk is stimulable on many of the collapses.
Increasing linguistic complexity	When Kirk can produce word targets accurately, including minimal pairs, shift production to phrases and then sentences. In addition, progress from targets occurring only once in a word or phrase to more complex productions involving more than one occurrence and competing sounds.	To reach the terminal objective of spontaneous use of appropriate speech sounds and patterns, Kirk must be able to use his new speech sounds and patterns in increasingly complex linguistic units.

TABLE 10.1	(Continued)	
Component	**Procedure**	**Rationale**
Situational generalization	Bring persons in the child's environment into activities to reinforce Kirk's new speech skills. Using target names, preschool vocabulary, and frequently used words as a focus could be helpful.	Focusing on situational generalization as early as possible will help this young client generalize the new language skills to his environment. The environment will very likely reinforce increased intelligibility.
	Arrange for Kirk to "use" his new speech in the classroom and home.	

QUESTIONS FOR CHAPTER 10

1. Outline a linguistic approach to speech sound intervention and specify for whom it is appropriate.

2. Discuss how one can use minimal pairs in phonological treatment.

3. Outline the procedures for a cycles approach to therapy.

4. Describe how a whole-language or naturalistic approach differs from most other treatment approaches.

5. What is the difference between minimal oppositions and maximal oppositions?

6. What is the difference between a motor-based treatment and a linguistic based treatment?

7. Describe multiple opposition treatment and when might it be appropriate to use with a child.

8. Describe metaphon treatment and when might it be appropriate to use with a child.

9. What is meant by a "top-down" approach to intervention?

10. Discuss how the broader language-based treatments differ from a minimal pairs approach.

CHAPTER 11

Language and Dialectal Variations

BRIAN A. GOLDSTEIN
La Salle University

AQUILES IGLESIAS
Temple University

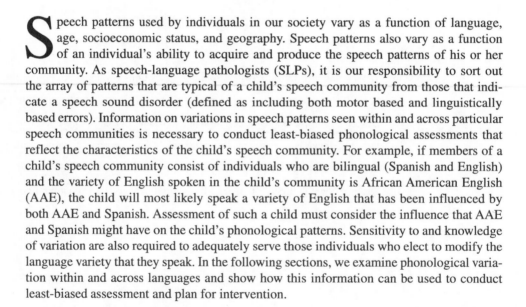

S peech patterns used by individuals in our society vary as a function of language, age, socioeconomic status, and geography. Speech patterns also vary as a function of an individual's ability to acquire and produce the speech patterns of his or her community. As speech-language pathologists (SLPs), it is our responsibility to sort out the array of patterns that are typical of a child's speech community from those that indicate a speech sound disorder (defined as including both motor based and linguistically based errors). Information on variations in speech patterns seen within and across particular speech communities is necessary to conduct least-biased phonological assessments that reflect the characteristics of the child's speech community. For example, if members of a child's speech community consist of individuals who are bilingual (Spanish and English) and the variety of English spoken in the child's community is African American English (AAE), the child will most likely speak a variety of English that has been influenced by both AAE and Spanish. Assessment of such a child must consider the influence that AAE and Spanish might have on the child's phonological patterns. Sensitivity to and knowledge of variation are also required to adequately serve those individuals who elect to modify the language variety that they speak. In the following sections, we examine phonological variation within and across languages and show how this information can be used to conduct least-biased assessment and plan for intervention.

DIALECT

Dialects are mutually intelligible forms of a language associated with a particular region, social class, or ethnic group. General American English, Southern White Standard, Appalachian English, Caribbean English, African American English, Eastern American English, and Spanish-influenced English are just some of the dialects spoken in the

United States. No dialect of any language is superior to any other because all thoughts can be expressed using any dialect of any language. This is not to say that all varieties of a language carry the same prestige. Some varieties of a language, specifically those used by the dominant groups in any socially stratified society, will be considered to have higher prestige (Wolfram, 1986), promulgated within the educational system (Adler, 1984), and valued by the private sector of the society (Shuy, 1972; Terrell and Terrell, 1983).

The promulgation of General American English (GAE; the prestige dialect in the United States) within the educational system and by contact through broadcast media between members of different regional dialects has decreased differences between dialects *(dialect leveling)*. At the same time, lack of linguistic contact among groups due to geographical or socioeconomic reasons has resulted in a linguistic isolation that has increased the distance between dialects (Labov, 1991). In addition, the increased immigration and ethnic isolation that have occurred among some subgroups have further increased the number and pervasiveness of dialects. The courts' acknowledgment of the rights of linguistic minority populations has resulted in more acceptance of varieties other than General American English. For example, *Martin Luther King Junior Elementary School Children et al.* v. *Ann Arbor School District* (1978) provided for the use of children's home language, including African American English, in the educational process. At least in terms of dialects, the "melting pot" hypothesis appears to be a myth for certain segments of our society.

Regardless of whether dialects are becoming more or less like each other, people hold many different myths about them. Wolfram and Schilling-Estes (1998) have indicated a number of myths held about dialects and have countered those myths with corresponding facts (see Table 11.1).

TABLE 11.1 Dialect Myths and Facts.

Myth	Fact	Example
A dialect is a variety spoken by someone else.	Everyone speaks some dialect of a language.	Although there is a dialect form often referred to as the "standard" (e.g., Standard or General American English), it is usually a form not actually spoken by anyone in an invariable form. There is variation to one extent or another used by all speakers.
Dialectal features are always distinct and noticeable.	Some dialectal features are shared by many different dialects.	The weakening of postvocalic "r" (e.g., /moɚ/ → [moə]) is exhibited by speakers of African American English, Eastern American English, and Southern American English.
Dialects arise from ineffective tries at speaking the correct form of the language.	Speakers of dialects acquire those features by interacting with members of the speech community in which they live.	Some native speakers of Spanish often use characteristics of African American English because speakers of both varieties live in the same community (Poplack, 1978).
Dialects are random changes from the "standard."	Dialects are precise and show regular patterns.	In many dialects of the American South, /ɪ/ and /ɛ/ are pronounced as [ɪ] before nasals; /pɪn/; /pɛn/ → [pɪn].
Dialects are always viewed negatively.	Dialects are not inherently viewed negatively (or positively, for that matter); prestige of any dialect is derived from the social prestige of its speakers.	Ramirez and Milk (1986) found that bilingual teachers rated the local Mexican dialect of Spanish as less prestigious than the general dialect of Spanish. The dialect of English spoken by the British monarchy, however, is often perceived as prestigious.

Speakers of a particular dialect do not always use all features present in their dialect. A speaker's use of particular features depends on the context and interlocutors (*register*). *Registral varieties* depend on the participants, setting, and topic. For example, one would typically use one register when talking to friends about an enjoyable weekend and use another variety when speaking to a police officer about a speeding violation. The extent to which particular individuals use the available features of their dialect (*dialect density*) can depend on factors such as socioeconomic status and geography (e.g., Oetting & McDonald, 2002). Sometimes the differences in dialect density are associated with socioeconomic status, a sociolinguistic phenomenon referred to by Wolfram (1986) as *social diagnosticity*. Wolfram observed the frequency of occurrence of selected AAE features among the speech of individuals representing four socioeconomic groups: upper middle class, lower middle class, upper working class, and lower working class. His research revealed that certain AAE linguistic features showed *gradient stratification* across the four groups. That is, individuals in lower socioeconomic groups used more of the available features of that dialect than individuals in higher socioeconomic groups. Washington and Craig (1998) found this same effect for 5- and 6-year-old AAE-speaking boys. For example, the lack of realization of postvocalic *r* (e.g., /sɪstɚ/ → [sɪstə]) is an example of gradient stratification because all socioeconomic groups use this phonological feature albeit with different levels of frequency. On the other hand, certain AAE features show a pattern of usage referred to as *sharp stratification*, which refers to linguistic features that more clearly differentiate socioeconomic groups based on significant differences in frequency of usage. One example of this type of stratification is the substitution of [f] for /θ/. The use of this feature contrasts middle-class with working-class groups because working-class groups use the feature much more frequently than middle-class speakers. Wolfram has indicated that features revealing sharp stratification are of greater social diagnosticity than those showing gradient stratification.

Geography may also play a role in the likelihood of a specific dialect feature being expressed. For example, Hinton and Pollock (1999) examined the occurrence of vocalic and postvocalic American English /ɹ/[*] in African American English speakers from two geographic regions (Davenport, Iowa, and Memphis, Tennessee). Overall, they found that speakers in Davenport were more likely than speakers in Memphis to maintain the rhotic quality of vocalic and postvocalic /ɹ/. Hinton and Pollock accounted for these results largely in terms of the demographic characteristics of the two communities. The African American community in Memphis accounts for nearly 50% of the city's population compared to only 5% in Davenport. Moreover, African American children in Memphis are much more likely to be taught by African American teachers compared to those in Davenport.

CHARACTERISTICS OF AMERICAN ENGLISH DIALECTS

In addition to GAE, a number of dialects of English are spoken in the United States. This chapter focuses on five common dialects: African American English, Eastern American English, Southern American English, Appalachian English, and Ozark English. Most of

---

[*]For purposes of this chapter only, the symbol /ɹ/ is used to represent the rhotic sound found in General American English and its dialects. The symbol /r/, as specified by the International Phonetic Alphabet Association, is used to designate the alveolar trill.

the available literature on these dialects focuses on their characteristics rather than on their development.

African American English

African American English (AAE) is a variety of American English that is spoken by many, but not all, African Americans. Other groups who have contact with AAE speakers also speak it. For example, English-speaking Puerto Rican teenagers in East Harlem, New York, have been found to use features of AAE (Wolfram, 1974). Wolfram found that the degree of contact that the teenagers had with AAE speakers greatly influenced the number of AAE features in their speech. Those individuals with the most contact showed the most features in their speech. Poplack (1978) examined the use of AAE, Puerto Rican Spanish, and Philadelphia English variants in the speech of sixth-grade Puerto Rican boys and girls. She found that the Puerto Rican boys tended to use more features of AAE, and the girls used more features of Philadelphia English. Poplack concluded that the specific variants used by the children were more related to "covert prestige" than to their linguistic environment, with the boys assigning more prestige to AAE speakers and the girls assigning more prestige to Philadelphia English. The results of both of these studies support the notion that use of dialect features is influenced by patterns in the speech community and that speech patterns are greatly affected by peer interaction.

Like all dialects, AAE is systematic with rule-governed phonological, semantic, syntactic, pragmatic, and proxemic systems (Wolfram, Adger, & Christian, 1999). There are two major hypotheses accounting for the origin of African American English (Poplack, 2000; Wolfram and Schilling-Estes, 1998). The Creole hypothesis assumes that AAE descended from Plantation Creole (Wolfram, 1994; Wolfram and Schilling-Estes), a language that developed from a mixture of languages brought into contact during the slave trade period. Plantation Creole was commonly used by African Americans on plantations in the South but was not spoken by European Americans at the time. Over time, AAE has spread and changed. The exodus of African Americans from the southeast to the northeast and other parts of the United States in the early 1900s brought AAE to the urban areas of the North (Stewart, 1971). In many cases, individuals from a particular state tended to migrate to particular cities (e.g., South Carolinians moving to Philadelphia). The restricted social environments in which many African Americans lived in addition to the continued contact with their southern families and communities reinforced the use of AAE. In its evolution, AAE has undergone a decreolization process showing fewer links to its creole past and acquiring features that are not traceable to the original Creole (e.g., stopping of interdental fricatives) (Wolfram and Schilling-Estes, 1998).

An alternative hypothesis, the (Neo-) Anglicist hypothesis, states that African American English is considered a dialect of English. That is, AAE can be traced to the varieties of English spoken in Britain (Wolfram and Schilling-Estes, 1998). Thus, slaves who were brought to the United States eventually "learned the regional and social varieties of surrounding white speakers" (Wolfram and Schilling-Estes, p. 176). Although the exact origins of AAE are unsettled, the prevailing view seems to be that AAE owes its current form to influences of both its dialect and Creole roots (Green, 2004).

A number of linguistic features distinguish AAE from General American English. The major phonological features that distinguish these two varieties are listed in Table 11.2

TABLE 11.2 Major Phonological Features Distinguishing African American English and General American English

Pattern	Example(s)
Word-final consonant cluster reduction (particularly when one of the two consonants is an alveolar)	/tɛst/ → [tɛs]
Deletion of /ɹ/	/sɪstɚ/ → [sɪstə]
	/kæɹəl/ → [kæəl]
	/pɹʌfɛsɚ/ → [pʌfɛsə]
Deletion of /l/ in word-final abutting consonants	/hɛlp/ → [hɛp]
Deletion of nasal consonant in word-final position with nasalization of preceding vowel	/mun/ → [mũ]
Substitution of [I] for /ɛ/ before nasals	"pin" /pɪn/ and "pen" /pɛn/ pronounced as [pɪn]
Substitution of [k] for /t/ in initial /stɹ/ clusters	/stɹit/ → [skɹit]
Realization of /θɹ/ as [θ]	/θɹo/ → [θo]
Substitution of f/θ and v/ð in intervocalic position	/nʌθiŋ/ → [nʌfiŋ]
	/beðiŋ/ → [beviŋ]
Substitution of f/θ in word-final position	/sɑʊθ/ → [sɑʊf]
Realization of /v/ as [b] and /z/ as [d], in word-internal position before syllabic nasals	/sɛvən/ → [sɛbən]
Stopping of word-initial interdentals	/ðe/ → [de]
	/θɑt/ → [tɑt]
Metathesis	/æsk/ → [æks]

(compiled from Bailey and Thomas, 1998; Craig, Thompson, Washington, and Potter, 2003; Hyter, 1996; Pollock and colleagues, 1998; Rickford, 1999; Stockman, 1996a; Velleman & Pearson, 2010; Wolfram and Schilling-Estes, 1998). These features are always optional, are not used in each possible phonetic context, and are not produced by all AAE speakers. For example, the simplification of word-final clusters tends to occur when one of the consonants is an alveolar and the other (i.e., the deleted consonant) is a morphological marker (Stockman). Hence, some AAE speakers may not differentiate between the present and past tense of the same verb (e.g., *miss* and *missed* are pronounced as [mɪs]), but would retain the cluster in a word such as *mist*. Moreover, the occurrence of phonological dialect features appears to change over time. Craig and Washington (2004) found a significant decline in the number of phonological dialect features produced between second and third grades in a group of 400 typically developing African American children in low- or middle-income households.

Features of AAE extend to suprasegmental phenomena as well (Hyter, 1996; Stockman, 1996a). For example, AAE speakers may place stress on the first rather than second syllable (Detróit → Détroit), use a wide range of intonation contours and vowel elongations, and produce more level and falling final contours than rising contours. Moreover, phonotactics and suprasegmental phenomena tend to interact. For example, AAE-speaking children tend to produce /d/ less accurately in unstressed syllables versus stressed ones and reduce clusters more often in unstressed versus stressed syllables (Burns, Velleman, Green, & Roeper, 2010).

Phonological Development in AAE

In comparison to the investigation of phonological skills in speakers of GAE, less information exists on the development of AAE phonology. Existing studies have examined phonological development in typically developing AAE-speaking children and AAE-speaking children with speech sound disorders. Major findings indicate that AAE-speaking children tend to produce the same phonetic inventory as speakers of GAE (Stockman, 1996a); show great intersubject variability; exhibit systematic error patterns; and demonstrate differences in both the type and quantity of speech errors exhibited by typically developing speakers and those with speech sound disorders (Stockman, 2010).

Preschoolers speaking AAE and GAE often exhibit similar phonological patterns although with different frequencies. Bland-Stewart (2003) examined the phonological skills of eight AAE-speaking 2-year-olds. She found that their phonological skills were similar to those exhibited by GAE-speaking peers. Seymour and Seymour (1981) compared the performance of 4- and 5-year-old African American and White children. They reported that both groups evidenced phonological variations typically associated with AAE (e.g., f/θ in medial and final positions; d/ð in initial and medial positions; b/v in initial and medial positions). The AAE features occurred more frequently, however, in the productions of the African American children. Thus, both groups produced the same type of substitutions, but the frequency of their use differed between the two groups. These results suggested that for the children they studied, the contrast between AAE and GAE was *qualitatively* undifferentiated at this age. The same result has also been demonstrated for phonological processes (i.e., patterns) (Haynes and Moran, 1989).

Stockman (2006a) examined the production of syllable-initial consonants in seven typically developing AAE-speaking children ages 2;8 to 3;0. All seven children produced 15 syllable-initial, singleton consonants (/m, n, p, b, t, d, k, g, w, j, l, ɹ, f, s, h/) at least four times in at least two different words. These 15 segments represent the minimal competency core of phonemes that are invariant in AAE and GAE (Stockman, 1996a). Accuracy for the group of segments in the minimal competency core exceeded 80 percent (range = 81 to 99 percent) compared to less than 80 percent (range = 14 to 76 percent) for sounds not in the core (i.e., the segments that vary between AAE and GAE). Error patterns included voicing errors, liquid gliding, stopping, and fronting. All seven children produced syllable-initial consonant clusters, totaling 19 types. Of the 19 types, 15 were of the oral stop + sonorant or fricative + sonorant variety. The children also produced /s/ + stop clusters and one 3-member cluster, /skr-/. Results show that the phonetic skills of young AAE-speaking children are similar to those of same-aged children speaking GAE. In a follow-up study with 120 African American children, Stockman (2008) corroborated findings from the earlier study. Results from this study also were commensurate with those examining the production of initial consonants in speakers of GAE (e.g., Smit and colleagues, 1990) and Standard British English (e.g., Dodd, Holm, Hua, and Crosbie, 2003).

Pearson, Velleman, Bryant, and Charko (2009) examined the phonological skills of 537 children ages 4 to 12 acquiring AAE and 317 children of the same age acquiring

Mainstream (i.e., General) American English (MAE). They found that children acquiring AAE and MAE showed commensurate mastery (accuracy of more than or equal to 90 percent) of most singleton consonants in initial position—(/b/, /t/, /k/, /g/, /m/, /n/, /h/, /j/, /w/, /dʒ/, /ʃ/, /t/, /l/). However, children acquiring AAE mastered some initial segments (e.g., /ɹ/ and /s/), initial clusters (/kl-, pl-, kɹ -, gɹ -, pɹ -, sp-, st-, sk ɹ -/), and some final singletons (/s/ and /z/) earlier than did children acquiring MAE. Finally, acquisition of /d/ and /ð/ by AAE speakers occurred after that of MAE speakers. In final position, results were similar in that speakers of AAE and MAE generally showed comparable skills. By 6 years of age, AAE speakers had mastered all consonants except /t/, /d/, /θ/, and /ð/; MAE speakers had mastered all consonants except /θ/ and /ð/. It should be noted that MAE speakers mastered /ð/ at age 8 compared with age 12 for AAE speakers. However, AAE speakers mastered /s/ and /z/ by age 4 compared to age 6 for MAE speakers. Finally, speakers of AAE tended to master a number of initial clusters (e.g., /kl/, pɹ/) earlier than MAE speakers, but MAE speakers mastered final clusters (e.g., /ks/, /nt/) before AAE speakers.

In a follow-up study with this same group of participants, Velleman, Pearson, Bryant, and Charko (2010) examined the relationship between phonetic and phonotactic (e.g., syllable structure) development in AAE and MAE speakers. Results indicated that AAE speakers showed more advanced phonological skills related to segments than to phonotactics. The authors had predicted this finding because AAE speakers have less overall exposure to structures such as final singleton consonants, final clusters, and iambic words (i.e., words such as *gi-RAFFE* that have a weak-strong stress pattern). Taken together, the results from these two studies indicate that AAE speakers may be placing more emphasis on segmental rather than phonotactic learning, which in turn leads to mastery of some later developing consonants by AAE speakers before MAE speakers.

Consonant accuracy also has been examined across contexts in AAE speakers. For typically developing children, Stockman (2008) found that accuracy averaged 81–82% in 3-year-olds on a spontaneous speech task. In elicited single words, it averaged 95–98% for children aged 3;7–6;1 (Pollock & Berni, 1997, as cited in Stockman, 2010).

Variability across children has been found to be a hallmark of AAE phonological development. Seymour and Seymour (1981) reported considerable interchild variability among AAE speakers. Not all of the target features were present in each AAE speaker nor were they equally distributed among the speakers. Although there is variability in phonological development between AAE-speaking children, the context for error patterns exhibited by these children has been found to be systematic. For example, although AAE-speaking children delete final consonants, they do not do so arbitrarily. Stockman (1996a, 2006b) noted that alveolar consonants were more likely than either labials or velars to be deleted; oral stops and nasals were more likely than fricatives to be deleted; and final consonants preceding a consonant were more likely to be deleted. In addition, the absence of final consonants might be marked by lengthening or nasalizing the vowel that preceded the absent consonant (Moran, 1993). Bryant, Velleman, Abdualkarim, and Seymour (2001) found that AAE-speaking children were more likely to delete one element of a word-final cluster if a more sonorous element preceded a less sonorous element. For example, words ending in /sk/ clusters (more sonorous element preceding less sonorous element) were more likely to undergo deletion than /ks/ clusters (less sonorous element preceding more sonorous element). In addition, their results indicated that in the clusters in which a more sonorous element preceded a less sonorous one, the most sonorous element was preserved. For example, AAE-speaking children would produce *desk* /dɛsk/ as [dɛs], not [dɛk].

Developmental differences between typically developing AAE speakers and those with speech sound disorders have been found to be quantitatively and qualitatively different. Bleile and Wallach (1992) compared the articulation of nonspeech-delayed and speech-delayed AAE-speaking children ranging in age from 3;6 to 5;5. Head Start teachers who shared the same racial and linguistic background as the children differentiated the two groups of children. Data analysis was based on non-AAE phonological patterns exhibited by the children in a picture-identification, single-word test. The delayed and nondelayed groups demonstrated differences in the type and quantity of their speech errors. Speech-delayed children had more (1) stop errors (especially velars), (2) fricative errors in all positions (especially fricatives other than /θ/), and (3) affricate errors in all positions. Nonspeech-delayed participants evidenced more devoicing of final /d/, sonorant errors, and errors related to /ɹ/. Both groups of children produced a large number of consonant cluster errors with the speech-delayed children exhibiting more cluster errors. Bleile and Wallach (1992) concluded that a combination of characteristics rather than a single indicator appears to be the most reliable index of speech delay in African American English speakers, just as it is with children who do not speak AAE. Velleman and Pearson (2010) examined the phonological skills of 76 AAE speakers with speech sound disorders (SSD) and 72 GAE speakers with SSD, all ages 4–12 years. Velleman and Pearson found that the features exhibited by both groups were similar. Moreover, the children "did not differ by dialect with respect to their overall number of mismatches to GAE targets in any position" (p. 184), indicating that dialect was largely neutralized in these groups of children with SSD. Finally, the AAE-speaking children with SSD mastered some consonants before their GAE counterparts—/s, tʃ, dʒ, ɹ/. Results from this study show the similarity and differences in the phonological skills of AAE- and GAE-speaking children and highlight the need to account for dialect features in children's speech.

Eastern American English and Southern American English

Eastern American English and Southern American English, described by Labov (1991) as northern and southern dialects, are two geographical variations of GAE. The Eastern American dialect runs generally from Vermont to the north, parts of Iowa and Minnesota to the west, and New Jersey to the south (Wolfram and Schilling-Estes, 1998). The Southern American dialect runs generally from Maryland to the north, Texas to the west, and Florida to the south (Wolfram and Schilling-Estes). Although these two dialects share many of the same features, they can also be differentiated from each other through differences in the production of both vowels and consonants (see Table 11.3) (compiled from Parker and Riley, 2000; Small, 2004; Wolfram and Schilling-Estes, 1998).

Appalachian English and Ozark English

Two other common geographical dialects of English are Appalachian English (AE) and Ozark English (OE). Christian, Wolfram, and Nube (1988) indicate that AE and OE are related linguistically with OE showing many similar features as AE. Given the phonological

TABLE 11.3 Common Dialectal Variations in English

Pattern	Example		Dialect
Vowels			
Tense → Lax	/i/ → [ɪ]	/rili/ → [rɪlɪ]	SAE
	/u/ → [ʊ]	/rut/ → [rʊt]	EAE
Lax → Tense	/ɪ/ → [i]	/fɪʃ/ → [fiʃ]	SAE
	/ɛ/ → [e]	/ɛg/ → [eg]	SAE
	/æ/ → [ɑ]	/hæf/ → [hɑf]	EAE
Vowel Neutralization	/ɪ/; /ɛ/ → [ɪ]	/pɪn/; /pɛn/ → [pɪn]	SAE
Diphthong Reduction	/ɑɪ/ → [ɑ]	/pɑɪ/ → [pɑ]	SAE
a/ɔ		[fɔt] → [fɑt]	SAE, EAE
Lowering	/ɔ/ → [ɑ]	/fɔɚ/ → [fɑɚ]	SAE, EAE
Derhoticization	/ɚ/ → [ə]	/fɔɚ/ → [fɔə]	SAE, EAE
"r" Deletion		/kɑɚ/ → [kɑ]	SAE, EAE
"r" Addition	/ə/ → [ɚ]	/lɪndə/ → [lɪndɚ]	EAE
Consonants			
Velar Fronting	/ŋ/ → [n]	/ɹʌnɪŋ/ → [ɹʌnɪn]	SAE
/j/ Addition		/nu/ → [nju]	SAE, EAE
Voicing Assimilation	/s/ → [z]	/gɹisi/ → [gɹizi]	SAE
Glottalization	/t/; /d/ → [ʔ]	/batəl/ → [baʔəl]	EAE
[t]; [d] for /θ/; /ð/	/θ/ → [t]	/θɪŋk/ → [tɪŋk]	EAE
	/ð/ → [d]	/dɪs/	EAE

Key: SAE = Southern American English; EAE = Eastern American English

similarities of these two dialects, they are discussed together. Appalachian English is spoken generally in the area of parts of Kentucky, Tennessee, Virginia, North Carolina, and West Virginia (parts of the Carolinas, Georgia, and Alabama may also be included). Ozark English is spoken in an area encompassing northern Arkansas, southern Missouri, and northwestern Oklahoma.

Christian, Wolfram, and Nube (1988, pp. 153–159) have outlined the characteristics of AE and OE; these are shown in Table 11.4. Only the most common features are outlined (see Christian, Wolfram, and Nube, 1988, and Flipsen, 2007, for more details).

As was the case for AAE in African American speakers, not all features of AE and OE are utilized by every speaker, used in every situation, or produced in every context. For example, the rule noted as *intrusive t* in which [t] may be added to words ending in /s/ or /f/ is usually limited to a small set of words. Most commonly, the rule takes effect on the words *once* and *twice*. In addition, the number of words exhibiting this rule seems to be more extensive in AE than OE.

TABLE 11.4	Characteristics of Appalachian English and Ozark English

Rule	Example
Epenthesis Following Clusters	
CCC# → CC↔C#	/gosts/ → [gostəs]
Intrusive *t* (more common in AE)	
/s/# → [st]	/wʌns/ → [wʌnst]
/f/# → [ft]	/klɪf/ → [klɪft]
Stopping of Fricatives	
/θ/ → [t]	/θɑt/ → [tɑt]
/ð/ → [d]	/ðe/ → [de]
Initial *w* Reduction	
/w/ → ø	/wɪl/ → [ɪl]
Initial Unstressed Syllables	
IUS → ø	/əlɑʊd/ → [lɑʊd]
h Retention	
ø → [h]	/ɪt/ → [hɪt]
Retroflex *r*	
/ɹ/ → ø (post-consonantal)	/θɹo/ → [θo]
/ɹ/ → ø (intervocalic)	/kæɹi/ → [kæi]
Lateral *l*	
/l/ → ø before labials	/wʊlf/ → [wʊf]

PHONOLOGY IN SPEAKERS OF LANGUAGE VARIETIES OTHER THAN ENGLISH

Prior to the arrival of Europeans, what is now the continental United States was a polyglot area in which more than 200 languages or dialects were spoken (Leap, 1981). Over the past 600 years, immigrants to this area have brought their cultures and languages. Historically, the general trend for most immigrants to the United States was to use their home language as their primary language of communication. By the third generation, though, immigrants tended to lose their language of origin (Veltman, 1988). Some immigrant groups, however, have maintained the use of their home language (also termed *first* or *primary language*) from generation to generation with reinforcement from new immigrants and travel to their country of origin. In total, more than 55 million individuals older than 5 years in the United States speak a language other than or in addition to English, 44 percent of whom speak English less than "very well" (U.S. Bureau of the Census, 2008a). Of those 55 million speakers, more than 34 million speak Spanish, and there are more than one million speakers of Chinese (including all dialects), French, German, Korean, Tagalog, and Vietnamese. It is estimated that by the year 2050, if birth rates and current immigration trends continue, the percentage of individuals of Asian descent will be almost 8 percent, of Hispanic/Latino descent will be 30 percent, and of Native American descent will increase to about 1.25 percent (for information on Native American languages, see Goldstein, 2000) (U.S. Bureau of the Census). Thus, the number of individuals speaking a language variety other than English in the United States is likely to increase in the coming years.

There has been a realization that, although English is the most common and dominant language spoken in the United States, other languages have a right to co-exist in our linguistically plural society. For example, *Lau* v. *Nichols* (1974) and the *Lau* Remedies (1975) mandated that federally funded schools must eliminate language barriers in school programs that excluded nonnative English speakers. The *Individuals with Disabilities Education Act* (IDEA, 2004) required that the native language commonly used in the home or learning environment be utilized in all contact with a child who has a disability.

The current number and future increase of individuals from culturally and linguistically diverse populations mean that SLPs will likely encounter speakers of languages and language varieties other than English. To complete appropriate phonological assessments that guide the intervention process for children whose home language is not English, SLPs need to gather segmental, prosodic, syllabic, and developmental information. The next section describes the characteristics of pidgins, creoles, and Spanish and Asian languages and presents information about phonological acquisition and development in speakers of Spanish and Asian languages. Although languages other than Spanish and those of Asia are spoken in the United States (e.g., Arabic) (Amayreh and Dyson, 1998, 2000; Dyson and Amayreh, 2000), we focus on those languages because the majority of children in the schools who speak other languages use them (Kindler, 2001).

Pidgins and Creoles

Language is always changing. Change occurs in all areas of language—phonology, syntax, semantics, lexicon, and pragmatics. These changes may take place because of a number of factors such as geography, social prestige, and the introduction of new vocabulary (Crystal, 1997). Pidgins and creoles are two examples of language change.

A *pidgin* is a communication system used by groups of people who wish and need to communicate with each other but have no means to do so. They use a limited vocabulary and "simplified" syntactic structure as compared to their two native languages (Crystal, 1997). Pidgins are not simply degraded natural languages but come to have rules all their own. In fact, some pidgins—for example, Tok Pisin in Papua New Guinea—have become the most widely used linguistic variety in the country. Crystal notes, however, that a pidgin often has a short life (perhaps a few years) and disappears when the need for a common communication system ceases to exist. He also suggests that a pidgin may develop into a creole.

A *creole* is a pidgin that becomes the mother tongue of a community. Thus, pidgins and creoles are two points on the same language development continuum (Crystal, 1997). In essence, a creole is a pidgin that serves as primary input to the next generation of speakers. That is, a pidgin becomes a creole when it is passed on to child speakers. Compared with pidgins, creoles show increased complexity in syntax, phonology, lexicon, semantics, and pragmatics (Muyksen and Smith, 1995). Creoles tend to show rules that were not exhibited in their pidgin ancestor (Holm, 1988).

Common Creoles in the United States

SLPs might encounter four main creoles: Gullah, Hawaiian Creole, Louisiana French Creole, and Haitian Creole. In this section, we briefly outline their phonological characteristics.

Gullah (or *Geechee* or *Sea Island Creole,* as it is sometimes called) is spoken by approximately 250,000 to 300,000 speakers mostly on the barrier islands off the coasts of South Carolina and Georgia (Holm, 1989). This English creole is closely related to other creoles such as Sierra Leone Krio, Cameroons Creole, Jamaican Creole, the Creole of British Guiana, and the Creoles of Surinam (Cunningham, 1992). The origin of this creole is debated. Some believe that Gullah arrived in the American colonies from the west coast of Africa as a fully developed creole (Nichols, 1981). Others link its development to a complex interaction of White British settlers, Africans, and Caribbeans (Holm). Some phonological features of Gullah (compared with General American English) include the use of [a] for /æ/, [t] for /θ/, [d] for /ð/, [ʤ] for /z/, and deletion of postvocalic /ɹ/.

Hawaiian Creole arose in the 19th century and culminates from the influence of many sources such as Polynesian, European, Asian, and pidgin languages (Holm, 1989). Some phonological features of Hawaiian Creole (compared with General American English) include [t] for /θ/, [d] for /ð/, backing in the environment of [ɹ] (/θɹ/→ [tʃɹ]; /tɹ/ → [tʃɹ]; /str/ → [ʃɹ]), deletion of postvocalic /ɹ/, and deletion of the second member of word-final abutting consonants—for example, /nɛst/ → [nɛs] (Bleile, 1996).

Louisiana French Creole evolved as the native language of descendants of West African slaves brought to southern Louisiana by French colonists (Dubois and Horvath, 2003; Nichols, 1981). The creole has also been influenced by features of Cajun, a variety of regional French brought from Canada (Holm, 1989). It is estimated that there are 60,000 to 80,000 speakers of this creole (although the number of speakers of French Creole in the U.S. is estimated to be approximately 629,000 [U.S. Census Bureau, 2007]). The vowel system consists of four front vowels, /i, e, ɛ, a/, four back vowels, /u, o, ɔ, a/, schwa /ə/, and three nasalized vowels /ɛ̃, ɔ̃, ã/ (Morgan, 1959; Nichols; Oetting, 2007). The consonant system contains six oral stops /b, d, g, p, t, k/, three nasals /m, n, ɲ/, seven fricatives /f, s, ʃ, v, z, ʒ, h/, two liquids /l, ɹ/, and one glide /j/. Common phonological patterns (Nichols; Oetting & Garrity, 2006) include these: (1) Abutting consonants across word boundaries are often assimilated to the voicing of the second member of the consonant pair, for example, /pæs ði/ → [pæz ði], (2) word-final consonants may be deleted, (3) word-final unstressed syllables are often weakened or deleted, (4) voiceless stops might be deaspirated, (5) substitution of [t, d] for /θ, ð/, (6) vowel raising may take place in which [i] is substituted for /ɛ/, and (7) monophthongization of /aɪ/.

Speech-language pathologists might also encounter speakers of *Haitian Creole*. This Caribbean creole, spoken in Haiti, has approximately six million speakers (Muyksen and Veenstra, 1995). There are three dialects of Haitian Creole: northern, central (including the capital Port-au-Prince), and southern. The Haitian Creole vowel system contains seven segments: /i, u, e, o, a/ and two front-rounded vowels /ø/ and /œ/. The creole also contains 17 consonants, six stops /b, d, g, p, t, k/, six fricatives /f, s, ʃ, v, z, ʒ/, three nasals /m, n, ɲ/, and two liquids /l/ and /r/.

Spanish

Spanish has become the second most common language spoken in the United States with approximately 35 million speakers, or 12.3 percent of the U.S. population over 5 years of age (U.S. Census Bureau, 2007). According to Hammond (2001), there are two main dialects of American Spanish: highland Spanish and coastal Spanish. Dialects are categorized by one of these two types based on the behavior of syllable- and word-final consonants. Dialects in which syllable- and word-final consonants are preserved are known as *conservative dialects;* those in which final consonants tend to be deleted are known as *radical dialects* (Guitart, 1978, 1996). Mexican Spanish exemplifies a conservative dialect, and Puerto Rican Spanish is emblematic of a radical dialect. In the following sections, we review Spanish phonology and phonological development in Spanish speakers.

Spanish Phonology

A brief overview of the Spanish consonant and vowel system is presented here (for a more complete description, see Goldstein, 1995, 2007a; Hammond, 2001; and Lipski, 2008). There are five primary vowels in Spanish: the two front vowels /i/ and /e/ and the three back vowels /u/, /o/, and /a/. There are 18 consonants in general Spanish (Núñez-Cedeño and Morales-Front, 1999): the voiceless unaspirated stops /p/, /t/, and /k/; the voiced stops /b/, /d/, and /g/; the voiceless fricatives /f/, /x/, and /s/; the affricate /tʃ/; the glides /w/ and /j/; the lateral /l/; the flap /ɾ/ and trill /r/; and the nasals /m/, /n/, and /ɲ/.

The existence of differences between Spanish dialects further complicates the process of characterizing phonological patterns in Spanish-speaking children. Unlike English, in which dialectal variations are generally defined by variations in vowels, Spanish dialectal differences primarily affect consonant sound classes rather than vowels or a few specific phonemes. The dialect differences primarily affect certain sound classes over others. Fricatives and liquids (in particular /s/, flap /r/, and trill /r/) tend to show more variation than stops, glides, or the affricate. The differences among Spanish dialects make it paramount that SLPs be aware of the dialect the children are speaking. Otherwise, the likelihood of misdiagnosis increases.

Phonological Development in Spanish-Speaking Children

Normative data (summarized in detail in Goldstein, 1995, 2000, 2007a) show that typically developing Spanish-speaking infants tend to produce CV syllables containing oral and nasal stops with front vowels (e.g., Oller and Eilers, 1982). By the time typically developing Spanish-speaking children reach 3 1/2 years of age, they are likely to use the dialect features of the community and to have mastered the vowel system and most of the consonant system (e.g., Anderson and Smith, 1987; Goldstein and Cintron, 2001; Pandolfi and Herrera, 1990). In terms of vowel development in Spanish-speaking children, Oller and Eilers found that the mean proportion occurrence of vowel-like productions in 12- to 14-month-old English- and Spanish-speaking children was remarkably similar. In general, they noted that the children were likely to produce more anteriorlike vowels than posteriorlike ones. The rank order of the first 10 vowels in Spanish-speaking infants was (1) [ɛ], (2) [æ], (3) [e], (4) [i], (5) [a], (6) [ʌ], (7) [ʊ], (8) [u], (9) [ɪ], and (10) [o] (p. 573).

Maez (1981) indicated that by 18 months, the three children in the study had mastered (i.e., produced correctly at least 90 percent of the time) the five basic Spanish vowels, [i], [e], [u], [o], and [a]. Maez's study, however, focused on consonant development but did not indicate whether any vowel errors occurred.

Goldstein and Pollock (2000) examined vowel productions in 23 Spanish-speaking children (10 three-year-olds and 13 four-year-olds) with speech sound disorders. Of the 23 children in the study, 14 exhibited vowel errors. Only 1 child exhibited more than one vowel error (five errors). The other 13 children each exhibited only one vowel error. Across all children, the results indicated that there were only 18 total vowel errors. Almost half the errors were on the vowel /o/.

In terms of consonant production, typically developing children exhibit some difficulty by the end of preschool with consonant clusters and a few phones, specifically, [ð], [x], [s], [ʃ], [tʃ], [ɾ], [r], and [l] (e.g., Acevedo, 1991; Jimenez, 1987). These children might exhibit low percentages of occurrence of the following phonological patterns: cluster reduction, unstressed syllable deletion, stridency deletion, and tap/trill deviation but are likely to have suppressed phonological patterns such as velar and palatal fronting, prevocalic singleton omission, stopping, and assimilation (e.g., Goldstein and Iglesias, 1996a; Stepanof, 1990). For some Spanish-speaking children, phonetic mastery continues into the early elementary school years when they continue to show some, although infrequent, errors on the fricatives [x] and [s], the affricate [tʃ], the flap [ɾ], the trill [r], the lateral [l], and consonant clusters (e.g., Bailey, 1982; De la Fuente, 1985).

Speech Sound Disorders in Spanish-Speaking Children

Although there have been quite a number of studies describing phonological patterns in typically developing children, similar data remain scarce for Spanish-speaking children with speech sound disorders. Data indicated that the percentage of Spanish-speaking children with speech sound disorders who exhibit specific phonological patterns was similar across studies (e.g., Bichotte and colleagues, 1993; Goldstein and Iglesias, 1996b; Meza, 1983). Phonological patterns exhibited by a large percentage of children (>40 percent) included cluster reduction, unstressed syllable deletion, stopping, liquid simplification, and assimilation.

Finally, Goldstein (2007b) found that children speaking the Puerto Rican and Mexican dialects of Spanish show similar error types and error rates on vowel accuracy, consonant accuracy, sound class accuracy, percentage of occurrence of phonological patterns, and frequency and types of substitutions.

Asian Languages

In the year 2000, there were approximately seven million speakers of Asian languages in the United States, representing 2.7 percent of the total U.S. population over 5 years of age (U.S. Bureau of the Census, 2000). Three main families of languages are spoken in Asia (Crystal, 1997). The first is the more than 100 Austro-Asiatic languages, most of the languages spoken in Southeast Asia (the countries between China and Indonesia) including Khmer, Hmong, and Vietnamese. The second is the Tai family centered on Thailand and extending into Laos, North Vietnam, and parts of China. The third branch is Sino-Tibetan containing the languages of China, Tibet, and Burma, including Mandarin (also termed *Putonghua*) and Cantonese. Combined, these families contain more than 440 languages spoken by more than one billion people. Two other families, Austronesian and Papuan, contain languages spoken in the Pacific Islands (Cheng, 1993). Austronesian contains languages such as Hawaiian, Chamorro, Ilocano, and Tagalog. The Papuan family contains New Guinean.

There are a number of dialectal variations in Asian languages just as there are within English (e.g., Wang, 1990). For example, there are two main dialects of Chinese spoken in the United States: Mandarin and Cantonese (Cheng, 1987). There are also a number of subdialects within those two main dialects. Japanese has a few dialects, but they are mutually unintelligible; however, Khmer's four dialects are mutually intelligible (Cheng, 1993). In the next two sections, Asian language phonology and phonological development in children speaking Asian languages are described.

Asian Language Phonology

The phonological structure of Asian languages varies greatly. In general, there are few syllable-final segments and few consonant clusters. For example, (1) the only syllable-final consonants in Mandarin Chinese are /n/ and /ŋ/, (2) there are no labiodental, interdental, or palatal fricatives in Korean, and (3) Hawaiian contains only five vowels and eight consonants. There are, however, segmental systems in Asian languages that are relatively complex. For example, Hmong (the language spoken by dwellers in mountainous areas of Indochina) contains 56 initial consonants, 13 or 14 vowels (depending on dialect), seven tones, and one final consonant /ŋ/ (Cheng, 1993). For segmental information on specific languages and dialects, consult the following sources: Cheng (1987, 1993), Hwa-Froelich, Hodson, and Edwards (2002), Tipton (1975), and Wang (1989).

Syllable structure in Asian languages also shows considerable variation. For example, Laotian contains three syllable types (CVC, CVVC, and CVV). Khmer exhibits eight syllable types (CVC, CCVC, CCCVC, CVVC, CCVVC, CCCVVC, CVV, CCVV); however, there are few polysyllabic words in Khmer (Cheng, 1987). Many Asian languages also show restrictions on the types of segments that may appear in certain syllable positions. Vietnamese has a limited number of final consonants (voiceless stops and nasals); the only final consonant in Hmong is / ŋ /; in Korean, there are no fricatives or affricates in word-final position. Stress also may be different in Asian languages compared with English. For example, there is no tonic word stress in Korean, so, to native English speakers, native speakers of Korean can sound somewhat "monotone" when speaking English (Cheng, 1993).

Many, but not all, Asian languages are tone languages. For example, Cantonese is a tone language, but Japanese is not. *Tone languages* are ones in which differences in word meaning are signified by differences in pitch. Tone languages are generally composed of register tones (typically two or three in a language) and contour tones (usually two or three per language) (O'Grady, Archibald, Aronoff, and Rees-Miller, 2010). *Register tones* are level tones, usually signaled by high, mid, and low tones. *Contour tones* are a combination of register tones over a single syllable. For example, in Mandarin Chinese, the phonetic string [ma] takes on different meanings, depending on the tone or tone sequence that is applied. If produced with a high, level tone, [ma] means "mother," but if that same phonetic form is produced with a high-fall, register tone (i.e., a high then low tone), it means "scold."

There have been few studies on tone acquisition in Asian languages. Existing studies have illustrated the developmental process of tone (Li and Thompson, 1977; So and Dodd, 1995; Tse, 1978; Zhu and Dodd, 2000a). For example, Tse found that perceptual discrimination of tone began as early as age 10 months. The results from all four studies found that (1) children acquired the correct tone system relatively quickly (in about 8 months), (2) mastery of tone occurred before segmental mastery, (3) high and falling tones were acquired earlier and more easily than rising and contour tones, and (4) substitution errors often exist for rising and contour tones during the two- and three-word stages.

Phonological Development in Speakers of Asian Languages

Of late, the number of studies of children acquiring the phonology of Asian languages has increased. Major findings from those studies are summarized here by language. Detail is included as well when it is available. For most languages, the summary includes speech sound acquisition, consonant accuracy, and occurrence of phonological processes/patterns.

Cantonese. So (2006, 2007) indicated that early-acquired speech sounds (typically by 2;6) in Cantonese are vowels, bilabial and alveolar stops, nasals, and glides. Aspirated stops are acquired around 3;6 followed by fricatives and affricates. Consonant accuracy is approximately 85% at age 2. By age 4;0, only cluster reduction and stopping are commonly occurring. So and Dodd (1994, 1995) investigated phonological development in typically developing Cantonese-speaking children and noted similar phoneme acquisition to English but at a more rapid rate. In general, anterior consonants were acquired before posterior ones, and oral and nasal stops and glides were acquired before fricatives and affricates. They also noted the presence of phonological processes (i.e., patterns) and found that by age 4 years, no process was exhibited over 15 percent of the time. Between the ages of 2;0 and 4;0, these children showed processes similar in quantity (>15 percent) and type to those of English-speaking children: assimilation, cluster reduction, stopping, fronting, affrication, and final consonant deletion.

So and Dodd (1994) also provided increased detail on the phonological patterns exhibited by the 13 children labeled as either "phonological delay" or "consistently disordered." Children with phonological delay tended to exhibit assimilation, cluster reduction, stopping, fronting, deaspiration, affrication, and final consonant deletion. Children with phonological disorder tended to exhibit final consonant deletion, final glide deletion, initial consonant deletion, aspiration, gliding, vowel rule, and backing.

Cheung and Abberton (2000) examined the phonological skills of 251 Cantonese-speaking children (ages 3;6 to 6;0) with speech sound disorders. They found that tones and vowels largely were produced accurately with consonants being most affected. The children showed most difficulty with /s/, aspirated consonants (e.g., /pʰ/), and labialized consonants (e.g., /kʷ/). Thus, deaspiration was a commonly occurring phonological pattern as were stopping and fronting of velars.

Japanese (Ota and Ueda, 2007). In Japanese, most consonants are acquired by 4;0 except [ç, s, ts, z, ɾ] with clusters being acquired by 4;6. Vowels are acquired by 3;0. There are few occurrences of phonological processes at age 5. By age 5, 94% of children produced syllables accurately (Sumio, 1978 in Ota and Ueda).

Korean (Kim and Pae, 2007).   By age 3, all consonants in Korean are acquired except [l], [ɾ], [s], and [s*] (voiceless fortis). Bilabials are acquired before velars and affricates. Intersyllabic clusters are acquired by age 4 years. Few phonological processes are exhibited by 6;5.

Putonghua (Modern Standard Chinese) (Hua, 2007).   Hua (2006, 2007) indicated that consonants in Putonghua are acquired by 4;6 with 92% accuracy. Vowels are acquired by 2;0. The following phonological patterns are still exhibited at age 4;6: fronting, backing, deaspiration, final /n/ deletion, and triphthong reduction. Zhu and Dodd (2000a) examined the phonological skills of 129 typically developing speakers of Putonghua ages 1;6 to 4;6. Their results indicated that tone was acquired first, followed by syllable-final consonants and vowels and finally syllable-initial consonants. By age 4;6, 90 percent of the children accurately produced all the syllable-initial consonants. Similar to typically developing children acquiring other languages, the Putonghua-speaking children exhibited syllabic and substitution phonological patterns such as unstressed syllable deletion, fronting, and gliding. The children also showed language-specific patterns such as deaspiration and triphthong reduction of vowels.

Thai (Lorwatanapongsa and Maroonroge, 2007).   In Thai, consonants except /s/ and /r/ are acquired by age 5;0. Thai-speaking children exhibit many of the same phonological patterns exhibited by children speaking other languages: backing, cluster reduction, final consonant deletion, fronting, stopping, and stridency deletion.

Vietnamese (Tang and Barlow, 2006).   Tang and Barlow investigated the phonological skills of four Vietnamese-speaking children (ages 4;4 to 5;5) with speech sound disorders. They found that tone was adultlike for all four children. The four children also produced all vowels and the majority of stops, nasals, and glides in syllable-initial and syllable-final positions. At least two of the children exhibited seven phonological patterns: gliding, fronting, glottal replacement, backing, velar assimilation, stopping, and final consonant deletion. Many of these patterns are common cross-linguistically (e.g., stopping, fronting, and final consonant deletion) although others are not (e.g., glottal replacement). Finally, final consonants were acquired before initial ones.

Speech Sound Disorders in Speakers of Asian Languages

A few studies have also investigated speakers of Asian languages with speech sound disorders. Zhu and Dodd (2000b) assessed 33 children learning Putonghua ages 2;8 to 7;6 with "atypical speech development" (p. 170). The largest subgroup of speakers (18 of 33 children) was characterized with "delayed phonological development" ("use of non-age-appropriate patterns and/or restricted phonetic or phonemic inventory," p. 168). Phonological patterns exhibited most commonly included fronting and stopping. Children with speech sound disorders had less difficulty with syllable components described as having more "phonological saliency" (p. 180). Phonological saliency, according to the authors, is based on syllable structure and is specific to each ambient language. In the case of Putonghua, tones, vowels, and syllable-final consonants are more salient, and syllable-initial consonants are less salient. As predicted, children with disorders had most difficulty with less salient features (i.e., syllable-initial consonants). So and Dodd (1994, pp. 238–240) outlined and defined four subgroups of children with speech sound disorders: delayed phonological development ("rules or processes used by more than 10% of children acquiring phonology normally"), consistent use of one or more unusual rules ("rules not used by more than 10 percent of children acquiring phonology normally"), articulation disorder ("consistent distortion of a phoneme"), and the making of inconsistent errors ("production of specific words or particular phonological segments"). So and Dodd applied these categories to 17 Cantonese-speaking children with speech sound disorders ages 3;6 to 6;4. Their results revealed that 8 of 17 participants (47 %) displayed delayed phonological development, 5 of 17 (30 %) were categorized as consistent users of one or more unusual rules, 2 of 17 (12 %) had an articulation disorder, and another 2 of 17 (12 %) were defined as making inconsistent errors.

PHONOLOGICAL DEVELOPMENT IN BILINGUAL CHILDREN

Although there is no doubt that SLPs will be assessing and providing intervention services to monolingual speakers of Spanish and Asian languages, it is more likely that SLPs in the United States will be delivering clinical services to bilingual children acquiring a language in addition to English. The historical view of phonological development in bilingual children is that it is "slower" than that of monolingual children. That is, bilingual children exhibit negative transfer. More recent studies of bilingual children indicate that phonological development in these children is similar, although not identical, to that of monolingual speakers of either language (Goldstein, 2004; Goldstein and Gildersleeve-Neumann, 2012; for a detailed review, see Goldstein and McLeod, 2012, and Grech and McLeod, 2012).

Negative Transfer

Results from a number of studies of bilingual children have indicated that their phonological development is slower than that of monolingual peers. Dodd, So, and Li (1996) examined the phonology of 16 typically developing, Cantonese-speaking children who were acquiring English in preschool. The results indicated that the children differentiated the phonology of each language. They also found that the children's error patterns were atypical for monolingual speakers of either language and that they produced a high number of atypical error patterns (e.g., initial consonant deletion) in an amount usually associated with children evidencing speech sound disorders. Holm and Dodd (2000) examined the phonological skills of two Cantonese-English bilingual children from ages 2;3 to 3;1 and from ages 2;9 to 3;5. They found that the children maintained separate phonological systems of each language, and both exhibited phonological patterns that were not typical for monolingual speakers (e.g., atypical aspiration); however, these patterns were exhibited by Cantonese-English bilingual speakers in other studies (e.g., Dodd et al., 1996).

In a group of typically developing Spanish-English bilingual preschoolers, Gildersleeve-Neumann, Kester, Davis, and Peña (2008) found that the bilingual children exhibited lower overall accuracy and more errors than their English and Spanish monolingual counterparts. Compared with monolinguals, Goldstein and Washington (2001) found that typically developing Spanish-English bilingual children exhibited significantly lower accuracy on some sound classes (e.g., spirants, flap, and trill) but not on others (e.g., stops, nasals, and fricatives).

Positive Transfer

In addition to findings indicating negative transfer of phonological skills in bilinguals relative to monolinguals, results from other studies show positive transfer. In these studies, positive transfer was defined as bilinguals exhibiting either more advanced skills or commensurate skills in comparison to monolingual peers.

Studies of German-Spanish (Lleó and Kehoe, 2002; Lleó, Kuchenbrandt, Kehoe, and Trujillo, 2003) and Maltese-English (Grech and Dodd, 2008) bilingual children have indicated more advanced skills than their monolingual counterparts. Gildersleeve-Neumann and Davis (1998) demonstrated that although bilingual speakers exhibited different developmental patterns than their monolingual peers and exhibited more errors initially than monolingual speakers, these differences faded over time.

A number of studies of bilingual children indicate that their phonological development is commensurate with that of monolinguals (e.g., Fabiano-Smith and Goldstein, 2010). The children in Holm and Dodd's (2000) investigation of two Cantonese-English bilingual children showed phonetic development that was similar to that of monolingual children. Similarities in phonological skills between monolingual and bilingual speakers are also supported by the work of Goldstein and Washington (2001) and Goldstein, Fabiano, and Washington (2005). These researchers examined the Spanish and English phonological skills in typically developing 4- and 5-year-old bilingual (Spanish-English) children and found similarities in phonological skills between bilingual and monolingual children. Differences between groups were relegated to the accuracy of production of sounds in specific sound classes, especially in Spanish. Spirants, flap, and trill in Spanish were produced much less accurately in bilingual children than have been shown for monolingual Spanish-speaking children (Goldstein, 1988). Finally, in a group of Russian-English bilingual children ages 3;3 to 5;7, Gildersleeve-Neumann and Wright (2010) did not find differences across bilingual and monolingual children for syllable-level errors.

The results of these studies indicate that bilingual phonological development appears to proceed along the same course as that for monolingual speakers. That trajectory, however, is not entirely the same as it is for monolingual speakers. Bilingual children might exhibit error types that are less common in monolingual speakers, are likely to show cross-linguistic effects, and might be less accurate on some aspects of the phonological system in comparison to their monolingual peers. Those differences seem to diminish over time so that bilingual children are able to achieve adultlike phonological skills in both languages.

The Influence of One Language on Another

When there is contact between speakers of two or more languages, a tendency exists for one language to influence the other (Goldstein, 2007c; Goldstein and McLeod, 2012; Grech and McLeod, 2012). This influence is often bidirectional with each language influencing the other. For example, a native Spanish speaker acquiring English will exhibit characteristics of Spanish-influenced English and English-influenced Spanish. In a group of bilingual

(Spanish-English) children, Goldstein and Iglesias (1999) found that a few children substituted [tʃ] for /ʃ/; /ʃʌvəl/ (*shovel*) was produced as [tʃʌvəl] (Spanish-influenced English). The children also used the postvocalic "r" of General American English for the Spanish flap; /floɾ/ (*flower*) was produced as [floɚ] (English-influenced Spanish). In groups of Russian-English bilingual children and English children, Gildersleeve-Neumann and Wright (2010) found examples of Russian-influenced English. For example, the bilingual children produced palatalized consonants (e.g., /kʲ/) in their English.

For speakers acquiring more than one language, there are many ways that the phonology of one language can affect the phonology of another language (Goldstein, 2007c). First, the specific phonemes and allophones in the inventories of each language are not the same. For example, the alveo-palatal affricate [tʃ] found in English is not in the inventory of Cantonese (Cheng, 1993). A native Cantonese-speaking individual acquiring English might substitute [ts] for the alveo-palatal affricate, because [ts] exists in the inventory of Cantonese and is close to the place of articulation of the English affricate. Second, differences in the distribution of sounds exist across languages. For example, [ŋ] might be the only word-final sound realized in English by a native Hmong speaker, because it is the only word-final sound in Hmong (Cheng). Third, consonants can have different places of articulation in each language. For example, Spanish speakers acquiring English may produce /d/ with a dental place of articulation as is common in Spanish versus an alveolar place of articulation that is typical in English (Perez, 1994). Fourth, phonological rules may be different in each language. For example, the phrase *Cómo se llama su niño?* (What is your child's name?), which would be produced as [komo se jama su niɲo] in Spanish, might be realized as [koʊmoʊ se jama su niɲoʊ] in English-influenced Spanish because the speaker is diphthongizing vowels as is common in English. Finally, how and when pronunciation is acquired can contribute to the influence of one language on another. The major exposure for some individuals learning English as a second language might be in school where written language is being introduced. The lack of one-to-one correspondence between grapheme and phoneme in English may influence pronunciation (August, Calderón, and Carlo 2002). For example, the grapheme "s" in English is produced as [s] in *basin* and as [ʒ] in *measure* causing a speaker of Spanish-influenced English to produce both as [s].

ASSESSMENT CONSIDERATIONS FOR CHILDREN FROM CULTURALLY AND LINGUISTICALLY DIVERSE POPULATIONS

In assessing the speech and language skills of children from culturally and linguistically diverse populations, the same types of information are gathered as for all children: case history, oral-peripheral examination, hearing screening, language (e.g., syntax, semantics, pragmatics, and the lexicon), voice, fluency, and phonology. The analysis of speech sound productions by children from culturally and linguistically diverse populations requires a determination of whether the child's phonological system is within normal limits for his or her linguistic community (ASHA, 2004a). Thus, the assessment must be approached with an understanding of the social, cultural, and linguistic characteristics of that community and always guarding against stereotyping (Taylor, Payne, and Anderson, 1987). One cannot assume that any individual from any geographical area or ethnic/racial group is a speaker of a particular dialect. For example, although one African American's production of f/θ in the word *mouth* may be regarded as a dialect feature of AAE, it would be inappropriate to make the same clinical judgment for another African American who also produces f/θ. The first speaker may be an AAE speaker, but the second speaker may not be, and therefore the second speaker may have produced a true error.

Speech-language pathologists must also differentiate dialect differences from speech sound disorders. In ASHA's position papers on social dialects and communication disorders and variations, the association officially acknowledges the distinction between a speech-language difference and a speech-language disorder (ASHA, 1993, 1983). A few investigators have attempted to determine whether scoring dialectal features as "errors" would penalize children for patterns that are, in effect, dialect features, thus artificially inflating their severity ratings. In their examination of 10 AAE-speaking children ages 5;11 to 6;11, Cole and Taylor (1990) found that not taking dialect into account resulted in the misdiagnosis of speech sound disorder for half of the children, on average, across three phonological assessments. Two other studies, while advocating that dialect should be accounted for in phonological assessment, did not find the same significant results as Cole and Taylor. Fleming and Hartman (1989) examined 72 four-year-old AAE speakers using the *Computer Assessment of Phonological Processes* (*CAPP*; Hodson, 1985). They determined that although some test items are influenced by "Black English phonological rules," the assessment as a whole is not invalidated (p. 28). Moreover, they indicated that no typically developing child was labeled as having a disorder based solely on the factor of dialect. Washington and Craig (1992) examined 28 preschool AAE-speaking children ages 4;6 to 5;3. Their results indicated that dialect scoring changes did "not seem to penalize the BE-speaking preschooler to a degree that is clinically significant" (p. 23). Washington and Craig ascribed the contrast of their results to those of Cole and Taylor on the basis of geographical location. The participants in Cole and Taylor's study were from Mississippi, whereas the children in Washington and Craig's study resided in Detroit. Goldstein and Iglesias (2001) examined 54 typically developing Spanish-speaking children and 54 Spanish-speaking children with speech sound disorders to determine whether taking or not taking into account Puerto Rican Spanish dialect features altered the results of the analyses. The results indicated that had dialect features not been considered, almost 75 percent of typically developing children might have been erroneously characterized as exhibiting speech sound disorders. In addition, not considering dialect might have resulted in unnecessarily targeting for intervention phonological processes whose percentage of occurrence was inflated. Wing and Flipsen (2010) replicated the Goldstein and Iglesias (2001) study with speakers of a Mexican dialect of Spanish. Children in the study included 24 typically developing children (mean age = 5;0) and three children with phonological disorders (mean age = 4;10). Results from Goldstein and Iglesias were largely confirmed in that underidentification and overidentification occurred relative to the General Spanish Referent (i.e., not taking dialect into account). Accounting for dialect significantly increased classification accuracy.

Although the results of these studies reported somewhat different conclusions as to whether scoring dialectal features as "errors" affected the child's severity rating, these researchers all agreed that accounting for dialect features is a prime consideration in the assessment of children from culturally and linguistically diverse populations. Analysis of phonological information must be made by considering the child's dialect, especially because SLPs with less familiarity with a dialect yield less comprehensibility of that dialect (e.g., Robinson & Stockman, 2009). Thus, "errors" can be counted as such only when they conflict with the child's dialect. For example, in the Puerto Rican dialect of Spanish, the production of /dos/ (*"two"*) as [do:] would not be scored as an error because syllable-final /s/ is often deleted. The production of /floɾ/ (*"flower"*) as [flo] would be scored as an error because syllable-final deletion of /ɾ/ is not considered a typical feature of the dialect. Thus, to minimize the possibility of misdiagnosis, all phonological analyses should consider the features of that particular dialect which should not be scored as errors. To account for dialect features in any particular linguistic group, SLPs might (1) become thoroughly familiar with features of the dialects and language, (2) sample the adult speakers in the child's linguistic community, and (3) obtain information from interpreters/support personnel.

To minimize the effect that not accounting for dialect features might have on the phonological analysis of speakers from culturally and linguistically diverse populations, Stockman has suggested assessing a minimal competency core (MCC) developed to decrease bias in the assessment of AAE-speaking children (Stockman, 1996b, p. 358). *Minimal competency core* is defined as "the *least* amount of knowledge that one must exhibit to be judged as normal in a given age range" (p. 358, emphasis original). Stockman noted that MCC might best be used as a screening tool on a core subgroup of specific behaviors. The phonological features core includes the following word/syllable initial sounds that are invariable in GAE and AAE: /m, n, p, b, t, d, k, g, f, s, h, w, j, l, ɹ/. Wilcox and Anderson (1998) found that assessing these sounds along with clusters provided enough information to differentiate typical from atypical speech sound development in a group of African American English speakers.

Examiners must be aware of their own dialect and its effect on the assessment process. Seymour and Seymour (1977) noted that the client's perception of the formality of the situation affects dialect density. Casual speaking settings could increase dialect density by encouraging more frequent use of AAE, whereas a more formal setting may result in a decrease in dialect density by inhibiting and stigmatizing speech forms other than General American English. A similar issue could be encountered when a clinician uses Castilian Spanish (i.e., the dialect of Spanish spoken in some areas of Spain and taught in most educational systems in the United States) when conversing with a speaker of any of the other major Spanish dialects. This is not to say that one should force herself or himself to use the client's dialect. One must realize, however, the potential effect that one's particular dialect could have on a client and family.

The assessment of speakers of languages other than or in addition to English presents a challenge to the SLP who must determine the language or languages of assessment and then choose appropriate assessment tools. Even if the child seems to be a "dominant" English speaker, it is common practice to assess phonological skills in both languages because the child's phonological knowledge is distributed across the two languages (Goldstein, 2006). Analyses then should be completed in both languages. The speech-language pathologist must differentiate true speech sound errors from developmental errors from atypical/disordered patterns from cross-linguistic effects (Yavaş and Goldstein, 1998).

A detailed phonological assessment would include both formal measures (instruments standardized on speakers from a particular language group) and informal measures (such as a spontaneous language sample). The formal assessment tool should be designed specifically to assess productions in that language. Unfortunately, few formal measures covering a variety of languages are available. Using an assessment tool designed for any other linguistic group other than the one for which it was intended is likely to increase bias and lead to over-referral. In the absence of formal measures, the SLP might utilize informal client observations with siblings, peers, and/or parent(s) by asking a series of questions designed to determine the adequacy of the child's phonological system (Yavaş & Goldstein, 1998): Does the child sound like other children in his or her peer group (i.e., like other members of his or her speech community)? What consonants does the child produce (front versus back, syllable-initial versus syllable-final)? Does the child make any vowel errors? If appropriate, does the child use tone accurately? What percentage of the time is the child intelligible? Do the child's parents, family members, teachers, and friends understand the child all, some, or none of the time?

Role of the Monolingual Speech-Language Pathologist

Speech-language pathologists might have difficulty in assessing children who speak more than one language, because SLPs often are not bilingual themselves (Goldstein, 2001). Clinicians who do not speak the language of the individual they are assessing might consider alternatives such as hiring a bilingual consultant or bilingual diagnostician, training bilingual aides, or using interpreters/translators (I/Ts) (Langdon and Cheng, 2002). SLPs who use I/Ts should be sure they are trained, have exemplary bilingual/bidialectal communication skills, understand their responsibilities and act professionally, and can relate to members of the cultural group (Kayser; 1995; Langdon and Cheng). Interpreters/translators should assist the SLP in completing the assessment but not conduct it themselves. It might be tempting for SLPs to use family members of the client as I/Ts. Lynch (2004) advises against this practice because acting in this role may be burdensome to the family member, and family members may be reticent in discussing emotional matters, uncomfortable providing information to older or younger family members or to members of the opposite gender, and leave out information provided by the SLP.

In the absence of a bilingual speech-language pathologist at the site, monolingual SLPs could also play a role in the assessment of non-English-speaking children. If they have knowledge, skills, competencies, and training in providing services to individuals with limited- or non-English proficiency, monolingual SLPs can assess in English, administer an oral-peripheral examination, conduct a hearing screening, and administer nonverbal assessments (ASHA, 1985).

INTERVENTION FOR SPEECH SOUND DISORDERS IN CHILDREN FROM CULTURALLY AND LINGUISTICALLY DIVERSE POPULATIONS

Once the results of an assessment are gathered, SLPs must decide whether intervention is warranted. The traditional role of the SLP has been to provide clinical services for communication disorders but not for dialectal differences. However, ASHA's position paper on social dialects identifies the following expanded role for SLPs (ASHA, 1983):

> Aside from the traditionally recognized role, the speech-language pathologist may also be available to provide *elective* clinical services to nonstandard English speakers who do not present a disorder. The role of the speech-language pathologist for these individuals is to

prepare the desired competency in Standard English without jeopardizing the integrity of the individual's first dialect. The approach must be functional and based on context-specific appropriateness of the given dialect. (p. 24)

If elective services are to take place, it is important to remember that elective therapy does not mean necessarily that the client wants to eliminate the first dialect (D1). More often, the client prefers to be bidialectal. Taylor (1986) suggested a number of principles for SLPs who seek to guide speakers who want to acquire a second dialect: (1) Develop a positive attitude toward the speaker's home dialect, (2) compare the features of the home dialect to the one being acquired, (3) select targets based on language acquisition norms, frequency of occurrence of the features, and the speaker's attitude toward the features, (4) know the rules of the speaker's home dialect and the ones to be acquired, (5) consider the speaker's learning style, and (6) integrate language issues into the larger culture of the speaker. Taylor also proposed a series of steps that must be followed to maintain both dialects. First, a positive attitude toward D1 must be established. Second, the client must learn to contrast the features of the first dialect and the second dialect (D2). Finally, the client uses D2 in controlled, structured, and eventually spontaneous situations with a focus on form, content, and use.

Modifying someone's dialect involves more than simply having the person produce consonant and vowels as a native speaker would pronounce them. Learning nonsegmental aspects of speech production such as stress, pitch, and intonation are equally important. There are likely to be differences between the person's home language/dialect and the variety being acquired as a second language/dialect. For example, stress in English is relatively more complicated than in other languages. Placement of stress depends on a number of factors, including syntactic category and weight of the syllable (i.e., whether the vowel is long or short and the number of consonants that follow the vowel) (Goodluck, 1991). Pitch also differs as a function of language. For example, pitch modulates less in Spanish than it does in English (Hadlich, Holton, and Montes, 1968). Finally, intonational contours for statements, questions, and exclamations may be different in English than in other languages. For example, in English, utterances (statements, questions, and exclamations) may begin at an overall higher pitch than in other languages.

Speech-language pathologists must also recognize how dialectal variation and speech sound disorders interact (Wolfram, 1994). Wolfram has suggested the following guiding principles. He divided impairments into three types. *Type I* impairments were judged to be atypical patterns regardless of the speaker's dialect, for example, initial consonant deletion (e.g., [it] for /mit/) or velar fronting (e.g., [dot] for /got/). *Type II* impairments have a cross-dialectal difference in the normative (or underlying) form. For example, the normative form for the word *bathing* would be /beðɪŋ/ for speakers of GAE but /bevɪŋ/ for AAE speakers even though speakers from both dialect groups might misarticulate that word as [bezɪŋ]. *Type III* impairments influence forms that are shared across dialects but applied with different frequency. For example, syllable-final cluster reduction was exhibited in many dialects. In AAE, this pattern was observed more frequently than in other dialects. Wolfram noted that treating a type I impairment would not necessitate gathering different norms across dialect groups. The treatment of type II and type III impairments, however, would involve considering both qualitative and quantitative differences between dialect groups. Velleman and Pearson (2010, p. 185–187) have made a number of suggestions relative to providing intervention to AAE-speaking children with SSD:

■ Early developing sounds (except /j/) are not likely to be intervention targets because AAE speakers with SSD tend to produce them accurately.

■ /ð/ is not likely to be an intervention target because its status as a phoneme in AAE is questionable (Stockman, 2006a).

■ Syllable and word structure rules (i.e., phonotactics) need to be considered in the development of intervention targets and stimuli because obstruents and nasals are often optional in final position, clusters are typically reduced in final position, and initial, unstressed syllables are often omitted.

■ Target /j, f, s, v, tʃ, dʒ, ɹ/ and / ɹ / clusters earlier in the intervention sequence and /t, g, k, ʃ, ð/ and /s/ + stop clusters later in the intervention sequence.

Intervention for Bilingual Children with Speech Sound Disorders

Little information is available regarding direct intervention for individuals with speech sound disorders who speak a language other than or in addition to English. Available data indicate that principles guiding intervention choices for these children are both similar to and different from those for monolingual children. As with all children, the intervention process begins with the completion of a comprehensively broad and deep assessment. Once this information has been collected, SLPs need to compare those results with the appropriate database. Speech-language pathologists should remember neither to use normative data gathered from English-speaking children to assess children who speak a language other than or in addition to English nor to generalize developmental phonological data from one dialect group to another. That is, phonological skills in the bilingual child being assessed need to be compared to those of other, similar bilingual children.

Once the assessment is completed, the next step should be to determine the intervention goal and the intervention approach (Goldstein, 2006). Choosing the goal and approach will guide the SLP in determining the language of intervention. Kohnert and Derr (2012) and Kohnert and colleagues (2005) have proposed two main approaches for providing intervention to bilingual children. In the *bilingual approach*, they propose that SLPs should improve skills common to both languages. For example, initial goals would be to focus on constructs common to both languages (e.g., the phoneme /s/, final consonant deletion). To extend that approach, Gildersleeve-Neumann and Goldstein (2012) and Yavas͵ and Goldstein (1998) suggested that for a bilingual child with at least a moderate speech sound disorder, SLPs should choose intervention targets based on the error rates in both languages. Initially, error patterns that were exhibited with similar error rates in both languages should be targeted. For example, a pattern such as unstressed syllable deletion would be an initial intervention target because it would likely show similar error rates and greatly affect intelligibility in both languages. Treating errors that occur frequently in both languages are likely to improve intelligibility in both languages rather than in only one of them. Using this approach, however, requires frequently monitoring generalization across both languages although generalization across languages is not guaranteed. For example,

Holm, Dodd, and Ozanne (1997) found that intervention on one sound in English did generalize to Cantonese, but intervention on a phonological pattern did not. Subsequent to treating errors occurring with similar frequency in both languages, error patterns that are exhibited in both languages with unequal frequency should be treated. For example, final consonant deletion is a phonological pattern that is likely to be exhibited in English with a high percentage of occurrences but with a low percentage of occurrences in Spanish (Goldstein and Iglesias, 1996a). Finally, phonological patterns exhibited in only one language should be targeted. For example, final consonant devoicing may be exhibited in English but not in Spanish (Goldstein and Washington, 2001).

In the *cross-linguistic approach*, Kohnert and colleagues suggest that clinicians focus on skills distinct in each constituent language. This approach also is necessary (likely in conjunction with the bilingual approach) because of the differences in the phonological structures of the two languages. For example, labialized consonants exist in Cantonese, but not in English, and thus can be remediated in only one language. As an adjunct, SLPs might utilize the cross-linguistic approach based on types of errors and/ or error rates (Gildersleeve-Neumann and Goldstein, 2012; Yavaş and Goldstein, 1998). For example, the frequency of occurrence of final consonant deletion in Spanish-English bilingual children is higher in their English than in their Spanish (Goldstein, Fabiano, and Washington, 2005). Thus, intervention to decrease the use of final consonant deletion is likely to occur in English but not in Spanish. Finally, errors occurring in only one language would be targets for phonological intervention (e.g., final devoicing in language B but not in language A).

Adapting Intervention Approaches to Individuals from Culturally and Linguistically Diverse Populations

Although little specific information is available to guide the intervention of speech sound disorders in speakers of languages other than or in addition to English, specific intervention approaches developed for English-speaking children might be adapted for use with those from culturally and linguistically diverse populations. A number of different methods for remediating speech sound errors have been categorized into two main types: motor-based (see Chapter 9) and linguistic based (see Chapter 10). *Phonetic approaches*, such as the traditional approach (Van Riper, 1972) and the multiple phoneme approach (Bradley, 1985), and *phonemic approaches*, such as the cycles approach (Hodson and Paden, 1991) and language-based approaches (Hoffman, Norris, and Monjure, 1990), can be adapted for use with individuals from culturally and linguistically diverse populations.

Utilizing a motor-based approach poses several difficulties unless the speech-language pathologist speaks the child's native/home language. First, the SLP must be able to carry out the perceptual training phase of this approach. This includes the ability to produce an auditory model for the child. Second, the SLP must discern the segments in the child's home language, the segments in the child's repertoire, the order of acquisition of the sounds, the ease of production for the sounds, the frequency of occurrence of each phone in the language, and phonetic contexts that may facilitate production of the target sound (Stoel-Gammon and Dunn, 1985).

A linguistically based approach also raises issues for the SLP. First, each specific program would have to be adapted to the child's language and dialect. For example, English has about 25 consonants, but Hmong has about 60 as noted previously. Although English and Hmong both have affricates in their inventories, Hmong has a set of aspirated affricates, which English does not. Second, if the particular approach is based on patterns rather than individual sound segments, the SLP would need to differentiate a series of unrelated errors from a single phonological rule (Williams, 2001). Third, to apply this type of approach, the SLP should be able to identify errors most affecting intelligibility, errors that cut across sound classes, and errors that disappear at the earliest age from typically developing children (Stoel-Gammon and Dunn, 1985). In bilingual children, an error might occur in one language but not in the other (Gildersleeve-Neumann and Goldstein, 2012). Finally, the order of intervention advocated by the approach might need to be altered for a speaker of a language other than English. For example, Hodson and Paden (1991) in their cycles approach suggest treating syllabicity early in the remediation process. That is, if the child does not use two-syllable words, increasing the child's production of multisyllabic words might be warranted. For example, in a language such as Khmer, which has complex syllable types but few polysyllabic words, this might not be the initial target of choice.

A number of linguistically based approaches advocate the use of contrastive word pairs (i.e., minimal opposition pairs, *so/toe*, or maximal opposition pairs, *beet/seat*). Approaches using contrastive word-pairs include the *paired stimuli approach* (Weston and Irwin, 1985), *minimal phonemic contrast approach* (Cooper, 1985), *minimal "triads"* (Nelson, 1995), *metaphon* (Howell and Dean, 1991), *maximal opposition* (Gierut, 1989), and *multiple oppositions* (Williams, 2000a, 2000b). Contrastive word-pairs, however, may be difficult to adapt to speakers of languages other than English because it, unlike other languages, is replete with minimal pairs. It could be more difficult to apply this methodology to languages other than English if those languages lack a significant number of contrastive word-pairs that are appropriate for children.

SUMMARY

To provide least-biased assessment and evidence-based intervention to linguistically diverse individuals, SLPs must complete a number of steps. First, they should gather information about the cultural and linguistic norms of the individuals to whom they are providing service. These norms include the phonological rules of the dialects/languages spoken by the client, remembering that not all speakers of a particular dialect show or use every characteristic of it. Second, SLPs should complete a comprehensive phonological assessment that includes a wide array of independent and relational analyses. For these analyses, SLPs should consider dialect features that occur in all the client's languages. Finally, extensive information collected from the assessment should be used to plan intervention, remembering that intervention for a dialect difference should not occur unless elected by the client. For children acquiring more than one language, both the bilingual approach and the cross-linguistic approach are likely to be required. Following these steps can aid in providing appropriate services to children from culturally and linguistically diverse populations.

QUESTIONS FOR CHAPTER 11

1. What dialect do you speak? How do you think you acquired your dialect? If your dialect were to change, what dialect would you most/least like to have? Provide reasons for your decisions.

2. Administer a formal assessment to a speaker with a dialect other than your own. Score the assessment *not* considering the speaker's dialect features, and then score it considering the dialect features. Did the person's score change between each administration? Would the person have been labeled with a speech sound disorder if dialect features had not been considered?

3. How would you determine whether the phonological patterns exhibited by someone were characteristic of true errors or dialect features?

4. Design a protocol for using support personnel in the assessment of a preschool child who is bilingual in English and Vietnamese. You might consult the following ASHA papers to aid in your planning:

   American Speech-Language-Hearing Association. (2004). Knowledge and skills needed by speech-language pathologists and audiologists to provide culturally and linguistically appropriate services. *ASHA* (Suppl. 24).

   American Speech-Language-Hearing Association. (1996, Spring). Guidelines for the training, credentialing, use, and supervision of speech-language pathology assistants. *ASHA, 38* (Suppl. 16), pp. 21–34.

   American Speech-Language Hearing Association. (1994, March). ASHA policy regarding support personnel. *ASHA, 36* (Suppl. 13), p. 24.

5. Define *pidgin, creole, dialect*, and *language*. What are the similarities and differences between these language varieties?

6. Take an informal poll about myths and facts about dialect. Ask individuals to give you their opinion on people's dialects and how they feel about certain dialects. You might survey individuals who have a background in language studies and individuals who do not have such a background to compare their responses. Then write a paper listing those perceptions followed by facts that counter any myths that are mentioned by the people you interview.

7. Create a quick reference guide for phonological development in AAE, Spanish, Cantonese, Mandarin, and Hmong. You might list sounds in each of the inventories, age of acquisition for segments and tones (if appropriate), and age of suppression for phonological processes. Create a reference guide for a language/dialect not listed here.

8. Design a protocol for modifying the dialect of a native Spanish-speaking woman who wishes to sound "more like a native English speaker." List at least 10 questions you would ask her during the case history, enumerate the ways in which you would assess her speech, and outline your short-term and long-term goals, providing a rationale for each of those goals. What aspects of her speech do you think will be less difficult and more difficult to modify? Why?

9. Do you think newcomers to the United States who do not speak English should maintain their home language? Provide a rationale for your response. What are the advantages and disadvantages of immigrants to the United States maintaining/losing their native language?

10. Based on the following productions from an African American–speaking child, age 4:5, indicate whether the child's production is a dialect feature of AAE or a true error:

Gloss	Child's Production	AAE Feature	True Error
soap	[top]	No	Yes
mother	[mʌðə]		
mouth	[maʊf]		
tell	[tɪl]		
self	[sɛf]		
cool	[ku]		
bell	[bɛ]		
cool	[kũ]		
playing	[pejiŋ]		
fast	[fæs]		
stool	[tul]		

CHAPTER 12

Phonological Awareness: Description, Assessment, and Intervention

LAURA M. JUSTICE
Ohio State University

GAIL T. GILLON
University of Canterbury

BRIGID C. MCNEILL
University of Canterbury

C. MELANIE SCHUELE
Vanderbilt University

◆ ◆ ◆

Running speech consists of varying types of linguistic units that range in size from larger (sentences, words, syllables) to smaller (morphemes, phonemes). Most adult speakers of a language can readily and consciously recognize that speech comprises sentences, words, syllables, morphemes, and phonemes, and that these units are discrete and recurring elements of language. One's ability to consciously analyze the sound structure of speech called *phonological awareness* emerges in early childhood. Young children's phonological awareness is apparent when they successfully perform tasks requiring them to generate rhymes, identify the beginning sounds in words, or segment the individual phonemes comprising words. Children's successful performance on such tasks is consistently associated with performance on reading tasks—particularly those measuring word recognition—indicating that there are integrative linkages between phonological awareness and acquisition of word-level reading skills. Of particular importance to speech-language pathologists is evidence showing that children with speech sound difficulties often show lags in their development of phonological awareness and that such lags may pose specific risks for their timely development of skilled reading, writing, and spelling. This chapter provides a framework for understanding phonological awareness, recognizing why children with speech difficulties often have challenges in this area, and considering how such challenges may be addressed through clinical interventions.

WHAT IS PHONOLOGICAL AWARENESS?

Phonological awareness refers to an individual's awareness of the sound (phonological) structure of spoken words. Children exhibiting phonological awareness consciously recognize (or at least are sensitive to) the phonological units comprising a word. Often at relatively young ages (3 to 4 years), children become aware that spoken words contain syllables and that syllables within words contain smaller sound units. With increasing age, children become more aware of the intrasyllabic units of syllables and words, including onsets, rimes, and individual phonemes.

The intrasyllabic structure of a word in the English language can be distinguished on the basis of naturally occurring onset-rime units within a syllable (Anthony and Lonigan, 2004; Treiman et al., 1995). *Onset* refers to the consonant or consonant cluster that precedes the vowel in a syllable, whereas the *rime* encompasses the vowel and any subsequent consonants. For example, the onset of the word *hog* is "h" and the rime is "og." Likewise, the onset of *stripe* is "str" and the rime is "ipe." Studies have shown that the onset and rime compose natural boundaries governing the internal structure of the syllabic unit (Treiman and Zukowski, 1990).

With these terms in mind, *phonological awareness* describes a cluster of skills that includes an individual's awareness of the syllabic structure of words as well as the intrasyllabic structure; the latter includes attending to the onset and rime units within syllables and, at a more advanced level, recognizing that onset and rime units are composed of individual phonemes. This awareness of a word's phonological structure is *sublexical*, meaning that representation of these units occurs at a level distinct from meaning. This awareness is also viewed as being *metalinguistic* in nature because it requires an individual to focus on language as an object of thought. Phonological awareness is contingent on and mediated by the child's access to the phonology of his or her language (Wagner and Torgesen, 1987).

Other terms, such as *phonological processing, phonemic* and *phoneme awareness, phonological sensitivity, phoneme analysis, phonetic awareness,* and *linguistic awareness,* have been used more or less interchangeably with the term *phonological awareness.* Some scholars use the term only in reference to awareness at the level of the phoneme. Ball and Blachman (1991), for instance, describe phonological awareness as one's ability to represent spoken words and syllables as discrete sequences of individual sound segments at the level of the phoneme. In emphasizing only that level at which conscious, explicit awareness of phonemes is exhibited, this restricted use of the term *phonological awareness* does not encompass more implicit levels of sensitivity to the phonological structure of language (e.g., sensitivity to syllables and rime units in words). A more encompassing perspective of phonological awareness includes reference to skills ranging along a continuum of shallow to deep levels of awareness (Anthony et al., 2003; Stanovich, 2000).

Shallow Levels of Awareness

At more shallow levels of phonological awareness, children show sensitivity to the sound patterns that recur across and within words. At these levels, children may recognize, for instance, that the words *bell* and *tell* demonstrate certain phonological similarities (i.e., these words rhyme), and that *bell* can be divided into two components (i.e., its onset and rime: *b + ell*). They are also likely to be able to blend and segment multisyllabic words (e.g., *doorbell = door + bell, pancake = pan + cake*) and to identify when words share the same singleton onsets (e.g., *me* and *moon*).

Deep Levels of Awareness

At the opposite end of the continuum representing deeper levels of sensitivity, children demonstrate more conscious levels of awareness regarding the phonological structure of a word or syllable. With access to deeper levels of sensitivity, children are able to compare, contrast, and even manipulate phonological segments within and across syllables and words. For example, they can delete phonemes in words to create new words (such as deleting the first sound in the word *track* to create *rack*) and can count the number of sounds in individual words. Phoneme awareness is fully realized when children can recognize that each word or syllable consists of a series of discrete phonemes and can explicitly identify, blend, and segment these phonemes. A number of scholars have used the terms *phonemic* and *phoneme awareness* in reference to this sophisticated level of awareness.

A Developmental Perspective

Recognizing that the development of phonological awareness occurs along a continuum is consistent with the perspective that children's attainment of phonological awareness is developmental in nature (Stanovich, 2000). In general, children's development of phonological awareness follows a continuum along which they gain sensitivity first to words followed by syllables, onset/rimes, and then phonemes (Anthony et al., 2003; Lonigan et al., 2009). A considerable body of research supports a developmental trajectory in the growth of phonological awareness in both English and other alphabetic languages (Anthony et al.; Ziegler and Goswami, 2005). Some researchers use the term *quasi-parallel progression* to emphasize how children's sensitivity to words, syllables, onset/rimes, and phonemes emerges in overlapping rather than discrete stages (Anthony et al.). That is, children are developing awareness of onset/rimes simultaneously to developing awareness of phonemes although they might be closer to mastery for the former. Understanding the quasi-parallel nature of phonological awareness development suggests that children need not "master" one ability (e.g., rhyming) before another (e.g., identifying initial sounds in words). Both language abilities and experiences highly mediate children's growth in phonological awareness (Lonigan, Burgess, Anthony, and Barker, 1998; Stahl and Murray, 1994). In particular, growth in vocabulary development and letter knowledge are considered influential variables on children's early phonological awareness development during the preschool years (Burgess and Lonigan, 1998).

PHONOLOGICAL AWARENESS AS LITERACY DEVELOPMENT

Phonological awareness has often been studied within the context of children's literacy development. Although children's ability to represent and manipulate the phonological structure of words consciously is highly mediated by their linguistic abilities and experiences, the fundamental (and potentially causal) role that phonological awareness plays in reading development has encouraged many scientists and practitioners to study phonological awareness within the framework of literacy development. The term *literacy* is used here in a general sense to describe children's attainment of both emergent and conventional literacy skills; *emergent literacy* refers to skills and knowledge serving as prerequisites to reading and writing, whereas *conventional literacy* refers to fluent and skilled reading and writing.

More specifically, emergent literacy describes precursory reading and writing skills that are acquired by most children within the preschool and early kindergarten period. These skills lay the foundation for later skilled and fluent reading (van Kleeck, 1998). The two primary domains of development within this preliterate period are print knowledge (knowledge about forms and functions of written language; Justice and Ezell, 2004) and phonological awareness. Children's development of both print knowledge and phonological awareness is viewed as legitimate and critical elements of literacy development (Whitehurst and Lonigan, 1998) and provide the foundation for their eventual attainment of conventional literacy. To this end, preschool children with sophisticated levels of print knowledge and phonological awareness are more likely to develop into proficient conventional readers and writers as compared to preschoolers with low levels of awareness (Badian, 2000; Christensen, 2000; Storch and Whitehurst, 2002). Conventional literacy is typically acquired within the context of formal instruction, usually beginning in late kindergarten and first grade, or at about 6 to 7 years of age.

Historical perspectives of literacy development took the view—in both theoretical and practical terms—that children's acquisition of literacy skills began with formal literacy instruction. Relatively recently, researchers began to study literacy development in very young children and found that preschool children as young as 2 and 3 years of age possess considerable knowledge about reading and writing. A substantial number of researchers in the last two decades have described what young children know about literacy as well as determining how this knowledge is mediated by linguistic, cognitive, and environmental influences (e.g., Justice, Pence, Bowles, and Wiggins, 2006; Storch and Whitehurst, 2002). Across numerous studies of literacy development in young children, a single set of variables—those representing phonological awareness—has stood out in terms of its robust value in predicting reading achievement (e.g., Hogan, Catts, and Little, 2005; Torgesen, Wagner, and Rashotte, 1994). Awareness of the phonological structure of spoken language helps children decode printed text, recognize words in print, and spell words (see Gillon, 2004, for a review).

THE DEVELOPMENT OF PHONOLOGICAL AWARENESS

Serendipitously, the first author overheard the following conversation between a father and his son (who appeared to be about 4 years old) during the preparation of this chapter. The conversation took place in a local bookstore where father and son were looking at the cover of a magazine.

SON: Is that a butterfly?
DAD: Yes, that's a butterfly.

Son: But-ter-fly. Hey Dad, is *but* a word?

Dad: Yes, *but* is a word.

Son: Is *ter* a word?

Dad: No, *ter* is not a word.

Son: Is *fly* a word?

Dad: Yes, *fly* is a word.

Son: Dad, is *ter* a word?

Dad: Didn't we just go through this?

This dialogue provides a perfect preface to a brief discussion of how young children gradually acquire the ability to analyze words into smaller components. In this particular instance, the child decomposed a multisyllabic word at the level of the syllable; the conversation suggests that the child was trying to make sense of how these smaller units (i.e., the syllables) fit into his existing knowledge of language structure (e.g., Are these smaller units words? Do these smaller units carry meaning?).

As we previously noted, children's development of phonological awareness occurs on a continuum representing a hierarchy of sensitivity to the linguistic units that compose words (Hempenstall, 1997). The order of the linguistic units to which children become increasingly sensitive appears to be based on the size of the unit (Treiman and Zukowski, 1996). Children's early sensitivity to larger units, such as syllables and rime units, represents shallow levels of awareness, whereas later sensitivity to phonemes represents deep or higher levels of awareness (Burgess and Lonigan, 1998). Evidence for this developmental continuum comes from a substantial literature base indicating that sensitivity to syllable structure occurs considerably earlier than sensitivity to phonemes (e.g., Anthony et al., 2005; Lonigan et al., 1998, 2009). Boys and girls show similar patterns of early phonological awareness development, but children from middle-income backgrounds demonstrate stronger phonological awareness knowledge at 4 and 5 years of age compared to children from lower-income backgrounds (Lonigan et al., 1998). A plausible explanation for the socioeconomic differences observed is the quality of the language and literacy environments these children are exposed to in their early years.

Awareness of Rhyme

Sensitivity to rhyme is often viewed as one of the earliest benchmarks in the growth of phonological awareness because awareness of rhyme is contingent on one's ability to represent words as discrete units that can be analyzed on a distinctly phonological basis (Bryant, MacLean, and Bradley, 1990). The ability to detect and produce patterns of rhyme across words observed in children as young as 2 years of age has been viewed as a critical entry point in the development of phonological awareness (Hempenstall, 1997).

Sensitivity to rhyme begins to emerge in some children not long after they exhibit productive use of oral language. Large-scale laboratory studies of early phonological awareness development suggest that some children can perform above chance level on tasks tapping rhyming knowledge as young as 2 years, and the percentage of children demonstrating rhyming knowledge rapidly increases with age. Laboratory findings have been supported by more naturalistic observations of spontaneous use of rhyme by preschool children. Dowker (1989) elicited poems from 133 children, ages 2 to 6 years. Many of the children's poems exhibited rhyme, even those of the youngest children: 32 percent of the poems produced by children under 3 years of age exhibited rhyming patterns as compared to 46 percent of 6-year-old children. The majority of children from middle-income backgrounds can show competency on simple rhyming tasks by age 5. Table 12.1 provides examples of the performance of various age groups on some common tasks used to evaluate young children's awareness of or sensitivity to rhyming words.

Awareness of Syllables

Initially, children begin to recognize that multisyllabic words can be segmented at the level of the syllable (e.g., that *butterfly* can be broken into three parts). Usually around 4 years of age, children begin to exhibit explicit awareness of syllabic distinctions within multisyllabic words (i.e., that *hotdog* can be readily divided into *hot* and *dog*, or that *baby* can be segmented into *ba-by*) (see Table 12.1). Subsequently, children show increased sensitivity

TABLE 12.1   Examples of Research Findings Concerning Phonological Awareness Proficiency in Young Children

Task	Example	Age Group	Proficiency	Reference
Syllable counting	"How many syllables are in the word *puppy?*"	4 years 5 years	50% of children successful 90% of children successful	Moats, 2000
Rhyme matching	Which word rhymes with *sail: nail* or *boot?*	2 and 3 years 4 and 5 years	Average: 52% accuracy Average: 70% accuracy	Lonigan, et al. 2009
Rhyme oddity	Which word does not rhyme: *sail, nail, boot?*	2 and 3 years 4 and 5 years	Average: 38% accuracy Average: 48% accuracy	Lonigan, et al. 2009
Rhyme production	What rhymes with *boot?*	3 years	35% could generate at least one rhyming word	Chaney, 1992
Alliteration oddity	Which word does not start the same: *bed, hair, bell?*	3 years	Low- and middle-income groups: 9% scored above chance level*	Lonigan et al., 1998
		5 years	Middle income: 49% scored above chance* Low income: 13% scored above chance	
Phoneme elision (deletion)	Say *time* without saying /m/	3 years	Low- and middle-income groups: Less than 11% scored above zero	Lonigan et al., 1998
		5 years	Middle income: 72% scored 1 or more correct Low income: Only 7% scored 1 or more correct	

*Indicates the percentage of children within that age group whose accurate rate significantly exceeded what would be expected by chance.

to distinctions within intrasyllabic units. Specific patterns govern children's growth in sensitivity to intrasyllabic units within the syllable. In the early stages of sensitivity to syllable structure (when children are not yet perceiving phonemes as the basic linguistic unit), children show more facility in segmenting syllables into onsets and rimes when onsets occur as singleton consonants rather than consonant clusters (Treiman, 1983). For instance, children are more likely to be able to segment *tar* into an onset and rime as compared to *star*. Sensitivity to the onset-rime distinction appears to facilitate children's phoneme awareness, providing the framework for word and syllable analyses at the level of the phoneme

Awareness of Alliteration

Alliteration describes the sharing of a phoneme across two words or syllables, such as *bad* and *big*. Sensitivity to alliteration is also an early indicator of the advent of phonological awareness. By age 3, a few children begin to show sensitivity to alliteration across words, and by age 5, many children from advantaged backgrounds demonstrate this level of phonological awareness (see Table 12.1).

Dowker (1989) described the propensity toward alliteration by very young children in a naturalistic study of phonological awareness of young children. Examining the elicited poems of children ranging from 2 to 6 years of age, Dowker found that even 2-year-old children used alliteration with some frequency in their poems (27 percent of her 2-year-old sample used alliterative devices).

Children are more proficient at comparing and contrasting initial phonemes across two words if the words share a common vowel, such as *cup/cut* versus *cup/cat;* the identification of a similarity across the latter pair would be more difficult (Kirtley et al., 1989). In addition, children show substantially greater performance at comparing and contrasting final phonemes across syllables or monosyllabic words if the two words share a common vowel (in other words, the two words share a rime or rhyme; Kirtley et al.). For instance, children are much better at identifying a final phoneme commonality for *map* and *tap* than for *map* and *tip*.

Awareness of Phonemes

Phoneme awareness—the ability to identify phonemes as the units comprising syllables and words—is not exhibited with mastery by many children until about 6 or 7 years of age (Ball, 1993) although Lonigan and colleagues (1998) found that 5-year-old children from advantaged backgrounds could complete at least 1 item successfully on a phoneme-deletion task (see Table 12.1). Phoneme awareness comprises two areas of growth: phoneme segmentation (analysis or elision) and phoneme blending (or synthesis) (Torgesen, Morgan, and Davis, 1992). *Phoneme segmentation* is the ability to sequentially isolate all the individual sounds in a syllable or word or to segment (elide) a sound from a word or syllable. Using the word *pond,* for example, a phoneme segmentation task requires a child to break the word into its component phonemes and express those four phonemes in sequence: /p/ . . . /ɑ/ . . . /n/ . . . /d. In contrast to phoneme segmentation, a *phoneme-blending* task involves the ability to take a sequence of phonemes and build them into a larger linguistic unit. A task in this area would involve presenting a series of four phonemes (in the case of pond, /p/, /ɑ/, /n/, and /d/) and asking the child to combine the sounds into a word. Skills in both phoneme segmentation and blending are critical requisites for learning to read.

There is a developmental trend in children's performance on phoneme segmentation and blending tasks. In general, performance on phoneme-blending tasks is superior to that on segmentation and elision tasks (e.g., Lonigan et al., 2009). Phoneme segmentation and manipulation skills are highly mediated by the complexity of the linguistic units being analyzed. Segmenting simple consonant-vowel-consonant (CVC) words is much easier that segmenting words with blends (e.g., CCVC words) (Treiman, 1983).

Phoneme awareness requires children to have acquired adequate representations of phonemes as the discrete elements of syllables and words (Nittrouer, 1996); that is, to engage in phoneme awareness tasks, children must have a well-developed phonological system comprising robust representations of the phonemes within their language. In fact, examining children's abilities to manipulate phonemes demonstrates the depth and robustness of their phoneme representations. In their seminal work, Calfee, Lindamood, and Lindamood (1973) examined the attainment of relatively sophisticated levels of phoneme awareness in a study of 660 children from kindergarten through 12th grade. These researchers asked children to manipulate colored blocks representing the phoneme arrangements of nonsense syllables. Although children showed gradual improvement on phoneme manipulation across the grades, 12th-grade students showed only about 60 percent accuracy on complex tasks. Although these students undoubtedly were able to produce phonemes accurately, their receptive performance showed that mastery was elusive in more advanced tasks of phoneme awareness. Such findings indicate that although young children gradually increase their ability to represent words as discrete phonemes, the ability to manipulate words at the phoneme level requires more advanced representational skills. Some children (particularly if they are poor readers) may never acquire proficiency on complex phoneme manipulation tasks.

PHONOLOGICAL AWARENESS DEVELOPMENT AND READING

There is considerable overlap between children's development of phonological awareness and learning to read. However, we must note that there is controversy regarding the nature of the relationship between phonological awareness and reading instruction (Johnston, Anderson, and Holligan, 1996; Morais, Cary, Alegria, and Bertelson, 1979; Vandervelden and Siegel, 1995). Some researchers contend that reading development is driven by phonological awareness, particularly at the phoneme level, a view that asserts a causal relationship between phoneme awareness and reading ability. Research demonstrating that performance on phoneme segmentation and phoneme-blending tasks is a strong predictor of early reading development supports this position (see Christensen, 1997). Other researchers assert that phoneme awareness and reading skill develop in a reciprocal, rather than causal, manner. Evidence showing that phonological awareness increases reciprocally and concomitantly with reading proficiency provides support for this argument (see Stanovich, 2000). A position representing both perspectives is that a certain level of phonological awareness is required for the development of reading skill but that phoneme awareness and reading ability subsequently develop in a reciprocal and interrelated manner (Figure 12.1).

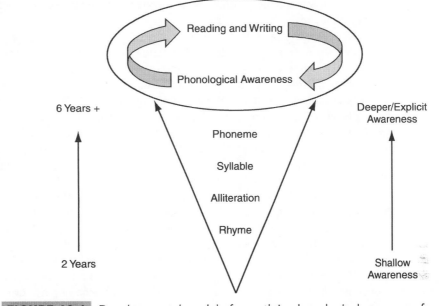

FIGURE 12.1 Developmental model of growth in phonological awareness from early childhood to the number of years of schooling.

Bradley and Bryant (1983) were among the first researchers to demonstrate a relationship between phonological awareness at a preschool age and subsequent reading performance. In their seminal work, they tested the ability of 403 children ages 4 and 5 to categorize sounds—that is, their skills in determining which word of three or four words presented did not share a common initial phoneme (e.g., *hill, pig, pen*). This measure of children's sensitivity to alliteration accounted for a significant and substantial proportion of variance in these children's reading skills 3 years later. O'Connor and Jenkins (1999) reported similar findings. In their study, measures of phonological awareness (e.g., initial sound identification, rhyme production, phoneme segmentation) collected at kindergarten predicted differences in reading achievement at the end of first grade and identified children who would later have a reading disability.

The relationship between phonological awareness and reading is best understood by considering the skills that are most critical for the beginning reader. Faced with the task of decoding a novel word, the novice reader must know the distinguishing features and names of alphabet letters in the word and must know its phoneme structure. In addition, and most importantly, the novice reader must bridge these two areas of knowledge by recognizing the systematic relationships between letters and phonemes (Hulme et al., 2007). Skill in recognizing and using the systematic correspondence between letters and phonemes is usually referred to as *phonological recoding* (Vandervelden and Siegel, 1995) or *phonological recoding in lexical access* (Wagner and Torgesen, 1987). The successful integration of these two areas of knowledge allows the child to decode novel words. Children with limited awareness of letter names and/or deficits in phoneme awareness are prone to difficulties in reading (Stanovich, 1986).

Stahl and Murray (1994) sought to determine the amount of phonological awareness necessary for a beginning reader to negotiate novel words. These researchers found that the ability to represent onset-rime distinctions and to isolate phonemes at the beginning and end of words were prerequisites for beginning reading. In other words, children who did not have these requisite abilities were unable to achieve or surpass preprimer instructional levels. These findings emphasize the importance of intrasyllabic awareness over word and syllable awareness to reading development (see Gillon, 2004) and converge with other reports showing that phoneme awareness skills exhibit a stronger predictive relationship with reading than rhyme awareness skills (Christensen, 1997, 2000; Muter, Hulme, Snowling, and Stevenson, 2004).

For children who are already readers, phoneme awareness ability reliably distinguishes between children who are proficient at reading and those who are struggling (Catts, Fey, Zhang, and Tomblin, 2001; Muter, Hulme, Snowling, and Stevenson 2004). In a seminal study, Calfee, Lindamood, and Lindamood (1973) found that many older and struggling readers show consistent deficits in their ability to represent and manipulate words at the phoneme level. For instance, fifth-grade students who were struggling readers performed phoneme manipulation tasks with about 37 percent accuracy as compared to about 80 percent accuracy for peers who were above-average readers. Stanovich (2000) referred to this phenomenon as the *Matthew effect*—such that "the poor get poorer and the rich get richer"—in that the gap separating children who are proficient readers from those who are failing gets larger over time.

In a classic study following a group of 54 children from first through fourth grades, Juel (1988) supported this contention. Juel found remarkable stability in reading achievement across these grades: "The probability that a child would remain a poor reader at the end of fourth grade, if the child was a poor reader at the end of first grade, was .88" (p. 440). In other words, children who experienced reading failure in first grade continued to experience failure in the next three grades. Deficits in phoneme awareness were important explanatory variables in distinguishing children who failed at reading from those who experienced success. At entry to first grade, children who subsequently experienced reading failure showed no skills in segmenting words into phonemes and analyzing words on the basis of phoneme properties. Such findings implicate the strong and reciprocal relationship between deficits in phonological awareness and the circumstances surrounding reading failure.

PHONOLOGICAL AWARENESS AND SPEECH SOUND DISORDERS

Let us now turn to considering the relationship between phonological awareness and disorders of speech production. Among typically developing children, relationships exist between speech production performance and phonological awareness (Foy and Mann, 2001; Mann and Foy, 2007) with increased speech sound errors being associated with lower scores on measures of phonological awareness. Neurocognitive research also supports this link, showing that reading utilizes areas of the brain that are initially developed for speech production during the preschool years (Frost et al., 2009). It makes sense, then, that children with speech sound disorders face increased risks for experiencing difficulty in phonological awareness and subsequent reading and spelling impairment (for a review, see Schuele, 2004). This does not mean, however, that all children who exhibit speech sound problems will have literacy difficulties. Children with speech production problems specific to deficits in phonological rules are most prone to experiencing difficulties with phonological awareness and reading. We refer to these children as having a *phonological disorder* (*PD;* Schuele). Children with PD often have multiple speech sound production errors and compromised intelligibility. They may or may not have concomitant language difficulties in other domains (e.g., vocabulary, grammar). The speech sound difficulties of children with PD tend to be more pronounced than those of children with articulation problems who might exhibit distortions or substitutions of a relatively small set of sounds. As mentioned earlier in this book, phonological disorder is often conceptualized as a cognitive-linguistic disorder rather than an articulatory or motoric disorder, resulting from underspecified or faulty phonological representations. For some children at least, difficulties with phonological development affect both expression (a speech sound production problem) and reception (a phonological awareness problem).

Children with PD, as a group, face an elevated risk for phonological awareness impairment, particularly when this is accompanied by more widespread language difficulties (Bird, Bishop, and Freeman, 1995; Catts, Fey, Tomblin, and Zhang, 2002; Larrivee and Catts, 1999; Snowling, Bishop, and Stothard, 2000). However, even having a phonological disorder in isolation is linked with early reading difficulties (Nathan, Stackhouse, Goulandris, and Snowling, 2004), and the presence of phonological awareness weakness in preschool children with speech disorders is independent of whether these children have language impairment (Rvachew, Ohberg, Grawburg, and Heyding, 2003). Factors such as genetic risk and low socioeconomic status will also increase these children's risk for reading difficulties (Chatterji, 2006; Lewis et al., 2006; Samuelsson et al., 2007).

Phonological awareness difficulty in preschool-aged children with speech sound disorder can interact with other important cognitive variables in determining their reading ability. Peterson, Pennington, Shriberg, and Boada (2009) concluded from their follow-up study of preschool children with speech sound disorder that phonological awareness interacts with children's syntactic oral language ability and nonverbal IQ in determining reading performance at 8 years of age. The "multiple deficit hypothesis" that literacy outcome in children with speech sound disorder is determined by a complex interaction between risk and protective factors is consistent with research evaluating potential genetic influences on comorbidity in speech disorder (Lewis et al., 2011).

Understanding the nature of children's speech difficulties may also be important for understanding their risk for literacy problems, including difficulties in phonological awareness (Dodd, 2005; Schuele, 2004). Children with speech production problems that are articulatory rather than phonological in nature may not display difficulties in attaining phonological awareness (Bishop and Adams, 1990; Catts, 1993; Levi, Capozzi, Fabrizi, and Sechi, 1982). Catts, for instance, found that first-graders with disorders of articulation performed similarly to a comparison group of typically developing peers on a variety of phonological awareness tasks. Children whose speech production problems are phonological in nature and accompanied by language difficulties (PD + language) face the greatest risks for failing to achieve good phonological awareness and, by extension, skilled reading (Lewis, Freebairn, and Taylor, 2000). By some estimates, nearly 50 percent of these children (PD + language) will fail to be good readers by third or fourth grade. These estimates suggest that growth in phonological awareness and reading achievement needs to be diligently tracked for children with PD, particularly those youngsters who exhibit concomitant language problems.

The nature of children's speech errors has also been found to influence phonological awareness (and literacy) development within groups of children with PD (Dodd, 2005; Preston and Edwards, 2010; Rvachew, Chiang, and Evans, 2007). Preston and Edwards found that the use of atypical speech errors predicted unique variance in phonological awareness (i.e., beyond that predicted by vocabulary and age) in 43 preschoolers with PD. Similarly, Rvachew, Chiang, and Evans reported that preschool children with PD who exhibited atypical segmental errors were more likely to perform poorly on phonological awareness testing than children with PD marked by typical speech errors. Children with childhood apraxia of speech are another group of children who exhibit atypical speech errors, among other risk factors for literacy impairment, and who are likely to experience phonological awareness deficits (Gillon and Moriarty, 2007; Marquardt, Sussman, Snow, and Jacks, 2002; McNeill, Gillon, and Dodd, 2009).

Bird, Bishop, and Freeman (1995) assert that problems in phonological awareness for children with PD can be attributed to their inability to master the phonological system, which translates into difficulties representing the phonological structure of language in both expression (i.e., speech intelligibility) and awareness tasks. These children have particular difficulties perceiving phonemes as the basic phonological building blocks of syllables and are therefore unable to break syllables into phoneme elements (Bird and Bishop, 1992). This hypothesis is supported by a number of studies that have shown that children with PD perform poorly on tasks designed to assess the strength of their phonological representations when compared to their typically developing peers (Anthony et al., 2011; Johnson, Pennington, Lowenstein, and Nittrouer, 2011; Sutherland and Gillon, 2005, 2007). The importance of access to distinct phonological representations to support early literacy development in children with PD exists regardless of the presence of concomitant language delays. Anthony et al. (2011) reported that 3- to -5-year-old children with speech disorder ($n = 68$) exhibited weaknesses in tasks assessing the distinctiveness and accessibility of phonological representations when compared to language (i.e., receptive vocabulary) matched and age matched comparison groups. Furthermore, performance on the phonological representation measures accounted for the phonological awareness and reading deficits also exhibited by the PD group.

Collectively, the research on phonological awareness for children with *phonological disorders* suggests the following conclusions, although further research on this population is warranted to better understand the impact of speech production difficulties on phonological awareness and literacy.

1. Children with phonological disorder are more likely than their peers with typical development to experience difficulties with phonological awareness and literacy achievement. Children who are most at risk for such problems are those whose speech difficulties are still pronounced at the onset of literacy instruction (e.g., kindergarten

and first grade) and who have limited phoneme awareness (Nathan, Stackhouse, Goulandris, and Snowling, 2004).

2. Children with phonological disorder who have concomitant receptive and/or expressive language difficulties are at greater risk than those with phonological disorder alone (Bird, Bishop, and Freeman, 1995; Larrivee and Catts, 1999; Lewis, O'Donnell, Freebairn, and Taylor. 1998).

3. Some children with phonological disorder might evidence problems in acquiring phonological awareness, but these problems do not present challenges to the early development of literacy (Peterson, Pennington, Shriberg, and Boada, 2009). These children may, for example, use strengths in visual memory and semantic or syntactic knowledge to compensate for limited ability to use phonological cues in the reading process (Gillon and Dodd, 2005). However, as demands in the curriculum increase over the elementary period, difficulties in inefficient word decoding as a result of poor phoneme awareness can become evident or more pronounced. Phonological awareness deficits can have their greatest impact on spelling, particularly around third grade and beyond (Clark-Klein and Hodson, 1995).

THE ROLE OF THE SPEECH-LANGUAGE PATHOLOGIST

Internationally, professional associations of speech-language pathology endorse the important and critical role speech-language pathologists should play in promoting phonological awareness (and literacy skills in general), particularly for children who experience communication disorders (American Speech-Language-Hearing Association, 2001; Royal College of Speech & Language Therapists, 2006; The Canadian Association of Speech-Language Pathologists and Audiologists, 2008; Speech Pathology Australia, 2011; New Zealand Speech-Language Therapists' Association, 2011; Irish Association of Speech & Language Therapists, 2011). Language consists of both written and oral dimensions and the role of SLPs does not stop with oral language. Moreover, we must also recognize that phonological abilities represent an important bridge between written and oral language because of the alphabetic principle, which relies on systematic relationships between sounds and letters. Children who experience problems with phonology—whether it manifests itself as a speech production problem—are more likely than other children to struggle with reading. Consequently, if SLPs are to promote children's success in schooling and in life, we must take a broad view toward identifying specific goals for treatment so that we expand beyond the traditional dimensions that only consider children's production of individual speech sounds or use of specific phonological processes. We must carefully study children's underlying sensitivities to the way in which spoken language is organized to ensure that the children are developing phonological awareness in a timely manner.

ASHA (2001) has encouraged SLPs to play a "critical and direct role in the development of literacy for children and adolescents with communication disorders" (p. 3). Primary roles and responsibilities include (1) prevention, (2) identification, (3) assessment, and (4) intervention. See Table 12.2 for an overview of these roles and responsibilities with respect to phonological awareness specifically. We discuss in further detail the SLP's role in assessment and intervention in the next sections.

TABLE 12.2	Roles and Responsibilities of Speech-Language Pathologies for Addressing Phonological Awareness

Role	Responsibility
Prevention	Encourage development of phonological awareness in young children at risk. These activities focus on precluding problems with phonological awareness and so necessarily focus on younger children. Primary focus is on high-frequency engagement of children in naturalistic exposure to phonological properties of oral language (e.g., listening to nursery rhymes).
Identification	Recognize children who are experiencing difficulties in phonological awareness attainment by (1) observing children in phonological awareness activities and (2) educating other professionals on strategies for identifying early problems with phonological awareness.
Assessment	Adopt a speech-language evaluation protocol that includes phonological awareness. Preschool assessment includes rhyme and alliteration awareness and emphasizes informal observation; school-age assessment includes syllable and phoneme awareness and can be accomplished using standardized or criterion-based measures.
Intervention	Implement curriculum-relevant and collaborative interventions that are individualized to target those aspects of phonological awareness that require attention for particular children. Intervention activities are developmentally appropriate following the normal developmental sequence for phonological awareness (e.g., for preschool and kindergarten children, focus first on awareness of rhyme and alliteration and only later target analysis at the level of the syllable and phoneme). For elementary students, training in phonological awareness should be combined with explicit alphabetic principle instruction.

Source: Adapted from American Speech-Language-Hearing Association (2001).

ASSESSMENT

Phonological awareness should be routinely assessed in children with a suspected or identified a speech sound disorder as part of a comprehensive assessment battery. Assessment materials vary depending on the child's developmental stage. The aim of phonological awareness assessment in a 3-year-old child with a speech sound disorder, for example, is not to diagnose the child with a phonological awareness deficit. The wide variability in phonological awareness development in children with typical development at this age would suggest such an assessment aim is inappropriate. Rather, phonological awareness assessment is required in such cases to establish their current levels of awareness and to monitor their growth in phonological awareness over time in response to home and preschool language experiences or specific therapy interventions. In contrast, the assessment aim for a school-age child with speech sound disorder is to profile his or her strengths and needs in phonological awareness. Assessment is also used to ascertain whether deficits in phonological awareness, particularly at the phoneme level, are contributing to any current reading or spelling difficulties and whether phonological awareness is sufficiently well developed for the current demands of the child's reading and spelling curriculum. A phonological awareness assessment is also necessary to track the effects of phonological awareness intervention so that its effects can be documented.

A range of phonological awareness assessment tasks, including norm-referenced and criterion-referenced measures as well as dynamic assessment, can be implemented.

Norm-Referenced Measures: Preschool Years

Several norm-referenced measures for assessing phonological awareness in preschool children are available. When considering the use of such tools, the clinician needs to consider the normative sample used for developing the instrument and its relevance to the child being assessed. Early language and preschool experiences influence a child's phonological awareness development. In some early education environments, children receive extensive and explicit guidance in letter-sound knowledge (e.g., the sound /g/ goes with the letter *G*) whereas in other educational facilities, the focus could be on rhyme and letter naming with little attention directed at facilitating other levels of phonological awareness or print knowledge. Thus, children's performance on phonological awareness tasks is likely to be influenced by early instructional methods that can vary across different educational settings. The use of local norms for phonological awareness skill development could be one strategy to help reduce this problem. However, given the general pattern of consistency in phonological awareness development that is evident across countries and across alphabetic languages, norm-referenced assessments with strong psychometric properties can provide a useful guide against which to compare phonological awareness development in preschool and kindergarten children with phonological disorder.

It is also important that the clinician consider the type of assessment task(s) included in measures designed for young children. Many measures were not designed with the child with speech production problems in mind. Consequently, measures that ask children to produce rhyming words, for instance, are nearly impossible to use with children with speech sound disorders. For instance, a rhyming production task might ask children to "produce a word that rhymes with *cat*" and a child with a speech disorder says "tat." If this child uses a fronting pattern, it is hard to know whether the child is saying "tat" or "cat"—for which the latter would not be correct. Likewise, a child with speech production problems who is asked to produce several words that rhyme with *cat* might say "tat, tat, and tat." For a child who represents many initial sounds (e.g., /g/, /k/, /d/, and /t/) with a single phoneme (e.g., /t/), this might be a correct answer, but it is impossible to know. Consequently, measures that rely on receptive tasks (in which the child points, for instance) may provide the most valid approach to assessing phonological awareness in children with speech difficulties. Gillon (2004) provides a comprehensive examination of phonological awareness assessment instruments and their psychometric properties (see also Schuele, Skibbe, and Rao, 2007).

Norm-Referenced Measures: School-Age Children

Several norm-referenced instruments for evaluating phonological awareness in school-age children have been developed in recent years. Table 12.3 provides a summary of several instruments widely used to assess phonological awareness in school-age children. With one exception (Torgesen and Bryant, 2004), these measures use age norms rather than grade norms; thus, one should be cautious when applying these norms to children who are young or old for their grade because their experiences might not be similar to that of age-matched peers. In addition, interpretation must consider that educational experiences in the early elementary years can vary widely across schools. Norm-referenced measures such as these may prove useful in delineating the extent to which a child exhibits phonological

TABLE 12.3 Examples of Norm-Referenced Phonological Awareness Measures	
Measure Name	**Age/Grade Range**
Clinical Evaluation of Language Fundamentals Preschool – 2 (includes phonological awareness subtest) (Wiig, Semel, and Secord, 2004).	3 to 6 years
Pre Reading Inventory of Phonological Awareness (Dodd, Crosbie, McIntosh, Teitzel, and Ozanne, 2003)	4 to 7 years
Test of Phonological Awareness–Second Edition: PLUS (Torgesen and Bryant, 2004)	K to grade 3
Phonological Awareness Test 2 (Robertson and Salter, 2007)	5 to 9 years
Test of Phonological Awareness Skills (Newcomer and Barenbaum, 2003)	5 to 10 years
Clinical Evaluation of Language Fundamentals – 4 (includes phonological awareness subtest) (Semel, Wiig, and Secord, 2003).	5 to 21 years
Comprehensive Test of Phonological Processing (Wagner, Torgesen, and Rashotte, 1999)	5 to 24 years

awareness difficulties compared to a cohort of age-matched peers. They can be particularly useful for identifying children for whom intensive phonological awareness intervention is needed (Heath and Hogben, 2004). With some of these measures, information about potential intervention targets may be gleaned from careful analysis of a child's pattern of performance. However, such targets must also be educationally relevant and developmentally appropriate.

Criterion-Referenced Procedures

Criterion-referenced measures are used to determine a child's performance against a specific criterion (McCauley, 2001). The child's performance is not compared to a cohort of age-matched peers but to a particular local or curriculum-based standard. Several criterion-referenced instruments are available commercially for evaluating phonological awareness (e.g., Lindamood and Lindamood, 1971; Sawyer, 1987). In addition, the research literature also contains several descriptions of useful criterion-referenced tools (e.g., Ball, 1993; Ball and Blachman, 1991; Murray, Smith, and Murray, 2000; Swank and Catts, 1994; Yopp, 1988). These can be used at no cost by clinicians. Dynamic Indicators of Basic Early Literacy Skills (DIBELS; Good and Kaminski, 2002), Phonological Awareness and Literacy Screening (PALS:K; Invernizzi, Meier, Swank, and Juel, 2001), and PALS:1–3 (Invernizzi and Meier, 2002–2003) are frequently used measures in schools that include criterion-based measures of phonological awareness.

Catts, Fey, Zhang, and Tomblin (2001) provide an excellent tool to identify kindergartners who may be at risk for later reading problems. A set of 21 words is presented to the child one at a time (**base**ball, **hair**cut, **Sun**day, **rail**road, **some**time, **re**turn, **a**round, **mo**tel, **al**most, **help**ful, **ba**by, **per**son, **mon**key, **f**at, **s**eat, **sh**out, **t**all, **d**oor, **f**ew, **s**nail, **th**read). For each word, the child is then asked to say the word without the underlined part. Used in combination with measures of oral language ability, alphabet knowledge, processing speed, and maternal education, the researchers were able to identify with a high level of precision those kindergartners in their study most likely to go on to be successful readers.

Computer-administered assessment is also a promising form of criterion-referenced phonological awareness assessment. In a pilot study, Carson, Gillon, and Boustead (2011a) compared computer-based and paper-based phonological awareness assessment for preschool children with typical development ($n = 21$) and children with speech sound disorder ($n = 12$). The researchers found comparable performance across assessment modalities for both groups. The computer-based version was faster to administer, had strong concurrent validity with a standardized phonological awareness measure, and eliminated examiner bias from the assessment process.

The goal of criterion-referenced measures is to determine children's competency in a specific area of phonological awareness, and clinicians can devise their own criterion-referenced tasks to use for screening and diagnostic purposes. These more informal tasks can be used to identify children who are deficient relative to an established criterion, describe children's current level of performance (strengths and needs), delineate intervention goals, document treatment progress, and determine when intervention is no longer warranted.

Dynamic Assessment

Dynamic assessment examines children's performance in response to varying types of cues or prompts provided by the clinician; it offers a method for obtaining a clearer picture of children's underlying competencies as well as their potential for learning new skills (Bain and Olswang, 1995). The goal is to determine how much and what type of assistance is required to encourage higher levels of performance by the child (Justice and Ezell, 1999). Knowledge gained from dynamic assessments can identify children's underlying competencies and their short- and long-term propensity for change.

The use of dynamic assessment in combination with static screening measures may be an important approach to improve the accuracy of early identification of children with phoneme awareness and reading difficulty. Catts et al. (2009) reported floor effects at initial assessment points that led to the overidentification of children at risk of reading disability in an analysis of the performance of 18,667 children in the DIBELS assessment from kindergarten to third grade. The presence of floor effects during assessment that takes place in the early stages of formal literacy instruction is likely because of the limited instructional experience of children at this age. The addition of dynamic assessment measures is preferable for improving the accuracy of screening measures rather than delaying administration until later in the school year because the latter approach is likely to compromise the early intervention of children who are at risk of reading disability.

Spector (1992) described the use of dynamic assessment to determine how much assistance children needed to segment words consisting of two or three phonemes. The dynamic assessment procedure was reported as more useful for predicting children's later phonological awareness and reading skills than were normative or criterion-referenced assessments. Refer to Table 12.4 for a description of this procedure. For each word that a child is asked to segment, the clinician begins with the first prompting. If the child is not successful, subsequent prompts (2 through 7) are given until the child is successful or all seven prompts have been provided. The clinician records the level of prompt necessary for successful segmentation of each word. To interpret the findings, clinicians would be interested in the extent to which a child who needs strong prompts (e.g., prompts 5 through 7) at the outset of the task

TABLE 12.4	Dynamic Assessment Task
Prompt 1	*Listen while I say the word very slowly.* Model slow pronunciation. *Now can you tell me each sound?*
Prompt 2	*What's the first sound you hear in _____?*
	If first sound is correct: *Now can you tell me each of the sounds?*
	If incorrect or no response: *Try to tell me just a little bit of the word.*
	If child still does not isolate first sound, skip Prompts 3 and 4. Go to Prompt 5.
Prompt 3	If child correctly identified first sound but not next sound(s):
	_____ *is the first sound in _____.*
	What sound comes next?
	Now can you tell me each sound?
Prompt 4	*There are 2 [or 3] sounds in _____. What are they?*
Prompt 5	*Watch me.* Model segmentation of word: Place a token in a square as each sound is spoken. Then repeat word as a whole. After demo say the following: *Try to do what I just did.*
	Score response as correct if child can imitate correct segmentation.
Prompt 6	*Let's try together.* Model segmentation of word with child. Work hand-over-hand with child, and ask child to pronounce segments along with you.
	Now try to do it yourself. Do what we just did together.
Prompt 7	Model again with child (as in Prompt 6). *Now try again to do it yourself.*

Source: Spector (1992).

becomes successful with weaker prompts (e.g., prompts 1 through 4) on the later presented words. Cunningham and Carroll (2011) reported that a dynamic phoneme segmentation task (adapted from Spector) provided a more sensitive measure than static assessment of phoneme segmentation and deletion when disentangling age and schooling effects in phoneme awareness development in the first year of schooling.

Children's responses to the various prompts can provide insights into teaching strategies for therapy. Dynamic assessment can thus be used in conjunction with more static evaluation strategies to derive more sensitive profiles of children's phonological awareness development and to determine therapy goals and strategies.

INTERVENTION

Speech-language pathologists who work with preschool and school-age children should give careful attention to phonological awareness in both their assessment and intervention practices. Several effective practice guidelines for phonological awareness instruction can be gleaned from research over the last two decades (Ehri, 2001; Gillon, 2004; Gillon and McNeill, 2009; Torgesen and Mathes, 2000). These practice guidelines stem from findings showing only a small percentage of children (less than 5 percent) would struggle with reading if we rigorously supported literacy development from preschool forward (e.g., Moats, 2000). The SLP should play an integral role in promoting effective practice by collaborating with other specialists, including classroom teachers.

1. For preschoolers and kindergartners, clinicians should provide phonological awareness experiences (and literacy experiences in general) as an integral part of therapy. Attention to phonological awareness can be embedded within speech production activities, and clinicians should work collaboratively with classroom teachers and reading specialists to ensure that classroom curricula provide adequate classroom-based phonological awareness experiences.

2. Children who have not attained adequate levels of performance at the end of kindergarten or the beginning of first grade should be provided small-group intensive intervention that includes phonological awareness instruction as a core objective (Torgesen, 1999).

3. Children for whom small-group instructional intervention is not sufficient should be provided intensive one-on-one instruction; phonological awareness as well as other key reading objectives are addressed (e.g., vocabulary, reading fluency).

Promoting Phonological Awareness in Preschool Children with Phonological Disorders

Speech-language pathologists need to ensure that young children with a phonological disorder whose assessment profile suggests that they are at risk for written language (i.e., literacy) difficulties develop strong phonological awareness. Preliminary evidence suggests that it is possible to *simultaneously* improve both speech and phonological awareness development in children with speech sound disorders (Gillon, 2005; Major and Bernhardt, 1998) and children with concomitant speech and language impairment (for review, see Otaiba, Puranik, Ziolkowski, and Montgomery, 2009, and Tyler, Gillon, Macrae, and Roberta, 2011).

In a longitudinal study, Gillon (2005; Kirk and Gillon, 2007) demonstrated significant benefits for later reading and spelling development by facilitating children's phonological awareness and letter knowledge from children as young as 3 years. In this study, 12 children (mean age 3.5 years) with moderate or severe speech sound disorders enrolled in school at 5 years of age with strong phoneme awareness and emerging letter knowledge following approximately 25 hours of intervention between the ages of 3 and 5 years. The intervention sought to improve speech intelligibility, phoneme awareness, and letter knowledge. Results showed that the children accelerated quickly in reading development and that 80 percent of the group demonstrated above-average reading ability by the end of the first year. In contrast, 60 percent of children in a control group with speech disorder who received intervention to improve speech intelligibility but who did not receive any explicit instruction in phonological awareness showed delayed reading development and poor spelling ability over time.

Other studies have also shown that phonological awareness can be readily facilitated in young children with phonological disorder. Van Kleeck, Gillam, and McFadden (1998) evaluated the effectiveness of a 9-month classroom-based phonological awareness training program for preschool children. Of the 16 children participating in the experimental classrooms, 11 exhibited speech impairment (9 of whom also exhibited language impairment). Over the course of intervention, children participated in approximately 45 minutes of phonological awareness activities daily; the target for the first 12 weeks of the program was rhyming skills, and in the final 12 weeks targets were initial and final phoneme awareness within and across words. The children in the intervention classrooms made significant gains on measures of phonological awareness (e.g., scores on rhyme detection and production tasks nearly doubled) when compared to the control group over the 9-month period. Hesketh, Dima, and Nelson, et al. (2007) showed that phoneme awareness intervention stimulated superior growth in the early phoneme awareness skills of 4-year-old children with speech sound disorders than intervention focused on general language stimulation. However, reading and spelling outcomes were not measured in any of these studies.

Intervention Goals

Although a primary goal of intervention for children with phonological disorder is to improve their speech intelligibility, a secondary goal should seek to facilitate these children's phonological awareness, particularly at the phoneme level. Research evidence suggests that to give preschool children with phonological disorder the optimum chance for reading success, intervention should seek to achieve the following prior to formal literacy instruction or at least by the end of the first year of schooling:

- Resolve or significantly improve the child's speech disorder (and any co-occurring language impairment) (Nathan, Stackhouse, Goulandris, and Snowling, 2004).
- Facilitate phonological awareness, including early developing awareness of phonemes in words (Gillon, 2005; Kirk and Gillon, 2007).
- Facilitate at least some letter sound knowledge and stimulate the child's understanding of the relationship between spoken and written words (Hulme et al., 2007).

Achieving these goals may require relatively intensive periods of intervention during the preschool years, particularly for children with severe speech sound disorder. If such intervention is successful in preventing reading problems in addition to improving speech intelligibility, it will prove both efficient and cost effective.

Intervention Models

Intervention models that involve collaboration between the SLP, teacher, and parents are considered best practice when attempting to improve the phonological awareness of children with speech or language impairment (Roth and Paul, 2006). Thus, literacy skills should be addressed in speech therapy in the classroom and in the home.

Phonological Awareness Instruction Embedded into Therapy

A variety of activities that stimulate phonological awareness and knowledge of letter sounds can be integrated into therapy for preschool children. Many relatively inexpensive manuals can be examined for activity suggestions (Table 12.5). Also, some reputable Internet sites have useful resources, including the University of Virginia PALS website (http://pals.virginia.edu/) and the National Center for Learning Disabilities Get Ready to Read website (www.getreadytoread.org/). Gillon and McNeill's (2007) integrated phonological awareness program and resources for preschoolers with speech sound disorders can

TABLE 12.5 Examples of Published Manualized Programs for Delivering Phonological Awareness Instruction	
Program (Author, Year)	**Program Overview**
Road to the Code (Blachman, Ball, Black, and Tangel, 2000)	44 of 15- to 20-minute lessons in spiral-bound book; organized as an 11-week program (4 lessons per week); appropriate for small groups or one-on-one; recommended for kindergartners and first-graders
Phonemic Awareness in Young Children (Adams, Foorman, Lundberg, and Beeler, 1998)	51 of 15- to 20-minute lessons in spiral-bound book; organized as an 8-month program for kindergartners or 8-week program for first-graders; appropriate for whole class or small groups; includes pre- and posttest assessment tools
The Sounds Abound Program (Lenchner and Podhajski, 1998)	20 lessons and variety of accompanying materials in kit (games, DVD, stickers); organized to provide sequenced classroom-based instruction and supplemental supports for children who struggle; specified for ages preschool to third grade
Sounds Abound: Listening, Rhyming, and Reading (Catts and Olsen, 1993)	Variety of lesson plans for teaching rhyme, alliteration, and phoneme segmenting and blending; appropriate for whole classroom, small groups, or one-on-one; includes pre- and posttest assessment tools

also be freely downloaded online at http://www.education.canterbury.ac.nz/people/gillon/. See also Justice, Kaderavek, Bowles, and Grimm (2005) and Ukrainetz et al. (2000) for details of intervention activities.

Some practical suggestions for embedding phonological awareness into therapy include the following:

1. Write words clearly and in large font underneath stimulus pictures for speech production goals. Specifically draw children's attention to the printed word (rather than the picture) when practicing the speech target words.
2. Regularly employ alliteration activities that ask children to attend to the initial sounds in words; for instance, at the start of therapy, children might have to sort a pile of picture cards into those starting with one sound (e.g., /s/) and those starting with another (/t/).
3. Use an alphabet chart or letter cards to practice target speech sounds and make explicit for the child the link between the letter and the speech sound that it represents.
4. Model segmentation of target speech words that have two or three phonemes, as in: "Let's break the word *key* into its two sounds: /key/. . ./k/. . ./i/. . . . Now you say it just the way I did, /k/. . ./i/."
5. Read storybooks that feature rhyme and alliteration patterns, and explicitly bring the child's attention to these phonological patterns.
6. Ask children to draw pictures associated with their speech production goals and write a word or sentence underneath their picture. Explicitly identify and discuss the letter sound relationships when writing the words.

Written letters and words can serve as visual prompts or reminders of particular speech targets for children. For example, if the child is attempting to say *sun* but says *tun*, the clinician can point to the written word under a picture of the sun and use the initial letter "s" to cue the child: "Oops. You forgot this /s/ sound at the beginning of the word [pointing to the letter s]. Put the /s/ at the beginning." Such activities do not necessarily require that the child understand the alphabetic references to produce accurate speech. Rather, the comments the clinicians make with reference to print and sound structure are provided in addition to the typical cues and prompts used to elicit accurate speech production (e.g., target models, phonetic placement cues). The pairing of letters with their corresponding sounds can provide children extra exposure to the phonological structure of language. Astute clinicians take advantage of teachable moments to scaffold children's attainment of higher levels of phonological awareness.

PHONOLOGICAL AWARENESS EXPERIENCES FOR PRESCHOOL CHILDREN

The SLP can collaborate with children's teachers and parents to help them identify methods they can use to stimulate phonological awareness across the full range of childhood education settings. Teachers and parents can use many of the same activities discussed above for therapeutic techniques. For teachers, however, it might be most important for them to adopt a classroom prereading curriculum that includes systematic and explicit attention to phonological awareness development during the academic year. Lonigan, Farver, Phillips, and Clancy-Menchetti, (2011) evaluated the effectiveness of a literacy-focused curriculum in stimulating phonological awareness, vocabulary, and print knowledge in 739 children across 48 preschools. They also examined the success of two professional development models (i.e., workshop attendance and workshop attendance plus mentoring) to support teacher implementation of the curriculum. Findings showed that children receiving the literacy-focused curriculum outperformed those receiving the comparison curriculum by about one-third of a standard deviation in emergent literacy measures. There was an additional effect of the professional development model with children who attended "mentored" classrooms producing the best scores. Similarly, Justice et al. (2010) examined the effects of introducing a language and literacy focus (including phonological awareness) into the curriculum for preschoolers at risk. Immediately following the intervention, children receiving the additional language-literacy focus exhibited superior emergent literacy skills when contrasted with the comparison group who received only the established curriculum. Brady, Fowler, Stone, and Winbury (1994) showed that the positive effects of an enhanced kindergarten literacy curriculum continued to be exhibited in the reading scores of participants at the end of first grade.

Support for the effectiveness of small-group intervention for preschoolers who have not responded to quality classroom instruction is also growing. Koutsoftas, Harmon, and Gray (2009) reported that a small-group phoneme awareness intervention for 34 low-income preschoolers implemented over 6 weeks was effective for more than 71 percent of participants. Ukrainetz, Ross, and Harm (2009) compared concentrated and dispersed scheduling of small-group phoneme awareness intervention for at-risk kindergarteners. Results showed no difference across the conditions with participants in both groups showing comparable growth in their response to the intervention. It is critical to follow literacy development in at-risk preschoolers who have participated in early phonological awareness intervention, because gains made in preschool might not translate into successful acquisition of later literacy skills (e.g., O'Connor, Arnott, McIntosh, and Dodd, 2009)

Parents and teachers can also benefit from information regarding ways to build phonological awareness in a less formal manner. Suggestions include encouraging parents and teachers to:

1. Read storybooks that include interesting sound patterns (e.g., rhyme, alliteration) with children regularly; draw children's attention to these patterns.
2. Engage children in reciting nursery rhymes together and clap out the beat in the rhymes.
3. Find toys or objects in the house or preschool that start with the same sound and comment on the sounds that are the same. For example: "*Light* and *lid* both start with the /l/ sound. Listen to the /l/ sound at the beginning of these words: *light, lid*. Hear the /l/ sound at the beginning?"
4. Identify the first phoneme in the child's name and family members' names.
5. Clap out the syllables in children's names or segment short names (e.g., *Kim*) into their respective phonemes (e.g., /k/ /ɪ/ /m/).
6. Say words as a series of sounds (e.g., /b/ /ɪ/ /g/) and ask children to guess the word being said.

It is important to remember that the focus of phonological awareness intervention during this preschool period is to facilitate awareness of the sound structure of spoken language, *not to teach skills to mastery level*. The process of learning to read and write following school entry will rapidly develop more advanced levels of phonological awareness and alphabetic knowledge (Perfetti, Beck, Bell, and Hughes, 1987). What is most important for preschool children with a phonological disorder is that their phonological awareness is at a level where they can readily respond to the rigors of formal reading instruction (which typically begins in later kindergarten and early first grade).

Promoting Phonological Awareness in School-Age Children with Speech Sound Disorders

School-age children with speech sound disorders who are experiencing reading and spelling difficulties can require direct and intensive periods of intervention specifically focused at enhancing phonological awareness with the greatest attention focused on facilitating phoneme awareness. Numerous studies indicate that intensive small-group or individual phonological awareness intervention results in improved phonological awareness and reading ability for school-age children who are at risk, children experiencing reading difficulties, and children with speech-language impairments (e.g., Ball and Blachman, 1991; Byrne and Fielding-Barnsley, 1991, 1993, 1995; Dayton and Schuele, 1997; Gillon and Dodd, 1995, 1997; Lundberg, Frost, and Peterson, 1988; Schuele, Paul, and Mazzaferri, 1998; van Kleeck, Gillam, and McFadden, 1998; Warrick and Rubin, 1992; Warrick, Rubin, and Rowe-Walsh, 1993). Ehri and colleagues (2001) concluded from a meta-analysis of 52 controlled research studies that phonological awareness has a statistically significant effect on developing reading accuracy and reading comprehension for children with typical development and children at risk. Interventions that focused at the phoneme level and integrate instruction on letter knowledge have shown the best results for reading development.

Some studies have specifically considered the effectiveness of phonological awareness intervention for school-age children with phonological disorder. Gillon (2000a) demonstrated that 20 hours of structured phonological awareness intervention (Gillon Phonological Awareness Training Programme for Children at Risk; Gillon, 2000b, http://www.education.canterbury.ac.nz/people/gillon/) was successful in accelerating phonological awareness development in 5- to 7-year-old children with speech sound disorders commensurate to the level of their peers. This intervention resulted in significantly superior reading and spelling development that was maintained over time (Gillon, 2002) compared to a control group of children who received other types of speech and language intervention. The phonological awareness intervention also resulted in improvements in speech production. The intervention was administered by an SLP to the child individually twice weekly for a 10-week period, or until 20 hours of intervention had been implemented. The activities predominantly focused at the phoneme level (e.g., phoneme identification, phoneme segmentation, phoneme blending, and phoneme manipulation) and used a variety of materials and games to help maintain the child's interest. The link between the spoken and written form of the word was made explicit for the child in each teaching session through the manipulation of letter blocks to form words.

The inclusion of adequate intervention time appears to be an important factor in determining the outcomes of children participating in therapy designed to simultaneously promote speech and phonological awareness development. Denne, Langdown, Pring, and Roy (2005) evaluated the effects of 12 hours of the Gillon Phonological Awareness program in 5- to 7-year old children with speech sound disorders (versus the recommended 20 hours of intervention). Although participants improved their phonological awareness skills, gains in speech and literacy skills were not exhibited. Additional research is required to determine the optimal service delivery model for providing integrated phonological awareness therapy for children with speech sound disorders.

Intervention Goals

The goals of phonological awareness intervention for school-age children with phonological disorder are to:

1. Enhance phonological awareness development commensurate to that of their peers with typical development
2. Ensure that children have strong phoneme awareness as demonstrated on tasks requiring phoneme segmentation, phoneme blending, and phoneme manipulation
3. Enable children to use phonological knowledge to help understand the relationship between a spoken and written representation of a word
4. Enhance transfer of phonological awareness to the reading and spelling process.

Intervention Models

For school-age children with speech sound disorders, the most prevalent models of phonological awareness intervention are small-group intensive intervention, classroom-based intervention, and integration of phonological awareness goals into conventional therapy.

Small-Group Intensive Phonological Awareness Intervention

Increasingly, elementary schools are organizing small-group instruction focused explicitly on phonological awareness for its kindergartners and first-graders who struggle in this area. Led by a speech-language pathologist (SLP), reading specialist, or other school staff member, children who are identified as at risk for literacy problems meet in small groups of three to six children one or more times per week for small-group sessions. These sessions can focus exclusively on phonological awareness or include attention to other literacy goals as needed (e.g., reading fluency, vocabulary).

A number of available curricula exist for organizing small-group intensive phonological awareness programs. One option is to adopt a general instructional sequence and to increase the frequency and intensity of instruction within the highly individualized context provided by small-group instruction. Two commercially available small-group intensive intervention programs that provide explicit guidelines for implementation and thus can be easily and efficiently implemented are the following: *Road to the Code* (Blachman, Ball, Black, and Tangel, 2000) and the *Intensive Phonological Awareness Program* (Schuele and Dayton, 2000). Torgesen and Mathes (2000) provide a description and critique of additional programs. These programs are recommended for 5- and 6-year-old children. The program provides small groups of about six children instruction several times weekly for an extended period of time (e.g., 4 or 5 months). SLPs, reading specialists, and regular or special educators can provide the instruction.

The program *Road to the Code* (Blachman, Ball, Black, and Tangel, 2000) provides a detailed curriculum for intensive phonological awareness instruction. Lessons are delivered four times weekly in 15-minute sessions for an 11-week period. The program was designed for children who are generally at risk for difficulties in early literacy achievement. The program consists of 44 detailed lesson plans with scripts to guide implementation. Each lesson includes a phonological awareness (e.g., rhyme production), phoneme segmentation, and letter-sound correspondence activity. Investigators indicated that with kindergarten children (e.g., Ball and Blachman, 1988, 1991), this program significantly improved phonological awareness and word decoding skills.

The Intensive Phonological Awareness Program (Schuele and Dayton, 2000) was designed to meet the needs of children with language impairments. Intervention (30-minute) sessions are held three times a week for a 12-week period. Skills that are targeted in 3-week blocks include rhyme, initial sounds, final sounds, and phoneme analysis and synthesis. Thirty-six lesson plans describe activities and provide detailed guidance on teaching strategies. Pilot studies (Dayton and Schuele, 1997; Schuele et al., 2008) have suggested that the program is effective in increasing phonological awareness and word decoding skills in children with language impairment and in a broad sample of kindergartners. However, the efficacy of this program for children with speech impairments still needs to be established.

Classroom-Based Phonological Awareness Instruction

Increasingly, explicit phonological awareness activities are found in the daily activities of kindergarten, first-, and second-grade classrooms. Providing phonological awareness instruction within the classroom can be an efficient and effective means for promoting these skills in all children, including those with speech difficulties (Fuchs et al., 2001; Shapiro and Solity, 2008)

SLPs have a dual role in ensuring the successful implementation of classwide phonological awareness teaching. First, clinicians should review the school's curriculum to familiarize themselves with the way phonological awareness is targeted. In the primary grades of school phonological awareness instruction should be based primarily at the phoneme level and explicitly connect speech and print (Gillon, 2004). SLPs might need to provide supplemental activities if the curriculum does not met this requirement. The clinicians' second role lies in assisting with the successful implementation of an evidenced-based classroom program. A large body of research now shows that teachers tend to have a poor understanding of linguistic structure, including phonological awareness, that limits their ability to provide explicit instruction in these skills (for a review, see Moats, 2009). SLPs can provide professional development and ongoing coaching to support the use of explicit phonological awareness teaching. It is important that this is done in a collaborative manner in which the teacher's knowledge of literacy development is acknowledged and links to other aspects of the classroom curriculum are emphasized.

Preliminary evidence suggests that the implementation of quality literacy curricula by teachers with the appropriate professional support dramatically reduces the number of students who need specialist literacy support. Shapiro and Solity (2008) examined the effects of integrating phoneme awareness and phonics instruction into classwide reading lessons in the first two years of schooling. Following the program, children who received the phoneme awareness instruction ($n = 251$) exhibited superior reading ability, and benefits of the program were maintained at 1 year after completion of the program. Reading difficulty was reported for 5 percent of students in intervention schools versus 20 percent in comparison schools. Similarly, Carson, Gillon, and Boustead (2011b) reported an incidence of reading difficulty of 6 percent in students receiving a classroom-based phoneme awareness program versus 26 percent in students receiving an established curriculum. Refer to Table 12.6 for a summary of the classroom program and professional development support for the Shaprio and Solity study.

Phonological Awareness Integrated into Conventional Speech Therapy

Children with speech sound disorders who appear not to have benefited from classroom or small-group phonological awareness programs or for whom these programs are not available for some reason may require explicit phonological awareness instruction embedded into their (one-on-one or small-group) conventional speech therapy. Clinicians can include activities in every session to stimulate children's awareness at the phoneme level and facilitate their generalization of phonological awareness knowledge in reading and in spelling. Twenty hours of intervention (administered by an SLP twice weekly) has proven effective in ensuring long-term gains from phonological awareness to reading and spelling for children with speech impairment (Gillon, 2002). The phonological awareness intervention may be structured to simultaneously target speech goals and phonological awareness knowledge at the phoneme level. An example of integrating speech targets and phonological awareness for a 6-year-old child is discussed below (see also Gillon, 2004).

TABLE 12.6 Example of Classroom-Based Phonological Awareness Training

Component	Content	Length
Classwide (12 minutes, 3 times per day)	Phoneme blending (synthesizing sounds together to form a word)	2 minutes
	Phoneme segmentation (breaking down a word into its sounds)	2 minutes
	Phonics (letter-sound knowledge)	2 minutes
	Sight-reading	2 minutes
	Application of phonological reading strategies in shared "big-book" reading,	4 minutes
Individual supervised reading	Encouragement of children to use phonological strategies when attempting to decode an unknown word	2–3 times per week
Professional support	Plenary sessions	5 half days
	Regular school visits	Around 4 per term

Source: Adapted from Shapiro and Solity (2008).

Teaching Example

Speech Goal: Reduce speech error pattern of cluster reduction for "st" cluster.

Phonological Awareness Goals: Increase awareness of phonemes in words and make explicit the link between phonemes and graphemes.

Target Speech Words for Lesson: star, sty, stop, step, Stan

Stimulus Items: Picture cards of target speech items with the words printed underneath in large, clear font (e.g., font size 48).

Prompt: Prompt the correct articulation of the target cluster through integrating phonological awareness and letter knowledge. For example, the child articulates the word *star* as *tar* and the clinician prompts: "When you say *tar,* I can't hear the /s/ sound at the beginning [pointing to the letter *s* in the word *star*]. Listen to the /s/ sound at the beginning of the word *star.* Let's try again with the /s/ sound at the beginning *star* [pointing to the letter *s* at the beginning of the word]."

Appendix B provides illustrations of various phoneme awareness activities that can be used to promote children's phoneme awareness. Activities such as these can be readily integrated into conventional therapies focused on speech intelligibility.

Intervention with Older Children

Research suggests that older children can increase their phonological awareness with direct instruction in phonological awareness (Gillon and Dodd, 1995, 1997; Swanson, Hodson, and Schommer-Aikins, 2005; Torgesen et al., 1997). Thus, older children experiencing reading difficulties in combination with phonological disorder could benefit from explicit phonological awareness intervention delivered by the SLP; indeed, deficits in phonological awareness can contribute substantially to many of these children's problems with reading and writing (Preston and Edwards, 2007). In addition, some children who have moved beyond the early elementary grades might never have developed an adequate phonological awareness foundation. Other children might have rudimentary skills but fail to develop more complex phonological awareness skills (e.g., phoneme analysis and synthesis). For some children who have histories of phonologic impairment, this weakness can be most evident in poor spelling ability (Clark-Klein and Hodson, 1995). A thorough multidisciplinary evaluation of reading, writing, and phonological awareness should clarify children's needs (Gentry, 1988; Masterson and Crede, 1999). Subsequently, clinicians can provide systematic instruction with specific goals and activities designed to meet these children's individual needs.

We can expect that explicit phonological awareness intervention that facilitates children's awareness of phonemes in words and facilitates understanding of the link between spoken and written words will lead to improved phonological awareness, reading, and spelling for many children with disorders of speech production. However, continued research is necessary to more clearly understand the relationship between phonological disorder, phonological awareness, and reading development. Of greatest need is to identify treatment approaches that are most effective and efficient for addressing speech difficulties simultaneously with phonological awareness challenges. Of particular importance is identifying a sufficient array of approaches so that children who do not respond adequately to one approach can be provided another. In this regard, the educational outcomes and literacy potential of children who exhibit developmental vulnerabilities in both speech and reading can be maximized.

QUESTIONS FOR CHAPTER 12

1. What are some key indicators of phonological awareness that emerge during the preschool period?

2. What is the relationship between phonological awareness and reading ability?

3. Why are children with expressive phonological disorders at increased risk for problems with phonological awareness?

4. What is the speech-language pathologist's role with respect to phonological awareness?

5. What are specific strategies that the speech-language pathologist can use to promote phonological awareness for preschool-age children?

6. What might a classroom-based or intensive small-group phonological awareness intervention program look like?

Procedures for Teaching Sounds

SPECIFIC INSTRUCTIONAL TECHNIQUES

As a supplement to the establishment procedures presented in Chapter 9, the following methods for teaching sounds are presented. Clinicians must be familiar not only with general approaches to the establishment of phonemes but also with specific suggestions for teaching sounds. Material presented on the following pages represents a potpourri of ideas that may be helpful to those who are beginning to develop a repertoire of techniques for evoking and establishing consonant sounds frequently in error. Sources such as Bosley (1981) and Secord and colleagues (2007) include more extensive instruction for phonetic placement and successive approximation approaches to sound teaching. Clinicians who need word lists, pictures, and/or treatment materials are referred to CD-ROM productions such as *Articulation I: Consonant Phonemes* (Scarry-Larkin, 2001) and materials available from commercial vendors: e.g., *Target Words for Contextual Training,* Secord and Shine, 1997b); *Contrasts: The Use of Minimal Pairs in Articulation Training* (Elbert, Rockman, and Saltzman, 1980); *Phonetic Context Drill Book* (Griffith and Miner, 1979); *Articulation* (Lanza and Flahive, 2000); *Phonological Processing* (Flahive and Lanza, 1998); and *Manual of Articulation and Phonological Disorders* (Bleile, 1995).

Instructions for Correction of an Interdental Lisp

It is important to remember that /s/ may be taught by having the client place his or her tongue behind either the upper teeth or the lower teeth.

1. Instruct the client to protrude the tongue between the teeth and produce a /θ/, and then push the tip of his or her tongue inward with a thin instrument, such as a tongue blade. As a variation, instruct the client to slowly and gradually withdraw the tongue while saying /θ/ and, while still attempting to make /θ/, scrape the tongue tip along the back of the front teeth and upward.
2. Instruct the client to produce /t/ in a word such as tea. Have him or her pronounce it with a strong aspiration after release of the /t/ prior to the vowel. Instruct the client to slowly slide the tip of the tongue backward from the alveolar ridge following a prolonged release. The result should be [ts]. Then prolong the [s] portion of [ts].

3. Instruct the client to say the following word-pairs, pointing out that the tongue is in a similar position for /t/ and /s/.

tea—sea	*teal—seal*	*tell—sell*	*told—sold*	*tame—same*	*tip—sip*
top—sop	*tight—sight*	*too—Sue*	*tub—sub*	*turf—surf*	*till—sill*

4. Instruct the client to open his or her mouth, put the tongue in position for /t/, drop the tip of the tongue slightly, and send the airstream through the passage. The client can sometimes feel the emission of air by placing a finger in front of his or her mouth.
5. Instruct the client to produce /ʃ/ and then retract his or her lips (smile) and push the tongue slightly forward.
6. Instruct the client to say /i/ and blow through the teeth to produce /s/.
7. Insert a straw in the groove of the tongue and have the client blow to produce /s/.
8. Instruct the client to use the following phonetic placement cues:
   a. Raise the tongue so that the sides are firmly in contact with the inner surface of the upper back teeth.
   b. Groove the tongue slightly along the midline.
   c. Place the tip of the tongue about a quarter of an inch behind the upper teeth.
   d. Bring the teeth together.
   e. Direct the airstream along the groove of the tongue toward the cutting edges of the lower teeth.

Instructions for Correction of a Lateral Lisp

1. Position a straw so that it protrudes from the side of the mouth. When a lateral [s] is made, the straw should resonate on the side of the mouth where the airstream is directed. When the straw is inserted into the front of the mouth and a correct /s/ is made, the straw will resonate in the front of the mouth.
2. Direct attention to a central emission of the airstream by holding a feather, a strip of paper, or a finger in front of the center of the mouth, or have the client tap the incisor gently with his or her forefinger while producing [s]. If the sound is being emitted through a central aperture, a break in continuity of the outflow of the breath will be noted. If the sound is being emitted laterally, no break in the continuity of the airstream will be noted. Instructing the client to inhale air and directing his or her attention to the cool sensation from the intake of air can also develop an awareness of central emission. Then instruct the client to exhale the air through the same aperture by which air entered upon inhalation.
3. Instruct the client to put a tongue blade down the midline of the tongue in order to establish a groove for the airstream.
4. Instruct the client to retract the lips sharply and push the tongue forward, attempting to say /s/.
5. Instruct the client to make /t/, holding the release position for a relatively long time, and then retract the lips and drop the jaw slightly. A [ts] should be heard if grooving was maintained properly. Then extend the duration of the [ts], gradually decreasing

the release phase of [t] until /s/ is approximated. Saying a word that ends with /ts/, such as /kæts/ or /lɛts/ might be useful.

Instructions for Production of the /ɝ/

1. Instruct the client to growl like a tiger (grrr), crow like a rooster (r-rr-rr) or sound like a race car (rrr).
2. Instruct the client to lower the jaw, say /l/, and push the tongue back until [ɝ] is produced. One can also move from [n] to [nɚ] or [d] to [dɚ].
3. Instruct the client to produce /l/. Then, using a tongue blade, gently push the tip of the tongue back until the depressor can be inserted between the tongue tip and teeth ridge so that an /ɝ/ is produced.
4. Instruct the client to imitate a trilled tongue plus /ɝ/ sound with the tongue tip on the alveolar ridge. Stop the trill but continue producing /ɝ/.
5. Instruct the client to produce /a/ as in the word *father*. As he or she produces the [a], instruct him or her to raise the tongue tip and blade, arching the tongue toward the palate but not touching the palate.
6. Instruct the client to produce /i/ and then lift and retract the tongue tip to produce /ɝ/.
7. Instruct the client to place the tongue lightly between the incisors as in /θ/ and then retract the tip quickly into the /ɝ/. Instruct the client to keep the tip of the tongue near the alveolar ridge to avoid the intrusion of a vowel sound.
8. Instruct the client to say /z/ and to continue to do so while dropping the jaw and saying /ɝ/.
9. Instruct the client to position the tongue for /d/ and then retract it slightly, at the same time dropping the tongue tip and saying /ɝ/. Other clusters such as /tr/, /θr/, and /gr/ may also be used.
10. Spread the sides of the child's mouth with his or her finger, and then ask him or her to produce a prolonged /n/ and then curl the tongue backward, continuing to make the sound.
11. Contrast pairs of words beginning with /w/ and /r/. This task may make the distinction between these two sounds more obvious for the client who substitutes /w/ for /r/.

   Practice word-pairs might include:

wipe—ripe	*woo—rue*	*wing—ring*	*way—ray*	*wake—rake*
wag—rag	*wail—rail*	*woe—roe*	*weep—reap*	*wed—red*

Instructions for Production of /l/

1. Instruct the client to produce /l/ with the mouth open in front of a mirror.
2. Instruct the client to position the tongue for /l/ and then lower it to produce /a/. Alternate these movements. The result should be [la], [la], [la]. This procedure can be varied by using /i/ and /u/ instead of /a/.

3. Instruct the client to imitate the clinician's singing of the nonsense syllables [leɪ], [li], [laɪ].

4. Using a lollipop, peanut butter, or tongue blade, touch the place on the client's alveolar ridge where the tongue tip makes contact to produce a correct /l/. Then tell the client to place the tongue at that point and say /l/.

5. Instruct the client to pretend that the tongue is one part of a bird's beak and the roof of the mouth is the other part of the beak. Tell him or her to put the tongue directly behind the teeth and move it up and down quickly, as a bird's beak might move when it is chirping, and say /a/.

Instructions for Production of /f/ and /v/

1. Instruct the client to touch the lower lip with the upper front teeth and blow. The breath stream may be directed by placing a feather or strip of paper in front of his or her mouth while /f/ or /v/ is being produced.

2. Instruct the client to say [a], place the lower lip under the edge of the upper teeth, and blow the breath stream between the lip and teeth so that frication is audible.

Instructions for Production of /k/ and /g/

1. Press underneath the posterior portion of the child's chin and ask him or her to say [kʌ] in a whisper as the pressure is suddenly released.

2. Hold the tongue tip behind the lower teeth, using a tongue blade if necessary. Instruct the client to hump the back of the tongue and build up oral pressure. The tongue contact should be released quickly, thus releasing the pressure built up behind the constriction.

3. Instruct the client to imitate the clinician as the clinician pretends to shoot a gun, producing a lingua-fricative, as in [ka].

4. Instruct the client to alternate the raising of the back and front of the tongue in a rocking movement from [k] to [t].

Instructions for Production of /t/ and /d/

1. Instruct the client to press the tongue tip firmly against the upper dental ridge in front of a mirror. Then have him or her quickly lower the tongue; air pressure will be released, producing approximations of /t/ or /d/.

2. Instruct the client to make a /p/. Then ask him or her to place the tongue tip between the lips and again to try to say /p/. This gives the tactual sensation of a stop made with the tip of the tongue but is not the correct position for /t/ or /d/. Finally, instruct the client to make a similar sound with the tongue tip in contact with the upper lip only. Repeat with the tongue tip touching the alveolar ridge.

Activities for Facilitating Phonemic Awareness in School-Age Children

PHONEME IDENTITY

Teach the child to identify the initial sounds in words. Find pictures that start with /s/ (with words written clearly under them). Prompt the child as necessary to articulate each word by "reading" the word under the picture. Ask the child to identify those words that begin with the sound /s/. Initially, introduce distracter items that have wide initial phonological and visual contrasts. An initial set of words might include *star, moon, step, box, Stan, Carl, stop, go, sty,* and *barn.*

After several experiences with the preceding activity, repeat it, but remove the picture stimuli and focus the child's attention on the print. Place words written in a large, clear font in front of the child or on a computer screen and ask the her or him to find the words that start with /s/. A fun alternative is to put the words on the floor (as below) and ask the child to jump onto the words that start with /s/. As the child reads the words aloud, prompt for the correct articulation of the /s/ cluster.

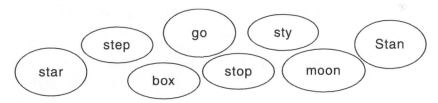

Use the same activity to teach any other initial sounds in words.

PHONEME SEGMENTATION

Teach the child that words can be segmented into phonemes. Use blocks of different colors to represent each sound in a word to help the child understand the concept of segmentation. Require the child to articulate each phoneme using one block for each color.

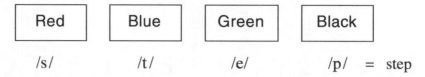

/s/   /t/   /e/   /p/   =   step

The child moves a colored block as she or he produces each sound in a word. This can be repeated for many different words, as in:

Stop: s- t- o- p (4 different colored blocks)

Star: s- t- a- r (3 different colored blocks)

Stan: s- t- a -n (4 different colored blocks)

Sty: s- t- y (3 different colored blocks)

PHONEME MANIPULATION

Similar to the preceding activity, this teaches the child that the phonemes in words can be rearranged to make new words. Colored blocks or cards featuring individual letters can serve this purpose. The child is asked to manipulate phonemes in words to form new words using blocks or cards; encourage the child to articulate each new word and to reflect on the sound change that is being made. Prompt the child as necessary to ensure success and gradually reduce the prompts. Here is an example:

THERAPIST: "If this word says 'top,' show me 'stop.'"

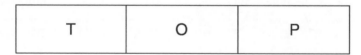

Child adds a new block to the beginning of the word and says, "stop."

THERAPIST: "Now, then, turn "stop" into "tops.""

Child moves the initial block to the end of the word and says, "tops."

SPELLING

Practice spelling target speech words by putting letters into boxes that represent the number of phonemes in the word. Begin by modeling the activity for the child and articulate the phonemes as you write each letter in a box for the child. Repeat the activity and encourage the child to write the letters in each box as she or he segments the word and articulates the phonemes. If the child is unable to write the letters easily, use letter cards or letter blocks to spell the word. Prompt as necessary to ensure success.

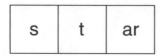

References

Aase, D., C. Hovre, K. Krause, S. Schelfhout, J. Smith, and L. Carpenter, *Contextual Test of Articulation*. Eau Claire, WI: Thinking Publications, 2000.

Acevedo, M., "Spanish consonants among two groups of Head Start children." Paper presented at the convention of the American Speech-Language-Hearing Association, Atlanta, GA, 1991.

Acevedo, M. A., "Development of Spanish consonants in preschool children." *Journal of Childhood Communication Disorders, 15* (1993): 9–15.

Ackerman, J. L., A. L. Ackerman, and A. B. Ackerman, "Taurodont, pyramidal and fused molar roots associated with other anomalies in a kindred." *American Journal of Physical Anthropology, 38* (1973): 681–694.

Adams, M. J., B. R. Foorman, I. Lunberg, and T. Beeler, *Phonemic awareness in young children*." Baltimore, MD: Brookes, 1998.

Adams, P. F., and V. Benson, "Current estimates from the National Health Interview Survey." Hyattsville, MD: National Center for Health Statistics. *Vital Health Statistics, 10*, 181 (1991).

Adams, S. G., "Rate and clarity of speech: An x-ray microbeam study."Unpublished doctoral dissertation, University of Wisconsin–Madison, 1990.

Adams, S. G., G. Weismer, and R. D. Kent, "Speaking rate and speech movement velocity profiles." *Journal of Speech and Hearing Research, 36* (1993): 41–54.

Adler, S., *Cultural Language Differences: Their Educational and Clinical-Professional Implications*. Springfield, IL: Charles Thomas, 1984.

Adler-Bock, M., B. M. Bernhardt, B. Gick, and P. Bacsfalvi, "The use of ultrasound in remediation of North American English /r/ in 2 adolescents." *American Journal of Speech-Language Pathology, 16* (2007). 128–139.

Allen, G., and S. Hawkins, "Phonological rhythm: Definition and development." In G. Yeni-Komshian, J. Kavanagh, and C. Ferguson (Eds.), *Child Phonology*, Volume 1 (pp. 227–256). New York: Academic Press, 1980.

Almost, D., and P. Rosenbaum, "Effectiveness of speech intervention for phonological disorders: A randomized control trial." *Developmental Medicine and Child Neurology, 40* (1998): 319–325.

Amayreh, M., and A. Dyson, "The acquisition of Arabic consonants." *Journal of Speech, Language, and Hearing Research, 41* (1998): 642–653.

Amayreh, M., and A. Dyson, "Phonetic inventories of young Arabic-speaking children." *Clinical Linguistics and Phonetics, 14* (2000): 193–215.

American Speech-Language-Hearing Association, "Social dialects: A position paper." *ASHA* (1983): 23–27.

American Speech-Language, Hearing Association, "Clinical management of communicatively handicapped minority language populations." *ASHA* (1985): 29–32.

American Speech-Language-Hearing Association, "The role of the speech-language pathologist in management of oral myofunctional disorders." *ASHA, 33*, Suppl. 5 (1991): 7.

American Speech-Language-Hearing Association, "Definitions of communication disorders and variations." *ASHA*, Suppl. 10 (1993): 40–41.

American Speech-Language-Hearing Association, "Roles and responsibilities of speech-language pathologists with respect to reading and writing in children and adolescents (position statement, executive summary of guidelines, technical report)." *ASHA,* Suppl. 21 (2001): 17–27.

American Speech-Language-Hearing Association, "Knowledge and skills needed by speech-language pathologists and audiologists to provide culturally and linguistically appropriate services." Rockville, MD: ASHA, 2004a.

American Speech-Language-Hearing Association, "Evidence-Based Practice in Communication Disorders: An Introduction [technical report]." Rockville, MD: ASHA, 2004b.

American Speech-Language-Hearing Association, "Evidence-Based Practice in Communication Disorders [position statement]." Rockville, MD: ASHA, 2005.

American Speech-Language-Hearing Association, "Childhood apraxia of speech [position statement]." Rockville, MD: ASHA, 2007a.

American Speech-Language-Hearing Association, "Childhood apraxia of speech [technical report]." Rockville, MD: ASHA, 2007b.

American Speech-Language-Hearing Association, "Schools Survey: Caseload Characteristics Trends 1995–2008." Rockville, MD: ASHA, 2008.

Anderson, E. E., "Examining conversational prosody and intelligibility in children with cochlear implants." Unpublished master's thesis, Meridian, ID: Idaho State University, 2011.

Anderson, R., "Onset clusters and the sonority sequencing principle in Spanish: A treatment efficacy study." Poster presented at the VIIIth International Clinical Phonetics and Linguistics Association Conference, Edinburgh, 2000.

Anderson, R. T., "Phonological acquisition in preschoolers learning a second language via immersion: A longitudinal study." *Clinical Linguistics and Phonetics, 18* (2004): 183–210.

Anderson, R., and B. Smith, "Phonological development of two-year-old monolingual Puerto Rican Spanish-speaking children." *Journal of Child Language, 14* (1987): 57–78.

Anthony, A., D. Bogle, T. T. S. Ingram, and M. W. McIsaac, *The Edinburgh Articulation Test.* Edinburgh, UK: E. and S. Livingstone, 1971.

Anthony, J., and C. Lonigan, "The nature of phonological awareness: Converging evidence from four studies of preschool and early grade school children." *Journal of Educational Psychology, 96* (2004): 43–55.

Anthony, J. L., C. J. Lonigan, K. Driscoll, B. M. Phillips, and S. R. Burgess, "Phonological sensitivity: A quasi-parallel progression of word structure units and cognitive operations." *Reading Research Quarterly, 38* (2003): 470–487.

Anthony, J. L., R. G. Aghara, M. J. Dunkelberger, T. I. Anthony, J. M. Williams, and Z. Zhang, "What factors place children with speech sound disorders at risk for reading problems?" *American Journal of Speech-Language Pathology, 20* (2011): 146–160.

Aram, D. M., and S. J. Horwitz, "Sequential and non-speech praxic abilities in developmental verbal apraxia." *Developmental Medicine and Child Neurology, 25* (1983): 197–206.

Arlt, P. B., and M. T. Goodban, "A comparative study of articulation acquisition as based on a study of 240 normals, aged three to six." *Language, Speech, and Hearing Services in Schools, 7* (1976): 173–180.

Arndt, W., M. Elbert, and R. Shelton, "Standardization of a test of oral stereognosis." In J. Bosma (Ed.), *Second Symposium on Oral Sensation and Perception* (pp. 379–383). Springfield, IL: Charles C Thomas, 1970.

Arndt, J., and E. C. Healey, "Concomitant disorders in school-age children who stutter." *Language, Speech, and Hearing Services in Schools, 32* (2001): 68–78.

Arnst, D., and D. Fucci, "Vibrotactile sensitivity of the tongue in hearing impaired subjects." *Journal of Auditory Research, 15* (1975): 115–118.

Aslin, R. N., D. B. Pisoni, and P. W. Jusczyk, "Auditory development and speech perception in infancy." In M. M. Haith and J. J. Campos (Eds.), *Infancy and Psychobiology* (pp. 573–687). New York: Wiley, 1983.

August, D., M. Calderón, and M. Carlo, "Transfer of skills from Spanish to English: A study of young learners." Washington, DC: Center for Applied Linguistics, 2002.

Augustyn, M., and B. Zuckerman, "From mother's mouth to infant's brain." *Archives of Disease in Childhood: Fetal and Neonatal Edition, 92,* 2 (2007): F82.

Aungst, L., and J. Frick, "Auditory discrimination ability and consistency of articulation of /r/." *Journal of Speech and Hearing Disorders, 29* (1964): 76–85.

AVAAZ Innovations, Inc. *Speech Assessment and Interactive Learning Systems (Version 1.2)* [computer software]. London, Ontario, Canada: Author, 1994.

Backus, O., "Speech rehabilitation following excision of tip of the tongue." *American Journal of the Disabled Child, 60* (1940): 368–370.

Badian, N. A., "Do preschool orthographic skills contribute to prediction of reading?" In N. A. Badian (Ed.), *Prediction and Prevention of Reading Failure* (pp. 31–56). Timonium, MD: York, 2000.

Bailey, G., and E. Thomas, "Some aspects of African-American Vernacular English phonology." In S. Mufwene, J. Rickford, G. Bailey, and J. Baugh (Eds.), *African American English: History and Use* (pp. 85–109). London: Routledge, 1998.

Bailey, S., "Normative data for Spanish articulatory skills of Mexican children between the ages of six and seven." Unpublished master's thesis, San Diego State University, San Diego, CA, 1982.

Bain, B., and L. Olswang, "Examining readiness for learning two-word utterances by children with specific expressive language impairment: Dynamic assessment validation." *American Journal of Speech-Language Pathology, 4,* 1 (1995): 81–91.

Baker, E., "Changing nail to snail: A treatment efficacy study of phonological impairment in children." Unpublished doctoral thesis, The University of Sydney, Australia. 2000.

Baker, E., "The pros and cons of dummies." *Acquiring Knowledge in Speech, Language, and Hearing, 4* (2002): 134–136.

Baker, E., "The experience of discharging children from phonological intervention." *International Journal of Speech-Language Pathology, 12* (2010a): 325–328.

Baker, E., "Minimal pair intervention." In A. L. Williams, S. McLeod, and R. J. McCauley (Eds.), *Interventions for Speech Sound Disorders in Children* (pp. 41–72), Baltimore, MD: Brookes, 2010b.

Baker, E., K. Croot, S. McLeod, and R. Paul, "Psycholinguistic models of speech development and their application to clinical practice." *Journal of Speech, Language, and Hearing Research, 44* (2001): 685–702.

Baker, E., and S. McLeod, "Evidence-based practice for children with speech-sound disorders: Part 1 narrative review." *Language, Speech, and Hearing Services in Schools, 42* (2011a): 102–139.

Baker, E., and S. McLeod, "Evidence-based practice for children with speech-sound disorders: Part 2 application to clinical practice." *Language, Speech, and Hearing Services in Schools, 42* (2011b): 140–151.

Ball, E., "Assessing phoneme awareness." *Language, Speech, and Hearing Services in Schools, 24* (1993): 130–139.

Ball, E., and B. Blachman, "Phoneme segmentation training: Effect on reading readiness." *Annals of Dyslexia, 38* (1988): 208–225.

Ball, E., and B. Blachman, "Does phoneme awareness training in kindergarten make a difference in early word recognition and developmental spelling?" *Reading Research Quarterly, 26* (1991): 49–66.

Ball, L., "Communication characteristics of children with developmental apraxia of speech." Unpublished doctoral dissertation, University of Nebraska–Lincoln, 1999.

Ball, M. J., and F. Gibbon (Eds.), *Vowel Disorders.* Woburn, MA: Butterworth Heineman, 2001.

Ball, M. J., and R. D. Kent (Eds.), *The New Phonologies: Developments in Clinical Linguistics.* San Diego, CA: Singular Publishing, 1997.

Ball, M. J., and N. Müller, "Sonority as an explanation in clinical phonology." Paper presented at the 9th meeting of the International Clinical Phonetics and Linguistics Association, Hong Kong, 2002.

Bankson, N. W., and J. E. Bernthal, *Quick Screen of Phonology.* Chicago: Riverside Press, 1990a.

Bankson, N. W., and J. E. Bernthal, *Bankson-Bernthal Test of Phonology.* San Antonio, TX: Special Press, 1990b.

Bankson, N. W., and M. Byrne, "The relationship between missing teeth and selected consonant sounds." *Journal of Speech and Hearing Disorders, 24* (1962): 341–348.

Bankson, N. W., and M. C. Byrne, "The effect of a timed correct sound production task on carryover." *Journal of Speech and Hearing Research, 15* (1972): 160–168.

Barbosa, C., S. Vasquez, M. A. Parada, J. C. V. Gonzalez, C. Jackson, N. D. Yanez, B. Gelaye, and A. L Fitzpatrick, "The relationship of bottle feeding and other sucking behaviors with speech disorder in Patagonian preschoolers." *BMC Pediatrics, 9* (2009): 66.

Barkovich, A. J., B. O. Kjos, D. E. Jackson Jr., and D. Norman, "Normal maturation of the neonatal and infant brain: MR imaging at 1.5 T." *Radiology, 166* (1988): 173–180.

Barlow, J. A., "Variability and phonological knowledge." In T. W. Powell (Ed.), *Pathologies of Speech and Language: Contributions of Clinical Phonetics and Linguistics* (pp. 125–133) New Orleans, LA: International Clinical Phonetics and Linguistics Association, 1996.

Barlow, J. A., and J. A. Gierut, "Optimality theory in phonological acquisition." *Journal of Speech, Language and Hearing Research, 42* (1999): 1482–1498.

Barnes, E., J. Roberts, S. H Long, G. E. Martin, M. C. Berni, K. C. Mandulak, and J. Sideris, "Phonological accuracy and intelligibility in connected speech of boys with Fragile X or Down syndrome." *Journal of Speech, Language, and Hearing Research, 52* (2009): 1048–1061.

Bashir, A., F. Grahamjones, and R. Bostwick, "A touch-cue method of therapy for developmental apraxia." *Seminars in Speech and Language, 5* (1984): 127–137.

Bates, E., P. S. Dale, and D. Thal, "Individual differences and their implications for theories of language development." In P. Fletcher and B. MacWhinney (Eds.), *The Handbook of Child Language* (pp. 96–151) Oxford, UK: Blackwell, 1995.

Bauman-Waengler, J., *Articulatory and Phonological Impairments: A Clinical Focus* (3rd ed.). Boston: Allyn and Bacon, 2008.

Behne, D., "Acoustic effects of focus and sentence position on stress in English and French." Unpublished doctoral dissertation, University of Wisconsin–Madison, 1989.

Bennett, B., C. Bennett, and C. James, "Phonological development from concept to classroom." Paper presented at the Speech-Language-Hearing Association of Virginia Annual Conference, Roanoke, VA, 1996.

Berg, T., "Sound change in child language: A study of inter-word variation." *Language and Speech, 38* (1995): 331–363.

Bernhardt, B., "Developmental implications of nonlinear phonological theory." *Clinical Linguistics and Phonetics, 6* (1992a): 259–281.

Bernhardt, B., "The application of nonlinear phonological theory to intervention with one phonologically disordered child." *Clinical Linguistics and Phonetics, 6* (1992b): 283–316.

Bernhardt, B. M., K. D. Bopp, B. Daudlin, S. M. Edwards, and S. E. Wastie, "Nonlinear phonological intervention." In A. L. Williams, S. McLeod, and R. J. McCauley (Eds.), *Interventions for Speech Sound Disorders in Children* (pp. 315–331). Baltimore, MD: Paul H. Brookes, 2010.

Bernhardt, B. H., and J. Stemberger, *Handbook of Phonological Development from the Perspective of Constraint-Based Nonlinear Phonology.* San Diego, CA: Academic Press, 1998.

Bernhardt, B. H., and C. Stoel-Gammon, "Nonlinear phonology: Introduction and clinical application." *Journal of Speech and Hearing Research, 37* (1994): 123–143.

Bernstein, M., "The relation of speech defects and malocclusion." *American Journal of Orthodontia, 40* (1954): 149–150.

Bernstein-Ratner, N., "Interactive influences on phonological behaviour: A case study." *Journal of Child Language, 20* (1993): 191–197.

Bernthal, J. E., and N. W. Bankson (Eds.), *Articulation and Phonological Disorders* (4th ed.). Boston: Allyn and Bacon, 1998.

Bernthal, J. E., and D. R. Beukelman, "Intraoral air pressures during the production of *p* and *b* by children, youths, and adults." *Journal of Speech and Hearing Research, 21* (1978): 361–371.

Bertolini, M. M., and J. R. Paschoal, "Prevalence of adapted swallowing in a population of school children." *International Journal of Orofacial Myology, 27* (2001): 33–43.

Bertoncini, J., and J. Mehler, "Syllables as units in infant speech perception." *Infant Behavior and Development, 4* (1981): 247–260.

Bichotte, M., B. Dunn, L. Gonzalez, J. Orpi, and C. Nye, "Assessing phonological performance of bilingual school-age Puerto Rican children." Paper presented at the annual convention of the American Speech-Language-Hearing Association, Anaheim, CA, 1993.

Biever, A., and D. Kelsall, "Impact of bilateral pediatric cochlear implantation on speech perception abilities in quiet and noise." Paper presented at the 11th International Conference on Cochlear Implants in Children, Charlotte, NC: 2007.

Bird, A., and A. Higgins, *Minimal Pair Cards*. Austin, TX: Pro-Ed, 1990.

Bird, J., and D. Bishop, "Perception and awareness of phonemes in phonologically impaired children." *European Journal of Disorders of Communication, 27* (1992): 289–311.

Bird, J., D. Bishop, and N. H. Freeman, "Phonological awareness and literacy development in children with expressive phonological impairments." *Journal of Speech and Hearing Research, 38* (1995): 446–462.

Bishop, D., and C. Adams, "A prospective study of the relationship between specific language impairment, phonological disorders and reading retardation." *Journal of Child Psychology and Psychiatry, 31* (1990): 1027–1050.

Bishop, M., R. Ringel, and H. House, "Orosensory perception, speech production and deafness." *Journal of Speech and Hearing Research, 16* (1973): 257–266.

Blachman, B., E. Ball, R. Black, and D. Tangel, *Road to the Code: A Phonological Awareness Program for Young Children*. Baltimore, MD: Brookes, 2000.

Blakely, R., *Screening Test for Developmental Apraxia of Speech* (2nd ed.). Austin, TX: Pro-Ed, 2001.

Bland-Stewart, L., "Phonetic inventories and phonological patterns of African American two-year-olds: A preliminary investigation." *Communication Disorders Quarterly, 24* (2003): 109–120.

Bleile, K., "Consonant ordering in Down's Syndrome." *Journal of Communicative Disorders, 15* (1982): 275–285.

Bleile, K. M., "Individual differences." In K. M. Bleile (Ed.), *Child Phonology: A Book of Exercises for Students* (pp. 57–71). San Diego, CA: Singular Publishing, 1991.

Bleile, K. M., *Manual of Articulation and Phonological Disorders*. San Diego, CA: Singular Publishing, 1995.

Bleile, K. M., *Articulation and Phonological Disorders: A Book of Exercises* (2nd ed.). San Diego, CA: Singular Publishing, 1996.

Bleile, K. M., *Manual of Articulation and Phonological Disorders: Infancy through Adulthood* (2nd ed.). Clifton Park, NY: Thomson Delmar Learning, 2004.

Bleile, K. M., *The Late Eight*. San Diego, CA: Plural Publishing, 2006.

Bleile, K. M., "Neurological foundations of speech acquisition." In S. McLeod (Ed.), *The International Guide to Speech Acquisition* (pp. 14–18). Clifton Park, NY: Thomson Delmar Learning, 2007.

Bleile, K. M., and H. Wallach, "A sociolinguistic investigation of the speech of African-American preschoolers." *American Journal of Speech-Language Pathology, 1* (1992): 44–52.

Bloch, R., and L. Goodstein, "Functional speech disorders and personality: A decade of research." *Journal of Speech and Hearing Disorders, 36* (1971): 295–314.

Blood, G. W., and R. Seider, "The concomitant problems of young stutterers." *Journal of Speech and Hearing Disorders, 46* (1981): 31–33.

Bloodstein, O., "Early stuttering as a type of language difficulty." *Journal of Fluency Disorders, 27* (2002): 163–167.

Bock, J. K., "Toward a cognitive psychology of syntax: Information processing contributions to sentence formulation." *Psychological Review, 89* (1982): 1–47.

Bonvillian, J. D., V. P. Raeburn, and E. A. Horan, "Talking to children: The effects of rate, intonation, and length on children's sentence imitation." *Journal of Child Language, 6* (1979): 459–467.

Bordon, G., "Consideration of motor-sensory targets and a problem of perception." In H. Winitz (Ed.), *Treating Articulation Disorders: For Clinicians by Clinicians* (pp. 51–65). Austin, TX: Pro-Ed, 1984.

Bowen, C., "Parents and children together (PACT): Intervention." In A. L. Williams, S. McLeod, and R. J. McCauley (Eds.), *Interventions for Speech Sound Disorders in Children* (pp. 407–426). Baltimore, MD: Brookes, 2010.

Bowen, C., and L. Cupples, "Parents and children together (PACT): A collaborative approach to phonological therapy." *International Journal of Language and Communication Disorders, 34* (1999): 35–83.

Bradford, A., B. Murdoch, E. Thompson, and P. Stokes, "Lip and tongue function in children with developmental speech disorders: A preliminary investigation." *Clinical Linguistics and Phonetics, 11* (1997): 363–387.

Bradley, D., "A systematic multiple-phoneme approach to articulation treatment." In P. Newman, N. Creaghead, and W. Secord (Eds.), *Assessment and Remediation of Articulatory and Phonological Disorders* (pp. 315–335). Columbus, OH: Merrill, 1985.

Bradley, L., and P. E. Bryant, "Categorizing sounds and learning to read—A causal connection." *Nature, 301* (1983): 419–421.

Brady, S., A. Fowler, B. Stone, and N. Winbury, "Training phonological awareness: A study with inner-city kindergarten children." *Annals of Dyslexia, 44* (1994): 26–59.

Braine, M. D. S., *On What Might Constitute Learnable Phonology.* San Diego, CA: College Hill, 1979.

Branigan, G., "Syllabic structure and the acquisition of consonants: The great conspiracy in word formation." *Journal of Psycholinguistic Research, 5* (1976): 117–133.

Branigan, G., "Some reasons why successive single word utterances are not." *Journal of Child Language, 6* (1979): 411–421.

Bressmann, T., R. Sader, T. L. Whitehill, and N. Samman, "Consonant intelligibility and tongue mobility in patients with partial glossectomy." *Journal of Oral and Maxillofacial Surgery, 62* (2004): 298–303.

Broomfield, J., and B. Dodd, "The nature of referred subtypes of primary speech disability." *Child Language Teaching and Therapy, 20* (2004): 135–151.

Bryan, A., and D. Howard, "Frozen phonology thawed: The analysis and remediation of a developmental disorder of real word phonology." *European Journal of Disorders of Communication, 27* (1992): 343–365.

Bryant, P., M. MacLean, and L. Bradley, "Rhyme, language, and children's reading." *Applied Psycholinguistics, 11* (1990): 237–252.

Bryant, T., S. Velleman, L. Abdualkarim, and H. Seymour, "A sonority account of consonant cluster reduction in AAE." Paper presented at the Child Phonology Conference, Boston, 2001.

Burgess, S. R., and C. J. Lonigan, "Bidirectional relations of phonological sensitivity and prereading abilities: Evidence from a preschool sample." *Journal of Experimental Child Psychology, 70* (1998): 117–141.

Burns, F., S. Velleman, L. Green, and T. Roeper, "New branches from old roots: Experts respond to questions about African American English development and language intervention." *Topics in Language Disorders, 30* (2010): 253–264.

Burt, L., A. Holm, and B. Dodd, "Phonological awareness skills of 4-year-old British children: An assessment and developmental data." *International Journal of Language and Communication Disorders, 34*, 3 (1999): 311–335.

Byrne, B., and R. Fielding-Barnsley, "Evaluation of a program to teach phonemic awareness to young children." *Journal of Educational Psychology, 83* (1991): 451–455.

Byrne, B., and R. Fielding-Barnsley, "Evaluation of a program to teach phonemic awareness to young children: A 1-year follow-up." *Journal of Educational Psychology, 85* (1993): 104–111.

Byrne, B., and R. Fielding-Barnsley, "Evaluation of a program to teach phonemic awareness to young children: A 2- and 3-year follow-up and a new preschool trial." *Journal of Educational Psychology, 87* (1995): 488–503.

Bzoch, K. R., *Communicative Disorders Related to Cleft Lip and Palate* (5th ed.). Austin, TX: Pro-Ed, 2004.

Calfee, R. C., P. Lindamood, and C. Lindamood, "Acoustic-phonetic skills and reading—Kindergarten through twelfth grade." *Journal of Educational Psychology, 64* (1973): 293–298.

Calvert, D., "Articulation and hearing impairments." In L. Lass, J. Northern, D. Yoder, and L. McReynolds (Eds.), *Speech, Language and Hearing*, Volume 2 (pp. 638–651). Philadelphia: Saunders, 1982.

Camarata, S., "Final consonant repetition: A linguistic perspective." *Journal of Speech and Hearing Disorders, 54* (1989): 159–162.

Camarata, S., "The application of naturalistic conversation training to speech production in children with speech disabilities." *Journal of Applied Behavior Analysis, 26* (1993): 173–182.

Camarata, S. M., "Naturalistic intervention for speech intelligibility and speech accuracy." In A. L. Williams, S. McLeod, and R. J. McCauley (Eds.), *Interventions for Speech Sound Disorders in Children* (pp. 381–406), Baltimore, MD: Brookes, 2010.

Camarata, S., and J. Gandour, "Rule invention in the acquisition of morphology by a language-impaired child." *Journal of Speech and Hearing Disorders, 50* (1985): 40–45.

Camarata, S., and R. Schwartz, "Production of object words and action words: Evidence for a relationship between phonology and semantics." *Journal of Speech and Hearing Research, 26* (1985): 50–53.

Campbell, T. F., C. A. Dollaghan, H. E. Rockette, J. L. Paradise, H. M. Feldman, L. D. Shriberg, et al., "Risk factors for speech delay of unknown origin in 3-year-old children." *Child Development, 74* (2003): 346–357.

Canadian Association of Speech-Language Pathologists and Audiologists (CASLPA), "Scope of Practice for Speech-Language Pathology." Available from http://www.caslpa.ca/english/resources/scopes.asp, 2008.

Canning, B., and M. Rose, "Clinical measurements of the speech, tongue and lip movements in British children with normal speech." *British Journal of Disorders of Communication, 9* (1974): 45–50.

Canoy, D., J. Pekkanen, P. Elliott, A. Pouta, J. Laitinen, A.-L. Hartikainen, P. Zitting, S. Patel, M. P. Little, and M.-R. Jarvelin, "Early growth and adult respiratory function in men and women followed from the fetal period to adulthood." *Thorax, 62*, 5 (2007): 396–402.

Cantwell, D. P., and L. Baker, "Clinical significance of childhood communication disorders: Perspectives from a longitudinal study." *Journal of Child Neurology, 2* (1987): 257–264.

Carrell, J., and K. Pendergast, "An experimental study of the possible relation between errors of speech and spelling." *Journal of Speech and Hearing Disorders, 19* (1954): 327–334.

Carrier, J. K., "A program of articulation therapy administered by mothers." *Journal of Speech and Hearing Disorders, 33* (1970): 344–353.

Carroll, J. M., M. J. Snowling, C. Hulme, and J. Stevenson, "The development of phonological awareness in preschool children." *Developmental Psychology, 39* (2003): 913–923.

Carson, K., G. T. Gillon, and T. Boustead, "Computer-administered versus paper-based assessment of school entry phonological awareness ability." *Asia Pacific Journal of Speech, Language, and Hearing, 14* (2011a): 85–101.

Carson, K., G. Gillon, and T. Boustead. "Introducing phonological awareness instruction into classroom reading programs." Speech Pathology Australia National Conference: Diversity and Development, Darwin, Australia, 26–29 June (2011b).

Carter, E., and M. Buck, "Prognostic testing for functional articulation disorders among children in the first grade." *Journal of Speech and Hearing Disorders, 23* (1958): 124–133.

Carter, P., and S. Edwards, "EPG therapy for children with long-standing speech disorders: Predictions and outcomes." *Clinical Linguistics and Phonetics, 18* (2004): 359–372.

Carterette, E., and M. Jones, *Informal Speech: Alphabetic and Phonemic Texts with Statistical Analyses and Tables.* Berkeley: University of California Press, 1974.

Catts, H. W., "Speech, production/phonological deficits in reading-disordered children." *Learning Disabilities, 19* (1986): 504–508.

Catts, H. W., "The relationship between speech-language impairments and reading disabilities." *Journal of Speech and Hearing Research, 36* (1993): 948–958.

Catts, H. W., M. E. Fey, J. B. Tomblin, and X. Y. Zhang, "A longitudinal investigation of reading outcomes in children with language impairments." *Journal of Speech Language, and Hearing Research, 45* (2002): 1142–1157.

Catts, H. W., M. E. Fey, X. Zhang, and J. B. Tomblin, "Estimating the risk of future reading difficulties in kindergarten children: A research-based model and its clinical implementation." *Language, Speech, and Hearing Services in Schools, 32* (2001): 38–50.

Catts, H. W., and T. Olsen, *Sounds Abound: Listening, Rhyming, and Reading.* East Moline, IL: Linguisystems, 1993.

Catts, H. W., Y. Petscher, C. Schatschneider, M. S. Bridges, and K. Mendoza, "Floor effects associated with universal screening and their impact on the early identification of reading disabilities." *Journal of Learning Disabilities, 42* (2009): 163–176.

Cavagna, G. A., and R. Margaria, "Airflow rates and efficiency changes during phonation: Sound production in man." *Annals of the New York Academy of Sciences, 155* (1968): 152–164.

Chaney, C., "Language development, metalinguistic skills, and print awareness in 3-year-old children." *Applied Psycholinguistics, 13* (1992): 485–514.

Chaney, C., and P. Menyuk, "Production and identification of /w, l, r/ in normal and articulation-impaired children." Paper presented at the convention of the American Speech and Hearing Association, Washington, DC, 1975.

Chatterji, M., "Reading achievement gaps, correlates, and moderators of early reading achievement: Evidence from the Early Childhood Longitudinal Study (ECLS) kindergarten to first grade sample." *Journal of Educational Psychology 98* (2006): 489–507.

Cheng, H. Y., B. E. Murdoch, and J. V. Goozee, "Temporal features of articulation from childhood to adolescence: An electropalatographic investigation." *Clinical Linguistics and Phonetics, 21*, 6 (2007): 481–499.

Cheng, H. Y., B. E. Murdoch, J. V. Goozee, and D. Scott, "Electropalatographic assessment of tongue-to-palate contact patterns and variability in children, adolescents, and adults." *Journal of Speech, Language, and Hearing Research, 50*, 2 (2007a): 375–392.

Cheng, H. Y., B. E. Murdoch, J. V. Goozee, and D. Scott, "Physiologic development of tongue-jaw coordination from childhood to adulthood." *Journal of Speech, Language, and Hearing Research, 50*, 2 (2007b): 352–360.

Cheng, L. R. L., *Assessing Asian Language Performance: Guidelines for Evaluating Limited-English-Proficient Students.* Rockville, MD: Aspen, 1987.

Cheng, L. R. L., "Asian-American cultures." In D. Battle (Ed.), *Communication Disorders in Multicultural*

Populations (pp. 38–77). Boston: Andover Medical Publishers, 1993.

Chervela, N., "Medial consonant cluster acquisition by Telugu children." *Journal of Child Language, 8* (1981): 63–73.

Cheung, P., and E. Abberton, "Patterns of phonological disability in Cantonese-speaking children in Hong Kong." *International Journal of Language and Communication Disorders, 35* (2000): 451–473.

Chiat, S., "From lexical access to lexical output: What is the problem for children with impaired phonology?" In M. Yavas, (Ed.), *First and Second Language Pathology* (pp. 107–133). San Diego, CA: Singular Publishing, 1994.

Chin, S. B., "The role of the sonority hierarchy in delayed phonological systems." In T. Powell (Ed.), *Pathologies of Speech and Language: Contributions of Clinical Phonetics and Linguistics* (pp. 109–117). New Orleans, LA: International Clinical Phonetics and Linguistics Association, 1996.

Chin, S. B., and D. B. Pisoni, "A phonological system at 2 years after cochlear implantation." *Clinical Linguistics and Phonetics, 14* (2000): 53–73.

Ching, T. Y. C., P. Incerti, M. Hill, and E. van Wanrooy, "An overview of binaural advantages for children and adults who use binaural/bimodal hearing devices." *Audiology and Neurotology, 11*, Supplement 1 (2006): 6–11.

Chirlian, N. S., and C. F. Sharpley, "Children's articulation development: Some regional differences." *Australian Journal of Human Communication Disorders, 10* (1982): 23–30.

Chomsky, N., and M. Hallé, *The Sound Pattern of English.* New York: Harper & Row, 1968.

Christian, D., W. Wolfram, and N. Nube, *Variation and Change in Geographically Isolated Communities: Appalachian English and Ozark English.* Tuscaloosa, AL: The University of Alabama Press, 1988.

Christensen, C. A., "Onset, rhymes, and phonemes in learning to read." *Scientific Studies of Reading, 1* (1997): 341–358.

Christensen, C. A., "Preschool phonological awareness and success in reading." In N. A. Badian (Ed.), *Prediction and Prevention of Reading Failure* (pp. 153–178). Timonium, MD: York, 2000.

Chumpelik, D., "The prompt system of therapy: Theoretical framework and applications for developmental apraxia of speech." *Seminars in Speech and Language, 5* (1984): 139–155.

Clark, C. E., I. E. Schwarz, and R. W. Blakeley, "The removable r-appliance as a practice device to facilitate correct production of /r/." *American Journal of Speech-Language Pathology, 3* (1993): 84–92.

Clark, R., "Maturation and speech development." *Logos, 2* (1959): 49–54.

Clark-Klein, S., and B. Hodson, "A phonologically based analysis of misspellings by third graders with disordered-phonology histories." *Journal of Speech and Hearing Research, 38* (1995): 839–849.

Clements, G. N., "The role of the sonority cycle in core syllabification." In J. Kingston and M. Beckman (Eds.), *Papers in Laboratory Phonology 1: Between the Grammar and Physics of Speech.* (pp. 283–333). Cambridge, UK: Cambridge University Press, 1990.

Cohen, A., R. Collier, and J. t'Hart, "Declination: Construct or intrinsic feature of speech pitch?" *Phonetica, 39* (1982): 254–273.

Cole, P., and Taylor, O., "Performance of working class African-American children on three tests of articulation." *Language, Speech, and Hearing Services in Schools, 21* (1990): 171–176.

Cooper, R., "The method of meaningful minimal contrasts." In P. Newman, N. Creaghead, and W. Secord (Eds.), *Assessment and Remediation of Articulatory and Phonological Disorders* (pp. 369–382). Columbus, OH: Merrill, 1985.

Cooper, R. P., and R. N. Aslin, "Preference for infant-directed speech in the first month after birth." *Child Development, 61* (1990): 1584–1595.

Coplan, J., and J. R. Gleason, "Unclear speech: Recognition and significance of unintelligible speech in preschool children." *Pediatrics, 82* (1988): 447–452.

Costello, J., and C. Bosler, "Generalization and articulation instruction." *Journal of Speech and Hearing Disorders, 41* (1976): 359–373.

Courchesne, E., H. J. Chisum, J. Townsend, A. Cowles, J. Covington, B. Egaas, M. Harwood, S. Hinds, and G. A. Press, "Normal brain development and aging: Quantitative analysis at in vivo MR imaging in healthy volunteers." *Radiology, 216* (2000): 672–682.

Craig, H., C. Thompson, J. Washington, and S. Potter, "Phonological features of child African American English." *Journal of Speech, Language, and Hearing Research, 46* (2003): 623–635.

Craig, H., and J. Washington, "Grade-related changes in the production of African American English." *Journal of Speech, Language, and Hearing Research, 47* (2004): 450–463.

Crosbie, S., A. Holm, and B. Dodd, "Intervention for children with severe speech disorder: A comparison of two approaches." *International Journal of Language and Communication Disorders, 40* (2005): 467–491.

Crosbie, S., C. Pine, A. Holm, and B. Dodd, "Treating Jarrod: A core vocabulary approach." *Advances in Speech-Language Pathology, 8*, 3 (2006): 316–321.

Crowe-Hall, B. J., "Attitudes of fourth and sixth graders toward peers with mild articulation disorders." *Language, Speech, and Hearing Services in Schools, 22* (1991): 334–340.

Crystal, D., *Prosodic Systems and Intonation in English.* Cambridge, UK: Cambridge University Press, 1969.

Crystal, D., "Non-segmental phonology in language acquisition: A review of the issues." *Lingua, 32* (1973): 1–45.

Crystal, D., "Prosodic development." In P. J. Fletcher and M. Garman (Eds.), *Studies in First Language Development* (pp. 174–197) New York: Cambridge University Press, 1986.

Crystal, D., "Towards a 'bucket' theory of language disability: Taking account of interaction between linguistic levels." *Clinical Linguistics and Phonetics, 1* (1987): 7–22.

Crystal, D. *The Cambridge Encyclopedia of Language* (2nd ed.) Cambridge, UK: Cambridge University Press, 1997.

Cumley, G. D., and S. Swanson, "Augmentative and alternative communication options for children with developmental apraxia of speech: Three case studies." *Augmentative and Alternative Communication, 15* (1999): 110–125.

Cunningham, A., and J. Carroll, "Age and schooling effects on early literacy and phoneme awareness." *Journal of Experimental Child Psychology, 109* (2011): 248–255.

Cunningham, I., *A Syntactic Analysis of Sea Island Creole.* Tuscaloosa: The University of Alabama Press, 1992.

Curtis, J., and J. Hardy, "A phonetic study of misarticulations of /r/." *Journal of Speech and Hearing Research, 2* (1959): 224–257.

Dagenais, P. A., P. Critz-Crosby, and J. B. Adams, "Defining and remediating persistent lateral lisps in children using electropalatography: Preliminary findings." *American Journal of Speech-Language Pathology, 3* (1994): 67–76.

Daniloff, R. G., and K. L. Moll, "Coarticulation of lip rounding." *Journal of Speech and Hearing Research, 11* (1968): 707–721.

Darley, F., A. Aronson, and J. Brown, *Motor Speech Disorders.* Philadelphia: Saunders, 1975.

Davis, B. L., "Goal and target selection for developmental speech disorders." In K. E. Pollock and A. G. Kamhi (Eds.), *Phonological Disorders in Children: Clinical Decision Making in Assessment and Intervention* (pp. 89–100). Baltimore, MD: Brookes, 2005.

Davis, B. L., K. J. Jakielski, and T. P. Marquardt, "Developmental apraxia of speech: Determiners of differential diagnosis." *Clinical Linguistics and Phonetics, 12* (1998): 25–45.

Davis, B. L., and P. F. MacNeilage, "The articulatory basis of babbling." *Journal of Speech and Hearing Research, 38* (1995): 1199–1211.

Davis, E., "The development of linguistic skills in twins, singletons with siblings, and only children from age five to ten years." *Institute of Child Welfare Monograph Series 14.* Minneapolis: University of Minnesota Press, 1937.

Dawson, J. I., and P. J. Tattersall, *Structured Photographic Articulation Test–II.* DeKalb, IL: Janelle Publications, 2001.

Dawson, L., "A study of the development of the rate of articulation." *Elementary School Journal, 29* (1929): 610–615.

Dayton, N., and C. Schuele, "Effects of phonological awareness training on young children with specific language impairment." Paper presented at the annual convention of the American Speech-Language-Hearing Association, Boston, 1997.

DeCasper, A. J., and W. P. Fifer, "Of human bonding: Newborns prefer their mothers' voices." *Science, 208* (1980): 1174–1176.

DeCasper, A. J., J.-P. LeCanuet, M.-C. Busnel, C. Granier-Deferre, and R. Maugeais, "Fetal reactions to recurrent maternal speech." *Infant Behavior and Development, 17* (1994): 159–164.

de Jong, K. J. "The oral articulation of English stress accent." Unpublished doctoral dissertation, The Ohio State University, Columbus, OH, 1991.

De la Fuente, M. T., "The order of acquisition of Spanish consonant phonemes by monolingual Spanish speaking children between the ages of 2.0 and 6.5." Unpublished doctoral dissertation, Georgetown University, Washington, DC, 1985.

Denne, M., N. Langdown, T. Pring, and P. Roy, "Treating children with expressive phonological disorders: Does phonological awareness therapy work in the clinic?" *International Journal of Language and Communication Disorders, 40* (2005): 493–504.

Dewey, G., *Relative Frequency of English Speech Sounds.* Cambridge, MA: Harvard University Press, 1923.

Diedrich, W. M., "Procedures for counting and charting a target phoneme." *Language, Speech, and Hearing Services in Schools, 2* (1971): 18–32.

Diedrich, W. M., "Stimulability and articulation disorders." In J. Locke (Ed.), *Assessing and Treating Phonological Disorders: Current Approaches. Seminars in Speech and Language, 4.* (1983): 297–311.

Diedrich, W. M., and J. Bangert, "Training and speech clinicians in recording and analysis of articulatory behavior." Washington, D.C.: U.S. Office of Education Grant No. OEG-0-70-1689 and OEG-0-71-1689, 1976.

Dinnsen, D. A., J. A. Barlow, and M. L. Morrisette, "Long-distance place assimilation with an interacting error pattern in phonological acquisition." *Clinical Linguistics and Phonetics, 11* (1997): 319–338.

Dinnsen, D. A., S. B. Chin, M. Elbert, and T. Powell, "Some constraints on functionally disordered phonologies: Phonetic inventories and phonotactics." *Journal of Speech and Hearing Research, 33* (1990): 28–37.

Dinnsen, D., and M. Elbert, "On the relationship between phonology and learning." In M. Elbert, D. Dinnsen, and G. Weismer (Eds.), *Phonological Theory and the*

Misarticulating Child, ASHA Monographs, 22 (1984): 59–68). Rockville, MD: ASHA, 1984.

Dodd, B., "Children's acquisition of phonology." In B. Dodd (Ed.), *Differential Diagnosis and Treatment of Children with Speech Disorder* (pp. 21–48). San Diego, CA: Singular Publishing, 1995a.

Dodd, B., "Procedures for classification of sub groups of speech disorder." In B. Dodd (Ed.), *Differential Diagnosis and Treatment of Children with Speech Disorder* (pp. 49–64). San Diego, CA: Singular Publishing, 1995b.

Dodd, B., *Differential Diagnosis and Treatment of Children with Speech Disorder* (2nd ed.). London: Whurr Publishers, 2005.

Dodd, B., "Differentiating speech delay from disorder. Does it matter?" *Topics in Language Disorders, 31* (2011): 96–111.

Dodd, B., and A. Bradford, "A comparison of three therapy methods for children with different types of developmental phonological disorder." *International Journal of Language and Communication Disorders, 35* (2000): 189–209.

Dodd, B., S. Crosbie, and A. Holm, *Core Vocabulary Therapy: An Intervention for Children with Inconsistent Speech Disorders.* Brisbane, Australia: Perinatal Research Centre, Royal Brisbane & Women's Hospital, University of Queensland, 2004.

Dodd, B., S. Crosbie, B. MCintosh, A. Holm, C. Harvey, M. Liddy, K. Fontyne, B. Pinchin, and H. Rigy, "The impact of selecting different contrasts in phonological therapy." *International Journal of Speech-Language Pathology, 10* (2008): 334–345.

Dodd, B., S. Crosbie, B. McIntosh, T. Teitzel, and A. Ozanne. *Pre-Reading Inventory of Phonological Awareness.* San Antonio, TX: Harcourt, 2003.

Dodd, B., and G. Gillon, "Exploring the relationship between phonological awareness, speech impairment, and literacy." *Advances in Speech-Language Pathology, 3* (2001): 139–147.

Dodd, B., A. Holm, S. Crosbie, and P. McCormack, "Differential diagnosis of phonological disorders." In B. Dodd (Ed.), *Differential Diagnosis and Treatment of Children with Speech Disorder* (2nd ed., pp. 44–70). London: Whurr Publishers, 2005.

Dodd, B., A. Holm, S. Crosbie, and B. McIntosh, "A core vocabulary approach for management of inconsistent speech disorder." *Advances in Speech-Language Pathology, 8* (2006): 220–230.

Dodd, B., A. Holm, Z. Hua, and S. Crosbie, "Phonological development: A normative study of British English-speaking children." *Clinical Linguistics and Phonetics, 17* (2003): 617–643.

Dodd, B., Z. Hua, S. Crosbie, A. Holm, and A. Ozanne, *Diagnostic Evaluation of Articulation and Phonology (DEAP).* London: Psychological Corporation, 2002.

Dodd, B., Z. Hua, S. Crosbie, A. Holm, and A. Ozanne, *Diagnostic Evaluation of Articulation and Phonology (DEAP).* San Antonio, TX: Harcourt Assessment, 2006.

Dodd, B., L. So, and W. Li, "Symptoms of disorder without impairment: The written and spoken errors of bilinguals." In B. Dodd, R. Campbell, and L. Worrall (Eds.), *Evaluating Theories of Language: Evidence from Disorder* (pp. 119–136). London: Whurr Publishers, 1996.

Dollaghan, C. A., *The Handbook for Evidence-Based Practice in Communication Disorders.* Baltimore, MD: Brookes, 2007.

Donegan, P., "Normal vowel development." In M. J. Ball and F. E. Gibbon (Eds.), *Vowel Disorders* (pp. 1–35). Woburn, MA: Butterworth-Heinemann, 2002.

Dore, J., "Holophrases, speech acts and language universals." *Journal of Child Language, 2,* 1 (1975): 21–40.

Dowker, A., "Rhyme and alliteration in poems elicited from young children." *Journal of Child Language 16* (1989): 181–202.

Dubois, E., and J. Bernthal, "A comparison of three methods for obtaining articulatory responses." *Journal of Speech and Hearing Disorders, 43* (1978): 295–305.

Dubois, S., and B. Horvath, "The English vernaculars of the Creoles of Louisiana." *Language Variation and Change, 15* (2003): 255–288.

Duff, M. C., A. Proctor, and E. Yairi, "Prevalence of voice disorders in African American and European American preschoolers." *Journal of Voice, 18* (2004): 348–353.

Duffy, J. R., *Motor Speech Disorders. Substrates, Differential Diagnosis, and Management* (2nd ed.). St. Louis, MO: Elsevier Mosby, 2005.

Dunn, C. and C. Barron, "A treatment program for disordered phonology: Phonetic and linguistic considerations." *Language, Speech, and Hearing Services in Schools, 13* (1982): 100–109.

Dunn, C., and L. Newton, "A comprehensive model for speech development in hearing-impaired children." *Topics in Language Disorders, 6* (1986): 25–46.

Dworkin, J., "Protrusive lingual force and lingual diadochokinetic rates: A comparative analysis between normal and lisping speakers." *Language, Speech, and Hearing Services in Schools, 9* (1978): 8–16.

Dworkin, J. P., and R. A. Culatta, "Oral structural and neuromuscular characteristics in children with normal and disordered articulation." *Journal of Speech and Hearing Disorders, 50* (1985): 150–156.

Dyson, A. T., "Development of velar consonants among normal two-year-olds." *Journal of Speech and Hearing Research, 29* (1986): 493–498.

Dyson, A. T., "Phonetic inventories of 2- and 3- year old children." *Journal of Speech and Hearing Disorders, 53* (1988): 89–93.

Dyson, A. T., and M. Amayreh, "Phonological errors and sound changes in Arabic-speaking children." *Clinical Linguistics and Phonetics, 14* (2000): 79–109.

Dyson, A. T., and E. P. Paden, "Some phonological acquisition strategies used by two-year-olds." *Journal of Childhood Communication Disorders, 7* (1983): 6–18.

Edeal, D. M., and C. E. Gildersleeve-Neumann, "The importance of production frequency in therapy for childhood apraxia of speech." *American Journal of Speech-Language Pathology, 20* (2011): 95–110.

Edwards, J., R. A. Fox, and C. L. Rogers, "Final consonant discrimination in children: Effects of phonological disorder, vocabulary size and articulatory accuracy." *Journal of Speech, Language, and Hearing Research, 45* (2002): 231–242.

Edwards, M. L., "Issues in phonological assessment." *Seminars in Speech and Language, 4* (1983): 351–374.

Edwards, M. L., "Phonological theories." In B. W. Hodson (Ed.), *Evaluating and Enhancing Children's Phonological Systems* (pp. 145–170). Greenville, SC: Thinking Publications, 2007.

Eguchi, S., and I. J. Hirsh, "Development of speech sounds in children." *Acta Orolaryngologica,* Suppl. 257 (1969).

Ehri, L. C., S. R. Nunes, D. M. Willows, B. V. Schuster, Z. Yaghoub-Zadeh, and T. Shanahan, "Phonemic awareness instruction helps children learn to read: Evidence from the National Reading Panel's meta-analysis." *Reading Research Quarterly 36* (2001): 250–287.

Eilers, R. E., and D. K. Oller, "The role of speech discrimination in developmental sound substitutions." *Journal of Child Language, 3* (1976): 319–329.

Eilers, R. E., W. R. Wilson, and J. M. Moore, "Developmental changes in speech discrimination in infants." *Journal of Speech and Hearing Research, 20* (1977): 766–780.

Eimas, P., "Auditory and linguistic units of processing of cues for place of articulation by infants." *Perception and Psychophysics, 16* (1974): 341–347.

Eimas, P., E. Siqueland, P. Jusczyk, and J. Vigorito, "Speech perception in infants." *Science, 171* (1971): 303–306.

Elbers, L., and J. Ton, "Play pen monologues: The interplay of words and babbles in the first words period." *Journal of Child Language, 12* (1985): 551–565.

Elbert, M., "Dismissal criteria from therapy." Unpublished Manuscript, 1967.

Elbert, M., D. A. Dinnsen, P. Swartzlander, and S. B. Chin, "Generalization to conversational speech." *Journal of Speech and Hearing Disorders, 55* (1990): 694–699.

Elbert, M., and J. Gierut, *Handbook of Clinical Phonology: Approaches to Assessment and Treatment*. San Diego, CA: College-Hill Press, 1986.

Elbert, M., and L. V. McReynolds, "Transfer of /r/ across contexts." *Journal of Speech and Hearing Disorders, 40* (1975): 380–387.

Elbert, M., and L. V. McReynolds, "An experimental analysis of misarticulating children's generalization." *Journal of Speech and Hearing Research, 21* (1978): 136–149.

Elbert, M., T. W. Powell, and P. Swartzlander, "Toward a technology of generalization: How many exemplars are sufficient?" *Journal of Speech and Hearing Research, 34* (1991): 81–87.

Elbert, M., R. L. Shelton, and W. B. Arndt, "A task for education of articulation change." *Journal of Speech and Hearing Research, 10* (1967): 281–288.

Engel, D. C., and L. R. Groth, "Case studies of the effect on carry-over of reinforcing postarticulation responses based on feedback." *Language, Speech, and Hearing Services in Schools, 7* (1976): 93–101.

Eski, M., M. Nisanci, A. Aktas, and M. Sengezer, "Congenital double lip: Review of 5 cases." *British Journal of Oral and Maxillofacial Surgery, 45* (2007): 68–70.

Everhart, R., "The relationship between articulation and other developmental factors in children." *Journal of Speech and Hearing Disorders, 18* (1953): 332–338.

Everhart, R., "Paternal occupational classification and the maturation of articulation." *Speech Monographs, 23* (1956): 75–77.

Everhart, R., "Literature survey of growth and developmental factors in articulation maturation." *Journal of Speech and Hearing Disorders, 25* (1960): 59–69.

Fabiano-Smith, L., and B. Goldstein, "Phonological acquisition in bilingual Spanish-English speaking children." *Journal of Speech, Language, and Hearing Research, 53* (2010): 160–178.

Fairbanks, G., and E. Green, "A study of minor organic deviations in 'functional' disorders of articulation; 2. Dimension and relationships of the lips." *Journal of Speech and Hearing Disorders, 15* (1950): 165–168.

Fairbanks, G., and M. Lintner, "A study of minor organic deviations in functional disorders of articulation." *Journal of Speech and Hearing Disorders, 16* (1951): 273–279.

Farquhar, M. S., "Prognostic value of imitative and auditory discrimination tests." *Journal of Speech and Hearing Disorders, 26* (1961): 342–347.

Fee, E. J., "Segments and syllables in early language acquisition." In J. Archibald (Ed.), *Phonological Acquisition and Phonological Theory* (pp. 43–61) Hillsdale, NJ: Erlbaum, 1995.

Fee, J., and D. Ingram, "Reproduction as a strategy of phonological development." *Journal of Child Language, 9* (1982): 41–54.

Felsenfeld, S., M. McGue, and P. A. Broen, "Familial aggregation of phonological disorders: Results from a 28-year follow-up." *Journal of Speech and Hearing Research, 38* (1995): 1091–1107.

Ferguson, C. A., "Learning to pronounce: The earliest stages of phonological development." In F. D. Minifie and L. L. Lloyd (Eds.), *Communicative and Cognitive Abilities: Early Behavioral Assessment* (pp. 273–297) Baltimore, MD: University Park Press, 1978.

Ferguson, C. A., and C. B. Farwell, "Words and sounds in early language acquisition." *Language, 51* (1975): 419–439.

Fey, M. E., *Language Intervention with Young Children.* San Diego, CA: College Hill Press/Little Brown, 1986.

Fey, M. E., *Language Intervention with Young Children.* Boston, MA: Allyn & Bacon, 1991.

Fey, M. E., "Articulation and phonology: Inextricable constructs in speech pathology." *Language, Speech, and Hearing Services in Schools, 23* (1992): 225–232.

Fey, M. E., P. L. Cleave, A. I. Ravida, S. H. Long, A. E. Dejmal, and D. L. Easton, "Effects of grammar facilitation on the phonological performance of children with speech and language impairments." *Journal of Speech and Hearing Research, 37* (1994): 594–607.

Fey, M. E., and J. Gandour, "Rule discovery in phonological acquisition." *Journal of Child Language, 9* (1982): 71–81.

Field, T. M., R. Woodson, R. Greenberg, and D. Cohen, "Discrimination and imitation of facial expression by neonates." *Science, 218,* 4568 (1982): 179–181.

Fields, D., and K. Polmanteer, "Effectiveness of oral motor techniques in articulation and phonology therapy." Poster presentation at the annual convention of the American Speech-Language-Hearing Association, Atlanta, GA.

Fitch, W. T., and J. Giedd, "Morphology and development of the human vocal tract: A study using magnetic resonance imaging." *The Journal of the Acoustical Society of America, 106,* 3 (1999): 1511–1522.

Fitzsimons, R., "Developmental, psychosocial and educational factors in children with nonorganic articulation problems." *Child Development, 29* (1958): 481–489.

Fleming, K., and J. Hartman, "Establishing cultural validity of the computer analysis of phonological processes." *Florida Educational Research Council Bulletin, 22* (1989): 8–32.

Fletcher, S., "Time-by-count measurement of diadochokinetic syllable rate." *Journal of Speech and Hearing Research, 15* (1972): 763–780.

Fletcher, S. G. *Articulation. A Physiological Approach.* San Diego, CA: Singular, 1992.

Fletcher, S., R. Casteel, and D. Bradley, "Tongue thrust swallow, speech articulation and age." *Journal of Speech and Hearing Disorders, 26* (1961): 201–208.

Fletcher, S., and J. Meldrum, "Lingual function and relative length of the lingual frenulum." *Journal of Speech and Hearing Research, 11* (1968): 382–399.

Flipsen, P., Jr., "Speaker-listener familiarity: Parents as judges of delayed speech intelligibility." *Journal of Communication Disorders, 28* (1995): 3–19.

Flipsen, P., Jr., "Longitudinal changes in articulation rate and phonetic phrase length in children with speech delay." *Journal of Speech, Language, and Hearing Research, 45,* 1 (2002a): 100–110.

Flipsen, P., Jr., "Causes and speech sound disorders. Why worry?" Paper presented at the Speech Pathology Australia National Conference, Alice Springs, Australia, 2002b.

Flipsen, P., Jr., "Syllables per word in typical and delayed speech acquisition." *Clinical Linguistics and Phonetics, 20,* 4 (2006a): 293–301.

Flipsen, P., Jr., "Measuring the intelligibility of conversational speech in children." *Clinical Linguistics and Phonetics, 20,* 4 (2006b): 303–312.

Flipsen, P., Jr., "Appalachian English speech acquisition." In S. McLeod (Ed.), *The International Guide to Speech Acquisition* (pp. 161–168). Clifton Park, NY: Thomson Delmar Learning, 2007.

Flipsen, P., Jr., "Intelligibility of spontaneous conversational speech produced by children with cochlear implants: A review." *International Journal of Pediatric Otorhinolaryngology, 72* (2008): 559–564.

Flipsen, P., Jr., J. B. Hammer, and K. M. Yost, "Measuring severity of involvement in speech delay: Segmental and whole-word measures." *American Journal of Speech-Language Pathology, 14* (2005): 298–312.

Flipsen, P., Jr., and R. G. Parker, "Phonological patterns in the speech of children with cochlear implants." *Journal of Communication Disorders, 41* (2008): 337–357.

Fluharty, N., *Fluharty Preschool Speech and Language Screening Test–Second Edition.* Austin, TX: Pro-Ed, 2001.

Flynn, P., and M. Byrne, "Relationship between reading and selected auditory abilities of third-grade children." *Journal of Speech and Hearing Research, 13* (1970): 731–740.

Forrest, K., "Are oral-motor exercises useful in the treatment of phonological/articulatory disorders?" *Seminars in Speech and Language, 23* (2002): 15–25.

Fox, A. V., B. Dodd, and D. Howard, "Risk factors for speech disorders in children." *International Journal of Language and Communication Disorders, 37* (2002): 117–131.

Foy, J. G., and V. Mann, "Does strength of phonological representations predict phonological awareness?" *Applied Psycholinguistics, 22* (2001): 301–325.

French, A., "The systematic acquisition of word forms by a child during the first fifty word stage." *Journal of Child Language, 16* (1989): 69–90.

Frost, S. J., N. Landi, W. E. Mencl, R. Sandak, R. K. Fulbright, and E. T. Tejada et al., "Phonological awareness predicts activation patterns for print and speech." *Annals of Dyslexia, 59* (2009): 78–97.

Fry, D., "Duration and intensity as physical correlates of linguistic stress." *Journal of the Acoustical Society of America, 27* (1955): 765–768.

Fucci, D., "Oral vibrotactile sensation: An evaluation of normal and defective speakers." *Journal of Speech and Hearing Research, 15* (1972): 179–184.

Fuchs, D., L. Fuchs, A. Thompson, S. Al Otaiba, L. Yen, and N. Yang, et al., "Is reading important in reading-readiness programs? A randomized field trial with teachers as program implementers." *Journal of Educational Psychology, 93* (2001): 251–267.

Furia, C. L. B., L. P. Kowalski, M. R. D. O. Latorre, E. C. Angelis, N. M. S. Mastins, A. P. B. Barros, and K. C. B. Ribeiro, "Speech intelligibility after glossectomy and speech rehabilitation." *Archives of Otolaryngology: Head and Neck Surgery, 127* (2001): 877–883.

Gable, T. O., A. W. Kummer, L. Lee, N. A. Creaghead, and L. J. Moore, "Premature loss of the maxillary incisors: Effect on speech production." *Journal of Dentistry for Children, 62* (1995): 173–179.

Gallagher, R., and T. Shriner, "Contextual variables related to inconsistent /s/ and /z/ production in the spontaneous speech of children." *Journal of Speech and Hearing Research, 18* (1975): 623–633.

Galvin, K., M. Mok, and R. Dowell, "Sequential bilateral implants for young children: Subjective outcomes, left versus right localization and speech detection results." Paper presented at the 11th International Conference on Cochlear Implants in Children, Charlotte, NC, 2007.

Gammon, S., P. Smith, R. Daniloff, and C. Kim, "Articulation and stress juncture production under oral anesthetization and masking." *Journal of Speech and Hearing Research, 14* (1971): 271–282.

Garrett, R., "A study of children's discrimination of phonetic variations of the /s/ phoneme." Ph.D. dissertation, Ohio University, 1969.

Geers, A. E., "Factors influencing spoken language outcomes in children following early cochlear implantation." *Advances in Otorhinolaryngology, 64* (2006): 50–65.

Gentry, J., "Developmental spelling and the speech-language pathologist." *National Student Speech-Language-Hearing Association, XX* (1988): 50–60.

Gerken, L., and K. McGregor, "An overview of prosody and its role in normal and disordered child language." *American Journal of Speech-Language Pathology, 7* (1998): 38–48.

Gibbon, F. E., and S. E. Wood. "Visual feedback therapy with electropalatography." In A. L. Williams, S. McLeod, and R. J. McCauley (Eds.), *Interventions for Speech Sound Disorders* (pp. 509–536). Baltimore, MD: Brookes Publishing Co., 2010.

Gierut, J., "Maximal opposition approach to phonological treatment." *Journal of Speech and Hearing Disorders, 54* (1989): 9–19.

Gierut, J. A., "Differential learning of phonological oppositions." *Journal of Speech and Hearing Research, 33* (1990): 540–549.

Gierut, J. A., "Homonymy in phonological changes." *Clinical Linguistics and Phonetics, 5* (1991): 119–137.

Gierut, J. A., "The conditions and courses of clinically-induced phonological changes." *Journal of Speech and Hearing Research, 35* (1992): 1049–1063.

Gierut, J. A., "Natural domains of cyclicity in phonological acquisition." *Clinical Linguistics and Phonetics, 12* (1998): 481–499.

Gierut, J. A., "Syllable onsets: Clusters and adjuncts in acquisition." *Journal of Speech, Language, and Hearing Research, 42* (1999): 708–726.

Gierut, J. A., "Complexity in phonological treatment: Clinical factors." *Language, Speech, and Hearing Services in Schools, 32* (2001): 229–241.

Gierut, J. A., and A. Champion, "Syllable onsets II: Three-element clusters in phonological treatment." *Journal of Speech, Language, and Hearing Research, 44* (2001): 886–904.

Gierut, J. A., M. Elbert, and D. A. Dinnsen, "A functional analysis of phonological knowledge and generalization learning in misarticulating children." *Journal of Speech and Hearing Research, 30* (1987): 462–479.

Gierut, J. A., M. L. Morrisette, M. T. Hughes, and S. Rowland, "Phonological treatment efficacy and developmental norms." *Language, Speech, and Hearing Services in Schools, 27* (1996): 215–230.

Gierut, J. A., M. L. Morrisette, and S. M. Ziemer, "Nonwords and generalization in children with phonological disorders." *American Journal of Speech-Language Pathology, 19* (2010): 167–177.

Gierut, J. A., and H. J. Neumann, "Teaching and learning /θ/: A nonconfound." *Clinical Linguistics and Phonetics, 6* (1992): 191–200.

Gildersleeve-Neumann, C., and B. Davis, "Learning English in a bilingual preschool environment: Change over time." Paper presented at the annual convention of the American Speech-Language-Hearing Association, San Antonio, TX, 1998.

Gildersleeve-Neumann, C. E., and B. Goldstein, "Intervention for multilingual children with speech sound disorders." In S. McLeod and B. Goldstein (Eds.), *Multilingual aspects of speech sound disorders* (pp. 214–227). Clevedon, UK: Multilingual Matters, 2012.

Gildersleeve-Neumann, C. E., and K. E. Wright, "English phonological acquisition in 3- to 5-year-old children learning Russian and English." *Language, Speech, and Hearing Services in Schools, 41* (2010): 429–444.

Giles, S. B., "A study of articulatory characteristics of /l/ allophones in English." Unpublished Ph.D. dissertation, University of Iowa, 1971.

Gillon, G. T., "The efficacy of phonological awareness intervention for children with spoken language impairment." *Language, Speech, and Hearing Services in Schools, 31* (2000a): 126–141.

Gillon, G. T., *The Gillon Phonological Awareness Training Programme* (2nd ed.). Christchurch, New Zealand: Canterprise, University of Canterbury. www.cmds. canterbury.ac.nz/people/gillon.shtml, 2000b.

Gillon, G. T., "Follow-up study investigating benefits of phonological awareness intervention for children with spoken language impairment." *International Journal of Language and Communication Disorders, 37* (2002): 381–400.

Gillon, G. T., *Phonological Awareness: From Research to Practice.* New York: Guilford Press, 2004.

Gillon, G. T., "Facilitating phoneme awareness development in 3- and 4-year-old children with speech impairment." *Language, Speech, and Hearing Services in Schools, 36* (2005): 308–324.

Gillon, G. T., and B. Dodd, "The effects of training phonological, semantic, and syntactic processing skills in spoken language on reading ability." *Language, Speech, and Hearing Services in Schools, 26* (1995): 58–68.

Gillon, G. T., and B. Dodd, "Enhancing the phonological processing skills of children with specific reading disability." *European Journal of Disorders of Communication, 32* (1997): 67–90.

Gillon, G. T., and B. Dodd, "Understanding the relationship between speech-language impairment and literacy difficulties: The central role of phonology." In B. Dodd (Ed.), *Differential Diagnosis and Treatment of Children with Speech Disorder* (2nd ed., pp. 289–304). London: Whurr Publishers, 2005.

Gillon, G. T., and B. C. McNeill, "An integrated phonological awareness programme for preschool children with speech disorder." Available from http:// www.education.canterbury.ac.nz/people/gillon/ integrated_phonological_awareness.shtml, 2007.

Gillon, G. T., and B. C. McNeill, "Effective practices in phonological awareness assessment and intervention." *ACQuiring Knowledge in Speech, Language and Hearing,* 11 (2009): 72–76.

Gillon, G. T., and B. C. Moriarty, "Childhood apraxia of speech: Children at risk for persistent reading and spelling disorder." *Seminars in Speech and Language, 28* (2007): 48–57.

Gillon, G. T., and I. E. Schwarz, "Screening New Zealand children's spoken language skills for academic success." In L. Wilson and S. Hewat (Eds.), *Proceedings of the 2001 Speech Pathology Australia National Conference* (pp. 207–214). Melbourne: Speech Pathology Australia, 2001.

Glaspey, A., and C. Stoel-Gammon, "Dynamic assessment in phonological disorders." *Topics in Language Disorders, 25* (2005): 220–230.

Gold, T., "Speech production in hearing-impaired children." *Journal of Communication Disorders, 13* (1980): 397–418.

Goldman, R., and M. Fristoe, *Goldman-Fristoe Test of Articulation.* Circle Pines, MN: American Guidance Service, 2000.

Goldman, R., M. Fristoe, and R. Woodcock, *The Goldman-Fristoe-Woodcock Test of Auditory Discrimination.* Circle Pines, MN: American Guidance Service, 1970.

Goldsmith, J., *Autosegmental Phonology.* New York: Garland Press, 1979.

Goldsmith, J. A., *Autosegmental and Metrical Phonology.* Oxford, UK: Blackwell, 1990.

Goldstein, B., "The evidence of phonological processes of 3- and 4-year-old Spanish speakers." Unpublished master's thesis, Temple University, 1988.

Goldstein, B., "Spanish phonological development." In H. Kayser (Ed.), *Bilingual Speech-Language Pathology: An Hispanic focus* (pp. 17–38). San Diego, CA: Singular Publishing, 1995.

Goldstein, B., *Cultural and Linguistic Diversity Resource Guide for Speech-Language Pathology.* San Diego, CA: Singular Publishing, 2000.

Goldstein, B., "Assessing phonological skills in Hispanic/ Latino children." *Seminars in Speech and Language, 22* (2001): 39–49.

Goldstein, B., "Phonological development and disorders in bilingual children." In B. Goldstein (Ed.), *Bilingual Language Development and Disorders in Spanish-English Speakers* (pp. 257–286). Baltimore, MD: Brookes, 2004.

Goldstein, B., "Clinical implications of research on language development and disorders in bilingual children." *Topics in Language Disorders, 26* (2006): 318–334.

Goldstein, B., "Spanish speech acquisition." In S. McLeod (Ed.), *The International Guide to Speech Acquisition* (pp. 539–553). Clifton Park, NY: Thomson Delmar Learning, 2007a.

Goldstein, B., "Phonological skills in Puerto Rican- and Mexican-Spanish speaking children with phonological disorders." *Clinical Linguistics and Phonetics, 21* (2007b): 93–109.

Goldstein, B., "Speech acquisition across the world: Spanish Influenced English." In S. McLeod (Ed.), *The International Guide to Speech Acquisition* (pp. 345–356). Clifton Park, NY: Thomson Delmar Learning, 2007c.

Goldstein, B., and P. Cintron, "An investigation of phonological skills in Puerto Rican Spanish-speaking 2-year-olds." *Clinical Linguistics and Phonetics, 15* (2001): 343–361.

Goldstein, B., L. Fabiano, and P. Washington, "Phonological skills in predominantly English, predominantly

Spanish, and Spanish-English bilingual children." *Language, Speech, and Hearing Services in Schools, 36* (2005): 201–218.

Goldstein, B., and C. Gildersleeve-Neumann, "Phonological development and disorders." In B. Goldstein (Ed.), *Bilingual language development and disorders in Spanish-English speakers* (2nd edition; pp. 285–309). Baltimore: Brookes, 2012.

Goldstein, B., and A. Iglesias, "Phonological patterns in normally developing Spanish-speaking 3- and 4-year-olds of Puerto Rican descent. *Language, Speech, and Hearing Services in Schools, 27* (1996a): 82–90.

Goldstein, B., and A. Iglesias, "Phonological patterns in Puerto Rican Spanish-speaking children with phonological disorders." *Journal of Communication Disorders, 29* (1996b): 367–387.

Goldstein, B., and A. Iglesias, "Phonological patterns in bilingual (Spanish-English) children." Seminar presented at the Texas Research Symposium on Language Diversity, Austin, TX, 1999.

Goldstein, B., and A. Iglesias, "The effect of dialect on phonological analysis: Evidence from Spanish-speaking children." *American Journal of Speech-Language Pathology, 10* (2001): 394–406.

Goldstein, B., and S. McLeod, "Typical and atypical multilingual speech acquisition." In S. McLeod and B. Goldstein (Eds.), *Multilingual aspects of speech sound disorders* (pp. 84–100). Clevedon, UK: Multilingual Matters, 2012.

Goldstein, B., and K. Pollock, "Vowel errors in Spanish-speaking children with phonological disorders: A retrospective, comparative study." *Clinical Linguistics and Phonetics, 14* (2000): 217–234.

Goldstein, B., and P. Washington, "An initial investigation of phonological patterns in 4-year-old typically developing Spanish-English bilingual children." *Language, Speech, and Hearing Services in Schools, 10* (2001): 153–164.

Good, R., and R. Kaminski, *Dynamic Indicators of Basic Early Literacy Skills* (6th ed.). Eugene OR: Institute for the Development of Educational Achievement, 2002.

Goodluck, H., *Language Acquisition: A Linguistic Introduction*. Oxford: Blackwell, 1991.

Goodsitt, J., P. Morse, and J. Ver Hoeve, "Infant speech recognition in multisyllabic contexts." *Child Development, 55* (1984): 903–910.

Gordon-Brannan, M., "Assessing intelligibility: Children's expressive phonologies." *Topics in Language Disorders, 14* (1994): 17–25.

Gordon-Brannan, M., B. Hodson, and M. Wynne, "Remediating unintelligible utterances of a child with a mild hearing loss." *American Journal of Speech-Language Pathology, 1*, 4 (1992): 28–38.

Goswami, U., and P. E. Bryant, *Phonological Skills and Learning to Read*. Hove, East Sussex, UK: Psychology Press, 1990.

Gratier, M., and E. Devouche, "Imitation and repetition of prosodic contour in vocal interaction at 3 months." *Developmental Psychology, 47* (2011): 67–76.

Gray, B., "A field study on programmed articulation therapy." *Language, Speech, and Hearing Services in Schools, 5* (1974): 119–131.

Gray, B., and B. Ryan, *A Language Program for the Nonlanguage Child*. Champaign, IL: Research Press, 1973.

Gray, S. I., and R. L. Shelton, "Self-monitoring effects on articulation carryover in school-age children." *Language, Speech, and Hearing Services in Schools, 23* (1992): 334–342.

Grech, H., and B. Dodd, "Phonological acquisition in Malta: A bilingual learning context." *International Journal of Bilingualism, 12* (2008): 155–171.

Grech, H., and S. McLeod, "Multilingual speech and language development and disorders." In D. Battle (Ed.), *Communication Disorders and Development in Multicultural Populations* (pp. 120–147). Salt Lake City, UT: Academic Press, 2012.

Green, J. R., C. A. Moore, and K. J. Reilly, "The sequential development of jaw and lip control for speech." *Journal of Speech, Language, and Hearing Research, 45* (2002): 66–79.

Green, L., Research on African American English since 1998: Origins, description, theory, and practice. *Journal of English Linguistics, 32* (2004): 210–229.

Greenlee, M., "Interacting processes in the child's acquisition of stop-liquid clusters." *Papers and Reports on Child Language Disorders, Stanford University, 7* (1974): 85–100.

Grogan, M. L., E. J. Barker, S. J. Dettman, and P. J. Blamey, "Phonetic and phonologic changes in the connected speech of children using a cochlear implant." *Annals of Otology, Rhinology, and Laryngology,* Suppl. 166 (1995): 390–393.

Gruber, F. A., S. D. Lowery, H.-K. Seung, and R. E. Deal, "Approaches to speech-language intervention and the true believer." *Journal of Medical Speech-Language Pathology, 11* (2003): 95–104.

Grunwell, P., "The development of phonology: A descriptive profile." *First Language, 3* (1981): 161–191.

Grunwell, P., *Clinical Phonology*. Rockville, MD: Aspen, 1982.

Grunwell, P., *Phonological Assessment of Child Speech (PACS)*. Windsor, UK: NFER-Nelson, 1985.

Grunwell, P., *Clinical Phonology* (2nd ed.). London: Croom Helm, 1987.

Grunwell, P., and M. Yavas, "Phonotactic restrictions in disordered child phonology: A case study." *Clinical Linguistics and Phonetics, 2* (1988): 1–16.

Guitart, J., "Conservative versus radical dialects in American Spanish: Implications for language instruction." *Bilingual Review, 5* (1978): 57–64.

Guitart, J., "Spanish in contact with itself and the phonological characterization of conservative and radical styles." In A. Roca and J. Jensen (Eds.), *Spanish in Contact: Issues in Bilingualism* (pp. 151–157). Somerville, MA: Cascadilla, Press, 1996.

Hadlich, R., J. Holton, and M. Montes, *A Drillbook of Spanish Pronunciation.* New York: Harper & Row, 1968.

Haelsig, P. C., and C. L. Madison, "A study of phonological processes exhibited by 3-, 4-, and 5-year-old children." *Language, Speech, and Hearing Services in Schools, 17* (1986): 107–114.

Hall, M., "Auditory factors in functional articulatory speech defects." *Journal of Experimental Education, 7* (1938): 110–132.

Hammond, R., *The Sounds of Spanish: Analysis and Application (with special reference to American English).* Somerville, MA: Cascadilla Press, 2001.

Hanson, M. L., "Orofacial myofunctional disorders: Guidelines for assessment and treatment." *International Journal of Orofacial Myology, 14* (1988a): 27–32.

Hanson, M. L., "Orofacial myofunctional therapy: Historical and philosophical considerations." *International Journal of Orofacial Myology, 14* (1988b): 3–10.

Hanson, M. L., "Oral myofunctional disorders and articulatory patterns." In J. Bernthal and N. Bankson (Eds.), *Child Phonology: Characteristics, Assessment, and Intervention with Special Populations* (pp. 29–53). New York: Thieme Medical Publishers, 1994.

Hardcastle, W. J., *Physiology of Speech Production.* London: Academic Press, 1976.

Harrington, J., I. Lux, and R. Higgins, "Identification of error types as related to stimuli in articulation tests." Paper presented at the annual convention of the American Speech-Language-Hearing Association, San Francisco, 1984.

Hauner, K. K. Y., L. D. Shriberg, J. Kwiatkowski, and C. T. Allen, "A subtype of speech delay associated with developmental psychosocial involvement." *Journal of Speech, Language and Hearing Research, 48* (2005): 635–650.

Haynes, W., and M. Moran, "A cross-sectional developmental study of final consonant production in Southern Black children from preschool through third grade." *Language, Speech, and Hearing Services in Schools, 20* (1989): 400–406.

Hazan, V., and S. Barrett, "The development of phonemic categorization in children aged 6–12." *Journal of Phonetics, 28* (2000): 377–396.

Heath, S. M., and J. H. Hogben, "Cost-effective prediction of reading difficulties." *Journal of Speech, Language, and Hearing Research, 47* (2004): 751–765.

Hedrick, D., E. Prather, and A. Tobin, *Sequenced Inventory of Consonant Development.* Seattle: University of Washington Press, 1975.

Helfrich-Miller, K., "Melodic intonation therapy with developmentally apraxic children." *Seminars in Speech and Language, 5* (1984): 119–126.

Heller, J., J. Gabbay, C. O'Hara, M. Heller, and J. P. Bradley, "Improved ankyloglossia correction with four-flap z-frenuloplasty." *Annals of Plastic Surgery, 54* (2005): 623–628.

Hempenstall, K., "The role of phonemic awareness in beginning reading: A review." *Behaviour Change 14* (1997): 201–214.

Hepper, P. G., and S. Shahidullah, "Development of fetal hearing." *Archives of Disease in Childhood, 71*, 2 (1994): F81–F87.

Hesketh, A., E. Dima, and V. Nelson, "Teaching phoneme awareness to pre-literate children with speech disorder: A randomized controlled trial." *International Journal of Language and Communication Disorders, 42* (2007): 251–271.

Hetrick, R. D., and R. K. Sommers, "Unisensory and bisensory processing skills of children having misarticulations and normally speaking peers." *Journal of Speech and Hearing Research, 31* (1988): 575–581.

Hewlett, N., "Processes of development and production." In P. Grunwell (Ed.), *Developmental Speech Disorders* (pp. 15–38) Edinburgh, UK: Churchill Livingstone, 1990.

Hewlett, N., F. Gibbon, and W. Cohen-McKenzie, "When is a velar an alveolar? Evidence supporting a revised psycholinguistic model of speech production in children." *International Journal of Language and Communication Disorders, 33* (1998): 161–176.

Hickman, L., *The Apraxia Profile.* San Antonio, TX: Psychological Corporation, 1997.

Higgs, J. A. W., "The phonetic development of word initial /s/ plus stop clusters in a group of young children." *British Journal of Disorders of Communication, 3* (1968): 130–138.

Hilton, L., "Treatment of deviant phonologic systems: Tongue thrust." In W. Perkins (Ed.), *Phonological-Articulatory Disorders* (pp. 47–54). New York: Thieme-Stratton, 1984.

Hinton, L., and K. Pollock, "Regional variations in the phonological characteristics of African American Vernacular English (AAVE) speakers." Paper presented at the Texas Research Symposium on Language Diversity, Austin, TX, 1999.

Hixon, T. J., "Mechanical aspects of speech production." Paper read at Annual Convention of the American Speech and Hearing Association, Chicago, 1971.

Hockett, C. F., "A manual of phonology." *International Journal of American Linguistics (Memoir II).* Baltimore, MD: Waverly Press, 1955.

Hodson, B., *Computer Analysis of Phonological Processes (CAPP)*. Stonington, IL: Phonocomp, 1985.

Hodson, B., "Phonological remediation: A cycles approach." In N. Creaghead, P. Newman, and W. Secord (Eds.), *Assessment and Remediation of Articulatory and Phonological Disorders* (pp. 323–333). Columbus, OH: Merrill, 1989.

Hodson, B. W., *Computerized Analysis of Phonological Patterns (HCAPP)*. Wichita, KS: Phonomp Software, 2003.

Hodson, B. W., *Hodson Assessment of Phonological Patterns* (3rd ed.). Austin, TX: Pro-Ed, 2004.

Hodson, B. W., *Evaluating and Enhancing Children's Phonological Systems*. Greenville, SC: Thinking Publications, 2007a.

Hodson, B. W., "Overview of the diagnostic evaluation process for children with highly unintelligible speech." In B. W. Hodson (Ed.), *Evaluating and Enhancing Children's Phonological Systems* (pp. 45–64). Greenville, SC: Thinking Publications, 2007b.

Hodson, B. W., L. Chin, B. Redmond, and R. Simpson, "Phonological evaluation and remediation of speech deviations of a child with a repaired cleft palate: A case study." *Journal of Speech and Hearing Disorders, 48* (1983): 93–98.

Hodson, B. W., and E. P. Paden, *Targeting Intelligible Speech: A Phonological Approach to Remediation* (2nd ed.). Austin, TX: Pro-Ed, 1991.

Hoffman, P., "Spelling, phonology, and the speech pathologist: A whole language perspective." *Language, Speech, and Hearing Services in Schools, 21* (1990): 238–243.

Hoffman, P., and J. Norris, "On the nature of phonological development: Evidence from normal children's spelling errors." *Journal of Speech and Hearing Research, 32* (1989): 787–794.

Hoffman, P. R., and J. A. Norris, "Dynamic systems and whole language intervention." In A. L. Williams, S. McLeod, and R. J. McCauley (Eds.), *Interventions for Speech Sound Disorders in Children* (pp. 333–354). Baltimore, MD: Brookes, 2010.

Hoffman, P., J. Norris, and J. Monjure, "Comparison of process targeting and whole language treatments of phonologically delayed children." *Language, Speech, and Hearing Services in Schools, 21* (1990): 102–109.

Hoffman, P., and G. H. Schuckers, "Articulation remediation treatment models." In R. G. Daniloff (Ed.), *Articulation Assessment and Treatment Issues*. San Diego: College-Hill Press, 1984.

Hoffman, P., G. Schuckers, and R. Daniloff, *Children's Phonetic Disorders: Theory and Treatment*. Boston: Little, Brown, 1989.

Hoffmann, B., U. Wendel, and S. Schweitzer-Kranz, "Cross-sectional analysis of speech and cognitive performance in 32 patients with classic galactosemia." *Journal of Inherited Metabolic Disease, 34* (2011): 421–427.

Hoffmann, K. A., "Speech sound acquisition and natural process occurrence in the continuous speech of three- to six-year-old children." Unpublished master's thesis, University of Wisconsin–Madison, 1982.

Hogan, T., H. Catts, and T. Little, "The relationship between phonological awareness and reading: Implications for the assessment of phonological awareness." *Language, Speech, and Hearing Services in Schools, 36* (2005): 285–293.

Holland, A., "Training speech sound discrimination in children who misarticulate. A demonstration of teaching machine technique in speech correction [Project No. 5007]." Washington, DC: U.S. Department of Health, Education and Welfare, 1967.

Holm, A., S. Crosbie, and B. Dodd, "Differentiating normal variability from inconsistency in children's speech: Normative data." *International Journal of Language and Communication Disorders, 42* (2007): 467–486.

Holm, A., and B. Dodd, "A longitudinal study of the phonological development of two Cantonese-English bilingual children." *Applied Psycholinguistics, 20* (2000): 349–376.

Holm, A., B. Dodd, and A. Ozanne, "Efficacy of intervention for a bilingual child making articulation and phonological errors." *International Journal of Bilingualism, 1* (1997): 55–69.

Holm, A., F. Farrier, and B. Dodd, "Phonological awareness, reading accuracy and spelling ability of children with inconsistent phonological disorder." *International Journal of Language and Communication Disorders* (2007).

Holm, J., *Pidgins and Creoles, Volume I: Theory and Structure*. Cambridge, UK: Cambridge University Press, 1988.

Holm, J., *Pidgins and Creoles, Volume II: Reference Survey*. Cambridge, UK: Cambridge University Press, 1989.

Hong, P., D. Lago, J. Seargeant, L. Pellman, A. E. Magit, and S. M. Pransky, "Defining ankyloglossia: A case study of anterior and posterior tongue ties." *International Journal of Pediatric Otorhinolaryngology, 74* (2010): 1003–1006.

Howard, S., "English speech acquisition." In S. McLeod (Ed.), *The International Guide to Speech Acquisition* (pp. 188–203). Clifton Park, NY: Thomson Delmar Learning, 2007.

Howard, S. J., and B. C. Heselwood, "The contribution of phonetics to the study of vowel development and disorders." In M. J. Ball and F. E. Gibbon (Eds.), *Vowel Disorders* (pp. 37–82) New York: Butterworth-Heinemann, 2002.

Howell, J., and E. Dean, *Treating Phonological Disorders in Children: Metaphon—Theory to Practice*. San Diego: Singular Publishing, 1991.

Hull, F., P. Mielke, R. Timmons, and J. Willeford, "The national speech and hearing survey: Preliminary results." *ASHA, 13* (1971): 501–509.

Hua, Z., "The normal and disordered phonology of Putonghua (Modern Standard Chinese)-speaking children." In Z. Hua and B. Dodd (Eds.), *Phonological Development and Disorders: A Cross-Linguistic Perspective* (pp. 81–108). Clevedon, UK: Multilingual Matters, 2006.

Hua, Z., "Putonghua (Modern Standard Chinese) speech acquisition." In S. McLeod (Ed.), *The International Guide to Speech Acquisition* (pp. 516–527). Clifton Park, NY: Thomson/Delmar, 2007.

Hulme, C., K. Goetz, D. Gooch, J. Adams, and M. J. Snowling, "Paired-associate learning, phoneme awareness, and learning to read." *Journal of Experimental Child Psychology, 96* (2007): 150–166.

Humphreys, M., "A contribution to infantile linguistics." *Transactions of the American Philological Association, 11* (1880): 5–17.

Hwa-Froelich, D., B. Hodson, and H. Edwards, "Characteristics of Vietnamese phonology." *American Journal of Speech-Language Pathology, 11* (2002): 264–273.

Hyter, Y., "Ties that bind: The sounds of African American English." *ASHA Special Interest Division 14 Newsletter, 2,* (1996): 3–6.

Individuals with Disabilities Education Act Amendments of 2004, PL No. 108–446, 20 U.S.C. Section 1400 et seq.

Ingram, D., *Phonological Disability in Children*. London: Edward Arnold, 1976.

Ingram, D., *Phonological Disability in Children* (2nd ed.). London: Cole and Whurr, 1989a.

Ingram, D., *First Language Acquisition: Method, Description and Explanation*. Cambridge, UK: Cambridge University Press, 1989b.

Ingram, D., L. Christensen, S. Veach, and B. Webster, "The acquisition of word-initial fricatives and affricates in English by children between 2 and 6 years." In G. H. Yeni-Komshian, J. F. Kavanagh, and C. A. Ferguson (Eds.), *Child Phonology. Volume 1: Production* (pp. 169–192) New York: Academic Press, 1980.

Ingram, D., and K. D. Ingram, "A whole-word approach to phonological analysis and intervention." *Language, Speech, and Hearing Services in Schools, 32* (2001): 271–283.

Ingram, J., J. Pittman, and D. Newman, "Developmental and socio-linguistic variation in the speech of Brisbane school children." *Australian Journal of Linguistics, 5* (1985): 233–246.

Invernizzi, M., and J. Meier, *Phonological awareness literacy screening (PALS: 1–3)*. Charlottesville: The Virginia State Department of Education and The University of Virginia, 2002–2003.

Invernizzi, M., J. Meier, L. Swank, and C. Juel, *Phonological Awareness Literacy Screening (PALS-K)*. Charlottesville: The Virginia State Department of Education and The University of Virginia, 2001.

Irish Association of Speech and Language Therapists (IASLT). "Speech and Language Therapy Scope of Practice." Available from http://www.iaslt.ie/docs/members/policy/IASLT%20Scope%20of%20Practice%20.pdf, 2011.

Irwin, J. V., and S. P. Wong (Eds.), *Phonological Development in Children 18 to 72 Months*. Carbondale, IL: Southern Illinois University Press, 1983.

Irwin, R. B., J. F. West, and M. A. Trombetta, "Effectiveness of speech therapy for second grade children with misarticulations: Predictive factors." *Exceptional Children, 32* (1966): 471–479.

Jakobson, R., *Child Language Aphasia and Phonological Universals*. The Hague, The Netherlands: Mouton, 1968.

James, D., "The use of phonological processes in Australian children aged 2 to 7:11 years." *Advances in Speech-Language Pathology, 3* (2001): 109–128.

James, D., "Hippopotamus is so hard to say: Children's acquisition of polysyllabic words." Unpublished doctoral dissertation, The University of Sydney, Australia, 2007.

James, D., P. McCormack, and A. Butcher, "Children's use of phonological processes in the age range of five to seven years." In S. McLeod and L. McAllister (Eds.), *Proceedings of the 1999 Speech Pathology Australia National Conference* (pp. 48–57). Melbourne: Speech Pathology Australia, 1999.

James, D., J. van Doorn, and S. McLeod, "Vowel production in mono-, di- and poly-syllabic words in children 3;0 to 7;11 years." In L. Wilson and S. Hewat (Eds.), *Proceedings of the Speech Pathology Australia Conference* (pp. 127–136). Melbourne: Speech Pathology Australia, 2001.

James, D., J. van Doorn, and S. McLeod, "Segment production in mono-, di- and polysyllabic words in children aged 3–7 years." In F. Windsor, L. Kelly, and N. Hewlett (Eds.), *Themes in Clinical Phonetics and Linguistics* (pp. 287–298). Hillsdale, NJ: Erlbaum, 2002.

James, D., J. van Doorn, and S. McLeod, "The contribution of polysyllabic words in clinical decision making about children's speech." *Clinical Linguistics and Phonetics, 22* (2008): 345–353.

Jann, G., M. Ward, and H. Jann, "A longitudinal study of articulation, deglutition and malocclusion." *Journal of Speech and Hearing Disorders, 29* (1964): 424–435.

Jimenez, B. C., "Acquisition of Spanish consonants in children aged 3–5 years, 7 months." *Language, Speech, and Hearing Services in Schools, 18* (1987): 357–363.

Johns, D., and K. Salyer, "Surgical and prosthetic management of neurogenic speech disorders." In D. Johns (Ed.), *Clinical Management of Neurogenic Communicative Disorders* (pp. 311–331). Boston: Little, Brown, 1978.

Johnson, E. P., B. F. Pennington, J. H. Lowenstein, and S. Nittrouer, "Sensitivity to structure in the speech signal by children with speech sound disorder and reading disability." *Journal of Communication Disorders, 44* (2011): 294–314.

Johnson, C. A., A. D. Weston, and B. A. Bain, "An objective and time efficient method for determining severity of childhood speech delay." *American Journal of Speech-Language Pathology, 13* (2004): 55–65.

Johnston, R. S., M. Anderson, and C. Holligan, "Knowledge of the alphabet and explicit awareness of phonemes in pre-readers: The nature of the relationship." *Reading and Writing: An Interdisciplinary Journal, 8* (1996): 217–234.

Jordan, L., J. Hardy, and H. Morris, "Performance of children with good and poor articulation on tasks of tongue placement." *Journal of Speech and Hearing Research, 21* (1978): 429–439.

Juel, C., "Learning to read and write: A longitudinal study of 54 children from first through fourth grades." *Journal of Educational Psychology, 80* (1988): 437–447.

Jusczyk, P., and E. Thompson, "Perception of phonetic contrasts in multisyllabic utterances by 2 month old infants." *Perception and Psychophysics, 23* (1978): 105–109.

Justice, L., J. Kaderavek, R. Bowles, and K. Grim, "Language impairment, parent-child shared reading, and phonological awareness: A feasibility study." *Topics in Early Childhood Special Education, 25* (2005): 143–156.

Justice, L. M., and H. K. Ezell, "Print referencing: An emergent literacy enhancement strategy and its clinical applications." *Language, Speech, and Hearing Services in Schools, 35* (2004): 185–193.

Justice, L. M., A. S. McGinty, S. Q. Cabell, C. R. Kilday, K. Knighton, and G. Huffman, "Language and literacy curriculum support for preschoolers who are academically at risk: A feasibility study." *Language, Speech, and Hearing Services in Schools, 41* (2010): 161–178.

Justice, L. M., K. Pence, R. B. Bowles, and A. Wiggins, "An investigation of four hypotheses concerning the order by which 4-year-old children learn the alphabet letters." *Early Childhood Research Quarterly, 21* (2006): 374–389.

Kager, R., *Optimality Theory*. Cambridge, UK: Cambridge University Press, 1999.

Kamhi, A. G., R. Friemoth-Lee, and L. Nelson, "Word, syllable and sound awareness in language disordered children." *Journal of Speech and Hearing Disorders, 50* (1985): 207–212.

Kantner, C. E., and R. West, *Phonetics*. New York: Harper & Row, 1960.

Karlsson, H. B., L. D. Shriberg, P. Flipsen Jr., and J. L. McSweeny, "Acoustic phenotypes for speech-genetics studies: Toward an acoustic marker for residual /s/ distortions." *Clinical Linguistics and Phonetics, 16* (2002): 403–424.

Kaufman, N., *Kaufman Speech Praxis Test for Children*. Detroit, MI: Wayne State University Press, 1995.

Kayser, H., "Interpreters." In H. Kayser (Ed.), *Bilingual Speech-Language Pathology: An Hispanic Focus* (pp. 207–221). San Diego, CA: Singular Publishing, 1995.

Keating, D., G. Turrell, and A. Ozanne, "Childhood speech disorders: Reported prevalence, comorbidity and socioeconomic profile." *Journal of Pediatric Child Health, 37* (2001): 431–436.

Kehoe, M., "Stress error patterns in English-speaking children's word productions." *Clinical Linguistics and Phonetics, 11* (1997): 389–409.

Kehoe, M. M., "Prosodic patterns in children's multisyllabic word productions." *Language, Speech, and Hearing Services in Schools, 32* (2001): 284–294.

Kemaloglu, Y. K., T. Kobayashi, and T. Nakajima, "Analysis of the craniofacial skeleton in cleft children with otitis media with effusion." *International Journal of Pediatric Otorhinolaryngology, 47* (1999): 57–69.

Kenney, K., and E. Prather, "Articulation in preschool children: Consistency of productions." *Journal of Speech and Hearing Research, 29* (1986): 29–36.

Kent, R. D., "Anatomical and neuromuscular maturation of the speech mechanism: Evidence from acoustic studies." *Journal of Speech and Hearing Research, 19* (1976): 421–447.

Kent, R. D. "Contextual facilitation of correct sound production." *Language, Speech, and Hearing Services in Schools, 13* (1982): 66–76.

Kent, R. D., and H. R. Bauer, "Vocalizations of one year olds." *Journal of Child Language, 12* (1985): 491–526.

Kent, R. D., and L. L. Forner, "Speech segment durations in sentence recitations by children and adults." *Journal of Phonetics, 8* (1980): 157–168.

Kent, R. D., J. F. Kent, and J. C. Rosenbek, "Maximum performance tests of speech production." *Journal of Speech and Hearing Disorders, 52* (1987): 367–387.

Kent, R. D., R. E. Martin, and R. L. Sufit, "Oral sensation: A review and clinical prospective." In H. Winitz (Ed.), *Human Communication and Its Disorders: A Review—1990* (pp. 135–191). Norwood, NJ: Ablex, 1990.

Kent, R. D., and F. D. Minifie, "Coarticulation in recent speech production models." *Journal of Phonetics, 5* (1977): 115–133.

Kent, R. D., G. Miolo, and S. Bloedel, "The intelligibility of children's speech: A review of evaluation procedures." *American Journal of Speech-Language Pathology, 3* (1994): 81–95.

Kent, R. D., and K. L. Moll, "Cinefluorographic analyses of selected lingual consonants." *Journal of Speech and Hearing Research, 15* (1972): 453–473.

Kent, R. D., and K. L. Moll. "Articulatory timing in selected consonant sequences." *Brain and Language, 2* (1975): 304–323.

Kent, R. D., and R. Netsell, "Effects of stress contrasts on certain articulatory parameters." *Phonetica, 24* (1972): 23–44.

Kent, R. D., M. J. Osberger, R. Netsell, and C. G. Hustedde, "Phonetic development in identical twins differing in auditory function." *Journal of Speech and Hearing Disorders, 52* (1987): 64–75.

Kent, R. D., and C. Tilkens, "Oromotor foundations of speech acquisition." In S. McLeod (Ed.), *International Guide to Speech Acquisition* (pp. 8–13). Clifton Park, NY: Thomson Delmar Learning, 2007.

Khan, L. M., "Major phonological processes." *Language, Speech, and Hearing Services in Schools, 13* (1982): 77–85.

Khan, L. M., *Basics of Phonological Analysis: A Programmed Learning Test.* San Diego, CA: College Hill, 1985.

Khan, L. M., and N. P. Lewis, *Khan-Lewis Phonological Analysis.* Circle Pines, MN: American Guidance Service, 1986, 2002.

Khinda, V., and N. Grewal, "Relationship of tongue-thrust swallowing and anterior open bite with articulation disorders: A clinical study." *Journal of the Indian Society of Pedodontia and Preventive Dentistry, 17* (1999): 33–39.

Kilminster, M. G. E., and E. M. Laird, "Articulation development in children aged three to nine years." *Australian Journal of Human Communication Disorders, 6* (1978): 23–30.

Kim, M., and S. Pae, "Korean speech acquisition. In S. McLeod (Ed.), *The International Guide to Speech Acquisition* (pp. 472–482). Clifton Park, NY: Thomson/Delmar. 2007.

Kindler, A., "Survey of the states' LEP students 2000–2001 summary report." Washington, DC: National Clearinghouse for English Language Acquisition, 2001.

Kiparsky, P., and L. Menn, "On the acquisition of phonology." In J. MacNamara (Ed.), *Language Learning and Thought* (pp. 47–78). New York: Academic Press, 1977.

Kirk, C., and G. T. Gillon, "Longitudinal effects of phonological awareness intervention on morphological awareness in children with speech impairment."

Language, Speech, and Hearing Services in Schools, 38 (2007): 342–252.

Kirtley, C., P. Bryant, M. MacLean, and L. Bradley, "Rhyme, rime, and the onset of reading." *Journal of Experimental Child Psychology, 48* (1989): 224–245.

Kisatsky, T., "The prognostic value of Carter-Buck tests in measuring articulation skills in selected kindergarten children." *Exceptional Children, 34* (1967): 81–85.

Klaiman, P., M. A. Witzel, F. Margar-Bacal, and I. R. Munro, "Changes in aesthetic appearance and intelligibility of speech after partial glossectomy in patients with Down Syndrome." *Plastic and Reconstructive Surgery, 82* (1988): 403–408.

Klatt, D. H., "Linguistic uses of segmental duration in English: Acoustic and perceptual evidence." *Journal of the Acoustical Society of America, 59* (1976): 1208–1221.

Kleffner, F., "A comparison of the reactions of a group of fourth grade children to recorded examples of defective and nondefective articulation." Unpublished Ph.D. Thesis, University of Wisconsin, 1952.

Klein, E. S., "Phonological/traditional approaches to articulation therapy: A retrospective group comparison." *Language, Speech, and Hearing Services in Schools, 27* (1996): 314–323.

Klein, H. B., and M. Liu-Shea, "Between word simplification patterns in the continuous speech of children with speech sound disorders." *Language, Speech, and Hearing Services in Schools, 40* (2009): 17–30.

Koch, H., "Sibling influence on children's speech." *Journal of Speech, language, and Hearing Disorders, 21* (1956): 322–329.

Koegel, L. K., R. L. Koegel, and J. C. Ingham, "Programming rapid generalization of correct articulation through self-monitoring procedures." *Journal of Speech and Hearing Disorders, 51* (1986): 24–32.

Koegel, R., L. Koegel, K. Van Voy, and J. Ingham, "Within-clinic versus outside-of-clinic self-monitoring of articulation to promote generalization." *Journal of Speech and Hearing Disorders, 53* (1988): 392–399.

Kohnert, K., and A. Derr, "Language intervention with bilingual children." In B. Goldstein (Ed.), *Bilingual Language Development and Disorders in Spanish-English Speakers* (2nd ed., pp. 311–342). Baltimore, MD: Brookes, 2012.

Kohnert, K., D. Yim, K. Nett, P. F. Kan, and L. Duran, "Intervention with linguistically diverse preschool children: A focus on developing home language(s)." *Language, Speech, and Hearing Services in Schools, 36* (2005): 251–263.

Koutsoftas, A., M. Harmon, and S. Gray, "The effect of tier 2 intervention for phonemic awareness in a response-to-intervention model in low-income preschool classrooms." *Language, Speech, and Hearing Services in Schools, 40* (2009): 116–130.

Kronvall, E., and C. Diehl, "The relationship of auditory discrimination to articulatory defects of children with no known organic impairment." *Journal of Speech and Hearing Disorders, 19* (1954): 335–338.

Kummer, A., "Ankyloglossia: An effect on speech . . . or not." Paper presented at the annual convention of the American Speech-Language-Hearing Association, New Orleans, LA, 2009.

Kumin, L., "Intelligibility of speech in children with Down Syndrome in natural settings: Parents' perspective." *Perceptual and Motor Skills, 78* (1994): 307–313.

Kumin, L., C. Council, and M. Goodman, "A longitudinal study of emergence of phonemes in children with Down syndrome." *Journal of Communication Disorders, 27* (1994): 293–303.

Kwiatkowski, J., and L. D. Shriberg, "Speech normalization in developmental phonological disorders: A retrospective study of capability-focus theory." *Language, Speech, and Hearing Services in Schools, 24* (1993): 10–18.

Kwiatkowski, J., and L. D. Shriberg, "The capability-focus treatment framework for child speech disorders." *American Journal of Speech-Language Pathology, 7* (1998): 27–38.

Labov, W., "The three dialects of English." In P. Eckert (Ed.), *New Ways of Analyzing Sound Change* (pp. 1–44). New York: Academic Press, 1991.

Ladefoged, P., *Preliminaries to Linguistic Phonetics.* Chicago: University of Chicago Press, 1971.

Ladefoged, P., *A Course in Phonetics.* New York: Harcourt Brace Jovanovich, 1975.

Ladefoged, P., *A Course in Phonetics* (3rd ed.). New York: Harcourt Brace, 1993.

Ladefoged, P., *Vowels and Consonants* (2nd ed.) Oxford, UK: Blackwell, 2005.

Laine, T., M. Jaroma, and A. L. Linnasalo, "Relationships between interincisal occlusion and articulatory components of speech." *Folia Phoniatrica, 39* (1987): 78–86.

Laitinen, J., M.-L. Haapanen, M. Paaso, J. Pulkkinen, A. Heltovaara, and R. Ranta, "Occurrence of dental consonant misarticulations in different cleft types." *Folia Phoniatrica et Logopedica, 50* (1998): 92–100.

Langdon, H., and L. R. L. Cheng, *Collaborating with Interpreters and Translators.* Eau Claire, WI: Thinking Publications, 2002.

Lapko, L., and N. Bankson, "Relationship between auditory discrimination, articulation stimulability and consistency of misarticulation." *Perceptual and Motor Skills, 40* (1975): 171–177.

Lapointe, L., and R. Wertz, "Oral-movement abilities and articulatory characteristics of brain-injured adults." *Perceptual Motor Skills, 39* (1974): 39–46.

LaRiviere, C., H. Winitz, J. Reeds, and E. Herriman, "The conceptual reality of selected distinctive features." *Journal of Speech and Hearing Research, 17* (1974): 122–133.

Larrivee, L., and H. Catts, "Early reading achievement in children with expressive phonological disorders." *American Journal of Speech-Language Pathology, 8* (1999): 118–128.

Lasky, R. E., and A. L. Williams, "The development of the auditory system from conception to term." *Neoreviews, 6*, 3 (2005): e141–e152.

Lass, N. J., and M. Pannbacker, "The application of evidence-based practice to nonspeech oral-motor treatments." *Language, Speech, and Hearing Services in Schools, 39* (2008): 408–421.

Lau v. Nichols, 414 U.S. 563 (1974).

Lau Remedies, Office of Civil Rights, task force findings specifying remedies available for eliminating past educational practices rules unlawful under *Lau* v. *Nichols,* IX, pt. 5, 1975.

Law, J., J. Boyle, F. Harris, A. Harkness, and C. Nye, "Screening for speech and language delay: A systematic review of the literature." *Health Technology and Assessment, 2,* 9 (1998): 1–183.

Law, J., Z. Garrett, and C. Nye, "The efficacy of treatment for children with developmental speech and language delay disorders: A meta-analysis." *Journal of Speech, Language, and Hearing Research* (2004): 924–943.

Leap, W., "American Indian languages." In C. Ferguson and S. Heath (Eds.), *Language in the USA* (pp. 116–144). Cambridge. UK: Cambridge University Press, 1981.

Lebrun, Y., "Tongue thrust, tongue tip position at rest, and stigmatism: A review." *Journal of Communication Disorders, 18* (1985): 305–312.

Leder, S., and J. W. Lerman, "Some acoustic evidence for vocal abuse in adult speakers with repaired cleft palate." *Laryngoscope, 95* (1985): 837–840.

Leder, S., and J. Spitzer., "A perceptual evaluation of the speech of adventitiously deaf adult males." *Ear and Hearing, 11* (1990): 169–175.

Lehiste, I., *Suprasegmentals.* Cambridge, MA: M.I.T. Press, 1970.

Leitão, S., and J. Fletcher, "Literacy outcomes for students with speech impairment: Long-term follow-up." *International Journal of Language and Communication Disorders, 39* (2004): 245–256.

Lenchner, O., and B. Podhajski, *The Sounds Abound Program.* East Moline, IL: Linguisystems, 1998.

Lenden, J. M., and P. Flipsen Jr., "Prosody and voice characteristics of children with cochlear implants." *Journal of Communication Disorders, 40* (2007): 66–81.

Leonard, L., "The nature of deviant articulation." *Journal of Speech and Hearing Disorders, 38* (1973): 156–161.

Leonard, L. B., and J. S. Leonard, "The contribution of phonetic context to an unusual phonological pattern: A case study." *Language, Speech, and Hearing Services in Schools, 16* (1985): 110–118.

Leonard, L. B., L. E. Rowan, B. Morris, and M. E. Fey, "Intra-word phonological variability in young children." *Journal of Child Language, 9* (1982): 55–69.

Leonard, R. J., "Characteristics of speech in speakers with oral/oralpharyngeal ablation." In J. Bernthal and N. Bankson (Eds.), *Child Phonology: Characteristics, Assessment, and Intervention with Special Populations* (pp. 54–78). New York: Thieme Medical Publishers, 1994.

Leopold, W., *Speech Development of a Bilingual Child: A Linguist's Record.* Volume 2, *Sound Learning in the First Two Years.* Evanston, IL: Northwestern University Press, 1947.

Leopold, W., *Speech Development of a Bilingual Child: A Linguist's Record.* Volume 1, *Vocabulary Growth in the First Two Years* (1939). Volume 3, *Grammar and General Problems in the First Two Years* (1949). Volume 4, *Diary from Age Two* (1949). Evanston, IL: Northwestern University Press, 1939–1949.

Levi, G., F. Capozzi, A. Fabrizi, and E. Sechi, "Language disorders and prognosis for reading disabilities in developmental age." *Perceptual and Motor Skills, 54* (1982): 1119–1122.

Levitt, H., and H. Stromberg, "Segmental characteristics of speech of hearing-impaired children: Factors affecting intelligibility." In I. Hochberg, H. Levitt, and M. Osberger (Eds.), *Speech of the Hearing Impaired* (pp. 53–73). Baltimore, MD: University Park Press, 1983.

Lewis, B. A., "Genetic influences on speech sound disorders." In R. Paul and P. Flipsen Jr. (Eds.), *Speech Sound Disorders in Children: In Honor of Lawrence D. Shriberg* (pp. 51–70). San Diego, CA: Plural Publishing, 2009.

Lewis, B. A., A. A. Avrich, L. A. Freebairn, H. G. Taylor, S. K. Iyengar, and C. M. Stein, "Subtyping children with speech sound disorders by endophenotypes." *Topics in Language Disorders, 31* (2011): 112–127.

Lewis, B. A., B. Ekelman, and D. Aram, "A familial study of severe phonological disorders." *Journal of Speech and Hearing Research, 32* (1989): 713–724.

Lewis, B. A., L. A. Freebairn, A. J. Hansen, l. Miscimarra, S. K. Iyengar, and H. G. Taylor, "Speech and language skills of parents of children with speech sound disorders." *American Journal of Speech-Language Pathology, 16* (2007): 108–118.

Lewis, B. A., L. A. Freebairn, A. J. Hansen, C. M. Stein, L. D. Shriberg, S. K. Iyengar, and H. G. Taylor, "Dimensions of early speech sound disorders: A factor analytic study." *Journal of Communication Disorders, 39* (2006): 139–157.

Lewis, B. A., L. A. Freebairn, and H. G. Taylor, "Follow-up of Children with Early Expressive Phonology Disorders." *Journal of Learning Disabilities 33* (2000): 433–444.

Lewis, B. A., and L. Freebairn-Farr, "Preschool phonology disorders at school age, adolescence, and adulthood." Paper presented at the annual convention of the American Speech-Language-Hearing Association, Atlanta, 1991.

Lewis, B. A., B. O'Donnell, L. Freebairn, and H. Taylor, "Spoken language and written expression-interplay of delays." *American Journal of Speech-Language Pathology, 7*, 3 (1998): 77–84.

Li, C., and S. Thompson, "The acquisition of tone in Mandarin-speaking children." *Journal of Child Language, 4* (1977): 185–199.

Liberman, I., and D. Shankweiler, "Phonology and problems of learning to read and write." *Remedial and Special Education, 6* (1985): 8–17.

Lieberman, P., *Intonation, Perception and Language.* Cambridge, MA: M.I.T. Press, 1967.

Lindamood, C., and P. Lindamood, *Lindamood Auditory Conceptualization Test.* Boston: Teaching Resources, 1971.

Lindblom, B., "Spectrographic study of vowel reduction." *Journal of the Acoustical Society of America, 35* (1963): 1773–1781.

Lindblom, B., "Explaining phonetic variation: A sketch of the H&H theory." In W. J. Hardcastle and A. Marchal (Eds.), *Speech Production and Speech Modeling* (pp. 403–439). Amsterdam, The Netherlands: Kluwer, 1990.

Lindblom, B., and R. Zetterström (Eds.), *Precursors of Early Speech Development.* New York: Stockton, 1986.

Ling, D., *Foundations of Spoken Language for Hearing-Impaired Children.* Washington, DC: Alexander Graham Bell Association for the Deaf, 1989.

Lipski, J. *Varieties of Spanish in the United States.* Washington, DC: Georgetown University Press, 2008.

Lleo, C., "Homonymy and reduplication: On the extended availability of two strategies in phonological acquisition." *Journal of Child Language, 17* (1990): 267–278.

Lleó, C., and M. Kehoe, "On the interaction of phonological systems in child bilingual acquisition." *International Journal of Bilingualism, 6* (2002): 233–237.

Lleó, C., I. Kuchenbrandt, M. Kehoe, and C. Trujillo, "Syllable final consonants in Spanish and German monolingual and bilingual acquisition." In N. Müller (Ed.), *(In)vulnerable domains in multilingualism* (pp. 191–220). Amsterdam, The Netherlands: John Benjamins, 2003.

Lleo, C., and M. Prinz, "Consonant clusters in child phonology and the directionality of syllable structure assignment." *Journal of Child Language, 23* (1996): 31–56.

Locke, J., "The inference of speech perception in the phonologically disordered child. Part I: A rationale, some criteria, the conventional tests." *Journal of Speech and Hearing Disorders, 45* (1980a): 431–444.

Locke, J., "The inference of speech perception in the phonologically disordered child. Part II: Some clinically novel procedures, their use, some findings." *Journal of Speech and Hearing Disorders, 45* (1980b): 445–468.

Locke, J., "Vocal development in the human infant: Functions and phonetics." In F. Windsor, M. L. Kelly, and N. Hewlett (Eds.), *Investigations in Clinical Phonetics and Linguistics* (pp. 243–256). Hillsdale, NJ: Erlbaum, 2002.

Locke, J., and K. Kutz, "Memory for speech and speech for memory." *Journal of Speech and Hearing Research, 18* (1975): 179–191.

Locke, J., and P. Mather, "Genetic factors in phonology. Evidence from monozygotic and dizygotic twins." Paper presented at the annual convention of the American Speech-Language-Hearing Association, New Orleans, 1987.

Lof, G., "A study of phoneme perception and speech stimulability." Unpublished Ph.D. dissertation, University of Wisconsin–Madison, 1994.

Lof, G. L., "Science-based practice and the speech-language pathologist." *International Journal of Speech-Language Pathology, 13* (2010): 189–196.

Lof, G., and S. Synan, "Is there a speech discrimination/perception link to disordered articulation and phonology? A review of 80 years of literature." *Contemporary Issues in Communication Science and Disorders, 24* (1997): 63–77.

Lof, G. L., and M. M Watson, "A nationwide survey of nonspeech oral motor exercise use: Implications for evidence-based practice." *Language, Speech, and Hearing Services in Schools, 39* (2008): 392–407.

Lonigan, C. J., J. L. Anthony, B. M. Phillips, D. J. Purpura, S. B. Wilson, and J. D. McQueen, "The nature of preschool phonological processing abilities and their relations to vocabulary, general cognitive abilities, and print knowledge." *Journal of Educational Psychology, 101* (2009): 345–358.

Lonigan, C. J., S. R. Burgess, J. L. Anthony, and T. A. Barker, "Development of phonological sensitivity in 2- to 5-year-old children." *Journal of Educational Psychology, 90* (1998): 294–311.

Lonigan, C. J., J. M. Farver, B. M. Phillips, and J. Clancy-Menchetti, "Promoting the development of preschool children's emergent literacy skills: A randomized evaluation of a literacy-focused curriculum and two professional development models." *Reading and Writing, 24* (2011): 305–337.

Long, S., "About time: A comparison of computerized and manual procedures for grammatical and phonological analysis." *Clinical Linguistics and Phonetics, 15* (2001): 399–426.

Long, S. H., M. E. Fey, and R. W. Channell, "Computerized profiling (Version CP941.exe)." Cleveland, OH: Case Western Reserve University, 2002.

Lorwatanapongsa, P., and S. Maroonroge, "Thai speech acquisition." In S. McLeod (Ed.), *The International Guide to Speech Acquisition* (pp. 554–565). Clifton Park, NY: Thomson/Delmar, 2007.

Lowe, R. J., P. J. Knutson, and M. A. Monson, "Incidence of fronting in preschool children." *Language, Speech, and Hearing Services in Schools, 16* (1985): 119–123.

Lundberg, I., J. Frost, and O. Peterson, "Effects of an extensive program for stimulating phonological awareness in preschool children." *Reading Research Quarterly, 23* (1988): 263–284.

Lynch, E., "Developing cross-cultural competence." In E. Lynch and M. Hanson (Eds.), *Developing Cross-Cultural Competence: A Guide for Working with Children and Their Families* (3rd ed., pp. 41–77). Baltimore, MD: Brookes, 2004.

Maas, E., D. A. Robin, S. N. Austermann Hula, S. E. Freedman, G. Wulf, K. J. Ballard, and R. A. Schmidt, "Principles of motor learning in treatment of motor speech disorders." *American Journal of Speech-Language Pathology, 17* (2008): 277–298.

Maassen, B., L. Nijland, and S. van der Meulen, "Coarticulation within and between syllables by children with developmental apraxia of speech." *Clinical Linguistics and Phonetics, 15* (2001): 145–150.

Macken, M., "Phonological acquisition." In J. A. Goldsmith (Ed.), *The Handbook of Phonological Theory* (pp. 671–696). Cambridge, MA: Blackwell, 1995.

Macken, M. A., "The child's lexical representation: The 'puzzle, puddle, pickle' evidence." *Journal of Linguistics, 16* (1980a): 1–17.

Macken, M. A., "Aspects of the acquisition of stop systems: A cross-linguistic perspective." In G. H. Yeni-Komshian, J. F. Kavanagh, and C. A. Ferguson (Eds.), *Child Phonology,* Volume 1, *Production* (pp. 143–168) New York: Academic Press, 1980b.

Maclagan, M., and G. T. Gillon, "New Zealand English speech acquisition." In S. McLeod (Ed.), *The International Guide to Speech Acquisition* (pp. 257–268). Clifton Park, NY: Thomson Delmar Learning, 2007.

MacNeilage, P. F., "Speech physiology." In H. H. Gilbert (Ed.), *Speech and Cortical Functioning* (pp. 1–72). New York: Academic Press, 1972.

Madell, J. R., N. Sislian, and R. Hoffman, "Speech perception for cochlear implant patients using hearing aids on the unimplanted ear." *International Congress Series, 1273* (2004): 223–226.

Maez, L., "Spanish as a first language." Unpublished doctoral dissertation, University of California–Santa Barbara. Santa Barbara, CA: 1981.

Majnemer, A., and B. Rosenblatt, "Reliability of parental recall of developmental milestones." *Pediatric Neurology, 10* (1994): 304–308.

Major, E. M., and B. H. Bernhardt, "Metaphonological skills of children with phonological disorders before and after phonological and metaphonological intervention." *International Journal of Language and Communication Disorders 33* (1998): 413–444.

Mann, V. A. and J. G. Foy, "Speech development patterns and phonological awareness in preschool children." *Annals of Dyslexia, 57* (2007): 51–74.

Marchant, C. D., P. A. Shurin, V. A. Turczyk, D. E. Wasikowski, M. A. Tutihasi, and S. E. Kinney, "Course and outcome of otitis media in early infancy: A prospective study." *The Journal of Pediatrics, 104* (1984): 826–831.

Marder, L., and C. N. Cholmain, "Promoting language development for children with Down's syndrome." *Current Pediatrics, 16* (2006): 495–500.

Margar-Bacal, F., M. A. Witzel, and I. Munro, "Speech intelligibility after partial glossectomy in children with Down's syndrome." *Plastic and Reconstructive Surgery, 79* (1988): 44–47.

Marquardt, T. P., A. Jacks, and B. L. Davis, "Token-to-token variability in developmental apraxia of speech: Three longitudinal case studies." *Clinical Linguistics and Phonetics, 18* (2004): 127–144.

Marquardt, T. P., H. M. Sussman, T. Snow, and A. Jacks, "The integrity of the syllable in developmental apraxia of speech." *Journal of Communication Disorders 35* (2002): 31–49.

Marshall, P., "Oral-motor techniques in articulation therapy [videotapes]." Seattle, WA: Innovative Concepts, 1992.

Martin Luther King Junior Elementary School Children, et al., v. Ann Arbor School District Board, Civil Action No. 7-71861, 451 F. Supp. 1324 (1978).

Marunick, M., and N. Tselios, "The efficacy of palatal augmentation prostheses for speech and swallowing in patients undergoing glossectomy: A review of the literature." *The Journal of Prosthetic Dentistry, 91* (2004): 67–74.

Mase, D., "Etiology of articulatory speech defects." *Teacher's College Contribution to Education, No. 921.* New York: Columbia University, 1946.

Mason, R., "Orthodontic perspectives on orofacial myofunctional therapy." *International Journal of Orofacial Myology, 14* (1988): 49–55.

Mason, R., and W. Proffit, "The tongue-thrust controversy: Background and recommendations." *Journal of Speech and Hearing Disorders, 39* (1974): 115–132.

Mason, R., and N. Wickwire, "Examining for orofacial variations." *Communiqué, 8* (1978): 2–26.

Masterson, J., "Classroom-based phonological intervention." *American Journal of Speech-Language Pathology, 2* (1993): 5–9.

Masterson, J., and B. H. Bernhardt, *CAPES: Computerized Articulation and Phonology Evaluation System* (Version 1.0.1). San Antonio, TX: Psychological Corporation, 2001.

Masterson, J., and L. Crede, "Learning to spell: Implications for assessment and intervention." *Language, Speech, and Hearing Services in Schools, 30* (1999): 243–254.

Masterson, J. J., and D. L. Daniels, "Motoric versus contrastive approaches to phonology therapy: A case study." *Child Language Teaching and Therapy, 7* (1991): 127–140.

Masterson, J., S. Long, and E. Buder, "Instrumentation in clinical phonology." In J. Bernthal and N. Bankson (Eds.), *Articulation and Phonological Disorders* (4th ed., pp. 378–406). Boston: Allyn and Bacon, 1998.

Masterson, J., and F. Pagan, *Interactive System for Phonological Analysis (ISPA).* San Antonio, TX: The Psychological Corporation, 1993.

Matheny, A., and C. Bruggeman, "Children's speech: Heredity components and sex differences." *Folia Phoniatrica, 25* (1973): 442–449.

Matheny, N., and J. Panagos, "Comparing the effects of articulation and syntax programs on syntax and articulation improvement." *Language, Speech, and Hearing Services in Schools, 9* (1978): 57–61.

Maxwell, E. M., "On determining underlying phonological representations of children: A critique of the current theories." *Phonological Theory and the Misarticulating Child, ASHA Monographs 22*: 18–29. Rockville, MD: ASHA, 1984.

Mayo, C., J. M. Scobbie, N. Hewlett, and D. Waters, "The influence of phonemic awareness development on acoustic cue weighting strategies in children's speech perception." *Journal of Speech, Language, and Hearing Research, 46,* 5 (2003): 1184–1196.

McAllister, A., "Voice disorders in children with oral motor dysfunction: Perceptual evaluation pre and post oral motor therapy." *Logopedics, Phoniatrics, and Vocology, 28* (2003): 117–125.

McAuliffe, M. J., and P. L. Cornwell, "Intervention for lateral /s/ using electropalatography (EPG) biofeedback and an intensive motor learning approach: A case report." *International Journal of Language and Communication Disorders, 43* (2008): 219–229.

McCauley, R., *Assessment of Language Disorders in Children.* Mahwah, NJ: Lawrence Erlbaum, 2001.

McCormack, P., "New approaches to the assessment of children's speech." *Australian Communication Quarterly* (Autumn 1997): 3–5.

McCormack, P. F., and T. Knighton, "Gender differences in the speech patterns of two and a half year old children." In P. McCormack and A. Russell (Eds.), *Speech Science and Technology: Sixth Australian International Conference* (pp. 337–341). Adelaide: Australian Speech Science and Technology Association, 1996.

McDermot, K. D., E. Bonora, N. Sykers, A. M. Coupe, C. S. Lai, S. C. Vernes, F. Vargha-Khadem, F. McKenzie, R. L. Smith, A. P. Monaco, and S. E. Fisher, "Identification of FOXP2 truncation as a novel cause of developmental speech and language deficits." *American Journal of Human Genetics, 76* (2005): 1074–1080.

McDonald, E. T., *Articulation Testing and Treatment: A Sensory Motor Approach.* Pittsburgh, PA: Stanwix House, 1964a.

McDonald, E. T., *A Deep Test of Articulation.* Pittsburgh, PA: Stanwix House, 1964b.

McEnery, E., and F. Gaines, "Tongue-tie in infants and children." *Journal of Pediatrics, 18* (1941): 252–255.

McGlaughlin, A., and A. Grayson, "A cross sectional and prospective study of crying in the first year of life." In S. P. Sohov (Ed.), *Advances in Psychology Research,* Volume 22 (pp. 37–58). New York: Nova Science, 2003.

McGregor, K. K., and R. G. Schwartz, "Converging evidence for underlying phonological representation in a child who misarticulates." *Journal of Speech and Hearing Research, 35* (1992): 596–603.

McInnes, A., "Phonemic awareness and sight word reading in toddlers." Unpublished doctoral dissertation, Baton Rouge, LA: Louisiana State University, 2008.

McKercher, M., L. McFarlane, and P. Schneider, "Phonological treatment dismissal: Optimal criteria." *Canadian Journal of Speech-Language Pathology and Audiology, 19* (1995): 115–123.

McKinnon, D. H., S. McLeod, and S. Reilly, "The prevalence of stuttering, voice and speech-sound disorders in primary school students in Australia." *Language, Speech, and Hearing Services in Schools, 38,* 1 (2007): 5–15.

McLeod, S. (Ed.), *The International Guide to Speech Acquisition.* Clifton Park, NY: Thomson Delmar Learning, 2007a.

McLeod, S., "Australian English speech acquisition." In S. McLeod (Ed.), *The International Guide to Speech Acquisition* (pp. 241–256) Clifton Park, NY: Thomson Delmar Learning, 2007b.

McLeod, S., "Laying the foundations for multilingual acquisition: An international overview of speech acquisition." In M. Cruz-Ferreira (Ed.), *Multilingual norms* (pp. 53–71). Frankfurt, Germany: Peter Lang Publishing, 2010.

McLeod, S., and J. Arciuli, "School-aged children's production of /s/ and /r/ consonant clusters." *Folia Phoniatrica et Logopaedica, 61* (2009): 336–341.

McLeod, S., L. J. Harrison, and J. McCormack, "The intelligibility in context scale: Validity and reliability of a subjective rating measure." *Journal of Speech, Language, and Hearing Research, 55* (2012): 648–656.

McLeod, S., and S. R. Hewett, "Variability in the production of words containing consonant clusters by typical two- and three-year-old children." *Folia Phoniatrica et Logopaedica, 60* (2008): 163–172.

McLeod, S., J. van Doorn, and V. A. Reed, "Homonyms in children's productions of consonant clusters." In W. Ziegler and K. Deger (Eds.), *Clinical Phonetics and Linguistics* (pp. 108–114) London: Whurr, 1998.

McLeod, S., J. van Doorn, and V. A. Reed, "Normal acquisition of consonant clusters." *American Journal of Speech-Language Pathology, 10* (2001a): 99–110.

McLeod, S., J. van Doorn, and V. A. Reed, "Consonant cluster development in two-year-olds: General trends and individual difference." *Journal of Speech, Language, Hearing Research, 44* (2001b): 1144–1171.

McLeod, S., J. van Doorn, and V. A. Reed, "Typological description of the normal acquisition of consonant clusters." In F. Windsor, L. Kelly, and N. Hewlett (Eds.), *Investigations in Clinical Phonetics and Linguistics* (pp. 185–200). Hillsdale, NJ: Erlbaum, 2002.

McNeill, B., "Advancing spoken and written language development in children with childhood apraxia of speech." Unpublished doctoral dissertation. Christchurch, NZ: University of Canterbury, 2007.

McNeill, B. C., G. T. Gillon, and B. Dodd, "Phonological awareness and early reading development in childhood apraxia of speech (CAS)." *International Journal of Language and Communication Disorders, 44* (2009): 175–192.

McNeill, D., "The two-fold way for speech." In *Problèmes Actuels en Psycholinguistique.* Paris: Editions du Centre National de la Recherche Scientifique, 1974.

McNutt, J., "Oral sensory and motor behaviors of children with /s/ or /r/ misarticulations." *Journal of Speech and Hearing Research, 20* (1977): 694–703.

McReynolds, L. V., "Articulation generalization during articulation training." *Language and Speech, 15* (1972): 149–155.

McReynolds, L. V., and M. Elbert, "An experimental analysis of misarticulating children's generalization." *Journal of Speech and Hearing Research, 21* (1978): 136–150.

Menn, L., "Phonotactic rules in beginning speech." *Lingua, 26* (1971): 225–241.

Menn, L., "Phonological units in beginning speech." In A. Bell and J. B. Hooper (Eds.), *Syllables and Segments* (pp. 157–171). Amsterdam: North Holland, 1978.

Menn, L., "Development of articulatory, phonetic, and phonological capabilities." In B. Butterworth (Ed.), *Language Production,* Volume. 2, (pp. 3–50). London: Academic Press, 1983.

Menn, L., "Perspective on research in first language developmental phonology." In M. Yavas, (Ed.), *First and Second Language Pathology* (pp. 3–8). San Diego, CA: Singular Publishing, 1994.

Menn, L., K. Markey, M. Mozer, and C. Lewis, "Connectionist modeling and the microstructure of phonological development: A progress report." In B. de Boysson-Bardies, S. de Schonen, P. Jusczyk, P. McNeilage, and J. Morton (Eds.), *Developmental Neurocognition: Speech and Face Processing in the First Year of Life* (pp. 421–433). Dordrecht, Netherlands: Kluwer Academic, 1993.

Menn, L., and E. Matthei, "The 'two lexicon' account of child phonology looking back, looking ahead." In C. A. Ferguson, L. Menn, and C. Stoel-Gammon (Eds.), *Phonological Development: Models, Research, Implications* (pp. 211–247). Timonium, MA: York, 1992.

Menn, L., and C. Stoel-Gammon, "Phonological development." In P. Fletcher and B. MacWhinney (Eds.), *The Handbook of Child Language* (pp. 335–359). Oxford, UK: Blackwell, 1995.

Menyuk, P., J. Liebergott, and M. Schultz, "Predicting phonological development." In B. Lindblom and R. Zetterström (Eds.), *Precursors of Early Speech* (pp. 79–93). Basingstoke, Hampshire, UK: MacMillan, 1986.

Messner, A. H., and M. L. Lalakea, "The effect of ankyloglossia on speech in children." *Otolaryngology—Head and Neck Surgery, 127* (2002): 539–545.

Meza, P., "Phonological analysis of Spanish utterances of highly unintelligible Mexican-American children." Unpublished master's thesis, San Diego State University, San Diego, CA, 1983.

Metz, D. E., V. J. Samar, N. Schiavetti, R. W. Sitler, and R. L. Whitehead, "Acoustic dimensions of hearing-impaired speakers' intelligibility." *Journal of Speech and Hearing Research, 28* (1985): 345–355.

Miccio, A., and M. Elbert, "Enhancing stimulability: A treatment program." *Journal of Communication Disorders, 29* (1996): 335–363.

Miccio, A. W., M. Elbert, and K. Forrest, "The relationship between stimulability and phonological acquisition in children with normally developing and disordered phonologies." *American Journal of Speech-Language Pathology, 8* (1999): 347–363.

Mills, A., and H. Streit, "Report of a speech survey, Holyoke, Massachusetts." *Journal of Speech Disorders, 7* (1942): 161–167.

Mines, M., B. Hanson, and J. Shoup, "Frequency of occurrence of phonemes in conversational English." *Language and Speech, 21* (1978): 221–241.

Moats, L., *Speech to Print*. Baltimore, MD: Brookes, 2000.

Moats, L. C., "Knowledge foundations for teaching reading and spelling." *Reading and Writing, 22* (2009): 379–399.

Moll, K. L., and R. G. Daniloff, "Investigation of the timing of velar movements during speech." *Journal of the Acoustical Society of America, 50* (1971): 678–684.

Moon, S. J., and B. Lindblom, "Formant undershoot in clear and citation-form speech: A second progress report." Royal Institute of Technology (Stockholm, Sweden). *Speech Transmission Laboratory, Quarterly Progress and Status Reports, 1* (1989): 121–123.

Moore, C. A., and J. L. Ruark, "Does speech emerge from earlier appearing oral motor behaviors?" *Journal of Speech and Hearing Research, 39* (1996): 1034–1047.

Morais, J., L. Cary, J. Alegria, and P. Bertelson, "Does awareness of speech as a sequence of phones arise spontaneously?" *Cognition, 7* (1979): 323–331.

Moran, M., "Final consonant deletion in African American English: A closer look." *Language, Speech, and Hearing Services in Schools, 24* (1993): 161–166.

Morgan, R., "Structural sketch of Saint Martin Creole." *Anthropological Linguistics, 1*, 8 (1959): 20–24.

Morley, D., "A ten-year survey of speech disorders among university students." *Journal of Speech and Hearing Disorders, 17* (1952): 25–31.

Morris, S. R., "Test-retest reliability of independent measures of phonology in the assessment of toddler speech." *Language, Speech, and Hearing Services in Schools, 40* (2009): 46–52.

Morris, S. R., "Clinical application of the mean babbling level and syllable structure level." *Language, Speech, and Hearing Service in Schools, 41* (2010): 223–230.

Morrison, J. A., and L. D. Shriberg, "Articulation testing versus conversational speech sampling." *Journal of Speech and Hearing Research, 35* (1992): 259–273.

Mowrer, D. E., *Methods of Modifying Speech Behaviors* (2nd ed.). Columbus, OH: Merrill, 1982.

Mowrer, D., R. Baker, and R. Schutz, "Operant procedures in the control of speech articulation." In H. Sloane and B. MacAulay (Eds.), *Operant Procedures in Remedial Speech and Language Training* (pp. 296–321). Boston: Houghton Mifflin, 1968.

Mullen, R. and T. Schooling, "The national outcomes measurement system for pediatric speech-language pathology." *Language, Speech, and Hearing Services in Schools, 41* (2010): 44–60.

Munson, B., E. M. Bjorum, and J. Windsor, "Acoustic and perceptual correlates of stress in nonwords produced by children with suspected developmental apraxia of speech and children with phonological disorder." *Journal of Speech, Language, and Hearing Research, 46* (2003): 189–202.

Murray, B. A., K. A. Smith, and G. G. Murray, "The test of phoneme identities: Predicting alphabetic insight in prealphabetic readers." *Journal of Literacy Research, 32* (2000): 421–447.

Muter, V., C. Hulme, M. J. Snowling, and J. Stevenson. "Phonemes, Rimes, Vocabulary, and Grammatical

Skills as Foundations of Early Reading Development: Evidence from a Longitudinal Study." *Developmental Psychology, 40* (2004): 665–681.

Muyksen, P., and N. Smith, "The study of pidgin and creole languages." In J. Arends, P. Muyksen, and N. Smith (Eds.), *Pidgins and Creoles: An Introduction* (pp. 3–14). Amsterdam, The Netherlands: John Benjamins Publishing, 1995.

Muyksen, P., and T. Veenstra, "Haitian." In J. Arends, P. Muyksen, and N. Smith (Eds.), *Pidgins and Creoles: An Introduction* (pp. 153–164). Amsterdam, The Netherlands: John Benjamins Publishing, 1995.

Naeser, M. A., "The American child's acquisition of differential vowel duration." Technical Report No. 144, Wisconsin Research and Development Center for Cognitive Learning, University of Wisconsin–Madison, 1970.

Nagy, J., *5–6 Éves Gyermekeink Iskolakészültsége (Preparedness for School of Five to Six Year Old Children)*. Budapest, Hungary: Akadémiai Kiadó, 1980.

Nakanishi, Y., K. Owada, and N. Fujita, "Köonkensa to sono kekka ni kansuru kösatsu." *Tokyo Gakugei Daigaku Tokushu Kyoiku Shisetsu Hokoku, 1* (1972): 1–19.

Nathan, L., J. Stackhouse, N. Goulandris, and M. Snowling, "The development of early literacy skills among children with speech difficulties: A test of the 'critical age hypothesis.'" *Journal of Speech, Language and Hearing Research, 47* (2004): 377–391.

Nathani, S., D. J. Ertmer, and R. E. Stark, "Assessing vocal development in infants and toddlers." *Clinical Linguistics and Phonetics, 20*, 5 (2006): 351–369.

Neils, J., and D. Aram, "Family history of children with developmental language disorders." *Perceptual and Motor Skills, 63* (1986): 655–658.

Neiva, F. S., and H. F. Wertzner, "A protocol for oral myofunctional assessment: For application with children." *International Journal of Orofacial Myology, 2* (1996): 8–19.

Nelson, H. D., P. Nygren, M. Walker, and R. Panoscha, "Screening for speech and language delay in preschool children: Systematic evidence review for the US preventive services task force." *Pediatrics, 117* (2006): e298–e319.

Nelson, L., "Establishing production of speech sound contrasts using minimal 'triads.'" *The Clinical Connection, 8*, 4 (1995): 16–19.

Netsell, R., *A Neurobiologic View of Speech Production and the Dysarthrias*. Boston: College-Hill Press, 1986.

Netsell, R., W. K. Lotz, J. E. Peters, and L. Schulte, "Developmental patterns of laryngeal and respiratory function for speech production." *Journal of Voice, 8* (1994): 123–131.

Nettleton, S., and P. R. Hoffman, "Phonic faces v animated literacy alphabets in preschool phonological intervention." Poster presentation at the annual convention of the American Speech-Language-Hearing Association, San Diego, CA., 2005.

Newcomer, P., and E. Barenbaum, *Test of Phonological Awareness Skills*. Austin, TX: Pro-Ed, 2003.

New Zealand Speech Language Therapy association (NZSTA)., "Scope of practice." Available from http://www.speechtherapy.org.nz/, 2011.

Nichols, P., "Creoles of the USA." In C. Ferguson and S. Heath (Eds.), *Language in the USA* (pp. 69–91). Cambridge. UK: Cambridge University Press, 1981.

Nippold, M. A., "Stuttering and phonology: Is there an interaction?" *American Journal of Speech, Language, Pathology, 11* (2002): 99–110.w

Nittrouer, S., "The relationship between speech perception and phonological awareness: Evidence from low SES Children and children with chronic OM." *Journal of Speech and Hearing Research, 39* (1996): 1059–1070.

Nittrouer, S., "Challenging the notion of innate phonetic boundaries." *Journal of the Acoustical Society of America, 110*, 3 (2001): 1598–1605.

Norris, J., and P. Hoffman, "Language intervention within naturalistic environments." *Language, Speech, and Hearing Services in Schools, 2* (1990): 72–84.

Norris, J. A., and P. R. Hoffman, "Goals and targets: Facilitating the self-organizing nature of a neuro-network." In A. Kamhi and K. Pollack (Eds.), *Phonological Disorders in Children: Clinical Decision Making in Assessment and Intervention* (pp. 77–87). Baltimore, MD: Brookes, 2005.

Nuffield Centre Dyspraxia Programme. London: Royal National Throat Nose and Ear Hospital, 1994.

Núñez-Cedeño, R., and Morales-Front, A., *Fonología generativa contemporánea de la lengua española (Contemporary generative phonology of the Spanish language)*. Washington, DC: Georgetown University Press, 1999.

O'Connor, M., W. Arnott, B. McIntosh, and B. Dodd, "Phonological awareness and language intervention in preschoolers from low socio-economic backgrounds: A longitudinal investigation." *British Journal of Developmental Psychology, 27* (2009): 767–782.

O'Conner, R., and J. R. Jenkins, "Prediction of reading disabilities in kindergarten and first grade." *Scientific Studies of Reading, 3* (1999): 159–197.

Oetting, J., "Cajun English speech acquisition." In S. McLeod (Ed.), *The International Guide to Speech Acquisition* (pp. 169–176). Clifton Park, NY: Thomson Delmar Learning, 2007.

Oetting, J., and A. Garrity, "Variation within dialects: A case of Cajun/Creole influence within child SAAE and SWE." *Journal of Speech, Language, and Hearing Research, 49* (2006): 16–26.

Oetting, J. B., and J. L. McDonald, "Methods for characterizing participants' nonmainstream dialect use in child language research." *Journal of Speech, Language, and Hearing Research, 45* (2002): 508–518.

O'Grady, W., J. Archibald, M. Aranoff, and J. Rees-Miller, *Contemporary Linguistics: An Introduction* (6th ed.). New York: St. Martin's Press, 2010.

Ohala, D., "The influence of sonority on children's cluster reductions." *Journal of Communication Disorders, 32* (1999): 397–421.

Oller, D. K., "Metaphonology of infant vocalizations." In B. Lindblom and R. Zetterström (Eds.), *Precursors of Early Speech* (pp. 21–35). Basingstoke, Hampshire, UK: Macmillan, 1986.

Oller, D. K., *The Emergence of the Speech Capacity.* Mahwah, NJ: Erlbaum, 2000.

Oller, D. K., and R. Eilers, "Similarity of babbling in Spanish- and English-learning babies." *Journal of Child Language, 9* (1982): 565–577.

Oller, D. K., and R. E. Eilers, "The role of audition in infant babbling." *Child Development, 59* (1988): 441–449.

Oller, D. K., R. E. Eilers, A. R. Neal, and H. K. Schwartz, "Precursors to speech in infancy: The prediction of speech and language disorders." *Journal of Communication Disorders, 32* (1999): 223–245.

Oller Jr., J. W., S. D. Oller, and L. C. Badon, *Milestones: Normal Speech and Language Development Across the Lifespan.* San Diego, CA: Plural Publishing, 2006.

Olmsted, D., *Out of the Mouth of Babes: Earliest Stages in Language Learning.* The Hague, The Netherlands: Mouton, 1971.

Olswang, L. B., and B. A. Bain, "The natural occurrence of generalization articulation treatment." *Journal of Communication Disorders, 18* (1985): 109–129.

Olswang, L. B., and B. Bain, "Data collection: Monitoring children's progress." *American Journal of Speech-Language Pathology, 3* (1994): 55–66.

Ota, M., and I. Ueda, "Japanese speech acquisition." In S. McLeod (Ed.), *The International Guide to Speech Acquisition* (pp. 457–471). Clifton Park, NY: Thomson/Delmar, 2007.

Otaiba, S., C. S. Puranik, R. A. Ziolkowski, and T. M. Montgomery, "Effectiveness of early phonological awareness interventions for students with speech or language impairments." *The Journal of Special Education, 43* (2009): 107–128.

Otomo, K., and C. Stoel-Gammon, "The acquisition of unrounded vowels in English." *Journal of Speech and Hearing Research, 35* (1992): 604–616.

Overby, M., "Relationships among speech sound perception, speech sound production, and phonological spelling in second grade children." Unpublished doctoral dissertation, University of Nebraska–Lincoln, 2007.

Overby, M., T. Carrell, and J. Bernthal, "Teachers' perceptions of students with speech sound disorders: A quantitative and qualitative analysis." *Language, Speech, and Hearing Services in Schools, 38* (2007): 327–341.

Overby, M. S., G. Trainin, A. Bosma Smit, J. E. Bernthal, and R. Nelson, "Preliteracy speech sound skills and later literacy outcomes: A study using the Templin archive." *Language, Speech, and Hearing Services in Schools, 43* (2012): 97–115.

Owens, R. E., *Language Development: An Introduction* (4th ed.). Boston: Allyn and Bacon, 1994.

Ozanne, A. E., "Normative data for sequenced oral movements and movements in context for children aged three to five years." *Australian Journal of Human Communication Disorders, 20* (1992): 47–63.

Pahkala, R., T. Laine, and S. Lammi, "Developmental stage of the dentition and speech sound production in a series of first-grade schoolchildren." *Journal of Craniofacial Genetics and Developmental Biology, 11* (1991): 170–175.

Palin, M., *Contrast Pairs for Phonological Training.* Austin, TX: Pro-Ed, 1992.

Palmer, J., "Tongue-thrusting: A clinical hypothesis." *Journal of Speech and Hearing Disorders, 27* (1962): 323–333.

Panagos, J., and P. Prelock, "Phonological constraints on the sentence productions of language disordered children." *Journal of Speech and Hearing Research, 25* (1982): 171–176.

Panagos, J., M. Quine, and R. Klich, "Syntactic and phonological influences on children's articulation." *Journal of Speech and Hearing Research, 22* (1979): 841–848.

Pandolfi, A. M., and M. O. Herrera, "Producción fonologica diastratica de niños menores de tres años (Phonological production in children less than three-years-old)." *Revista Teorica,* 1990.

Parker, F., "Distinctive features in speech pathology: Phonology or phonemics?" *Journal of Speech and Hearing Disorders, 41* (1976): 23–39.

Parker, F., and K. Riley, *Linguistics for Non-Linguists: A Primer with Exercises* (3rd ed.). Boston: Allyn and Bacon, 2000.

Parker, R. G., "Phonological process use in the speech of children fitted with cochlear implants." Unpublished master's thesis, University of Tennessee–Knoxville, 2005.

Parlour, S., and P. Broen, "Environmental factors in familial phonological disorders: Preliminary home scale results." Paper presented at the annual convention of the American Speech-Language-Hearing Association, Atlanta, 1991.

Parsons, C. L., T. A. Iacono, and L. Rozner, "Effect of tongue reduction on articulation in children with Down syndrome." *American Journal of Mental Deficiency, 91* (1987): 328–332.

Pascoe, M., J. Stackhouse, and B. Wells, "Phonological therapy within a psycholinguistic framework: Promoting change in a child with persisting speech difficulties." *International Journal of Language and Communication Disorders, 40* (2005): 189–220.

Pascoe, M., B. Wells, and J. Stackhouse, *Persisting Speech Difficulties in Children: Children's Speech and Literacy Difficulties Book 3.* London: Wiley and Sons, 2006.

Paterson, M., "Articulation and phonological disorders in hearing-impaired school-aged children with severe and profound sensorineural losses." In J. Bernthal and N. Bankson (Eds.), *Child Phonology: Characteristics, Assessment, and Intervention with Special Populations* (pp. 199–224). New York: Thieme Medical Publishers, 1994.

Paul, R., and P. Jennings, "Phonological behavior in toddlers with slow expressive language development." *Journal of Speech and Hearing Research, 35* (1992): 99–107.

Paul, R., and L. D. Shriberg, "Associations between phonology and syntax in speech delayed children." *Journal of Speech and Hearing Research, 25* (1982): 536–546.

Paul, R., and L. D. Shriberg, "Reply to Panagos and Prelock (Letter)." *Journal of Speech and Hearing Research, 27* (1984): 319–320.

Paus, T., A. Zijdenbos, K. Worsley, D. L. Collins, J. Blumenthal, J. N. Giedd, J. L. Rapoport, and A. C. Evans, "Structural maturation of neural pathways in children and adolescents: In vivo study." *Science, 28* (1999): 1908–1911.

Paynter, E. T., and N. A. Petty, "Articulatory sound acquisition of two-year-old children." *Perceptual and Motor Skills, 39* (1974): 1079–1085.

Paynter, W., and T. Bumpas, "Imitative and spontaneous articulatory assessment of three-year-old children." *Journal of Speech and Hearing Disorders, 42* (1977): 119–125.

Pearson, B. Z., S. L. Velleman, T. J. Bryant, and T. Charko, "Contrastive and non-contrastive phonological development in African American English-learning children." *Language, Speech, and Hearing Services in Schools, 40* (2009): 1–16.

Peña, E. D., T. J. Spaulding, and E. Plante, "The composition of normative groups and diagnostic decision making: Shooting ourselves in the foot." *American Journal of Speech-Language Pathology, 15* (2006): 247–254.

Peña-Brooks, A., and M. N. Hegde, *Assessment and Treatment of Articulation and Phonological Disorders in Children.* Austin, TX: Pro-Ed, 2000.

Perez, E., "Phonological differences among speakers of Spanish-influenced English." In J. Bernthal and

N. Bankson (Eds.), *Child phonology: Characteristics, Assessment, and Intervention with Special Populations* (pp. 245–254). New York: Thieme Medical Publishers, 1994.

Perfetti, C. A., I. Beck, L. C. Bell, and C. Hughes, "Phonemic knowledge and learning to read are reciprocal: A longitudinal study of first grade children." *Merrill-Palmer Quarterly, 33* (1987): 283–319.

Perkins, W., *Speech Pathology: An Applied Behavioral Science.* St. Louis: Mosby, 1977.

Peterson, R. L., B. F. Pennington, L. D. Shriberg, and R. Boada, "What influences literacy outcome in children with speech disorder?" *Journal of Speech, Language, and Hearing Research, 52* (2009): 1175–1188.

Picheny, M. A., N. I. Durlach, and L. D. Braida, "Speaking clearly for the hard of hearing. II: Acoustic characteristics of clear and conversational speech." *Journal of Speech and Hearing Research, 29* (1986): 434–446.

Pigott, T., J. Barry, B. Hughes, D. Eastin, P. Titus, H. Stensil, K. Metcalf, and B. Porter, *Speech-Ease Screening Inventory (K–1).* Austin, TX: Pro-Ed, 1985.

Pinborough-Zimmerman, J., R. Satterfield, J. Miller, D. Bilder, S. Hossain, and W. McMahon, "Communication disorders: Prevalence and comorbid intellectual disability, autism, and emotional / behavioral disorders." *American Journal of Speech-Language Pathology, 16* (2007): 359–367.

Polka, L., and O. Bohn, "Asymmetries in vowel perception." *Speech Communication, 41* (2003): 221–231.

Pollock, K., "The identification of vowel errors using transitional articulation or phonological process test stimuli." *Language, Speech, and Hearing Services in Schools, 22* (1991): 39–50.

Pollock, K., "Identification of vowel errors: Methodological issues and preliminary data from the Memphis Vowel Project." In M. J. Ball and F. E. Gibbon (Eds.), *Vowel Disorders* (pp. 83–113) Boston: Butterworth Heinemann, 2002.

Pollock, K., G. Bailey, M. Berni, D. Fletcher, L. Hinton, I. Johnson, and R. Weaver, "Phonological characteristics of African American English Vernacular (AAVE): An updated feature list." Seminar presented at the convention of the American Speech-Language Hearing Association, San Antonio, TX, 1998.

Pollock, K., and M. C. Berni, "Incidence of non-rhotic vowel errors in children: Data from the Memphis Vowel Project." *Clinical Linguistics and Phonetics, 17* (2003): 393–401.

Poole, E., "Genetic development of articulation of consonant sounds in speech." *Elementary English Review, 11* (1934): 159–161.

Poplack, S., "Dialect acquisition among Puerto Rican bilinguals." *Language in Society, 7* (1978): 89–103.

Poplack, S., "Introduction." In S. Poplack (Ed.), *The English History of African American English* (pp. 1–32). Oxford, UK: Blackwell, 2000.

Porter, J. H., and B. W. Hodson, "Collaborating to obtain phonological acquisition data for local schools." *Language, Speech, and Hearing Services in Schools, 32* (2001): 165–171.

Powell, J., and L. McReynolds, "A procedure for testing position generalization from articulation training." *Journal of Speech and Hearing Research, 12* (1969): 625–645.

Powell, T. W., and M. Elbert, "Generalization following the remediation of early- and later-developing consonant clusters." *Journal of Speech and Hearing Disorders, 49* (1984): 211–218.

Powell, T. W., M. Elbert, and D. A. Dinnsen, "Stimulability as a factor in the phonologic generalization of misarticulating preschool children." *Journal of Speech and Hearing Research, 34* (1991): 1318–1328.

Powers, M., "Functional disorders of articulation-symptomatology and etiology." In L. Travis (Ed.), *Handbook of Speech Pathology and Audiology*. Englewood Cliffs, NJ: Prentice-Hall, 1957, 1971.

Prather, E. M., D. L. Hedrick, and C. A. Kern, "Articulation development in children aged two to four years." *Journal of Speech and Hearing Disorders, 60* (1975): 179–191.

Preisser, D. A., B. W. Hodson, and E. P. Paden, "Developmental phonology: 18–29 months." *Journal of Speech and Hearing Disorders, 53* (1988): 125–130.

Preston, J., and M. Edwards, "Phonological processing skills of adolescents with residual speech sound errors." *Language, Speech, and Hearing Services in Schools, 38* (2007): 297–308.

Preston, J., and M. Edwards, "Phonological awareness and types of sound errors in preschoolers with speech sound disorders." *Journal of Speech, Language, and Hearing Research, 53* (2010): 44–60.

Price, E., and M. Scarry-Larkin, *Phonology* [CD-ROM]. San Luis Obispo, CA: LocuTour Multimedia, 1999.

Prince, A. S., and P. Smolensky, *Optimality Theory: Constraint Interaction in Generative Grammar. RUCCS Technical Report #2.* New Brunswick, NJ: Rutgers University Center for Cognitive Science, 1993.

Prins, D., "Analysis of correlations among various articulatory deviations." *Journal of Speech and Hearing Research, 5* (1962a): 151–160.

Prins, D., "Motor and auditory abilities in different groups of children with articulatory deviations." *Journal of Speech and Hearing Research, 5* (1962b): 161–168.

Proffit, W. R., *Contemporary Orthodontics*. St. Louis: Mosby, 1986.

Prosek, R., and A. House, "Intraoral air pressure as a feedback cue in consonant production." *Journal of Speech and Hearing Research, 18* (1975): 133–147.

Rabiner, L., H. Levitt, and A. Rosenberg, "Investigation of stress patterns for speech synthesis by rule." *Journal of the Acoustical Society of America, 45* (1969): 92–101.

Raitano, N. A., B. F. Penningtion, R. A. Tunick, R. Boada, and L. D. Shriberg, "Pre-literacy skills of subgroups of children with speech sound disorders." *Journal of Child Psychology and Psychiatry, 45* (2004): 821–835.

Ramirez, A., and R. Milk, "Notions of grammaticality among teachers of bilingual pupils." *TESOL Quarterly, 20* (1986): 495–513.

Read, C., and P. A. Schreiber, "Why short subjects are harder to find than long ones." In E. Wanner and L. Gleitman (Eds.), *Language Acquisition: The State of the Art* (pp. 78–101). Cambridge, UK: Cambridge University Press, 1982.

Reid, G., "The efficiency of speech re-education of functional articulatory defectives in elementary school." *Journal of Speech and Hearing Disorders, 12* (1947a): 301–313.

Reid, G., "The etiology and nature of functional articulatory defects in elementary school children." *Journal of Speech and Hearing Disorders, 12* (1947b): 143–150.

Rickford, J. (1999). *African American Vernacular English: Features, Evolution, Educational Implications*. Oxford, UK: Blackwell.

Ringel, R., K. Burk, and C. Scott, "Tactile perception: Form discrimination in the mouth." In J. Bosma (Ed.), *Second Symposium on Oral Sensation and Perception* (pp. 410–415). Springfield, IL: Charles C Thomas, 1970.

Ringel, R., and S. Ewanowski, "Oral perception: I. Two-point discrimination." *Journal of Speech and Hearing Research, 8* (1965): 389–400.

Ringel, R., A. House, K. Burk, J. Dolinsky, and C. Scott, "Some relations between orosensory discrimination and articulatory aspects of speech production." *Journal of Speech and Hearing Disorders, 35* (1970): 3–11.

Riski, J. E., and E. DeLong, "Articulation development in children with cleft lip/palate." *Cleft Palate Journal, 21* (1984): 57–64.

Robb, M. P., and K. M. Bleile, "Consonant inventories of young children from 8 to 25 months." *Clinical Linguistics and Phonetics, 8* (1994): 295–320.

Robb, M., H. Gilbert, V. Reed, and A. Bisson, "Speech rates in young Australian English-speaking children: A preliminary study." *Contemporary Issues in Communication Science and Disorders, 30* (2003): 84–91.

Robb, M. P., and G. T. Gillon, "Speech rates of New Zealand English- and American English-speaking children." *Advances in Speech-Language Pathology, 9*, 2 (2007): 173–180.

Robbins, J., and T. Klee, "Clinical assessment of oropharyngeal motor development in young children." *Journal of Speech and Hearing Disorders, 52* (1987): 271–277.

Roberts, J., S. H. Long, C. Malkin, E. Barnes, M. Skinner, E. A. Hennon, and K. Anderson, "A comparison of phonological skills of boys with Fragile X syndrome and Down syndrome." *Journal of Speech, Language, and Hearing Research, 48* (2005): 980–995.

Roberts, J. E., M. Burchinal, and M. M. Footo, "Phonological process decline from 2;6 to 8 years." *Journal of Communication Disorders, 23* (1990): 205–217.

Roberts, J. E., R. M. Rosenfeld, and S. A. Zeisel, "Otitis media and speech and language: A meta-analysis of prospective studies." *Pediatrics, 113* (2004): e238–e248.

Robertson, C., and W. Salter, *The Phonological Awareness Test 2.* East Moline, IL: Linguisystems, 2007.

Robin, D. A., L. B. Somodi, and E. S. Luschei, "Measurement of tongue strength and endurance in normal and articulation disordered subjects." In C. A. Moore, K. M. Yorkston, and D. R. Beukelman (Eds.), *Dysarthria and Apraxia of Speech: Perspectives on Management* (pp. 173–184). Baltimore, MD: Brookes, 1991.

Robinson, G., and I. Stockman, "Cross-dialectal perceptual experiences of speech-language pathologists in predominantly Caucasian American school districts." *Language, Speech, and Hearing Services in Schools, 40* (2009): 138–149.

Roca, I., and W. Johnson, *A Course in Phonology.* Oxford, UK: Blackwell, 1999.

Roe, V., and R. Milisen, "The effect of maturation upon defective articulation in elementary grades." *Journal of Speech Disorders, 7* (1942): 37–50.

Rosenbeck, J. C., R. D. Kent, and L. L. LaPointe, "Apraxia of speech: An overview and some perspectives." In J. C. Rosenbeck, M. R. McNeil, and A. E. Aronson (Eds.), *Apraxia of Speech: Physiology, Acoustics, Linguistics Management* (pp. 1–72). San Diego, CA: College Hill Press, 1984.

Rosin, M., E. Swift, D. Bless, and D. K. Vetter, "Communication profiles of adolescents with Down's Syndrome." *Journal of Childhood Communication Disorders, 12* (1988): 49–62.

Roth, F. P., and D. R. Paul, "Partnerships for literacy: Principles and practices [foreword]." *Topics in Language Disorders 26* (2006): 2–4.

Roulstone, S., S. Loader, K. Northstone, M. Beveridge, and the ALSPAC Team, "The speech and language of children aged 25 months: Descriptive data from the Avon Longitudinal Study of Parents and Children." *Early Child Development and Care, 172,* 3 (2002): 259–268.

Royal College of Speech and Language Therapists (RCSLT), "Communicating quality 3: RCSLT's guidance on best practice in service organisation and provision." London: Royal College of Speech and Language Therapists, 2006.

Ruark, J. L., and C. A. Moore, "Coordination of lip muscle activity by 2-year-old children during speech and nonspeech tasks." *Journal of Speech, Language, and Hearing Research, 40* (1997): 1373–1385.

Ruben, R. J., "A time frame of critical/sensitive periods of language development." *Acta Otolaryngology, 117* (1997): 202–205.

Ruffoli, R., M. A. Giambellica, M. C. Scavuzzo, D. Bonfigli, R. Cristofani, M. Gabriele, M. R. Giuca, and F. Giannessi, "Ankyloglossia: A morphofunctional investigation in children." *Oral Diseases, 11* (2005): 170–174.

Ruscellos, D., "Articulation improvement and oral tactile changes in children." Unpublished thesis, University of West Virginia, 1972.

Ruscello, D., "The importance of word position in articulation therapy." *Language, Speech, and Hearing Services in Schools, 6* (1975): 190–196.

Ruscello, D., "Motor learning as a model for articulation instruction." In J. Costello (Ed.), *Speech Disorders in Children* (pp. 129–156). San Diego, CA: College-Hill Press, 1984.

Ruscello, D. M., "Speech appliances in the treatment of phonological disorders." *Journal of Communication Disorders, 28* (1995): 331–353.

Ruscello, D. M., L. R. Cartwright, K. B. Haines, and L. I. Shuster, "The use of different service delivery models for children with phonological disorders." *Journal of Communication Disorders, 26* (1993): 193–203.

Ruscello, D. M., K. O. St. Louis, and N. Mason. "School-age children with phonological disorders: Coexistence with other speech/language disorders." *Journal of Speech and Hearing Research, 34* (1991): 236–242.

Rvachew, S., "Speech perception training can facilitate sound production learning." *Journal of Speech and Hearing Research, 37* (1994): 347–357.

Rvachew, S., "Perceptual foundations of speech acquisition." In S. McLeod (Ed.), *The International Guide to Speech Acquisition* (pp. 26–30). Clifton Park, NY: Thomson Delmar Learning, 2007a.

Rvachew, S., "Phonological processing and reading in children with speech sound disorders." *American Journal of Speech-Language Pathology, 16* (2007b): 260–270.

Rvachew, S., and F. Brosseau-Lapre, "Speech perception intervention." In A. L. Williams, S. McLeod, and R. J. McCauley (Eds.), *Interventions for Speech Sound Disorders in Children* (pp. 295–314), Baltimore, MD: Brookes, 2010.

Rvachew, S., P. Chiang, and N. Evans, "Characteristics of speech errors produced by children with and without delayed phonological awareness skills." *Language, Speech, and Hearing Services in Schools, 38* (2007): 60–71.

Rvachew, S., and M. Grawburg, "Correlates of phonological awareness in preschoolers with speech sound disorders." *Journal of Speech, Language, and Hearing Research, 49* (2006): 74–87.

Rvachew, S., and M. Nowak, "The effect of target-selection strategy on phonological learning." *Journal of Speech, Language, and Hearing Research, 44* (2001): 610–623.

Rvachew, S., M. Nowak, and G. Cloutier, "Effect of phonemic perception training on the speech production and phonological awareness skills of children with expressive phonological delay." *American Journal of Speech-Language Pathology, 13* (2004): 250–263.

Rvachew, S., A. Ohberg, M. Grawburg, and J. Heyding, "Phonological Awareness and Phonemic Perception in 4-Year-Old Children with Delayed Expressive Phonology Skills." *American Journal of Speech-Language Pathology 12* (2003): 463–471.

Rvachew, S., S. Rafaat, and M. Martin, "Stimulability, speech perception skills, and the treatment of phonological disorders." *American Journal of Speech-Language Pathology, 8* (1999): 33–43.

Sacks, S., and R. E. Shine, *SATPAC (Systematic Articulation Training Program Accessing Computers)*. Fresno, CA: SATPAC Speech, LLC, 2004.

Samuelsson, S., R. Olson, S. Wadsworth, R. Corley, J. C. DeFries, E. Willcutt, J. Hulslander, and B. Byrne, "Genetic and Environmental Influences on Prereading Skills and Early Reading and Spelling Development in the United States, Australia, and Scandinavia." *Reading and Writing 20*, (2007): 51–75.

Sander, E. K., "When are speech sounds learned?" *Journal of Speech and Hearing Disorders, 37* (1972): 55–63.

Sawyer, D., *Test of Awareness of Language Segments*. Austin, TX: Pro-Ed, 1987.

Sayler, H., "The effect of maturation upon defective articulation in grades seven through twelve." *Journal of Speech and Hearing Disorders, 14* (1949): 202–207.

Schery, T. K. "Correlates of language development in language-disordered children." *Journal of Speech and Hearing Disorders, 50*, (1985): 73–83.

Schiavettei, N., "Scaling procedures for the measurement of speech intelligibility." In R. D. Kent (Ed.), *Intelligibility in Speech Disorders* (pp. 11–34). Philadelphia: John Benjamin, 1992.

Schlanger, B., "Speech examination of a group of institutionalized mentally handicapped children." *Journal of Speech and Hearing Disorders, 18* (1953): 339–349.

Schlanger, B., and R. Gottsleben, "Analysis of speech defects among the institutionalized mentally retarded." *Journal of Speech and Hearing Disorders, 22* (1957): 98–103.

Schmauch, V., J. Panagos, and R. Klich, "Syntax influences the accuracy of consonant production in language-disordered children." *Journal of Communication Disorders, 11* (1978): 315–323.

Schmitt, L. S., B. H. Howard, and J. F. Schmitt, "Conversational speech sampling in the assessment of articulation proficiency." *Language, Speech, and Hearing Services in Schools, 14* (1983): 210–214.

Schuele, C. M., "The impact of developmental speech and language impairments on the acquisition of literacy skills." *Mental Retardation and Developmental Disabilities Research Reviews, 10* (2004): 176–183.

Schuele, C. M., and N. D. Dayton, *Intensive Phonological Awareness Program*. Cleveland, OH: Authors, 2000.

Schuele, C. M., L. Justice, S. Cabell, K. Knighton, B. Kingery, and M. Lee, "Field-based evaluation of two-tiered instruction for enhancing kindergarten phonological awareness." *Early Education and Development*, 19 (2008): 726–752.

Schuele, C. M., K. Paul, and K. Mazzaferri, "Phonological awareness training: Is it worth the time?" Paper presented at the annual convention of the American Speech-Language-Hearing Association, San Antonio, TX, 1998.

Schuele, C. M., L. Skibbe, and P. Rao, "Assessing phonological awareness." In K. Pence (Ed.), *Assessment in Emergent Literacy* (pp. 275–326). San Diego: Plural Publishing, 2007.

Schwartz, A., and R. Goldman, "Variables influencing performance on speech sound discrimination tests." *Journal of Speech and Hearing Research, 17* (1974): 25–32.

Schwartz, R. G., and L. B. Leonard, " 'Do children pick and choose?' An examination of phonological selection and avoidance in early lexical acquisition." *Journal of Child Language, 9* (1982): 319–336.

Schwartz, R. G., L. Leonard, M. K. Folger, and M. J. Wilcox, "Evidence for a synergistic view of linguistic disorders: Early phonological behavior in normal and language disordered children." *Journal of Speech and Hearing Disorders, 45* (1980): 357–377.

Schwartz, R. G., L. B. Leonard, M. J. Wilcox, and M. K. Folger, "Again and again: Reduplication in child phonology." *Journal of Child Language, 7* (1980): 75–87.

Scobbie, J. M., O. Gordeeva, and B. Matthews, "Scottish English speech acquisition." In S. McLeod (Ed.), *The International Guide to Speech Acquisition* (pp. 221–240). Clifton Park, NY: Thomson Delmar Learning, 2007.

Scott, C., and R. Ringel, "Articulation without oral sensory control." *Journal of Speech and Hearing Research, 14* (1971): 804–818.

Scripture, M. K., and E. Jackson, *A Manual of Exercises for the Correction of Speech Disorders*. Philadelphia: F. A. Davis, 1927.

Secord, W., "The traditional approach to treatment." In N. Creaghead, P. Newman, and W. Secord (Eds.), *Assessment and Remediation of Articulatory and Phonological Disorders* (pp. 129–159). Columbus, OH: Merrill, 1989.

Secord, W., S. E. Boyce, J. S. Donahue, R. A. Fox, and R. E. Shine, *Eliciting Sounds: Techniques and*

Strategies for Clinicians (2nd ed.). Greenville, SC: Super Duper Publications, 2007.

Secord, W. A., and J. S. Donohue, *Clinical Assessment of Articulation and Phonology.* Greenville, SC: Super Duper Publications, 2002.

Secord, W., and R. Shine, *Secord Contextual Articulation Tests (S-CAT).* Sedona, AZ: Red Rock Educational Publications, 1997.

Segal, L. M., R. Stephenson, M. Dawes, and P. Feldman, "Prevalence, diagnosis, and treatment of ankyloglossia." *Canadian Family Physician, 53* (2007): 1027–1033.

Selby, J. C., M. P. Robb, and H. R. Gilbert, "Normal vowel articulations between 15 and 36 months of age." *Clinical Linguistics and Phonetics, 14* (2000): 255–266.

Semel, E., E. Wiig, and W. Secord, *Clinical Evaluation of Language Fundamentals – 4.* San Antonio, TX: The Psychological Corporation, 2003.

Seymour, H., and C. Seymour, "A therapeutic model for communicative disorders among children who speak Black English Vernacular." *Journal of Speech and Hearing Disorders, 42* (1977): 247–256.

Seymour, H., and C. Seymour, "Black English and Standard American English contrasts in consonantal development of four- and five-year-old children." *Journal of Speech and Hearing Disorders, 46* (1981): 274–280.

Shafer, V. L., D. W. Shucard, J. L. Shucard, and L. Gerken, "An electrophysiological study of infants' sensitivity to the sound patterns of English speech." *Journal of Speech, Language, and Hearing Research, 41* (1998): 874–886.

Shahidullah, S., and P. G. Hepper, "Hearing in the fetus: Prenatal detection of deafness." *International Journal of Prenatal and Perinatal Studies, 4* 3/4 (1992): 235–240.

Shapiro, L. R., and J. Solity, "Delivering phonological and phonics training within whole-class teaching." *British Journal of Educational Psychology, 78* (2008): 597–620.

Sheahan, P., I. Miller, J. N. Sheahan, M. J. Earley, and A. W. Blayney, "Incidence and outcome of middle ear disease in cleft lip and/or cleft palate." *International Journal of Pediatric Otorhinolaryngology, 67* (2003): 758–793.

Shelton, R., "Disorders of articulation." In P. Skinner and R. Shelton (Eds.), *Speech, Language, and Hearing* (pp. 172–211). Reading, MA: Addison-Wesley, 1978.

Shelton, R., "Science, clinical art, and speech pathology." Paper presented at Kansas University, Spring 1989.

Shelton, R., A. F. Johnson, and W. B. Arndt, "Monitoring and reinforcement by parents as a means of automating articulatory responses." *Perceptual and Motor Skills, 35* (1972): 759–767.

Shelton, R., A. Johnson, and W. Arndt, "Delayed judgment speech sound discrimination and /r/ or /s/ articulation status and improvement." *Journal of Speech and Hearing Research, 20* (1977): 704–717.

Shelton, R., A. F. Johnson, V. Willis, and W. B. Arndt, "Monitoring and reinforcement by parents as a means of automating articulatory responses: II. Study of pre-school children." *Perceptual and Motor Skills, 40* (1975): 599–610.

Shelton, R., V. Willis, A. F. Johnson, and W. B. Arndt, "Oral form recognition training and articulation change." *Perceptual and Motor Skills, 36* (1973): 523–531.

Sherman, D., and A. Geith, "Speech sound discrimination and articulation skill." *Journal of Speech and Hearing Disorders, 10* (1967): 277–280.

Shprintzen, R. J. *Genetics, Syndromes, and Communication Disorders.* San Diego, CA: Singular Publishing, 1997.

Shriberg, L. D., "A response evocation program for /ɝ/." *Journal of Speech and Hearing Disorders, 40* (1975): 92–105.

Shriberg, L. D., "Toward classification of developmental phonological disorders" (pp. 1–18). In N. J. Lass (Ed.), *Speech and Language: Advances in Basic Research and Practice* [Volume 8]. Philadelphia: Saunders, 1982.

Shriberg, L. D., *Programs to Examine Phonetic and Phonologic Evaluation Records (PEPPER).* Hillsdale, NJ: Erlbaum, 1986.

Shriberg, L. D., "Directions for research in developmental phonological disorders." In J. Miller (Ed.), *Research on Child Language Disorders: A Decade of Progress* (pp. 267–276). Austin, TX: Pro-Ed, 1991.

Shriberg, L. D., "Four new speech and prosody-voice measures for genetics research and other studies in developmental phonological disorders." *Journal of Speech and Hearing Research, 36* (1993): 105–140.

Shriberg, L. D., "Childhood speech sound disorders: From post-behaviorism to the postgenomic era." In R. Paul and P. Flipsen Jr. (Eds.) *Speech Sound Disorders in Children: In Honor of Lawrence D. Shriberg* (pp. 1–34). San Diego, CA: Plural Publishing, 2009.

Shriberg, L. D., D. M. Aram, and J. Kwiatkowski, "Developmental apraxia of speech: I. Descriptive and theoretical perspectives." *Journal of Speech, Language, and Hearing Research, 40* (1997a): 273–285.

Shriberg, L. D., D. M. Aram, and J. Kwiatkowski, "Developmental apraxia of speech: II. Toward a diagnostic marker." *Journal of Speech, Language, and Hearing Research, 40* (1997b): 286–312.

Shriberg, L. D., and D. Austin, "Comorbidity of speech-language disorder. Implications for a phenotype marker for speech delay." In R. Paul (Ed.) *Exploring the Speech-Language Connection* (pp. 73–117). Baltimore, MD: Brookes. 1998.

Shriberg, L. D., D. Austin, B. A. Lewis, J. L. McSweeny, and D. L. Wilson, "The percentage of consonants correct (PCC) metric: Extensions and reliability data." *Journal of Speech, Language, and Hearing Research, 40* (1997a): 708–722.

Shriberg, L. D., D. Austin, B. A. Lewis, J. L. McSweeney, and D. L. Wilson, "The speech disorders classification system (SDCS): Extension and lifespan reference data." *Journal of Speech, Language, and Hearing Research, 40* (1997b): 723–740.

Shriberg, L. D., K. J. Ballard, J. B. Tomblin, J. R. Duffy, K. H. Odell, and C. A. Williams, "Speech, prosody, and voice characteristics of a mother and daughter with a 7:13 translocation affecting FOXP2." *Journal of Speech, Language, and Hearing Research, 49* (2006): 500–525.

Shriberg, L. D., P. Flipsen Jr., H. B. Karlsson, and J. L. McSweeny, "Acoustic phenotypes for speech-genetics studies: An acoustic marker for residual /ɝ/ distortions. *Clinical Linguistics and Phonetics, 15* (2001): 631–650.

Shriberg, L. D., P. Flipsen Jr., J. Kwiatkowski, and J. L. McSweeny, "A diagnostic marker for speech delay associated with otitis media with effusion: The intelligibility-speech gap." *Clinical Linguistics and Phonetics, 17* (2003): 507–528.

Shriberg, L. D., P. Flipsen Jr., H. Thielke, J. Kwiatkowski, M. Kertoy, R. Nellis, and M. Block, "Risk for speech disorder associated with early recurrent otitis media with effusion: Two retrospective studies." *Journal of Speech, Language, and Hearing Research, 43* (2000): 79–99.

Shriberg, L D., M. Folurakis, S. D. Hall, H. B. Karlsson, H. L. Lohmeier, J. L., McSweeny, N. L., Potter, A. R. Scheer-Cohen, E. A. Strand, C. M Tilkens, and D. Wilson, "Extensions to the speech disorders classification system (SDCS)." *Clinical Linguistics and Phonetics, 24* (2010): 795–824.

Shriberg, L. D., S. Friel-Patti, P. Flipsen Jr., and R. L. Brown, "Otitis media, fluctuant hearing loss and speech-language delay: A preliminary structural equation model." *Journal of Speech, Language, and Hearing Research, 43* (2000): 100–120.

Shriberg, L. D., R. D. Kent, H. B. Karlsson, C. J. Nadler, and R. L. Brown, "A diagnostic marker for speech delay associated with otitis media with effusion: Backing of obstruents." *Clinical Linguistics and Phonetics, 17* (2003): 529–547.

Shriberg, L. D., and J. Kwiatkowski, *Natural Process Analysis.* New York: Wiley, 1980.

Shriberg, L. D., and J. Kwiatkowski, "Phonological disorders III: A procedure for assessing severity of involvement." *Journal of Speech and Hearing Disorders, 42* (1982a): 242–256.

Shriberg, L. D., and J. Kwiatkowski, "Phonological disorders II: A conceptual framework for management." *Journal of Speech and Hearing Disorders, 42* (1982b): 242–256.

Shriberg, L. D., and J. Kwiatkowski, "Phonological disorders I: A diagnostic classification system." *Journal of Speech and Hearing Disorders, 42* (1982c): 226–241.

Shriberg, L. D., and J. Kwiatkowski, "Computer-assisted natural process analysis (NPA): Recent issues and data." *Seminars in Speech and Language, 4* (1983): 389–406.

Shriberg, L. D., and J. Kwiatkowski, "A retrospective study of spontaneous generalization in speech-delayed children." *Language, Speech, and Hearing Services in Schools, 18* (1987): 144–157.

Shriberg, L. D., and J. Kwiatkowski, "Self-monitoring and generalization in preschool speech-delayed children." *Language, Speech, and Hearing Services in Schools, 21* (1990): 157–170.

Shriberg, L. D., and J. Kwiatkowski, "Developmental phonological disorders I: A clinical profile." *Journal of Speech and Hearing Research, 37* (1994): 1100–1126.

Shriberg, L. D., J. Kwiatkowski, S. Best, J. Hengst, and B. Terselic-Weber, "Characteristics of children with phonologic disorders of unknown origin." *Journal of Speech and Hearing Disorders, 51* (1986): 140–161.

Shriberg, L. D., J. Kwiatkowski, and C. Rasmussen, *Prosody-Voice Screening Profile*, Tucson, AZ: Communication Skill Builders, 1990.

Shriberg, L. D., J. Kwiatkowski, C. Rasmussen, G. L. Lof, and J. F. Miller, "The prosody voice screening profile (PVSP): Psychometric data in reference information for children." *Phonology Project Technical Report No. 1*, Madison, WI: University of Wisconsin, 1992.

Shriberg, L. D., B. A. Lewis, J. B. Tomblin, J. L. McSweeny, H. B. Karlsson, and A. R. Scheer, "Toward diagnostic and phenotype markers for genetically transmitted speech delay." *Journal of Speech, Language and Hearing Research, 48* (2005): 834–852.

Shriberg, L. D., and G. L. Lof, "Reliability studies in broad and narrow phonetic transcription." *Clinical Linguistics and Phonetics, 5* (1991): 225–279.

Shriberg, L. D., N. L. Potter, and E. A. Strand, "Prevalence and phenotype of childhood apraxia of speech in youth with galactosemia." *Journal of Speech, Language, and Hearing Research, 54* (2011): 487–519.

Shriberg, L. D., J. B. Tomblin, and J. L. McSweeny "Prevalence of speech delay in 6-year-old children and comorbidity with language impairment." *Journal of Speech, Language, and Hearing Research, 42* (1999): 1461–1481.

Shriberg, L. D., and C. Widder, "Speech and prosody characteristics of adults with mental retardation."

Journal of Speech and Hearing Research, 33 (1990): 627–653.

Shriner, T., M. Holloway, and R. Daniloff, "The relationship between articulatory deficits and syntax in speech defective children." *Journal of Speech and Hearing Research, 12* (1969): 319–325.

Shuster, L. I., D. M. Ruscello, and A. R. Toth, "The use of visual feedback to elicit correct /r/." *American Journal of Speech-Language Pathology, 4* (1995): 37–44.

Shuy, R. "Social dialect and employability: Some pitfalls of good intentions." In L. Davis (Ed.), *Studies in Linguistics*. Birmingham: University of Alabama Press, 1972.

Siegel, R., H. Winitz, and H. Conkey, "The influence of testing instruments in articulatory responses of children." *Journal of Speech and Hearing Disorders, 28* (1963): 67–76.

Silverman, E., "Listeners' impressions of speakers with lateral lisps." *Journal of Speech and Hearing Disorders, 41* (1976): 547–552.

Siqueland, E. R., and C. A. Delucia, "Visual reinforcement of non-nutritive sucking in human infants." *Science, 165* (1969): 1144–1146.

Skelly, M., D. Spector, R. Donaldson, A. Brodeur, and F. Paletta, "Compensatory physiologic phonetics for the glossectomee." *Journal of Speech and Hearing Disorders, 36* (1971): 101–114.

Skelton, S. L., "Concurrent task sequencing in single-phoneme phonologic treatment and generalization." *Journal of Communication Disorders, 37* (2004): 131–155.

Skelton, S. L., and T. E. Funk, "Teaching speech sounds to young children using randomly ordered, variably complex task sequences." *Perceptual and Motor Skills, 99* (2004) 602–604.

Skinner, B. F., *Cumulative Record: A Selection of Papers* (3rd ed.). New York: Appleton-Century-Crofts, 1972.

Small, L. (2004). *Fundamentals of Phonetics: A Practical Guide for Students* (2nd ed.). Boston: Allyn and Bacon.

Smit, A. B., "Ages of speech sound acquisition: Comparisons and critiques of several normative studies." *Language, Speech, and Hearing Services in Schools, 17* (1986): 175–186.

Smit, A. B., "Phonologic error distributions in the Iowa-Nebraska articulation norms project: Consonant singletons." *Journal of Speech and Hearing Research, 36* (1993a): 533–547.

Smit, A. B., "Phonologic error distributions in the Iowa-Nebraska articulation norms project: Word-initial consonant clusters." *Journal of Speech and Hearing Research, 36* (1993b): 931–947.

Smit, A. B., "General American English speech acquisition." In S. McLeod (Ed.), *The International Guide to Speech Acquisition* (pp. 128–147) Clifton Park, NY: Thomson Delmar Learning, 2007.

Smit, A. B., and J. Bernthal, "Voicing contrasts and their phonological implications in the speech of articulation-disordered children." *Journal of Speech and Hearing Research, 26* (1983): 19–28.

Smit, A. B., and L. Hand, *Smit-Hand Articulation and Phonology Evaluation (SHAPE)*. Los Angeles: Western Psychological Services, 1997.

Smit, A. B., L. Hand, J. J. Freilinger, J. E. Bernthal, and A. Bird, "The Iowa articulation norms project and its Nebraska replication." *Journal of Speech and Hearing Disorders, 55* (1990): 779–798.

Smith, A. B., L. Goffman, H. N. Zelaznik, G. Ying, and C. McGillem, "Spatiotemporal stability and patterning of speech movement sequences." *Experimental Brain Research, 104* (1995): 493–501.

Smith, B. L., "Temporal aspects of English speech production: A developmental perspective." *Journal of Phonetics, 6* (1978): 37–67.

Smith, B. L., K. K. McGregor, and D. Demille, "Phonological development in lexically precocious 2-year-olds." *Applied Psycholinguistics, 27* (2006): 355–375.

Smith, B. L., and C. Stoel-Gammon, "A longitudinal study of the development of stop consonant production in normal and Down's syndrome children." *Journal of Speech and Hearing Disorders, 48* (1983): 114–118.

Smith, M. W., and S. Ainsworth, "The effect of three types of stimulation on articulatory responses of speech defective children." *Journal of Speech and Hearing Research, 10* (1967): 333–338.

Smith, N. V., *The Acquisition of Phonology: A Case Study*. New York: Cambridge University Press, 1973.

Snow, D., "Phrase-final syllable lengthening and intonation in early child speech." *Journal of Speech and Hearing Research, 37* (1994): 831–840.

Snow, J., and R. Milisen, "The influences of oral versus pictorial representation upon articulation testing results." *Journal of Speech and Hearing Disorders. Monograph, Suppl., 4* (1954): 29–36.

Snow, K., "Articulation proficiency in relation to certain dental abnormalities." *Journal of Speech and Hearing Disorders, 26* (1961): 209–212.

Snowling, M., D. V. M. Bishop, and S. E. Stothard, "Is Preschool Language Impairment a Risk Factor for Dyslexia in Adolescence?" *Journal of Child Psychology and Psychiatry and Allied Disciplines, 41* (2000): 587–600.

So, L., and B. Dodd, "Phonologically disordered Cantonese-speaking children." *Clinical Linguistics and Phonetics, 8* (1994): 235–255.

So, L. K. H., "Cantonese phonological development: Normal and Disordered." In Z. Hua and B. Dodd (Eds.), *Phonological Development and Disorders: A Cross-Linguistic Perspective* (pp. 109–134). Clevedon, UK: Multilingual Matters, 2006.

So, L. K. H., "Cantonese speech acquisition." In S. McLeod (Ed.), *The International Guide to Speech Acquisition* (pp. 313–326). Clifton Park, NY: Thomson/Delmar, 2007.

So, L. K. H., and B. J. Dodd, "The acquisition of phonology by Cantonese-speaking children." *Journal of Child Language, 22* (1995): 473–495.

Sommers, R. K., "Factors in the effectiveness of mothers trained to aid in speech correction." *Journal of Speech and Hearing Disorders, 27* (1962): 178–186.

Sommers, R. K., "The therapy program." In R. Van Hattum (Ed.), *Clinical Speech in the Schools* (pp. 277–334). Springfield, IL: Charles C. Thomas, 1969.

Sommers, R. K., A. K. Furlong, F. H. Rhodes, G. R. Fichter, D. C. Bowser, F. H. Copetas, and Z. G. Saunders, "Effects of maternal attitudes upon improvement in articulation when mothers are trained to assist in speech correction." *Journal of Speech and Hearing Disorders, 29* (1964): 126–132.

Sommers, R. K., R. Leiss, M. Delp, A. Gerber, D. Fundrella, R. Smith, M. Revucky, D. Ellis, and V. Haley, "Factors related to the effectiveness of articulation therapy for kindergarten, first- and second-grade children." *Journal of Speech and Hearing Research, 10* (1967): 428–437.

Sommers, R. K., R. Reinhart, and D. Sistrunk, "Traditional articulation measures of Down's syndrome speakers, ages 13–22." *Journal of Childhood Communication Disorders, 12* (1988): 93–108.

Sommers, R. K., M. H. Schaeffer, R. H. Leiss, A. J. Gerber, M. A. Bray, D. Fundrella, J. K. Olson, and E. R. Tomkins, "The effectiveness of group and individual therapy." *Journal of Speech and Hearing Research, 9* (1966): 219–225.

Sonderman, J., "An experimental study of clinical relationships between auditory discrimination and articulation skills." Paper presented at the annual convention of the American Speech and Hearing Association, San Francisco, 1971.

Sowell, E. R., P. M. Thompson, C. M. Leonard, S. E. Welcome, E. Kan, and A. W. Toga, "Longitudinal mapping of cortical thickness and brain growth in normal children." *Journal of Neuroscience, 24,* 38 (2004): 8223–8231.

Sowell, E. R., P. M. Thompson, and A. W. Toga, "Mapping changes in the human cortex throughout the span of life." *Neuroscientist, 10,* 4 (2004): 372–392.

Spector, J., "Predicting progress in beginning reading: Dynamic assessment of phonemic awareness." *Journal of Educational Psychology, 84* (1992): 353–363.

Speech Pathology Association of Australia (SPA)., "Scope of Practice." Available from http://www.speechpathologyaustralia.org.au/, 2011.

Speirs, R. L., and M. A. Maktabi, "Tongue skills and clearance of toffee in two age-groups and in children with problems of speech articulation." *Journal of Dentistry for Children, 57* (1990): 356–360.

Spencer, A., "Towards a theory of phonological development." *Lingua, 68* (1986): 3–38.

Spencer, A., "A phonological theory of phonological development." In M. J. Ball (Ed.), *Theoretical Linguistics and Disordered Language* (pp. 115–151). London: Croom Helm, 1988.

Spencer, A., *Phonology*. Oxford, UK: Blackwell, 1996.

Square, P., "Treatment of developmental apraxia of speech: Tactile-kinesthetic, rhythmic, and gestural approaches." In A. Caruso and E. Strand (Eds.), *Clinical Management of Motor Speech Disorders in Children* (pp. 149–185). New York: Thieme, 1999.

St. Louis, K., and D. Ruscello, *The Oral Speech Screening Examination*. Baltimore, MD: University Park Press, 2000.

St. Louis, K. O., D. M. Ruscello, and C. Lundeen, "Coexistence of communication disorders in schoolchildren." *Asha Monographs, 27* (1992).

Stackhouse, J., "Barriers to literacy development in children with speech and language difficulties." In D. Bishop and L. Leonard (Eds.), *Speech and Language Impairments in Children: Causes, Characteristics, Intervention and Outcome* (pp. 73–98). Hove, UK: Psychology Press, 2000.

Stackhouse, J., M. Pascoe, and H. Gardner, "Intervention for a child with persisting speech and literacy difficulties: A psycholinguistic approach." *Advances in Speech-Language Pathology, 8*(3) (2006): 231–244.

Stackhouse, J., M. Vance, M. Pascoe, and B. Wells, *Compendium of auditory and speech tasks. Children's Speech and Literacy Difficulties 4.* Chichester, UK: John Wiley and Sons, 2007.

Stackhouse, J., and B. Wells, "Psycholinguistic assessment of developmental speech disorders." *European Journal of Disorders of Communication, 28* (1993): 331–348.

Stackhouse, J., and B. Wells, *Children's Speech and Literacy Difficulties I: A Psycholinguistic Framework*. London: Whurr, 1997.

Stackhouse, J., and B. Wells, *Children's Speech and Literacy Difficulties: Identification and Intervention*. London: Whurr, 2001.

Stahl, S. A., and B. A. Murray, "Defining phonological awareness and its relationship to early reading." *Journal of Educational Psychology, 86* (1994): 221–234.

Stampe, D., "The Acquisition of Phonetic Representation." Paper presented at the Papers from the Fifth Regional Meeting of the Chicago Linguistic Society, Chicago, 1969.

Stampe, D. *A Dissertation on Natural Phonology*. New York: Garland, 1979.

Stanovich, K., "Matthew effects in reading: Some consequences of individual differences in the acquisition of literacy." *Reading Research Quarterly, 21* (1986): 360–407.

Stanovich, K., *Progress in Understanding Reading. Scientific Foundations and New Frontiers.* New York: Guilford Press, 2000.

Stark, R. E., L. E. Bernstein, and M. E. Demorest, "Vocal communication in the first 18 months of life." *Journal of Speech and Hearing Research, 36* (1983): 548–558.

Starr, C., "Dental and occlusal hazards to normal speech production." In K. Bzoch (Ed.), *Communicative Disorders Related to Cleft Lip and Palate* (pp. 670–680). Boston: Little, Brown, 1972.

Steeve, R. W., C. A. Moore, C. J. R. Green, K. J. Reilly, and J. Ruark McMurtrey, "Babbling, chewing, and sucking: Oromandibular coordination at 9 months." *Journal of Speech, Language and Hearing Research, 51* (2008): 1390–1404.

Stelcik, J., "An investigation of internal versus external discrimination and general versus phoneme-specific discrimination." Unpublished Thesis, University of Maryland, 1972.

Stemberger, J. P., "Between-word processes in child phonology." *Journal of Child Language, 15* (1988): 39–61.

Stepanof, E. R., "Procesos phonologicos de niños Puertorriqueños de 3 y 4 años evidenciado en la prueba APP-Spanish (Phonological processes evidenced on the APP-Spanish by 3- and 4-year-old Puerto Rican children)." *Opphla, 8,* 2 (1990): 15–20.

Stephens, M. I., P. Hoffman, and R. Daniloff, "Phonetic characteristics of delayed /s/ development." *Journal of Phonetics, 14* (1986): 247–256.

Stephens, N. S., "Implications of Beckwith-Wiedemann syndrome for the speech-language pathologist." Unpublished master's thesis. Idaho State University–Pocatello, 2011.

Steriade, D., "Greek prosodies and the nature of syllabification." Unpublished doctoral dissertation, Massachusetts Institute of Technology, 1990.

Stewart, S. R., and G. Weybright, "Articulation norms used by practicing speech-language pathologists in Oregon: Results of a survey." *Journal of Speech and Hearing Disorders, 45* (1980): 103–111.

Stewart, W., "Continuity and change in American Negro dialects." In W. Wolfram and N. Clarke (Eds.), *Black-White Speech Relationships* (pp. 51–73). Washington, DC: Center for Applied Linguistics, 1971.

Stockman, I., "Phonological development and disorders in African American children." In A. Kamhi, K. Pollock, and J. Harris (Eds.), *Communication Development and Disorders I in African American Children* (pp. 117–154). Baltimore, MD: Brookes, 1996a.

Stockman, I., "The promises and pitfalls of language sample analysis as an assessment tool for linguistic minority

children." *Language, Speech, and Hearing Services in Schools, 27* (1996b): 355–366.

Stockman, I., "Evidence for a minimal competence core of consonant sounds in the speech of African American children: A preliminary study." *Clinical Linguistics and Phonetics, 20* (2006a): 723–749.

Stockman, I., "Alveolar bias in the final consonant deletion patterns of African American children." *Language, Speech, and Hearing Services in Schools, 37* (2006b): 85–95.

Stockman, I., "Toward a validation of a minimal competence phonetic core for African American children." *Journal of Speech, Language, and Hearing Research, 51* (2008): 1244–1262.

Stockman, I., "A review of developmental and applied language research on African American children: From a deficit to difference perspective on dialect differences." *Journal of Speech, Language, and Hearing Research, 41* (2010): 123–38.

Stockman, I. J., and L. W. Stephenson, "Children's articulation of medial consonant clusters: Implications for syllabification. *Language and Speech, 24* (1981): 185–204.

Stoel-Gammon, C., "Phonetic inventories, 15–24 months: A longitudinal study." *Journal of Speech and Hearing Research, 28* (1985): 505–512.

Stoel-Gammon, C., "Phonological skills of 2-year-olds." *Language, Speech, and Hearing Services in Schools, 18* (1987): 323–329.

Stoel-Gammon, C., "Prespeech and early speech development of two late talkers." *First Language, 9* (1989): 207–224.

Stoel-Gammon, C., "Normal and disordered phonology in two-year-olds." *Topics in Language Disorders, 11* (1991): 21–32.

Stoel-Gammon, C., "Normal and disordered phonology in two-year olds." In K. Butler (Ed.), *Early Intervention: Working with Infants and Toddlers* (pp. 110–121). Rockville, MD: Aspen, 1994.

Stoel-Gammon, C., "Variability in the productions of young typically-developing children." Paper presented at the meeting of the International Clinical Linguistics and Phonetics Association, Lafayette, LA, 2004.

Stoel-Gammon, C., "Variability in speech acquisition." In S. McLeod (Ed.), *The International Guide to Speech Acquisition* (pp. 55–60). Clifton Park, NY: Thomson Delmar Learning, 2007.

Stoel-Gammon, C., "Relationships between lexical and phonological development in young children." *Journal of Child Language, 38* (2011): 1–34.

Stoel-Gammon, C., and C. Dunn, *Normal and Disordered Phonology in Children.* Baltimore, MD: University Park Press, 1985.

Stoel-Gammon, C., and P. B. Herrington, "Vowel systems of normally developing and phonologically disordered children." *Clinical Linguistics and Phonetics, 4* (1990): 145–160.

Stoel-Gammon, C., and M. Kehoe, "Hearing impairment in infants and toddlers: Identification, vocal development, and intervention in child phonology." In J. Bernthal and N. Bankson (Eds.), *Child Phonology: Characteristics, Assessment, and Intervention with Special Populations* (pp. 163–181). New York: Thieme Medical Publishers, 1994.

Stoel-Gammon, C., and K. Otomo, "Babbling development of hearing-impaired and normally hearing subjects." *Journal of Speech and Hearing Disorders, 51,* 1 (1986): 33–41.

Stokes, S. F., T. Klee, C. P. Carson, and D. Carson, "A phonemic implicational feature hierarchy of phonological contrasts for English-speaking children." *Journal of Speech, Language, and Hearing Research, 48,* 4 (2005): 817–833.

Stokes, T. F., and D. M. Baer, "An implicit technology of generalization." *Journal of Applied Behavior Analysis, 10* (1977): 349–367.

Storch, S. A., and G. J. Whitehurst, "Oral language and code-related precursors to reading: Evidence from a longitudinal structural model." *Developmental Psychology, 38* (2002): 934–947.

Storkel, H. L., "The emerging lexicon of children with phonological delays: Phonotactic constraints and probability in acquisition." *Journal of Speech, Language, and Hearing Research, 47* (2005): 1194–1212.

Storkel, H. L., "Do children still pick and choose? The relationship between phonological knowledge and lexical acquisition beyond 50 words." *Clinical Linguistics and Phonetics, 20,* 7/8 (2006): 523–529.

Storkel, H. L., and M. L. Morrisette, "The lexicon and phonology: Interactions in language acquisition." *Language, Speech, and Hearing Services in Schools, 33* (2002): 24–37.

Strand, E. A., and P. Debertine, "The efficacy of integral stimulation intervention with developmental apraxia of speech." *Journal of Medical Speech-Language Pathology, 8* (2000): 295–300.

Strand, E., and R. McCauley, "Assessment procedures for treatment planning in children with phonologic and motor speech disorders." In A. Caruso and E. Strand (Eds.), *Clinical Management of Motor Speech Disorders in Children* (pp. 73–107). New York: Thieme, 1999.

Strand, E., and A. Skindner, "Treatment of developmental apraxia of speech: Integral stimulation methods." In A. Caruso and E. Strand (Eds.), *Clinical Management of Motor Speech Disorders in Children* (pp. 109–148). New York: Thieme, 1999.

Strand, E. A., R. Stoeckel, and B. Baas, "Treatment of severe childhood apraxia of speech: A treatment efficacy study." *Journal of Medical Speech-Language Pathology, 14* (2006): 297–307.

Stringfellow, K., and S. McLeod, "Using a facilitating phonetic context to reduce an unusual form of gliding." *Language, Speech, and Hearing Services in Schools, 25* (1991): 191–193.

Subtelny, J., "Malocclusions, orthodontic corrections and orofacial muscle adaptation." *Angle Orthodontist, 40* (1970): 170.

Subtelny, J., J. Mestre, and J. Subtelny, "Comparative study of normal and defective articulation of /s/ as related to malocclusion and deglutition." *Journal of Speech and Hearing Disorders, 29* (1964): 269–285.

Subtelny, J., J. Worth, and M. Sakuda, "Intraoral pressure and rate of flow during speech." *Journal of Speech and Hearing Research, 9* (1966): 498–518.

Sullivan, M., C. Gaebler, D. Beukelman, G. Mahanna, J. Marshall, D. Lydiatt, and W. Lydiatt, "Impact of palatal prosthodontic intervention on communication performance of patients' maxillectomy defects: A multi-level outcome study." *Head and Neck, 24,* 6 (2002): 530–538.

Sun, J., Y. Weng, J. Li, G. Wang, and Z. Zhang, "Analysis of determinants on speech function after glossectomy." *Journal of Oral and Maxillofacial Surgery, 65* (2007): 1944–1950.

Sutherland, D., and G. T. Gillon, "Assessment of phonological representations in children with speech impairment." *Language, Speech, and Hearing Services in Schools, 36* (2005): 294–307.

Sutherland, D., and G. T. Gillon, "Development of phonological representations and phonological awareness in children with speech impairment." *International Journal of Language and Communication Disorders, 42,* 2 (2007): 229–250.

Swank, L., and H. Catts, "Phonological awareness and written word decoding." *Language, Speech, and Hearing Services in Schools, 25* (1994): 9–14.

Swanson, T. J., B. W. Hodson, and M. Schommer-Aikins, "An examination of phonological awareness treatment outcomes for 7th grade poor readers from a bilingual community." *Language, Speech, and Hearing Services in Schools, 36* (2005): 336–345.

Tang, G., and J. Barlow, "Characteristics of the sound systems of monolingual Vietnamese-speaking children with phonological impairment." *Clinical Linguistics and Phonetics, 20* (2006): 423–445.

Taylor, O., "Teaching standard English as a second dialect." In O. Taylor (Ed.), *Treatment of Communication Disorders in Culturally and Linguistically Diverse Populations* (pp. 153–178). San Diego, CA: College-Hill Press, 1986.

Taylor, O., K. Payne, and N. Anderson, "Distinguishing between communication disorders and differences." *Seminars in Speech and Language, 8* (1987): 415–427.

Teele, D. W., J. O. Klein, B. A. Rosner, and the Greater Boston Otitis Media Study Group, "Otitis media with effusion during the first three years of life and development of speech and language." *Pediatrics, 74* (1984): 282–287.

Terai, H., and M. Shimahara, "Evaluation of speech intelligibility after a secondary dehiscence operation using an artificial graft in patients with speech disorders after partial glossectomy." *British Journal of Oral and Maxillofacial Surgery, 42* (2004): 190–194.

Templin, M., "Spontaneous vs. imitated verbalization in testing pre-school children." *Journal of Speech and Hearing Disorders, 12* (1947): 293–300.

Templin, M., "Certain language skills in children." *Institute of Child Welfare Monograph Series 26.* Minneapolis: University of Minnesota, 1957.

Templin, M., "Development of speech." *Journal of Pediatrics, 62* (1963): 11–14.

Templin, M., and G. Glaman, "A longitudinal study of correlations of predictive measures obtained in prekindergarten and first grade with achievement measures through eleventh grade" [unpublished report #101]. Washington, DC: U.S. Department of Health, Education, and Welfare, Office of Education, 1976.

Terrell, P. A., "Alphabetic and phonemic awareness in toddlers." Unpublished doctoral dissertation. Louisiana State University–Baton Rouge, 2007.

Terrell, S., and F. Terrell, "Effects of speaking Black English upon employment opportunities." *ASHA, 25* (1983): 27–29.

Thomas, R. M., *Comparing Theories of Child Development* (5th ed.). Belmont, CA: Wadsworth, 2000.

Thompson, A. E., and T. J. Hixon, "Nasal air flow during speech production." *Cleft Palate Journal, 16* (1979): 412–420.

Tiffany, W., "Effects of syllable structure on diadochokinetic and reading rates." *Journal of Speech and Hearing Research, 23* (1980): 894–908.

Tingley, B. M., and G. D. Allen, "Development of speech timing control in children." *Child Development, 46* (1975): 186–194.

Tipton, G., "Non-cognate consonants of Mandarin and Cantonese." *Journal of the Chinese Language Teachers Association, 10,* 1 (1975): 1–13.

Tomblin, J. B., N. L. Records, P. Buckwalter, X. Zhang, E. Smith, and M. O'Brien, "Prevalence of specific language impairment in kindergarten children." *Journal of Speech, Language and Hearing Research, 40* (1997): 1245–1260.

Torgesen, J., "Assessment and instruction for phonemic awareness and word recognition skills." In H. Catts and A. Kamhi (Eds.), *Language and Reading Disabilities* (pp. 128–153). Boston: Allyn and Bacon, 1999.

Torgesen, J., and B. Bryant, *Test of Phonological Awareness—Second Edition: PLUS.* Austin, TX: Pro-Ed, 2004.

Torgesen, J., and P. Mathes, *A Basic Guide to Understanding, Assessing, and Teaching Phonological Awareness.* Austin, TX: Pro-Ed, 2000.

Torgesen, J., S. T. Morgan, and C. Davis, "Effects of two types of phonological awareness training on word learning in kindergarten children." *Journal of Educational Psychology, 84* (1992): 364–370.

Torgesen, J., R. Wagner, and C. Rashotte, "Longitudinal studies of phonological processing and reading." *Journal of Learning Disabilities, 27* (1994): 276–286.

Torgesen, J., R. Wagner, C. Rashotte, A. Alexander, and T. Conway, "Preventative and remedial interventions for children with severe reading disabilities." *Learning Disabilities: An Interdisciplinary Journal, 81* (1997): 51–62.

Travis, L., and B. Rasmus, "The speech sound discrimination ability of cases with functional disorders of articulation." *Quarterly Journal of Speech, 17* (1931): 217–226.

Trehub, S., "Infants' sensitivity to vowel and tonal contrasts." *Developmental Psychology, 9* (1973): 91–96.

Treiman, R., "The structure of spoken syllables: Evidence from novel word games." *Cognition, 15* (1983): 49–74.

Treiman, R., C. A. Fowler, J. Gross, D. Berch, and S. Weatherston, "Syllable structure or word structure? Evidence for onset and rime units with disyllabic and trisyllabic stimuli." *Journal of Memory and Language, 34* (1995): 132–155.

Treiman, R., and A. Zukowski, "Toward an understanding of English syllabification." *Journal of Memory and Language, 29* (1990): 66–85.

Treiman, R., and A. Zukowski, "Children's sensitivity to syllables, onsets, rimes, and phonemes." *Journal of Experimental Child Psychology, 61* (1996): 193–215.

Tse, J., "Tone acquisition in Cantonese: A longitudinal case study." *Journal of Child Language, 5* (1978): 191–204.

Tsao, F. M., H. M. Liu, and P. K. Kuhl, "Speech perception in infancy predicts language development in the second year of life: A longitudinal study." *Child Development, 75* (2004): 1067–1084.

Ttofari-Eecen, K., S. Reilly, and P. Eadie, "Parent report of speech sound development at 12 months of age: Evidence from a cohort study [unpublished manuscript]," 2007.

Tyler, A., "Planning and monitoring intervention programs." In K. E. Pollock and A. G. Kamhi (Eds.), *Phonological Disorders in Children: Clinical Decision Making in Assessment and Intervention* (pp. 123–138). Baltimore, MD: Brookes, 2005.

Tyler, A., M. Edwards, and J. Saxman, "Acoustic validation of phonological knowledge and its relationship to treatment." *Journal of Speech and Hearing Disorders, 55* (1990): 251–261.

Tyler, A., and G. R. Figurski, "Phonetic inventory changes after treating distinctions along an implicational hierarchy." *Clinical Linguistics and Phonetics, 8* (1994): 91–107.

Tyler, A. A., G. T. Gillon, T. Macrae, and L. Roberta, "Direct and indirect effects of stimulating phoneme awareness versus other linguistic skills in preschoolers with co-occurring speech and language impairments." *Topics in Language Disorders, 31* (2011): 128–144.

Tyler, A., K. E. Lewis, A. Haskill, and L. C. Tolbert, "Efficacy of cross-domain effects of a morphosyntax and a phonologic intervention." *Language, Speech, and Hearing Services in Schools, 33* (2002): 52–66.

Tyler, A., and K. Watterson, "Effects of phonological versus language intervention in preschoolers with both phonological and language impairment." *Child Language Teaching and Therapy, 7* (1991): 141–160.

Ukrainetz, T. A., M. H. Cooney, S. K. Dyer, A. J. Kysar, and T. J. Harris, "An investigation into teaching phonemic awareness through shared reading and writing." *Early Childhood Research Quarterly, 15* (2000): 331–355.

Ukrainetz, T. A., C. L. Ross, and H. M. Harm, "An investigation of treatment scheduling for phonemic awareness with kindergartners who are at risk for reading difficulties." *Language, Speech, and Hearing Services in Schools, 40* (2009): 86–100.

Umberger, F. G., and R. G. Johnston, "The efficacy of oral myofunctional and coarticulation therapy." *International Journal of Orofacial Myology, 23* (1997): 3–9.

U.S. Bureau of the Census, *Age by language spoken at home by ability to speak English for the population 5 years and over* (2000). www.census.gov/. Retrieved January 25, 2007

U.S. Bureau of the Census, *Detailed languages spoken at home and ability to speak English for the population 5 years and over for the United States: 2006–2008* (2008a). www.census.gov/hhes/socdemo/language/index.html. Retrieved June 29, 2011.

U.S. Bureau of the Census, *Projections of the Population by Sex, Race, and Hispanic Origin for the United States: 2010 to 2050* (2008b). www.census.gov/population/www/projections/summarytables.html. Retrieved June 29, 2011.

Vallino, L. D., R. Zuker, and J. A. Napoli, "A study of speech, language, hearing and dentition in children with cleft lip only." *Cleft Palate-Craniofacial Journal, 45* (2008): 485–494.

Vance, M., S. Rosen, and M. Coleman, "Assessing speech perception in young children and relationships with language skills." *International Journal of Audiology, 48* (2009): 708–717.

Vance, M., J. Stackhouse, and B. Wells, "Speech production skills in children aged 3–7 years." *International Journal of Language and Communication Disorders, 40* (2005): 29–48.

Vandervelden, M. C., and L. S. Siegel, "Phonological recording and phoneme awareness in early literacy: A developmental approach." *Reading Research Quarterly, 30* (1995): 854–875.

Van Beijsterveldt, C. E. M., S. Felsenfeld, and D. I. Boomsma, "Bivariate genetic analyses of stuttering and nonfluency in a large sample of 5-year-old twins." *Journal of Speech, Language, and Hearing Research, 53* (2010): 609–619.

Van Borsel, J., B. Morlion, K. Van Snick, and J. S. Leroy, "Articulation in Beckwith-Wiedemann syndrome: Two case studies." *American Journal of Speech-Language Pathology, 9* (2000): 202–213.

Van Borsel, J., and J. A. Tetnowski, "Fluency disorders in genetic syndromes." *Journal of Fluency Disorders, 32* (2007): 279–296.

Van Borsel, J., K. Van Snick, and J. Leroy, "Macxroglossia and speech in Bechwith-Wiedemann syndrome: A sample survey study." *International Journal of Language and Communication Disorders, 34* (1999): 209–221.

Van Hattum, R. J., "Program scheduling." In R. Van Hattum (Ed.), *Clinical Speech in the Schools* (pp. 163–195). Springfield, IL: Charles C. Thomas, 1969.

van Kleeck, A., "Preliteracy domains and stages: Laying the foundations for beginning reading." *Journal of Children's Communication Development, 20* (1998): 33–51.

van Kleeck, A., R. Gillam, and T. McFadden, "A study of classroom-based phonological awareness training for preschoolers with speech and/or language disorders." *American Journal of Speech-Language Pathology, 7*, 3 (1998): 65–76.

Van Lierde, K. M., G. Mortier, E. Huysman, and H. Vermeersch, "Long-term impact of tongue reduction on speech intelligibility, articulation and oromyofunctional behavior in a child with Beckwith-Wiedemann syndrome." *International Journal of Pediatric Otorhinolaryngology, 74* (2010): 309–318.

Van Riper, C., *Speech Correction: Principles and Methods*. Englewood Cliffs, NJ: Prentice-Hall, 1939.

Van Riper, C., *Speech Correction: Principles and Methods* (5th ed.). Englewood Cliffs, NJ: Prentice-Hall, 1972.

Van Riper, C., and L. Emerick, *Speech Correction: An Introduction to Speech Pathology and Audiology* (7th ed.). Englewood Cliffs, NJ: Prentice-Hall, 1984.

Van Riper, C., and R. Erickson, *Speech Correction: An Introduction to Speech Pathology and Audiology* (9th ed.). Englewood Cliffs, NJ: Prentice-Hall, 1996.

Van Riper, C., and J. V. Irwin, *Voice and Articulation*. Englewood Cliffs, NJ: Prentice-Hall, 1958.

Veatch, J., "An experimental investigation of a motor theory of auditory discrimination." Unpublished Ph.D. Dissertation, University of Idaho, 1970.

Velleman, S., *Childhood Apraxia of Speech, Resource Guide*. Clifton Park, NY: Thomson Delmar Learning, 2003.

Velleman, S. L., and B. Z. Pearson, "Differentiating speech sound disorders from phonological dialect differences: Implications for assessment and intervention." *Topics in Language Disorders, 30* (2010): 176–188.

Velleman, S., B. Z. Pearson, T. J. Bryant, and T. Charko, "Phonotactic versus phonetic development in African American English [manuscript]," 2010.

Velleman, S., and K. Strand, "Developmental verbal dyspraxia." In J. Bernthal, and N. Bankson (Eds.), *Child Phonology: Characteristics, Assessment, and Intervention with Special Populations* (pp. 110–139). New York: Thieme Publishers, 1994.

Velten, H., "The growth of phonemic and lexical patterns in infant language." *Language, 19* (1943): 281–292.

Veltman, C., *The Future of the Spanish Language in the United States*. Washington, DC: Hispanic Policy Development Project, 1988.

Vihman, M. M., "Early phonological development." In J. Bernthal and N. Bankson (Eds.), *Articulation and Phonological Disorders* (2nd ed.). Baltimore, MD: Williams and Wilkins, 1988.

Vihman, M. M., *Early Syllables and the Construction of Phonology*. Timonium, MD: York, 1992.

Vihman, M. M., *Phonological Development: The Origins of Language in the Child*. Cambridge, MA: Blackwell, 1996.

Vihman, M. M., "Early phonological development." In J. Bernthal and N. Bankson (Eds.), *Articulation and Phonological Disorders* (5th ed.; pp. 63–104). Boston: Allyn and Bacon, 2004.

Vihman, M. M., and M. Greenlee, "Individual differences in phonological development: Ages one and three years." *Journal of Speech and Hearing Research, 30* (1987): 503–521.

Vogel, J. E., J. B. Mulliken, and L. B. Kaban, "Macroglossia: A review of the condition and a new classification." *Plastic and Reconstructive Surgery, 78* (1986): 715–723.

Vogel Sosa, A., and C. Stoel-Gammon, "Patterns of intra-word phonological variability during the second year of life." *Journal of Child Language, 33* (2006): 31–50.

Vorperian, H., R. D. Kent, L. R. Gentry, and B. S. Yandell, "Magnetic resonance imaging procedures to study the concurrent anatomic development of vocal tract structures: Preliminary results." *International Journal of Pediatric Otorhinolaryngology, 49*, 3 (1999): 197–206.

Vorperian, H. K., S. Wang, M. K. Chung, E. M. Schimek, R. B. Durtschi, R. D. Kent, A. J. Ziegert, and L. R. Gentry, "Anatomic development of the oral and pharyngeal portions of the vocal tract." *Journal of the Acoustical Society of America, 125* (2009): 1666–1678.

Wadsworth, S. D., C. A. Maul, and E. J. Stevens, "The prevalence of orofacial myofunctional disorders among children identified with speech and language disorders in grades kindergarten through six." *International Journal of Orofacial Myology, 24* (1998): 1–19.

Wagner, R., and J. K. Torgesen, "The nature of phonological processing and its causal role in the acquisition of reading skills." *Psychological Bulletin, 101* (1987): 192–212.

Wagner, R., J. Torgesen, and C. Rashotte, *Comprehensive Test of Phonological Processing*. Austin, TX: Pro-Ed, 1999.

Walker, J. F., and L. M. D. Archibald, "Articulation rate in preschool children: A 3-year longitudinal study." *International Journal of Language and Communication Disorders, 41*, 5 (2006): 541–565.

Walsh, B., and A. Smith, "Articulatory movements in adolescents: Evidence for protracted development of speech motor control processes." *Journal of Speech, Language, and Hearing Research, 45*, 6 (2002): 1119–1133.

Walsh, H., "On certain practical inadequacies of distinctive feature systems." *Journal of Speech and Hearing Disorders, 39* (1974): 32–43.

Wang, W., *Languages and Dialects of Chinese*. Palo Alto, CA: Stanford University Press, 1989.

Wang, W., "Theoretical issues in studying Chinese dialects." *Journal of the Chinese Language Teachers Association, 25* (1990): 1–34.

Waring, R., J. Fisher, and N. Atkin, "The articulation survey: Putting numbers to it." In L. Wilson and S. Hewat (Eds.), *Proceedings of the 2001 Speech Pathology Australia National Conference: Evidence and innovation* (pp. 145–151). Melbourne, 2001.

Warrick, N., and H. Rubin, "Phonological awareness: Normally developing and language delayed children." *Journal of Speech-Language Pathology and Audiology, 16*, 1 (1992): 11–20.

Warrick, N., H. Rubin, and S. Rowe-Walsh, "Phoneme awareness in language-delayed children: Comparative studies and intervention." *Annals of Dyslexia, 43* (1993): 153–173.

Washington, J., and H. Craig, "Articulation test performances of low-income African American preschoolers with communication impairments." *Language, Speech, and Hearing Services in Schools, 23* (1992): 201–207.

Washington, J., and H. Craig, "Socioeconomic status and gender influences on children's dialectal variations." *Journal of Speech, Language, and Hearing Research, 41* (1998): 618–626.

Watson, J. B., "Psychology as a behaviorist views it." *Psychological Review, 101* (1913/1994): 248–253.

Watson, M. M., and G. P. Scukanec, "Phonological changes in the speech of two-year olds: A longitudinal investigation." *Infant-Toddler Intervention, 7* (1997a): 67–77.

Watson, M. M., and G. P. Scukanec, "Profiling the phonological abilities of 2-year-olds: A longitudinal investigation." *Child Language Teaching and Therapy, 13* (1997b): 3–14.

Weaver, C., C. Furbee, and R. Everhart, "Paternal occupational class and articulatory defects in children." *Journal of Speech and Hearing Disorders, 25* (1960) 171–175.

Weaver-Spurlock, S., and J. Brasseur, "Position training on the generalization training of [s]." *Language, Speech, and Hearing Services in Schools, 19* (1988): 259–271.

Weber, J., "Patterning of deviant articulation behavior." *Journal of Speech and Hearing Disorders, 35* (1970): 135–141.

Weikum, W. M., A. Vouloumanos, J. Navarra, S. Soto-Faraco, N. Sebastián-Gallés, and J. F. Werker, "Visual language discrimination in infancy." *Science, 316,* 25 (2007): 1159.

Weiner, F., *Phonological Process Analysis.* Baltimore, MD: University Park Press, 1979.

Weiner, F., "Systematic sound preference as a characteristic of phonological disability." *Journal of Speech and Hearing Disorders, 46* (1981a): 281–286.

Weiner, F., "Treatment of phonological disability using the method of meaningful minimal contrast: Two case studies." *Journal of Speech and Hearing Disorders, 46* (1981b): 97–103.

Weismer, G., D. Dinnsen, and M. Elbert, "A study of the voicing distinction associated with omitted, word-final stops." *Journal of Speech and Hearing Disorders, 46* (1981): 91–103.

Weiss, C. E., *Weiss Intelligibility Test.* Tigard, OR: CC Publications, 1982.

Wellman, B., I. Case, I. Mengert, and D. Bradbury, "Speech sounds of young children." *University of Iowa Studies in Child Welfare, 5* (1931).

Wells, B., and S. Peppé, "Intonation abilities of children with speech and language impairments." *Journal of Speech, Language, and Hearing Research, 46* (2003): 5–20.

Weston, A., and J. Irwin, "Paired stimuli treatment." In P. Newman, N. Creaghead, and W. Secord (Eds.), *Assessment and Remediation of Articulatory and Phonological Disorders* (pp. 337–368). Columbus, OH: Merrill, 1985.

Whitehurst, G. J., and C. J. Lonigan, "Child development and emergent literacy." *Child Development, 69* (1998): 848–872.

Wiig, E., E. Semel, and W. Secord, *"Clinical Evaluation of Language Fundamentals Preschool– 2."* San Antonio, TX: The Psychological Corporation, 2004.

Wilcox, K., and S. Morris, "Speech outcomes of the language-focused curriculum." In M. Rice and K. Wilcox (Eds.), *Building a Language-Focused Curriculum for the Preschool Classroom: A Foundation for Lifelong Communication* (pp. 73–79). Baltimore, MD: Brookes, 1995.

Wilcox, K., and S. Morris, *Children's Speech Intelligibility Measure.* San Antonio, TX: The Psychological Corporation, 1999.

Wilcox, L., and R. Anderson, "Distinguishing between phonological difference and disorder in children who speak African-American Vernacular English: An experimental testing instrument." *Journal of Communication Disorders, 31* (1998): 315–335.

Wilhelm, C. L., "The effects of oral form recognition training on articulation in children." Unpublished dissertation, University of Kansas, 1971.

Williams, A. L., "Generalization patterns associated with training least phonological knowledge." *Journal of Speech and Hearing Research, 34* (1991): 722–733.

Williams, A. L., "Phonological reorganization: A qualitative measure of phonological improvement." *American Journal of Speech-Language Pathology, 2* (1993): 44–51.

Williams, A. L., "A systemic approach to phonological assessment and intervention." Workshop presented at the Speech and Hearing Association of Virginia, Williamsburg, VA, 1999.

Williams, A. L., "Multiple oppositions: Case studies of variables in phonological intervention." *American Journal of Speech-Language Pathology, 9* (2000a): 289–299.

Williams, A. L., "Multiple oppositions: Theoretical foundations for an alternative contrastive intervention approach." *American Journal of Speech-Language Pathology, 9* (2000b): 282–288.

Williams, A. L., "Phonological assessment of child speech." In D. Ruscello (Ed.), *Tests and Measurements in Speech-Language Pathology* (pp. 31–76). Boston: Butterworth-Heinemann, 2001.

Williams, A. L., *Speech Disorders Resource Guide for Preschool Children.* Clifton Park, NY: Singular Publishing, 2003.

Williams, A. L., *SCIP: Sound Contrasts in Phonology* [Version 1.0]. Greenville, SC: Super-Duper Publications, 2006.

Williams, F., *Language and Speech: Introductory Perspectives.* Englewood Cliffs, NJ: Prentice-Hall, 1972.

Williams, G., and L. McReynolds, "The relationship between discrimination and articulation training in children with misarticulations." *Journal of Speech and Hearing Research, 18* (1975): 401–412.

Williams, P., and J. Stackhouse, "Diadochokinetic skills: Normal and atypical performance in children aged 3–5 years." *International Journal of Language and Communication Disorders, 33* (1998): 481–486.

Williams, P., and J. Stackhouse, "Rate, accuracy and consistency: Diadochokinetic performance of young, normally developing children." *Clinical Linguistics and Phonetics, 14* (2000): 267–294.

Wilson, F., "Efficacy of speech therapy with educable mentally retarded children." *Journal of Speech and Hearing Research, 9* (1966): 423–433.

Wing, K. and P. Flipsen Jr., "*Phonological disorders in Spanish-speaking children: Accounting for Mexican dialect.*" Poster presented at the convention of the American Speech-Language-Hearing Association, Philadelphia, PA, 2010).

Winitz, H., "Language skills of male and female kindergarten children." *Journal of Speech and Hearing Research, 2* (1959a): 377–386.

Winitz, H., "Relationship between language and nonlanguage measures of kindergarten children." *Journal of Speech and Hearing Research, 2* (1959b): 387–391.

Winitz, H., *Articulatory Acquisition and Behavior.* Englewood Cliffs, NJ: Prentice-Hall, 1969.

Winitz, H., *From Syllable to Conversation.* Baltimore, MD: University Park Press, 1975.

Winitz, H., "Auditory considerations in articulation training." In H. Winitz (Ed.), *Treating Articulation Disorders: For Clinicians by Clinicians* (pp. 21–49). Baltimore, MD: University Park Press, 1984.

Wise, C. M., *Introduction to Phonetics.* Englewood Cliffs, NJ: Prentice-Hall, 1957a.

Wise, C. M., *Applied Phonetics.* Englewood Cliffs, NJ: Prentice-Hall, 1957b.

Wolfe, V., and R. Irwin, "Sound discrimination ability of children with misarticulation of the /r/ sound." *Perceptual and Motor Skills, 37* (1973): 415–420.

Wolfe, V., C. Presley, and J. Mesaris, "The importance of sound identification training in phonological intervention." *American Journal of Speech-Language Pathology, 12* (2003): 282–288.

Wolfram, W., *Sociolinguistic Aspects of Assimilation: Puerto Rican English in New York City.* Arlington, VA: Center for Applied Linguistics, 1974.

Wolfram, W., "Language variation in the United States." In O. Taylor (Ed.), *Treatment of Communication Disorders in Culturally and Linguistically Diverse Populations* (pp. 73–116). San Diego, CA: College-Hill Press, 1986.

Wolfram, W., "The phonology of a sociocultural variety: The case of African American Vernacular English." In J. Bernthal and N. Bankson (Eds.), *Child Phonology: Characteristics, Assessment, and Intervention with Special Populations* (pp. 227–244). New York: Thieme Medical Publishers, 1994.

Wolfram, W., C. T. Adger, and D. Christian, *Dialects in schools and communities.* Mahwah, NJ: Erlbaum, 1999.

Wolfram, W., and N. Schilling-Estes, *American English: Dialects and Variation.* Oxford, UK: Blackwell, 1998.

Woolf, G., and M. Pilberg, "A comparison of three tests of auditory discrimination and their relationship to performance on a deep test of articulation." *Journal of Communication Disorders, 3* (1971): 239–249.

Wright, V., R. Shelton, and W. Arndt, "A task for evaluation of articulation change: III. Imitative task scores compared with scores for more spontaneous tasks." *Journal of Speech and Hearing Research, 12* (1969): 875–884.

Wyllie-Smith, L., S. McLeod, and M. J. Ball, "Typically developing and speech impaired children's adherence to the sonority hypothesis." *Clinical Linguistics and Phonetics, 20,* 4/5 (2006): 271–291.

Yaruss, J. S., and E. G. Conture, "Stuttering and phonological disorders in children: Examination of the covert repair hypothesis." *Journal of Speech and Hearing Research, 39* (1996): 349–364.

Yavaş, M., "Sonority effects of vowel nuclei in onset duration." Poster presented at VIIIth International Clinical Phonetics and Linguistics Association Conference, Edinburgh, 2000.

Yavaş, M., "Sonority and the acquisition of #sC clusters." *Journal of Multilingual Communication Disorders, 4,* 3 (2006): 159–168.

Yavaş, M., and C. Core, "Phonemic awareness of coda consonants and sonority in bi-lingual children." *Clinical Linguistics and Phonetics, 15* (2001): 35–39.

Yavaş, M., and L. Gogate, "Phoneme awareness in children: A function of sonority." *Journal of Psycholinguistic Research, 28* (1999): 245–260.

Yavaş, M., and B. Goldstein, "Phonological assessment and treatment of bilingual speakers." *American Journal of Speech-Language Pathology, 7* (1998): 49–60.

Yavaş, M., and S. McLeod, "Acquisition of /s/ clusters in English-speaking children with phonological disorders." *Clinical Linguistics and Phonetics, 24* (2010): 177–187.

Yin, R., *Case Study Research Design and Methods.* Newbury Park, CA: Sage, 1989.

Yoder, P., S. Camarata, and E. Gardner, "Treatment effects on speech intelligibility and length of utterance in children with specific language and intelligibility impairments." *Journal of Early Intervention, 28* (2005): 34–49.

Yopp, H., "The validity and reliability of phonemic awareness tests." *Reading Research Quarterly, 23* (1988): 159–177.

Yorkston, K. M., D. R. Beukelman, E. A. Strand, and M. Hakel, *Management of Motor Speech Disorders in Children and Adults* (3rd ed.). Austin, TX: Pro-Ed, 2010.

Yoss, K., and F. Darley, "Developmental apraxia of speech in children with defective articulation." *Journal of Speech and Hearing Research, 17* (1974): 399–416.

Young, E. C., "The effects of treatment on consonant cluster and weak syllable reduction processes in misarticulating children." *Language, Speech, and Hearing Services in Schools, 18* (1987): 23–33.

Zehel, Z., R. Shelton, W. Arndt, V. Wright, and M. Elbert, "Item context and /s/ phone articulation results." *Journal of Speech and Hearing Research, 15* (1972): 852–860.

Zhu, H., and B. Dodd, "The phonological acquisition of Putonghua (Modern Standard Chinese)." *Journal of Child Language, 27* (2000a): 3–42.

Zhu, H., and B. Dodd, "Putonghua (Modern Standard Chinese)-speaking children with speech disorder." *Clinical Linguistics and Phonetics, 14* (2000b): 165–191.

Ziegler, J. C., and U. Goswami, "Reading acquisition, developmental dyslexia, and skilled reading across languages: A psycholinguistic grain size theory." *Psychological Bulletin, 131* (2005): 3–29.

Zimmerman, I., V. Steiner, and R. Pond, *Preschool Language Scale–5th Edition*. Columbus, OH: Merrill, 2012.

Index

Academic performance, 169–172, 212, 234, 301
Ackerman syndrome, 151
Acoustic phonetics, 13, 50–51, 53, 54
    amplitude, 37, 38, 50
    and perception, 40, 106, 120
    duration, 17, 18, 37, 38, 39, 41, 42, 44, 45, 48, 50,
        51, 54, 55, 56, 67, 121, 122, 156, 198, 275,
        282, 311
    frequency, 37, 38, 41, 42, 50, 51, 80, 120
Additions (errors), 61, 66, 121, 122, 124, 216, 226,
    334
Aerodynamics of speech, 47–49
Affricates, 11, 23, 24, 25, 30, 31, 32, 34, 35, 50, 51,
    99, 100, 117, 145, 156, 190, 205, 221, 237,
    238, 239, 333, 338, 339, 340, 341, 342,
    345, 352
Affrication, 221
African American English (AAE), 233, 326, 328,
    329–333, 334, 337, 346, 347, 349, 350
    Anglicist hypothesis, 329
    characteristics, 329–331
    Creole hypothesis, 329
    phonological development, 331–333
Age and SSDs, 172–173
Age of acquisition, 89–96
    consonants, 90–93
    consonant clusters, 93
    gender and, 73, 108, 109–110
    vowels, 93–96
        paradigmatic, 95
        syntagmatic, 95, 96
Airflow (aerodynamics), 11, 12, 205
Air pressure (intraoral), 25, 47, 49, 156
Air pressure (subglottal), 47, 48, 49, 78
Alliteration, 107, 108, 109, 360, 361, 363, 368,
    375, 377
Allophone, 7–8, 29, 30, 46, 53, 217, 306, 345
    complementary distribution, 8
    free variation, 8

Alternative feedback approaches, 291–294
Alveolar consonants, 22, 29–30, 31, 33, 36, 37, 45,
    51, 85, 99, 132, 152, 165, 220, 229, 285,
    315, 328, 330, 332, 341, 345
Amplitude (loudness), 37, 38, 50
Analysis procedures of articulation/phonological
    assessments. See Assessment of
    articulation/phonology
Anglicist hypothesis, 329
Ankyloglossia, 154
Antecedent events, 243–244, 248, 304
Apraxia, 124–125. See also Childhood Apraxia of
    Speech
Apraxia Profile, 300
Appalachian English, 333–335
Approximation, 151, 243, 278, 279, 280,
    281–283, 299
Articulation,
    assessment of. See Articulatory tests/assessment
        procedures
    automatization, 243, 263, 288, 294
    consistency of, 79, 111, 148, 186, 193, 194, 206
    development/acquisition, 58–113
    error categories, 2, 63, 99–100, 103–105, 119,
        121–122, 123, 125, 128, 131, 132, 133,
        135, 220–222
    individual variability, 75, 84, 95, 108, 111–112,
        121, 200, 225, 227, 256, 331, 332, 368
    maintenance, 263–266, 270, 271, 284, 304
    related factors, 107–112, 144–179
Articulation (speaking) rate, 39, 55, 79, 117, 121,
    145, 156, 158, 159, 213
Articulators, 12, 13, 45, 46, 52, 79, 272
Articulatory phonetics, 11–42
Articulatory tests/assessment procedures, 63, 148,
    166, 170, 171, 183–201
Asian languages, 339–343
    and SSDs, 342–343
    acquisition of tone, 77, 340, 341, 342

433

Asian languages (*continued*)
  dialectal differences, 336, 340
  phonological development, 341–342
  phonology, 340–341
  syllable structure and stress, 340
  tone, 77, 340–341, 342, 348
Assessment of articulation/phonology, 180–241
  assessment in young children, 199–201, 228
  comprehensive, 184–201
  computer assisted, 234–235
  culturally and linguistically diverse populations,
      345–348
  related procedures, 201–210
      audiological screening, 206–207
      case history, 181, 202, 236, 298, 300, 345
      oral cavity examination, 202–206
      speech sound discrimination, 207–210
  sampling procedures, 180–181, 184–191
      connected speech, 184–186
      contextual testing, 193–195
      error pattern identification, 195–196
      single-word testing, 186–191
      sound inventories, 58, 85, 86, 186, 200, 201,
          235, 306, 322, 331, 339
      stimulability, 191–193
  screening, 181–184
  selecting assessment instruments, 196–197
  transcription and scoring procedures, 197–201
Assessment battery, 184–201
Assessment of phonological processes / patterns,
      99–103, 123, 193, 195–196, 213, 218–223
  theoretical considerations, 223
Assimilation, 44, 63, 99, 123, 220, 226, 315, 334,
      339, 341, 342
  consonant harmony, 99, 220
  alveolar, 101
  labial, 101, 220
  nasal, 44, 100, 220
  progressive, 220
  regressive, 220
  velar, 100, 220, 342
  voicing, 334
Atypical (unusual) pattern/process occurrence, 132,
      222, 227, 349
Audiological screening, 206–207
Auditory discrimination. *See* Speech sound
      discrimination

Auditory feedback, 10, 52
Automatic processing, 10
Automatization, 243, 263, 288, 294
Autosegmental theory, 63
Babbling, 55, 72, 82, 83–84, 86, 172
  and speech, 83–84, 86

Backing, 2, 63, 101, 123, 131, 132, 220,
      337, 341, 342
Bankson-Bernthal Test of Phonology (BBTOP), 63,
      224, 226, 227, 236, 238, 249
Behaviorist Models of Speech Acquisition,
      59, 60–61
Bifid uvula, 204
Bilabial sounds, 22, 23, 24, 25–26, 27, 33, 36, 44, 45,
      46, 51, 54, 151, 198, 292, 341, 342
Bilingual, 343–345, 348, 350–352
  assessment, 345–348
  development, 343–345
  intervention, 348–351
  language influence, 344–345
  negative transfer, 343–344
  positive transfer, 344
Bisyllabic, 156
Black English (BE). *See* African American
      English (AAE)
Blending, 107, 108, 110, 361, 362, 375, 378, 381
Block scheduling, 168, 245–246, 379
Broad transcription, *See* Transcription
Broader-based language approaches, 317–322

CAPES, 66, 234–235
Carryover. *See* Generalization
Case history, 181, 202, 236, 298, 300, 345
Case selection, 212–228
  developmental appropriateness, 224–227
  dialectal considerations, 232–233
  error patterns, 218
  guidelines, 227–228
  intelligibility, 213–215
  severity, 215–218
  social-vocational expectations, 233–234
  stimulability, 228–229
  types of patterns, 218–223
Case study, 235–240
  linguistic perspective, 323–325
  motor perspective, 303–305

Causative factors. *See* Articulation, related factors
Childhood Apraxia of Speech, 125–127, 132, 160,
      297–303
   assessment, 298–300
   characteristics, 126–127
   definition, 126
   inconsistency in, 126
   prevalence, 127
   prosodic deficits, 127
   transitions in, 126–127
   treatment, 301–303
   use of lexical stress in, 127
Children's Speech Intelligibility Measure (CSIM), 215
Citation-form (single word) sampling, 71, 165,
      186–191, 196, 215, 234
Classification, 114–136
   by etiology, 129–133
   by psycholinguistic deficit, 133–135
   by symptomatology, 135–136
   organically-based speech sound disorders,
      115–125
   speech sound disorders of unknown origin,
      127–136
Classroom model, 246–247, 259, 373, 375, 379–380,
      381
Clear speech, vs. conversational, 40
Cleft palate, 3, 49, 144, 202, 205, 206, 316
Clinical Assessment of Articulation and Phonology,
      249
Clinical change, 218, 249–254
   causes, 250–252
   extraneous effects, 250–252
   measurement, 249–254
   significance, 253–254
Closants, 82
Closed syllable, 65
Close (narrow) transcription, *See* Transcription
Cluster reduction, 62, 63, 67, 84, 85, 100, 101, 102,
      110, 123, 219, 226, 239, 307, 308, 330,
      339, 341, 342, 349, 381
Cluster simplification, 100, 219, 227
Coalescence, 61, 219
Coarticulation, 11, 42–47, 57, 127, 187, 257
   anticipatory, 43, 127
   overlapping, 44, 45, 46, 56, 193, 299
   retentive (perseverative), 43
Cochlear implants, *See* Hearing loss.

Cognates, 25, 49, 216, 258, 263
Cognitive-linguistic factors, 164–172
   academic performance, 169–172
   intelligence, 164–166
   language development, 166–169
Collapse, 232, 238, 239, 240, 308, 310, 311, 312,
      313, 323, 324
Combined Data-Collection Procedures, 76–77
Common mismatches, 103–105
Comorbidity, 126, 136–142, 365
   explanations, 136–138
   SSDs and emotional/psychiatric disorders,
      141–142
   SSDs and language disorders, 138–139
   SSDs and stuttering, 139–141
   SSDs and voice disorders, 141
Complementary distribution, 8
*Comprehensive Test of Phonological Processing
      (CTOPP)*, 370
Computer-assisted phonological analysis, 234–235
*Computerized Articulation and Phonology
      Evaluation System (CAPES)*, 66, 234–235
Computerized Profiling, 235, 237
Concurrent task sequencing,
Connected speech samples, 184–186
Consequent events, 243, 244, 305. *See also*
      Reinforcement
Consistency, of articulation, 79, 111, 125, 148, 186,
      193, 194, 206, 213, 214, 215, 227, 245,
      261, 295, 296, 298, 299, 300, 369
Consonant(s), 10, 12, 17, 20, 22–36
   acquisition, 90–93
   articulation, 12, 22–36
   assimilation, 44, 63, 99, 123, 220, 226, 315, 334,
      339, 341, 342
   by manner
      affricates, 11, 23, 24, 25, 30, 31, 32, 34, 35,
         50, 51
      fricatives, 11, 23, 24, 25, 26, 29, 30, 31, 32,
         33, 35, 36, 39, 45, 48, 49, 50, 51, 52
      glides, 11, 23, 24, 25, 26, 30, 32, 34, 35, 46,
         48, 49, 50
      lateral, 23, 25, 29, 35, 36
      liquids (/r/, /l/), 11, 29, 34, 35, 45, 48, 49, 50
      nasals, 8, 10, 12, 17, 19, 20, 23, 25, 29, 32,
         34, 35, 36, 43, 44, 45, 48, 49, 50, 51, 53,
         54, 57

Consonant(s) (*continued*)
    rhotic, 23, 24, 25, 31, 32
    stops, 10, 23, 24, 25, 29, 32, 33, 34, 35, 36, 40, 43, 44, 45, 48, 49, 50, 51, 52, 53, 54
   by place
    (lingua) alveolar, 22, 29–30, 31, 33, 36, 37, 45, 51
    bilabial, 22, 23, 24, 25–26, 27, 32, 35, 36, 44, 45, 46, 51
    glottal, 23, 24, 33, 44, 46
    (linguadental) interdental (dental), 22, 23, 24, 26–27, 28, 29, 30, 33, 35, 36, 37, 45, 46, 109, 152, 229, 292, 329, 330, 340
    labiodental, 22, 23, 26, 28, 33, 35, 36, 46
    (lingua) palatal, 23, 24, 25, 30–32, 33, 35, 36, 45, 46
    (lingua) velar, 22, 23, 24, 32, 33, 37, 43, 46, 51, 72, 99, 110, 132, 198, 218, 220, 231, 315, 332, 333, 342
   clusters, 44, 67, 68, 72, 74, 76, 77, 87, 89, 93, 94, 97–98, 100, 102, 103–104, 106, 107, 109, 110, 111, 165, 187, 188, 194, 196, 225, 231, 232, 237, 238, 240, 259, 261, 271, 276, 282, 283, 284, 285, 308, 315, 323, 330, 331, 332, 335, 339, 340, 341, 342, 347, 350, 361
   distinctive features, 19–22, 34–37, 60
   final deletion of, 63, 67, 85, 100, 101, 110, 123, 218, 223, 226, 227,232, 237, 239, 256, 263, 276, 304, 307, 308, 322, 341, 342, 350, 351
   frequency of occurrence, 33, 34, 55, 213, 217, 229, 230, 232, 328, 351
   frequency in conversation, 229
   inventories, 58, 75, 85, 86, 87–106, 167, 186, 188, 200, 201, 235, 306, 322, 331, 339, 342, 345
   percent correct, 87, 97
   syllabic, 22, 30, 38, 46, 231, 315, 330
   voiced vs. voiceless, 12, 17, 22, 24, 25, 26, 29, 30, 32, 34, 35, 36, 49, 52, 54, 65, 67, 80, 137
Consonantal, 19, 20, 34, 35, 45, 53, 54, 263
Contextual analysis, 194, 230–231
Contextual utilization approaches, 288–291
Contextual Probes of Articulation Competence (CPAC), 194
Contextual Test of Articulation, 194
Contextual testing, 193–194
Contextual utilization. *See* Phonetic context

Continuants, 35, 65, 128
Contour tones, 340, 341
Contrast testing, 210
Contrast training, 257, 274, 276, 283, 307–314
Contrastive stress, 41
Contrasts. *See also* Speech sound discrimination
   assessment, 210
   in treatment, 307–314
Controlled processing, 10
Conventional literacy, 358
Conversational speech, 91, 121, 132, 168, 184–186, 188, 257, 259, 260, 266, 284, 286, 291
   versus clear speech, 40
Core vocabulary approach, 294–296
CPAC, 194
Creole hypothesis, 329
Creoles, 329, 336–337
Criteria for selecting tests, 196–197
Cross-sectional studies, 73–75
CSIM, 215
CTOPP, 370
Culturally and linguistically diverse populations. *See* Nonstandard English
Customary production, 225
Cycles approach, 149, 275, 277–278, 304, 314–317, 351, 352
Cyclical goal attack strategy, 245

Deaffrication, 100, 101, 102, 221, 226
DEAP, 135, 183, 300
Declination, 41
Deep Test of Articulation, 148, 193–194
Deletion (omission), 61, 63, 66, 67, 84, 100, 101, 102, 105, 108, 110, 119, 121, 122, 123, 125, 131, 133, 149, 165, 199, 207, 216, 217, 218, 219, 226, 235, 237, 238, 239, 315, 320, 322, 334, 337, 339, 341, 342, 351
Denasalization, 198, 221
Dentalization, 29, 30, 45, 103, 198
Dental sounds, 22, 23, 24, 26–27, 28, 29, 30, 33, 35, 36, 37, 45, 46, 109, 152, 229, 292, 329, 330, 340
Dentition (teeth), 90, 152, 153, 162, 202, 203
Depalatalization, 222, 226
Derivation, 222
Developmental apraxia of speech, *See* Childhood Apraxia of Speech

Developmental appropriateness, 224–227
Developmental models, *See* Phonological
    Development Models
Developmental norms, 73, 224, 227, 238
Developmental sequence, 76, 77, 93, 190,
    231, 232
Developmental subclasses, 93
  Early 8, 93
  Middle 8, 93
  Late 8, 93
Developmental studies, 224
  Combined approaches, 76–77
  Cross-sectional, 71, 73–75
  Diary, 71, 72–73
  Longitudinal, 71, 73, 75–76
Developmental verbal dyspraxia, *See* Childhood
    Apraxia of Speech
Devoiced, 17, 44, 198, 222
Devoicing of final consonants, 45, 101, 222, 226,
    333, 351
Diacritics, 197, 198
Diadochokinesis (DDK), 79, 129, 158, 159, 160,
    206, 298, 299, 300
Diagnostic Evaluation of Articulation and Phonology
    (DEAP), 135, 183, 300
Diagnostic Screen, 183
Dialect density, 328, 347
Dialect leveling, 327
Dialect myths, 327–328
Dialectical considerations, 6, 181, 217, 232–233, 234
Dialects, 326–334. *See also* African American
    English; Appalachian English; Eastern
    American English; General American
    English; Hawaiian Creole; Louisiana
    French Creole; Native American languages;
    Nonstandard English; Ozark English;
    Southern American English; Spanish-
    influenced English
  characteristics, 328–335
Diary studies, 72–73
Diphthongs, 10, 17–19, 22, 82, 83, 95, 122, 123, 188,
    189, 196, 217, 231, 299, 300, 315, 334
Diphthongizing, 345
Discrimination. *See* Speech sound discrimination
Dismissal from instruction, 59, 245, 246, 263–266
  criteria, 265–266
  guidelines, 266

Distinctive features, 19–22, 34–37, 54, 59
Distortions, 125, 133, 153, 156, 162, 216, 217, 234,
    291, 365
Down syndrome, 116, 118–119, 139, 145,
    165–166, 205
Drill, 248, 291, 301, 303, 323, 324
Drill play, 248, 323, 324
Duration, 17, 18, 37, 38, 39, 41, 42, 44, 45, 48, 50,
    51, 54, 55, 56, 67, 121, 122, 156, 198, 275,
    282, 311
Dynamic Temporal and Tactile Cueing
    (DTTC), 302
Dysarthria, 117, 124, 125, 126, 131, 132,
    268, 298
Dyspraxia, *See* Apraxia.

Early 8, 93
Ear training. *See* Speech sound discrimination,
    training
Eastern American English, 333
Electropalatography (EPG), 79, 292, 293–294
Elicitation, 41, 76, 182, 183, 184, 185–186, 188–191,
    192–193, 194, 200, 234
Epenthesis, 102, 219, 226, 335
Emotional/psychiatric disorders and SSDs, 141–142
EPG, 79, 292, 293–294
Error(s), 96–98, 122, 123, 135–136, 180–181, 185,
    186, 187, 188, 189, 190 *See also* Common
    mismatches
  pattern identification, 195–196, 218–223
Establishment phase, 243, 255, 263, 270–283
  guidelines, 283
Etiology. *See* Classification, by etiology.
Evidence-based practice, 5, 249, 250, 252, 268–270
Exemplars, 195, 245, 256, 258, 306–307, 322
Expansion (stage of vocal development), 82, 83
Extraneous effects, 250–253, 268, 269
External discrimination, 148, 274, 287
External monitoring, 148, 243, 260, 277

Facilitating contexts, 194, 230–231, 256, 272, 282,
    285, 288, 290, 291, 301, 351
Factors affecting development, 107–112
  gender, 109–110
  individual variability, 111–112
  language development, 110
  socio-economic status, 110

Factors related to speech sound disorders, 144–179
   cognitive-linguistic factors, 164–172
   motor abilities, 158–164
   oral myofunctional disorders, 160–164
   psychosocial factors, 172–179
   structure and function of the mechanism, 144–158
Familial tendencies and SSDs, 175–176
Fauces, 204–205
Feature geometry, 63, 65
Feedback:
   Alternative approaches, 291–294
   internal, 10, 52, 155–158, 167
   external (from listeners), 59, 126, 137, 167, 243, 260, 273, 277, 295, 301, 318, 319, 320
Fifty-word stage, 84–85
Final consonant deletion, 63, 67, 85, 100, 101, 110, 123, 218, 223, 226, 227,232, 237, 239, 256, 263, 276, 304, 307, 308, 322, 341, 342, 350, 351
Fixed vocal signals, 82, 83
Fluency disorders and SSDs, 139–141
Fluharty Preschool Speech and Language Screening Test, 183
Fragile X syndrome, 119, 126, 139, 298
Free variation, 8
Frenum, 154, 206
Frequency, (Hz), 37, 38, 41, 42, 50, 51, 80, 120
Frequency of errors, 140. 168, 172, 188, 213, 214, 308, 339
Frequency of instruction. 232, 265, 271, 297, 368, 379
Frequency of occurrence, 33, 34, 55, 66, 217, 219, 230, 322, 328, 331, 349, 350, 351, 361
Fricatives, 11, 23, 24, 25, 26, 29, 30, 31, 32, 33, 35, 36, 39, 45, 48, 49, 50, 51, 52, 65, 67, 68, 85, 90, 93, 98, 99, 100, 101, 102, 109, 110, 116, 117, 122, 128, 144, 156, 190, 195, 196, 198, 205, 218, 221, 223, 228, 237, 238, 239, 240, 255, 256, 258, 259, 263, 276, 278, 322, 329, 331, 332, 333, 335, 337, 338, 339, 340, 341, 344
   acquisition, 85, 90, 93, 97–98, 99, 100, 101, 102, 109, 116
Frontal lisp, 2, 90, 149, 160–161, 203, 230, 234

Fronting, 62, 63, 99, 100, 101, 102, 123, 195, 218, 220, 222, 223, 226, 227, 254, 315, 331, 334, 339, 341, 342, 349, 369
   and tongue thrust, 161, 163, 164
Fully-resonant nuclei, 81–82
Fundamental frequency, 37, 38, 41, 42

Gates Silent Reading Test (GSRT), 170
Gender and SSDs, 173–174
General American English (GAE), 93, 233, 326, 327, 328, 329, 330, 337, 345, 347
Generalization, 254–263
   across linguistic-unit, 257
   across situations, 259–261
   across sound and feature, 195, 257–259
   across word position / context, 192, 231, 255–256
   and stimulability, 191, 192, 228
   cross-domain, 169
   facilitation of, 254–263
   guidelines for, 262–263
   parental assistance with, 262
   probes, 249, 252
   response generalization, 150
Generative phonology, 61–62
Genetic disorders, 118–120
Genetic syndromes, 118–120 *See also* Ackerman syndrome; Down syndrome, Fragile X syndrome, Rhett syndrome
GFTA, 166, 185, 191, 226, 249
GFWTAD, 207
Glides, 11, 23, 24, 25, 26, 30, 32, 34, 35, 46, 48, 49, 50, 65, 82, 84, 99, 117, 221, 239, 278, 284, 315, 337, 338, 341, 342
Gliding, 99, 100, 101, 102, 103, 195, 221, 226, 227, 239, 240, 315, 331, 341, 342
Glossectomy, 116, 155
Glottal replacement (substitution; glottalization), 101, 102, 123, 199, 221, 334, 342
Glottal sounds, 23, 24, 33, 44, 46, 83, 101, 102, 117, 123, 198, 199, 216, 221, 299, 342
Glottal stop, 117, 123, 198, 216, 221
Goal attack strategies, 244–245
Goldman-Fristoe Test of Articulation (GFTA), 166, 185, 191, 226, 249
Goldman-Fristoe-Woodcock Test of Auditory Discrimination (GFWTAD), 207
Goo or cooing (stage of vocal development), 83

Gradient stratification, 328
Grandfather passage, 182
GSRT, 170
Gullah, 337,

Haitian Creole, 337
HAPP, 63, 314
HCAPP, 235, 346
Hard palate, 117, 155, 203–204
Harmony processes. *See* Assimilation
Hawaiian Creole, 337, 340
Hawthorne effect, 251
Hearing loss, 120–123 *See also* Otitis media.
  cochlear implants, 121, 122, 123
Hearing screening, *See* Audiological screening
Hodson Assessment of Phonological Patterns
        (HAPP), 63, 314
Hodson Computer Assessment of Phonological
        Patterns (HCAPP), 235, 346
Home language, 110, 327, 335, 336, 349, 351
Homonyms, 85, 105, 235, 307
Homonymy, 72
Horizontal goal attack strategy, 244–245, 304
Hypernasality, 117, 118, 121, 122, 205

Idioglossia, 177
Idiosyncratic phonological process / pattern, 222,
        227, 228, 239
Imitation, 167–168, 184, 185–186, 189, 190, 196,
        200, 217, 229, 279, 282, 283, 288–289,
        299. *See also* Stimulability
Independent analysis, 200–201, 300
Individual variability, 75, 84, 95, 108, 111–112, 121,
        200, 225, 227, 256, 331, 332, 368
Individuals with Disabilities Education Act (IDEA), 336
Infant perception, 55–56, 79–81
  development, 79–81
  methods of study, 80
  visual, 81
Infant production, 81–84
  development, 81–84
  babbling and speech, 83–84
  Oller's stages, 83
  Stark's stages, 81–83
  vocalizations, 56, 81–83, 200
Information processing, 9
Intelligence, 164–166

Intelligibility, 40, 87–89, 116, 117, 119, 124, 141,
        156, 166, 169, 185, 186, 213–215, 227,
        228, 229, 232, 234, 296, 298, 300, 301,
        318, 320, 321, 322, 325, 350, 352, 365,
        366, 373, 374, 381
  development, 87–89
  factors, 156, 213–214
  interpretation, 214
  measurement, 213–215
Intelligibility Index (II), 215
Intelligibility-speech gap, 131, 132
Intensive Phonological Awareness Program, 379
Interactive System for Phonological Analysis
        (ISPA), 235
Interdental (dental) sounds, 22, 23, 24, 26–27, 28, 29,
        30, 33, 35, 36, 37, 45, 46, 109, 152, 229,
        292, 329, 330, 340
Interjudge reliability, 199
Intermittent scheduling, 245–246, 266
Internal discrimination/Internal monitoring, 148, 150
Internal (underlying) representations, 53, 61, 62, 66,
        68, 69, 70, 72, 127, 130, 134, 223, 229,
        356, 362, 365, 366
International Phonetic Alphabet (IPA), 37–38, 197,
        228, 288, 298, 327
Interpreters, 347, 348
Intervention. *See* Remediation systems and
        approaches.
Intervention style, 247–248
Intervocalic, 187, 192, 221, 231, 285, 330, 335
intonation, 38, 39, 85, 185, 273, 299, 300, 330, 349
  development, 105–106
Intrajudge reliability, 199
Intersyllabic clusters, 342
Inventories, 58, 75, 85, 86, 87–106, 167, 186, 188,
        200, 201, 235, 306, 322, 331, 339, 342,
        345, 352
  consonant, 75, 85, 86, 201
  growth of, 87–106
  syllable shape (phonotactic), 87, 201, 203
  vowel, 201
Iowa Silent Reading Test, 170
Iowa Test of Basic Skills, 170
Isolation, 51, 55, 95, 107, 108, 109, 156, 158, 191,
        192, 193, 224, 228, 236, 238, 239, 243,
        257, 273, 275, 278, 284
ISPA, 235

Jargon, 82, 83

Jaw (mandible), 12, 13, 14, 17, 25, 26, 28, 45, 46, 52, 53, 78. 79, 152, 158, 159, 161, 162, 203, 204, 280, 298, 302

Kaufman Speech Praxis Test for Children (KSPT), 300

Kinesthetic feedback, 51, 52, 120, 122, 155, 273, 275, 279, 290, 291, 302, 314

Labial assimilation, 101, 220

Labiodental sounds, 22, 23, 26, 28, 33, 35, 36, 46, 152, 229, 340

Language:

structure, 7–11

Language-based approaches, 306–325

Language development and SSDs, 166–169

Language disorders and SSDs, 138–139

Larynx, 12, 13, 19, 47, 48, 49

development, 78

Late 8, 93

Lateral, 23, 25, 29, 35, 36, 65, 335, 338, 339

Lateral lisp (lateralized fricative), 103, 197, 198, 227, 234, 294

Learning styles, 85, 349

Lexical stress, 41–42, 126, 131

Lexicalization, 9

Limb apraxia, 298, 299

Linguistic-based approaches to intervention, 306–322 *See also* Remediation systems and approaches

remediation guidelines, 322

Linguistic models of acquisition, 61–68

Linguistic perception, 68, 69, 79–81, 86, 95, 105, 106–107, 120–123, 146–151, 207–210

Lip(s), 12, 13, 14, 20, 22, 25, 26, 27, 32, 43, 45, 46, 53, 54, 115, 151, 158, 159, 203, 275, 280

position for speech sounds, 13, 14, 20, 22, 25, 26, 27, 32, 43, 45, 46

structural variations, 115, 151

Liquids (/r/, /l/), 11, 29, 34, 35, 45, 48, 49, 50, 63, 67, 90, 99, 100, 101, 102, 110, 117, 123, 145, 195, 208, 221, 226, 227, 231, 239, 259, 315, 331, 337, 338, 339

Longitudinal studies, 75–76

Loudness, *See* Amplitude

Louisiana French Creole, 237

Macroglossia, 116, 119, 145, 154–155, 205

relative, 116, 119, 205

true, 116, 119

Maintenance, 263–266, 270, 271, 284, 304

guidelines, 266

Malocclusion, 152–153

and tongue thrust, 160, 162, 164

Management. *See* Remediation systems and approaches

Manner of consonant production,

affricates, 11, 23, 24, 25, 30, 31, 32, 34, 35, 50, 51

fricatives, 11, 23, 24, 25, 26, 29, 30, 31, 32, 33, 35, 36, 39, 45, 48, 49, 50, 51, 52

glides, 11, 23, 24, 25, 26, 30, 32, 34, 35, 46, 48, 49, 50

lateral, 23, 25, 29, 35, 36

liquids (/r/, /l/), 11, 29, 34, 35, 45, 48, 49, 50

nasals, 8, 10, 12, 17, 19, 20, 23, 25, 29, 32, 34, 35, 36, 43, 44, 45, 48, 49, 50, 51, 53, 54, 57

rhotic, 23, 24, 25, 31, 32

stops, 10, 23, 24, 25, 29, 32, 33, 34, 35, 36, 40, 43, 44, 45, 48, 49, 50, 51, 52, 53, 54

Markedness, 66–67

Mastery of phonemes, 87, 90–96

Maximal oppositions, 307, 309–310, 313, 322, 324, 352

Melodic facilitation, 302

Melodic cueing (*DTTC*), 302

Melodic Intonation Therapy (*MIT*), 302

Metalinguistics, 87, 356

Metaphon, 311–313

Metathesis, 61, 102, 219, 330

Metrical theory, 63–66

Microglossia, 205

Middle 8, 93

Minimal competency core (*MCC*), 331

Minimal pair contrast therapy, 210, 276–277, 287, 307–314

Minimal pairs, 210, 274, 276, 283, 287, 296, 307, 308, 309–310, 317, 322, 352

Modified Templin Child-Rearing Questionnaire, 176

Models of speech acquisition, 59–71

Monophthongs, 10, 18, 337

Monosyllabic words, 95, 96, 97, 98, 99, 190, 285, 361

Morpheme, 7, 8, 93, 137, 194, 355

Motor (aspect of phonology), 2, 7, 60, 199–200

Motor abilities, 3, 56, 79, 123–125, 158–164, 229
Motor (traditional) approaches to treatment, 267–305 *See also* Remediation systems and approaches
Motor control, 40, 44, 54, 56, 123–125, 131, 166
Motor learning principles, 272–273
Motor programming / planning, 54, 69, 124, 127, 131, 134

Narrow (close) transcription, *See* Transcription
Nasal assimilation, 44, 100, 220
Nasality, 19, 117, 122, 198, 310
Nasals, 8, 10, 12, 17, 19, 20, 23, 25, 29, 32, 34, 35, 36, 43, 44, 45, 48, 49, 50, 51, 53, 54, 57, 61, 65, 67, 68, 85, 100, 116, 119, 121, 165, 220, 221, 222, 228, 229, 322, 327, 330, 332, 337, 338, 340, 341, 342, 344, 350
Native Americans, 146, 336
Native American languages, 336
Natural Phonology, 59, 62–63, 99, 127, 223
Natural Process Analysis, 63
Naturalistic intervention, 318, 320, 321–322
Neuromotor disorders, 123–125
    apraxia, 124–125
    developmental verbal dyspraxia, *See* Childhood Apraxia of Speech
    dysarthria, 117, 124, 125, 126, 131, 132, 268, 298
Nonlinear phonology, 59, 63–66
Nonsense syllables/words/utterances, 56, 68, 147, 148, 158, 192, 193, 257, 263, 264, 284–285, 289, 290, 362
Non-speech abilities, 125, 134, 205, 298
Non-speech oral motor activities, 126, 164, 205, 296–297
Non-speech vocalizations, 82, 83
Nonstandard English (dialects), 233, 345–350
    assessment, 345–348
    intervention, 348–350
Norms (developmental), 73, 74, 165, 182, 200, 223, 224, 225, 227, 238
Nuffield Centre Dyspraxia Programme, 303

Obstruents, 19, 34, 35, 40, 45, 194, 222, 315, 350
Occlusion, 152–153, 203
Oller's typology of infant phonations, 82, 83

Omissions (deletions), 61, 63, 66, 67, 84, 100, 101, 102, 105, 108, 110, 119, 121, 122, 123, 125, 131, 133, 149, 165, 199, 207, 216, 217, 218, 219, 226, 235, 237, 238, 239, 315, 320, 322, 334, 337, 339, 341, 342, 351
Open syllable, 65, 223, 307, 308
Optimality theory, 66–67
Oral anesthetization, 156
Oral appliances, 117, 202, 291, 292, 293
Oral apraxia, 125, 126, 298, 299
Oral cavity examination, 202–206
Oral facial motor skills, 158–160
Oral form recognition (stereognosis), 156–157
Oral mechanism development, 77–79
Oral-motor activities. *See* Non-speech oral motor activities.
Oral Myofunctional Disorders. *See* Tongue thrust
Oral-peripheral examination, *See* Oral cavity examination
Oral sensory function, 155–158
    and speech sound learning, 157
    oral anesthetization, 156
    oral form recognition, 156–157
    oral tactile sensitivity, 155–156
Oral stereognosis (oral form recognition), 156–157
Organically-based speech sound disorders, 115–125
Otitis media, 119, 131, 132, 145–146, 175, 316
Overall sequence of speech sound acquisition, 77
Ozark English, 328, 333–335

Pacifier use, 178–179
PACS, 63
PALS, 370, 374
Palatal fronting, 63, 100, 123, 339
Palatal sounds, 23, 24, 30–32, 33, 35, 36, 45, 46, 99, 132, 315, 340, 345
Palatalization, 45, 101, 222
Palate (hard), 30, 31, 117, 155, 203–204
Paralinguistics, 54, 55
Pattern analysis, error, 195–196, 218–223
    multiple pattern occurrence, 222
    phonological process / pattern analysis, 218–222
    place-manner-voice analysis, 218
    sound preferences, 222–223
    unusual pattern occurrence, 222
Peabody Picture Vocabulary Test (PPVT), 236
PEPPER, 235

Percentage correct, 87, 96–99
  consonants, 87, 96–97
  consonant clusters, 87, 97–98
  vowels, 87, 98–99
Percentage of consonants correct (PCC), 96–97
Perception, 68, 69, 79–81, 86, 95, 105, 106–107,
      120–123, 146–151, 207–210
  development, 105
  linguistic. *See* Linguistic perception; Speech sound
      discrimination
  prelinguistic. *See* Infant perception
Perceptual training, 149–150, 274–278, 287
Personality and SSDs, 178
Pharynx, 32, 204, 205
Phonation (stage of vocal development), 81–82
Phoneme, 7, 8, 13, 19, 52–53
Phonemic awareness, 68, 356, 357, 361–362, 364,
      367, 371, 372, 373, 374, 377, 380
Phonemic Awareness in Young Children, 375
Phonetic context, 43, 45, 193–194, 230–231
      See also *Facilitating Contexts*
  treatment, 282, 288–291
Phonetic placement, 279–281, 376
Phonetic symbols/transcription, 17, 23, 198
Phonological Assessment of Child Speech (PACS), 63
Phonological awareness:
  alliteration, 107, 108, 109, 360, 361, 363, 368,
      375, 377
  assessment, 368–372
      criterion-referenced, 370–371
      dynamic, 371–372
      norm-referenced, 369–370
  blending, 107, 108, 110, 361, 362, 375, 378, 381
  classroom, 379–380
  conventional therapy, and, 380–382
  deep, 357
  development, 106–107, 357, 358–362
  intervention, 372–376
  literacy, 357–358, 362–364
  onset, 64, 65, 83, 106, 107, 108, 150, 187, 356,
      357, 361, 364
  rhyme, 7, 64, 80, 106–107, 108, 109, 171, 355,
      356, 359–360, 361, 363, 364, 368, 369,
      374, 375, 377, 379
  rime, 64, 65, 73, 106, 107, 108, 356, 357, 359,
      361, 364, 373
  role of the speech-language pathologist, 367–368

segmentation, 106, 107, 108, 109, 171, 361, 362,
      363, 372, 375, 378, 381
  shallow, 356–357
  speech sound disorders, and, 364–367, 377–380
  syllable awareness, 107, 108, 360–361, 364
Phonological Awareness Literacy Screening (PALS),
      370, 374
Phonological Awareness Test, 370
Phonological contrast testing, 210
Phonological development models, 59–71
  autosegmental theory, 63
  behaviorist, 59, 60–61
  linguistic models, 61–68
      generative phonology, 59, 61–62
      natural phonology, 59, 62–63, 99, 223
      nonlinear phonology, 59, 63–66
      optimality theory, 59, 66–67
      sonority hypothesis, 67–68
  psycholinguistic, 60, 68–71, 105, 133–135
      single lexicon model, 69–70
      two lexicon model, 70
Phonological knowledge, 85–86, 230, 259, 261, 313
  and vocabulary acquisition, 85–86
Phonological patterns / processes, 59, 62, 63, 84, 85,
      87, 99–100, 101–103, 119, 218–222
  analysis, 195–196, 218–222
  assimilation (harmony) patterns/processes,
      99, 220
      alveolar assimilation, 101
      labial assimilation, 101, 220
      progressive assimilation, 220
      nasal assimilation, 44, 100, 220
      regressive (retentive) assimilation, 220
      velar assimilation, 100, 220, 342
  chronology, 101–103
  definitions, 99–100, 218–222
  multiple pattern occurrence, 222
  sound preference, 222–223
  substitution (segment change) patterns/processes,
      220–222
      affrication, 221
      backing, 2, 63, 101, 123, 131, 132, 220, 337,
          341, 342
      deaffrication, 100, 101, 102, 221, 226
      denasalization, 198, 221
      devoicing of final consonants, 45, 101, 222,
          226, 333, 351

(velar) fronting, 62, 63, 99, 100, 101, 102, 123, 195, 218, 220, 222, 223, 226, 227, 254, 315, 331, 334, 339, 341, 342, 349, 369

gliding, 99, 100, 101, 102, 103, 195, 221, 226, 227, 239, 240, 315, 331, 341, 342

glottal replacement, 101, 102, 123, 199, 221, 334, 342

prevocalic voicing, 101, 222, 226, 237, 238

stopping, 62, 63, 99, 100, 101, 102, 123, 128, 195, 196, 221, 222, 226, 227, 238, 239, 240, 304, 309, 311, 322, 329, 330, 331, 335, 339, 341, 342

vocalization, 101, 221, 226, 227

vowelization, 226

syllable (and whole word) structure changes, 100, 218–219

cluster reduction, 62, 63, 67, 84, 85, 100, 101, 102, 110, 123, 219, 226, 239, 307, 308, 330, 339, 341, 342, 349, 381

cluster simplification, 100, 219, 227

coalescence, 61, 219

epenthesis, 102, 219, 226, 335

final consonant deletion, 63, 67, 85, 100, 101, 110, 123, 218, 223, 226, 227, 232, 237, 239, 256, 263, 276, 304, 307, 308, 322, 341, 342, 350, 351

metathesis, 61, 102, 219, 330

reduplication, 84, 101, 195, 219, 226

unstressed (weak) syllable deletion, 63, 67, 100, 101, 102, 110, 123, 219, 226, 239, 342, 350

theoretical considerations, 223

unusual (atypical) pattern/process occurrence, 132, 222, 227, 349

Phonological perception. *See* Speech sound discrimination

Phonological recording, 197–198

Phonological reorganization, 40, 261, 313

Phonological rules, 2, 61–62, 66, 70, 233, 263, 267, 306, 313, 343, 345, 346, 352, 365

Phonological theories, *See* Phonological development models

Phonotactic, 106, 303, 306, 330, 332, 350

constraints, 85, 86

Phrase-final lengthening, 41

Pidgins, 336–337

Pitch, 38, 50, 51, 54, 55, 67, 121, 141, 288, 340, 349

Place of articulation,

(lingua) alveolar, 22, 29–30, 31, 33, 36, 37, 45, 51

bilabial, 22, 23, 24, 25–26, 27, 32, 35, 36, 44, 45, 46, 51

glottal, 23, 24, 33, 44, 46

(linguadental) interdental, 22, 23, 24, 26–27, 28, 29, 30, 33, 35, 36, 37, 45, 46, 109, 152, 229, 292, 329, 330, 340

labiodental, 22, 23, 26, 28, 33, 35, 36, 46

(lingua) palatal, 23, 24, 25, 30–32, 33, 35, 36, 45, 46

(lingua) velar, 22, 23, 24, 32, 33, 37, 43, 46, 51, 72, 99, 110, 132, 198, 218, 220, 231, 315, 332, 333, 342

Place-manner-voicing analysis, 195, 218, 235

Play, 348

PLS, 184

PPVT, 236

Polysyllabic, 58, 67, 77, 96, 97, 98, 99, 112, 340, 352

Postvocalic, 30, 56, 110, 187, 192, 216, 225, 231, 285, 289, 315, 327, 328, 337, 345

Practice principles, 273

Prepractice goals, 272–273

Pre-Reading Inventory of Phonological Awareness, 370

Preschool HOME Scale, 176

Preschool Language Scale (PLS), 184

Prevocalic, 30, 101, 225, 231

Prevocalic voicing, 101, 222, 226, 237, 238

Process (pattern) ordering, 222

Production training, 278–283

contextual utilization, 282–283

imitation, 167–168, 184, 185–186, 189, 190, 196, 200, 217, 229, 279, 282, 283, 288–289, 299. *See also* Stimulability

phonetic placement, 279–281, 282, 376

successive approximation, 279, 280, 281, 283

Prognosis, 161, 192

Programs to Examine Phonetic and Phonological Evaluation Records (PEPPER), 235

Progress in therapy, *See* Clinical change.

Prompts for Restructuring Oral Muscular Phonetic Targets (PROMPT), 302

Proprioceptive feedback, 51, 52, 273, 291, 302

Prosodic development, 105–106

Prosodic features. *See* Suprasegmentals

Psycholinguistic:
  approaches to classification, 133–135
  models of acquisition, 60, 62, 68–71
Psychosocial factors, 172–179
  age, 172–173
  familial tendencies, 175–176
  family background, 174–175
  gender, 173–174
  personality, 178
  siblings, 176–177
  socioeconomic status, 174–175, 177
Pull-out instruction, 246–247
Pure tone screening, 206
Pygmalion effect, 251

Quasi-resonant nuclei, 81, 82
Quasi-vowels, 82, 83

Rate (of speech), 39, 55, 79, 117, 121, 145, 156, 158,
    159, 213
Reduplication, 84, 101, 195, 219, 226
Referrals, 58, 127, 183, 201–202, 236, 299
Reflexive vocalizations, 81, 82
Register, 328
Register tones, 340
Registral varieties, 328
Regression, 264
Regression to the mean, 249, 251
Reinforcement, 60, 61, 243, 266, 273, 305
Relational analysis, 180, 201, 234, 352
Remediation. *See* Therapy/instruction/intervention/
    remediation/treatment
Remediation systems and approaches:
  core vocabulary, 136, 294–296, 301
  cycles approach, 275, 277, 314–317, 351, 352
  classroom model, 246–247
  dialectal considerations, 6, 181, 217, 232–233, 234
  dismissal from instruction, 59, 245, 246, 263–266
    criteria, 265–266
    guidelines, 266
  establishment phase, 243, 255, 263, 270–283
    guidelines, 283
  evidence, 268–270
  framework, 242–244
  generalization/transfer/carry-over. *See*
    Generalization
  goal attack strategies, 244–245

  intervention style, 247–248
  linguistic approaches, 306–325
    broader-based language-based approaches,
      317–322
    cycles approach, 314–317
    guidelines, 322
    maximal oppositions approach, 309–310
    metaphon therapy, 311–313
    minimal oppositions approach, 309–310
    minimal pair contrast therapy, 307–314
    multiple oppositions approach, 310–311
    naturalistic intervention, 320
    whole-language intervention, 317–320
  motor-based approaches, 267–305
    alternate feedback approaches, 291–294
    context utilization approaches, 288–291
    establishment of target behaviors, 273–283
    guidelines, 294
    motor learning principles, 272–273
    perceptual training, 274–278
    production training, 278–283
    traditional approach, 283–287
    treatment continuum, 270–272
    oral-motor exercises, 296–297
  pullout model, 246–247
  scheduling, 245–246
  social/vocational considerations, 233–234
  teaching sounds, 273–283
Respiratory system, 11–12, 13, 38, 49, 78, 299
Response generalization, 150, 255, 256 *See also*
    Generalization
Retention, 264–265, 266, 271
Rhett syndrome, 298
Rhotic, 23, 24, 25, 31, 32, 98, 99, 131, 133, 189, 328
Road to the Code, 375, 379

SAILS, 277
SATPAC, 290
S-CAT, 194, 249
Scheduling of instruction, 245–246
SCIP, 309, 311
Scoring of articulation errors, 197–199, 216
  diacritics, use in, 197–198
  dialect features, 346
Screening, 181–184
  formal, 183–184
  informal, 182–183

Screening Test for Developmental Apraxia of Speech (STDAS-2), 300

Secord Contextual Articulation Tests (S-CAT), 194, 249

Segment change pattern /process, 220

Segmental analysis, 237

Segmentation. *See* Phonological awareness

Self-monitoring, 150–151, 260–261, 263, 271

Semantics, 4, 8, 9, 56, 120, 180, 289, 318, 319, 320, 336, 345

Semivowels, 23, 25, 116

SESI, 183

Severity, 106, 129, 131, 157, 165, 169, 185, 186, 213, 215–218, 227, 228, 229, 245, 247, 318, 346

Shaping, 281–282, 283

Sharp stratification, 328

Sibilants, 31
    distortions (lisps), 2, 90, 119, 131, 133, 137, 162, 291
    vs. nonsibilants, 51

Sibling influences and SSDs. 176–177

Single words vs. connected speech, 185, 186, 187, 188, 218, 285

Single word sampling, 186–191, 218

Social diagnosticity, 328

Social-vocational expectations, 233–234

Socioeconomic status:
    and dialect, 327, 328, 359
    and normal development, 73, 110, 146
    and reading, 365
    and SSDs, 174–175, 177

Soft palate, 12, 117–118, 155, 204

Sonorants, 19, 20, 35, 65, 229

Sonority, 67–68

Sonority hypothesis, 67–68

Sonority sequencing principle, 67

Sound Contrast in Phonology (SCIP), 309, 311

Sound preference, 222–223

Sounds Abound: Listening, Rhyming, and Reading, 375

Southern American English, 333

SPAC, 194

Spanish, 338–339
    phonological development, 338–339
    phonology, 338
    and SSDs, 340

Spanish-influenced English, 326

Speaking rate, 39, 55, 79, 117, 121, 145, 156, 158, 159, 213

Spectrograms for treatment, 292, 293

Speech Assessment and Interactive Learning System (SAILS), 277

Speech-Ease Screening Inventory (SESI), 183

Speech perception, *See* Infant Perception.
    and SSDs, 146–151

Speech Production Perception Task (SP-PT), 207–210

Speech rate, 39, 55, 79, 117, 121, 145, 156, 158, 159, 213

Speech sound discrimination,
    acquisition. *See* Infant perception; Linguistic perception
    discrimination improvement, 274, 277
    external vs. internal, 148
    relationship between articulation and discrimination, 146–151
    testing, 207–210
    training, 274–278

Speech sound sampling, 180–181

Spirants, 344

Spontaneous speech, 124, 151, 168, 185, 187, 190, 213, 261, 263, 315, 322

SP-PT, 207–210

Stark Assessment of Early Vocal Development, 81–82, 83

Stark's Typology of Infant Phonation, 81–82

STDAS-2, 300

Stereognosis (oral form recognition), 156–157

Stimulability, 191–193, 224

Stimulus generalization, 254

Stopping, 62, 63, 99, 100, 101, 102, 123, 128, 195, 196, 221, 222, 226, 227, 238, 239, 240, 304, 309, 311, 322, 329, 330, 331, 335, 339, 341, 342

Stops, 10, 23, 24, 25, 29, 32, 33, 34, 35, 36, 40, 43, 44, 45, 48, 49, 50, 51, 52, 53, 54, 65, 66, 67, 68, 85, 93, 98, 99, 117, 122, 128, 144, 158, 165, 196, 198, 199, 205, 216, 218, 221, 228, 229, 231, 240, 258, 259, 278, 284, 307, 315, 322, 331, 332, 333, 337, 338, 340, 341, 342, 344, 350

Storytelling Probes of Articulation Competence (SPAC), 194

Stress, 37–38, 41–42, 45, 54, 55, 66, 67, 96, 105, 121, 122, 126, 127, 131, 185, 188, 190, 214, 216
  contrastive, 41
  lexical, 41–42,126, 127, 131
  syllable, 18, 37–38, 41–42, 45, 54, 67, 96, 100, 122, 188, 216
Stridency, 35, 50–51, 226, 315
Structural deviations (major), 115–118
Structural deviations (minor), 151–155
Structured play, 200, 248
Stuttering and SSDs, 139–141
Sublexical, 356
Substitutions, 38, 56, 61, 73, 85, 99, 115, 117, 121, 122, 123, 124, 125, 133, 135, 149, 195, 199, 216, 217, 218, 219, 220, 222, 235, 294, 315, 328, 330, 331, 337, 339, 341, 342, 365
  Patterns/processes, 220
  unusual, 117, 123
Successive approximation, , 280, 281–283, 299
Suprasegmentals, 37–42
  clear vs conversational speech, 40
  contrastive stress, 41
  declination, 41
  development, 105–106
  intonation, 38, 39, 85, 185, 273, 299, 300, 330, 349
  juncture, 38–39, 41
  lexical stress effects, 41–42, 126, 127, 131
  loudness, 38, 50, 67, 214, 299, 300
  new vs given information, 40–41
  phrase-final lengthening, 41
  pitch, 38, 50, 51, 54, 55, 67, 121, 141, 288, 340, 349
  speaking rate, 39, 55, 79, 117, 121, 145, 156, 158, 159, 213
  stress, 37–38, 41–42, 45, 54, 55, 66, 67, 96, 105, 121, 122, 126, 127, 131, 185, 188, 190, 214, 216
  vowel reduction, 39
Syllabic consonants, 22, 30, 38, 46, 231, 315, 330
Syllabicity, 352
Syllable, 4, 7, 13, 17, 22, 37, 38, 42, 46, 52, 53, 54, 55–56, 64–65, 66, 67, 82–83, 84, 87, 99
  canonical, 55, 82, 83
  development, 55–56

integrity, 52, 53
inventories, 87
nuclei (nucleus), 13, 17, 38, 54
shape, 22, 46, 55–56, 65, 66, 84
structure changes. *See* Phonological patterns / processes
tier, 64
Syntax, 2, 4, 8, 9, 56, 120, 137, 166, 167, 168, 236, 289, 317, 318, 319, 320, 336, 345
Systematic Articulation Training Program Accessing Computers (SATPAC), 290

Tactile feedback, 51, 52, 120, 122, 155–156, 157, 191, 273, 279, 280, 290, 291
Tactile feedback approaches to treatment, 292
Target speech sound/behavior, selection of:
  contextual analysis, 230–231
  developmental appropriateness, 229–230
  frequency of occurrence, 229
  guidelines, 231–232
  phonological pattern analysis, 231
  stimulability, 228–229
Teeth (dentition), 90, 152, 153, 162, 202, 203
Target Words for Contextual Training, 194
Templin Child Rearing Questionnaire, 176
Templin-Darley Tests of Articulation (TDTA), 170
Templin Prekindergarten Imitation Articulation Test, 171
Test(s). *See* Articulatory tests/assessment procedures
Test of Phonological Awareness (TPA), 370
Test of Phonological Awareness Skills (TPAS), 370
Therapy/instruction/intervention/remediation/treatment.
    See Remediation systems and approaches
The Sounds Abound Program, 375
Tones, 340, 341, 342
  contour, 340
  register, 340
Tongue, 12–13, 205–206
  frenum, 154, 206
  macroglossia, 116, 119, 145, 154–155, 205
    relative, 116, 119, 205
    true, 116, 119
  microglossia, 205
  position for consonants, 22–25
  position for vowels, 14–21
  removal (glossectomy), 116, 155
  size, 205
  strength, 129, 159–160

Tongue thrust, 160–164
   ASHA position statement, 163–164
   dentition,162
   treatment, 165
   speech sound errors, 164
Tongue-tie, 154
Touch cueing, 302
TPA, 370
TPAS, 370
TPIAT, 171
Traditional approach to treatment 283–287
Transcription, 3, 7, 197–199
   accuracy, 198–199
   broad, 197
   diacritics, 198
   International Phonetic Alphabet (IPA), 197
   narrow (close), 197, 216
   orthographic, 214
   phonetic vs. phonemic, 7
   recording responses, 197–198
   reliability, 199
Transcription and scoring procedures, 197–201
Transfer. *See* Generalization
Treatment approaches. *See* Remediation
     systems and approaches
Treatment continuum, 270–272

Ultrasound, 292, 293
Underlying (internal) representation, 10, 53,
     61, 62, 66, 68, 69, 70, 72, 105, 127,
     130, 134, 198, 223, 229, 356, 362, 365,
     366, 378
Unstressed (weak) syllable deletion, 63, 67,
     100, 101, 102, 110, 123, 219, 226, 239,
     342, 350
Unusual (atypical) phonological patterns / processes,
     132, 222, 227, 349

Van Riper method, 60–61, 274, 275, 283–287, 351
Variability and development, 56, 59, 70, 75, 84, 85,
     89, 90, 95, 108, 111–112, 121, 165, 200,
     225, 235, 332, 368
Vegetative sounds, 82, 83
Velar assimilation, 100, 220, 342

Velar fronting, 62, 63, 99, 100, 101, 102, 123, 195,
     218, 220, 222, 223, 226, 227, 254, 315,
     331, 334, 339, 341, 342, 349, 369
Velar sounds, 22, 23, 24, 32, 33, 37, 43, 46, 51, 72,
     99, 110, 132, 198, 218, 220, 231, 315, 332,
     333, 342
Velopharyngeal (in)competence, 49, 117, 205
Velopharyngeal mechanism (port), 25, 29, 32, 36, 43,
     48, 204, 205
Velopharynx, 12, 13, 26, 48, 53
Velum. *See* Soft palate
Verbal apraxia. *See* Apraxia; Childhood Apraxia of
     Speech
Vertical goal attack strategy, 244, 245
Visual feedback approaches to treatment, 292
Vocalic, 19–20, 34, 35, 117, 187, 231, 315, 328
Vocalizations, infant, 56, 81–83, 200
Vocants, 82
Voice disorders and SSDs, 141
Voice onset time (VOT), 106
Voiced consonants, 12, 17, 22, 24, 25, 26, 29, 30, 32,
     34, 35, 36, 49, 52, 54, 65, 67, 80, 137
Voiceless consonants, 22, 24, 34, 48, 65, 80
Voicing, 13, 19, 22, 23, 24, 45, 47, 67, 80
Vowels:
   acquisition of, 93–96
   articulation, 13–22
   central, 17
   diphthongs, 10, 17–19, 22
   distinctive features, 19–22
   front vs. back, 17, 20
   high vs. low, 17, 20
   mid, 17
   monophthongs, 10, 18
   quadrilateral, 15, 16
   rounded vs. unrounded, 13–14, 17, 20
   tense vs. lax,17, 20, 21–22

Weak (unstressed) syllable deletion, 63, 67, 100, 101,
     102, 110, 123, 219, 226, 239, 342, 350
Whole-language intervention, 317–320
Whole-word patterns / processes, 100, 218–219

Young children, assessment, 199–201